Women's Sexual Health

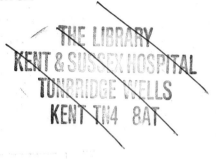

Senior Commissioning Editor: Ninette Premdas
Project Development Manager: Katrina Mather
Project Managers: Alasdair Deas, Cheryl Brant
Design: Judith Wright
Illustration: Antbits

Women's Sexual Health

Third Edition

Edited by

Gilly Andrews RGN ENB A08 8103
Clinical Nurse Specialist in Family Planning,
Kings College Hospital NHS Trust
Menopause and PMS Specialist Nurse
The Lister Hospital, London, UK

Foreword by

John Studd DSc MD FRCOG
Professor of Gynaecology
Chelsea and Westminster Hospital
The Lister Hospital, London, UK

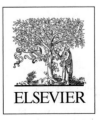

ELSEVIER

EDINBURGH   LONDON   NEW YORK   OXFORD   PHILADELPHIA   ST LOUIS   SYDNEY   TORONTO   2005

ELSEVIER

© 2005 Elsevier Ltd
© 2001 Harcourt publishers
Except Chapter 16, pp 451-483, Copyright © Kathy Abernethy

The right of Gilly Andrews to be identified as editor of this work has been asserted by her in accordance with the Copyright, Designs and Patents Act 1988.

First edition 1997
Second edition 2001
Third edition 2005

ISBN 0 70202762 6

British Library Cataloguing in Publication Data
A catalogue record for this book is available from the British Library

Library of Congress Cataloging in Publication Data
A catalog record for this book is available from the Library of Congress

Note
Medical knowledge is constantly changing. As new information becomes available, changes in treatment, procedures, equipment and the use of drugs become necessary. The editor/contributors and the publishers have taken care to ensure that the information given in this text is accurate and up to date. However, readers are strongly advised to confirm that the information, especially with regard to drug usage, complies with the latest legislation and standards of practice.

ELSEVIER

your source for books, journals and multimedia in the health sciences

www.elsevierhealth.com

The publisher's policy is to use **paper manufactured from sustainable forests**

Printed in China

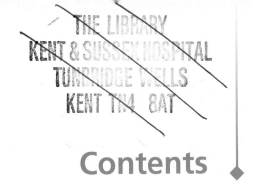

Contents

A colour plate section appears between pages 384 and 385.

Contributors

Kathy Abernethy RN ENB 900 225
Associate Director/Senior Nurse Specialist,
 The Menopause Clinical and Research Unit,
 North West London & St Mark's NHS Trust,
 Northwick Park Hospital, London, UK

Gilly Andrews RGN ENB A08 8103
Clinical Nurse Specialist, Department of
 Reproductive and Sexual Health,
 King's College Hospital NHS Trust,
 Menopause Nurse Specialist,
 The Lister Hospital, London, UK

Gillian Aston PhD MA RGN RM ADM PGCEA
Lecturer/Midwife Practitioner, King's College,
 University of London, London, UK

Karen Burnet RGN BSc MSc Onc Cert
 Advanced Breast Care Course
Lead Breast Care Nurse, Cambridge Breast Unit,
 Addenbrookes NHS Trust, Cambridge, UK

Mary Dolman RN ET NB978 BSc(Nurs)
Consultant Nurse Specialist, Urotherapy Clinic,
 Bath, UK

Catrina Donegan MSc RN
Senior Lecturer, Primary Public and Child
 Health, Middlesex University, School of
 Health and Social Sciences, London, UK

Alison Duffin RN ENB 998 901 276
Sexual and Reproductive Health Nurse/Sexual
 Health Community Nurse Educator,

Family Planning Victoria, The Action Centre,
 Melbourne, Australia

Suzanne Everett BSc(Hons) RGN RM ENB A08
 Advanced diploma in reproductive sexual
 health, PG Cert (HE)
Senior Lecturer, Middlesex University,
 Contraceptive Nurse Specialist,
 Margaret Pyke Centre, London, UK

Kati Gray Psychoanalyst RN RM BA(Hons)
Member of the Guild of Psychotherapists,
 Member of the Site for Contemporary
 Psychoanalysis, Member of the College
 of Psychoanalysts (UK), UKCP Registered
 Psychoanalyst. Elizabeth Garrett
 Anderson Hospital for Women,
 London, UK

Marjorie Hickerton RN BSc(Hons) Nurse
 Practitioner A36 FETC FP100 ENB 985,
 A08 Cert in Counselling
Senior Clinical Nurse, Specialist/Manager in
 Family Planning and Sexual Health,
 Wandsworth Primary Care Trust,
 London, UK

Liz Illman RN ENB 901 A08 998 N07
Nurse Specialist – Sexual and Reproductive
 Healthcare, Camden Primary Care Trust and
 Haringey Teaching Primary Care Trust;
 Smoking Cessation Specialist – Families
 and Parents-To-Be, Camden PCT,
 London UK

Shirley R Jones MA RGN RM ADM Cert Ed
(FE) ILT
Professor of Midwifery, Head of School of
Women's Health Studies, School of Women's
Health Studies, University of Central
England, Birmingham, UK

Lisa Lee RN ENB 225 998
Senior Nurse – Gynaecology, Princess Royal
University Hospital, Orpington, UK

Sandy Nelson MA Psychotherapist BEd,
Diploma in Systemic Management
Senior Lecturer, Thames Valley University,
London, UK

Vicky Padbury RGN, ENB 900 A08 998
Clinical Nurse Specialist in Family Planning,
East Surrey Primary Care Trust,
Redhill, UK

Mary Power RGN RM
Coordinator, Assisted Conception Unit,
The Lister Hospital, London, UK

Jane Selby RGN
Psychosexual seminar leader for the
Association of Psychosexual Nursing.

Jill Steele RN RHV
Formerly Research Nurse, Department of
Obstetrics and Gynaecology, UCL Hospitals
NHS Trust, London, UK

Catriona Sutherland RN ENB A08 A51 998
Clinical Nurse Specialist in Women's Health,
Paxton Green Group Practice, London, UK

Denise Tiran MSc RM RGN ADM PGCEA
Director, Expectancy Ltd; Visiting Lecturer,
University of Greenwich, London, UK

Acknowledgements

Editing such a comprehensive book as this third edition of *Women's Sexual Health* has been a mammoth task, and I am enormously grateful to all the contributors who gave their time and expertise in updating their chapters and in meeting all the editorial deadlines that I set. Without their hard work and professionalism my job would have been a lot more difficult. I would also like to thank their families, friends and colleagues who advised and supported them.

Gill Aston, author of the chapter on sexuality during and after pregnancy, wishes to thank Katie Lillington and Tamasine Ashcroft for their continuing help and support with her work. Mary Power would like to acknowledge Karen Hutchings for secretarial support in writing her chapter on the management of subfertility.

Alison Duffin, who wrote her chapter on sexually acquired infections whilst working in Australia (thank goodness for email!), says a big 'thank you' for the help and support that her parents and sister provided, both as personal secretaries and as administration assistants.

I would like to express my appreciation to Sue Bush for her help in reading through some chapters and to Professor John Studd for his generous encouragement and for writing the foreword to this third edition.

Finally, my last expression of thanks goes to my husband, Bob (despite his assurances that a third edition would be easy!), whose unstinting support, encouragement and proof-reading skills have been invaluable.

Foreword

The third edition of Gilly Andrew's highly successful *Women's Sexual Health* is an important, timely publication. Although it deals with women's sexual health, problems of libido, intercourse, young people and sex, contraception, sexual abuse and the use of complementary medicines, it is really much more. It is virtually a complete textbook of gynaecology written by highly experienced specialist nurses, which has produced a publication in my view better and more informative than most textbooks written by gynaecologists. It has been updated to bring in the large amount of new work concerning family planning, complications of HRT and the various ways of treating premenstrual depression. It also deals with fertility, breast cancer, menopause and psychosexual problems in a most informative and sensitive way. It even has a unique chapter on women with special needs, covering in some detail the cultural and religious aspects of sexuality and discussing the gynaecological problems that may be encountered in women of all major religions.

The knowledge behind the chapters really brings into question the old issue of job demarcation between doctor and nurse. We have a shamefully underfunded National Health Service and it is clearly the Government's intention to produce poorly paid nurses rather than doctors for much medical care. Whatever the political machinations behind this view, there is no doubt that nurses are at least as able as doctors in many areas of gynaecology. I am certainly aware that even in private practice there are many patients who are keen to be passed on to Gilly, a highly trained specialist nurse in family planning and the menopause, for clinical advice.

Gilly Andrews' chapter on premenstrual syndrome is superb, as is Kathy Abernethy's up-to-date chapter on the current conflicts relating to the menopause. Mary Power's chapter on subfertility, Alison Duffin on sexuality transmitted infections, Vicky Padbury on cervical screening, and breast screening by Karen Burnet are all products from nurses who have been involved in research and who lecture widely on their subjects, nationally and internationally. It is of course invidious to mention these few when the overall standard of expertise is quite overwhelming. I hope it does not seem patronizing when I say that it should not be a surprise that professional women write so well about women.

There is clearly a need for such a comprehensive view of women's sexual health and reproductive health written by women who understand the implications of these disorders. This unique book fills the gap.

For the health professional, there is everything that nurses need to know about women's health issues in one book. As I wrote in my foreword to the second edition, I believe that this book is so comprehensive and readable and it should be of huge benefit to the public and deserves to be a best seller from major book shops as it has such a great educational role. This is a book that should be for sale at stations and airports. After all, the title alone would make it a worthwhile purchase for a long journey.

John Studd

Preface

What is 'Sexual Health'? There is no doubt it is an increasingly high-profile subject, but the phrase is used in many different ways. To some it simply means medical and physical problems associated with sexual activity; to others it has broader connotations, concerned with self-esteem and mutual fulfilment.

The World Health Organization describes it in the following terms: 'a state of physical, emotional, mental and social well-being related to sexuality: it is not merely the absence of disease or infirmity. Sexual health requires a positive and respectful approach to sexuality and relationships, as well as the possibility of having pleasurable and safe sexual experiences free of coercion, discrimination and violence. For sexual health to be maintained the sexual rights of all persons must be respected, protected and fulfilled' (WHO, 2002).

Women's Sexual Health endorses this definition and covers the spectrum of reproductive life events from puberty to the post-menopausal years. It is written primarily for nurses who are involved or interested in women's health, whether in primary care or within a hospital environment, whether pre-registration or undertaking further training. Health professionals from other disciplines (including medical students) will also find it a comprehensive reference book and will encounter issues relevant to their own fields of work.

All the contributing authors are nurses who have been chosen for their skill, expertise and knowledge of their individual subjects. Topics are explained clearly, with a good use of diagrams and charts. Each chapter contains a list of learning objectives, considers how a woman's sexuality can be affected by a particular problem or disorder, and discusses how nurses can acknowledge these concerns whilst incorporating holistic care into their professional practice. All chapters include research findings, with comprehensive references, suggestions for further reading (for professionals and for clients) and a broad resource list for individual research. Two additional sections have been added to all chapters in this third edition, covering ideas for personal and professional development and patient education points.

Since the first edition of *Women's Sexual Health* was published in 1997 there have been many changes in female health care. New government initiatives and strategies have enhanced the provision of care for women and their partners, and advances in pharmacology and technology, and easier access to counselling, have improved health and sexual well-being. Many nurses have extended their roles and undergone specialized training within their own particular speciality. The programme for nurse prescribing is well established and nurse consultants are becoming increasingly common. This means that nurses are increasingly offering a 'one-stop service' with complete continuity of care. Some have argued that these advances in knowledge, analytical abilities and confidence will cause basic holistic care to become marginalized. *Women's Sexual Health* addresses these issues and has used the concept of holistic care throughout. Women are considered as individuals in the context of their physical, psychological, social and cultural needs.

xiii

The publication of this third edition has enabled all the chapters to be comprehensively revised and updated to reflect the latest research and developments in current thinking.

Women's Sexual Health is divided into three sections. Section One, 'Women Today', explores the concept of sexuality and well-being within physical, psychological and social dimensions. It discusses the premise that women's sexuality is not just about sex but is influenced throughout life by many factors, such as culture, ethnicity, environment, stress, sexual orientation and lifestyle. It also addresses some of the issues that can cause difficulties for health care professionals when dealing with the sexuality of their patients.

Section Two, 'Fertility', examines issues surrounding female fertility. For centuries women have tried to control their own fertility: a concept difficult to imagine a few decades ago, but now a reality due to the advances in contraceptive technology. Many women, however, still assume that conception will follow immediately after contraception is stopped, and have not considered the possibility of subfertility. Others, whether using contraception or not, find unplanned and unwanted pregnancies occur only too easily. This section explains and explores the options surrounding contraception, subfertility and unplanned pregnancy, and also focuses on sexuality during and after pregnancy.

Section Three, 'Women's Health Issues', concentrates on specific female health problems. Women's general health and their life expectancy have improved dramatically over the last century, yet in spite of these advances women continue to have health problems that are unique to them as women. This section explains what these disorders are and outlines many of the treatment options available. It provides referenced, up-to-date and accessible information, whilst adopting a health-oriented stance.

Widespread internet access, coupled with greater in-depth discussion of women's health issues by the media, means that women are increasingly likely to ask your advice about new research, treatment options and drug therapies of which you may have limited knowledge. *Women's Sexual Health* will provide a source of reference, enabling you to give an informed and positive response to their initial enquiries.

Women are becoming empowered to make free and responsible choices regarding their health, but to do so they need the advocacy and support of the nurses who care for them. As a nurse, you need to foster and build on the trust that your patients place in you: you are a key element in all health care teams and play a leading role in service provision.

In order to feel confident in dealing with the broad issues surrounding sexual health and well-being, you should think carefully about three basic areas where you might need further training: your own personal knowledge base, your own values and beliefs, and your own skills, whether of a clinical and technical nature or in the field of counselling and communication. *Women's Sexual Health* should stimulate your thoughts in all these areas.

Reference

World Health Organization (2002) Working definition: Gender and reproductive rights. Geneva: WHO. www.who.int.

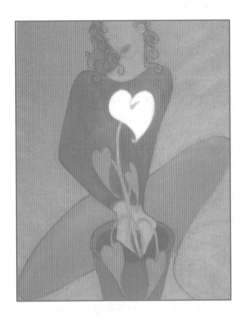

Women Today

1: Women's Sexuality

Sandy Nelson

OBJECTIVES

This chapter should help you understand:

- The relationship between gender and sexuality
- Theories of sexuality
- Female sexual development
- Bisexual and lesbian sexuality
- The relationship between culture, ethnicity, religion and sexuality.

Introduction

The purpose of this chapter is to explore female sexuality. The way we think about sexuality directly influences practice and has implications for the services we provide. It is necessary to understand women's sexuality in holistic terms, otherwise we are likely to be limited in the help we offer.

Nurses are expected to promote sexual health as part of holistic health care. Yet the definition of sexual health implicit in the services provided focuses narrowly on contraception, disease control and the treatment of dysfunction. The World Health Organization provides a much broader definition. It defines sexual health as: 'the integration of the somatic, emotional, intellectual and social aspects of sexual being, in ways that are positively enriching and that enhance personality, communication and love.'

It is essential to think about sexuality in these broader terms, so that the needs of each woman can be reflected in the care provided. However, sexuality is one of the most difficult areas of human experience to define. It is complex, varied and contradictory. It involves desire and excitement, intimacy and tenderness, risk and danger,

love and hate in sometimes confusing combinations. Historically, how we think about sexuality has changed over time, and within our own lives we are likely to think about, experience and express our sexuality in many different ways. The same sexual act can be experienced variously as unique and exciting, or mundane and repetitive, depending on expectations, mood and the circumstances that surround it.

It is the most intimate and private aspect of our lives, yet the Church and State have always been involved in controlling sexuality. Consequently, it is both intensely personal and a matter of public concern. It is learnt through interactions with others in the home, at school and through the media but also meaning is created individually. Hence, although we are influenced by the expectations of others we also experience our own desires, which may differ from theirs.

Moreover, the history of human sexuality has, in many senses, been the history of male sexuality. Women's sexuality has mostly been seen as mysterious and unknown. It is constructed in relation to male sexuality, as basically reactive and responsive. Women, particularly in the last three decades, have challenged this way of seeing female sexuality and have provided important new insights.

There are many competing theories of female sexuality, some of which are introduced in this chapter. What is of fundamental importance is to question the theories that inform current practices and to be aware of the assumptions made about women's sexuality as these affect sexual health in ways that are both subtle and powerful.

The relationship between gender and sexuality

A discussion of women's sexuality implies that female sexuality is distinct and separate from male sexuality. It seems evident that this is so and most sexual health services are predicated on that understanding. Indeed, it is almost impossible to separate gender and sexuality in our thinking. We think of biological sex and gender interchangeably. Biological sex refers to male or female physical characteristics, whereas gender refers to how we are expected to behave as men and women and has different meanings in different cultures and times. Biological sex itself is sometimes hard to determine, and transsexuals confound all our rigid assumptions about the relationship of gender to biology.

Gender and sexuality are fundamental to our sense of self, and because they are seen as natural, the beliefs and assumptions that are implicit in how we think about them are taken for granted. This has important implications when we consider sexual health care. It is imperative to look critically at both gender and sexuality and become aware of the way they are socially constructed.

How each woman constructs her own understanding of what it means to be a woman and to be sexual will influence her profoundly. Whether or not a woman uses contraception, or is able to negotiate safer sex, will necessarily involve how she thinks about her sexuality and herself as a woman. Apparently simple decisions, such as whether 'to go on the pill', will be imbued with meaning and will involve conscious and unconscious, rational and irrational elements, as well as social and cultural values. Barrier methods involve conscious negotiation and intrude upon sexual intercourse, whereas the pill allows

'passion' and 'spontaneity' and sex can take place without any reminders of the need for protection from pregnancy and disease. Verbal negotiation is not necessary, and assumptions can be made that it is her responsibility to take precautions. In research done by Thomson and Holland they state:

> Many of the young women to whom we spoke considered the 'spontaneity' enabled by the pill to be the central defining factor of sexual interaction and expressed opposition to condom use for reasons related to the disruption of this ideal.

> (Holland and Thomson, 1998, p. 66)

The relationship between gender and sexuality is complex and multifaceted. Consequently, it is possible that someone could see pregnancy as proof that she was a real woman. Indeed, many societies reinforce this view by according status to fecundity. This belief might then affect contraception use because of a conflict between a rational decision that pregnancy should be avoided, and a desire, not necessarily conscious, to get pregnant in order to affirm an insecure sense of gender identity or to attract social approval. This demonstrates how understanding a woman's belief about gender and sexuality can help to explain behaviour that may otherwise seem puzzling.

In the West, female sexuality has been constructed in terms of stereotypes of the whore and the Madonna. Women are seen sexually either as voracious and all consuming or pure and chaste. Women who are sexually active are often condemned for their behaviour and labelled as whores. Whilst this attitude has modified considerably it continues to affect women. Despite changes in the law, judges still question women who have been raped about their sexual histories, making their sexual behaviour as much on trial as the activities of the rapist. Young women may worry about their reputations and being called a 'slag' is a potent term of abuse (Holland *et al.*, 1990).

Women suffer the consequences of sexual activity through sanctions against them. In recent history women were placed in psychiatric hospitals because they were unmarried and pregnant.

Prostitutes have long been seen as a source of disease and blamed for their work. In the UK, the Contagious Diseases Acts from 1864 until 1883 were directed against women working as prostitutes and the language used was moralistic and condemnatory, whereas the examination of soldiers was abandoned in 1859 as 'repugnant to the feelings of the men' (Davenport-Hines, 1990).

More recently, Patton (1994) explored how prostitutes were seen by epidemiologists and policymakers as a source of HIV infection to heterosexual men rather than as at risk of infection *from* men. This was despite the probability that female sex workers are more at risk from men because of the greater risk of male to female transmission of HIV infection (Johnson and Johnstone, 1993).

At the other extreme female purity is venerated, and honour and virtue are connected with chastity. In the nineteenth century, sexologists promoted the idea that sexual desire amongst respectable women did not exist (Caplan, 1987). Although these ideas have changed they still have relevance. In the United States there is an increasing trend for young women to pledge that they will remain virgins until they marry and the traditional nuclear family is still revered by many as the ideal.

Of course, women's total experience of sexuality does not fit in with either of these extremes. Actual behaviour and consciously held attitudes and beliefs always lie in uneasy relationship with one another and never more so than in relation to sexuality. However, it can be seen from this how difficult it can be for women to see their sexuality as positive and healthy. Young women, in particular, may feel vulnerable as they attempt to create an identity for themselves as adult, sexual and female amidst the contradictory messages they receive.

Gender-specific expectations are a filter through which sexual encounters are endowed with meaning. For example, men are often expected to separate sex from love whereas women are expected to relate sex to love (Holland *et al.*, 1990). This can lead to very different ways of seeing the same sexual encounter and can cause distressing communication problems as couples struggle to understand one another.

Men are seen as active in sex, as the knowing sexual agent; women as innocent and passive. If being active sexually is defined as male then for women to carry condoms can seem to threaten femininity.

The construction of femininity as passive conflicts with women's ability to negotiate safer sex. This is evident in the research into young women's sexual practices conducted by the Women, Risk and AIDS Project. They provide illuminating examples of how young women know about safer sex and intend to use condoms but undermine themselves because of ideas of appropriate female sexual behaviour. One young woman described her boyfriend telling her that the condom should be blown up before use. She knew that this was wrong but felt unable to tell him because boys are supposed to know about sex whereas women are not. Penetrative sex is still regarded as the definitive sex act. As a result, although young women were aware that their pleasure in sex was not necessarily related to penetration, they continued to define sexual relationships as 'going the whole way' or not (Holland *et al.*, 1990).

Although women are expected to be passive, female sexuality is presented as powerful and dangerous, able to provoke uncontrollable lust in men. Men are not held responsible for their sexual behaviour because of the supposedly overwhelming nature of their sexual urges. Women are held responsible for controlling male sexual behaviour as well as their own. The threat of male sexual violence is used to justify women's need for protection and safety, and controls women's ability to freely express their sexuality. Men's frequent sexual irresponsibility is a contemporary problem because of the need to encourage men to use condoms to prevent the transmission of HIV infection.

Yet despite male sexual irresponsibility, the vast amount of research into teenage sexual health, for example, 'amounts to a relentless surveillance of female (but not male) adolescent sexual behaviour' (Tolman, 2002, p. 10). The focus is on risk, and the potential and actual harmful consequences for young women of sexual activity. Young men are under less scrutiny because of social constructions of their sexuality. The consequence of this for young women is to leave them fearful of their sexual desires and without any language or context in which it is safe to explore them. This might be seen as a small price to pay for their protection but Miller (1976) identifies sexual authenticity, 'this is, the ability to bring one's own real feelings of sexual desire and sexual pleasure meaningfully into intimate relationships – as a key feature of women's psychological health' (cited by Tolman, 2002, p. 20). Tolman (2002) goes on to research how teenage girls manage the dilemmas created by their sexual desires, and convincingly argues that an understanding of feelings of sexual desire helps girls to make responsible choices about sexual behaviour, and that, ironically, those girls who are most at risk are those who are out of touch with the messages their bodies send to them.

Women see their bodies and their sexuality presented everywhere in Western society as a commodity. Women's bodies are presented as objects, which must fit certain criteria in order to be seen as desirable. As a result, younger and younger women go on diets and become anorexic and older women resort to face lifts and plastic surgery in an attempt to fit the current definition of good looks. There is no place here for the ill or the elderly, and women who have had radical surgery, for example, have to find some way to come to terms with these pressures.

There are many subtle and complex connections between power and sexuality. The possession of money and power can determine the ability and ease of procuring and demanding sexual satisfaction. The lack of power women experience in patriarchal families may be partly responsible for the difficulty women have defining and insisting on their own sexual desires. Rape is an act of power over someone else where sex is used as the means of domination. Perpetrators of sexual abuse are attracted by the vulnerability of their victims. The need to empower women is, therefore, fundamental to sexual well-being.

A woman's sense of ownership of her own body, her understanding of her own sexuality and how she wishes to express it are essential preconditions for good sexual relationships.

Gender expectations may create considerable conflict for women and limit their capacity to enjoy a positive female sexuality.

The power of women to define their own sexuality is also crucial in that male definitions of female sexuality have prevailed throughout history. An example of this is the following quotation from the work of Van de Velde, a sexologist who wrote in 1928: 'The wife must be *taught* not only how to behave in coitus, but, above all, how and what to feel in this unique act!' (Caplan, 1987).

More pertinent, perhaps, is the influence the male perspective has had on medical practices. A well-known example of this is the way many gynaecologists used to insist that hysterectomies were good for women with the rationale that if women no longer needed a womb to bear children it would be better removed. A practice that came from a male perspective was presented as good medicine. Other practices can be seen to have more to do with male desire than female health. In the 1970s on billboards in California Caesareans were marketed for women with the slogan 'Keep your birth canal honeymoon fresh, have a caesar'. The 'marriage' stitch, which was an extra stitch given after birth to woman with episiotomies to tighten the vaginal canal for their male partners, was another example. Woman have challenged these practices and changes have resulted, but it is a useful reminder of the need to examine gender biases that might underpin current practices.

Theories of sexuality

The predominant view of sexuality is that it is natural and innate, yet what is taken as natural is by no means straightforward and uncontentious. The idea of sexuality as natural has implicit within it specific ideologies. Sexual behaviour is presented from a hierarchical value system with good, healthy, natural sex (heterosexual and for procreation) opposed to bad, unhealthy, unnatural sex (homosexual, depraved and diseased). Homosexuality and diverse forms of sexual expression occur throughout history and in all cultures.

In some senses, therefore, they must count as 'natural' behaviour but this is omitted from these theories.

Biologists have studied sexuality as a natural drive which reveals the animal nature of mankind. A basic premise of all their work is that men and women are fundamentally different in their sexual needs and desires because of their genital and reproductive differences. Theories that purport to describe human sexuality have been based on creatures as different from human beings as worms and sparrows! Their arguments fail to convince for many reasons. First, animal sexual behaviour varies so greatly that virtually any theory could be substantiated depending on what view you wished to promote. Second, supposedly scientific descriptions of animal behaviour use terms such as 'gang rape' and 'prostitution'. These descriptions are then presented as scientific evidence to support particular ideologies about sexuality.

Even the language used to describe the activity of sperm is gender coded. Thus it is described as thrusting, competitive, actively fighting its way to penetrate the passive, waiting ova.

Observed gender differences in human sexual behaviour are described as having a biological base:

> Because males have an almost infinite number of sperm, while women have a very restricted supply of eggs, it is deduced that men have an evolutionary propulsion towards spreading their seed to ensure diversity and reproductive success, and hence towards promiscuity, while women have an equal interest in reserving energy, an instinct for conservation and hence a leaning towards monogamy.
>
> (Weeks, 2003)

Biological theories have an appealing plausibility until we realize how much sexual behaviour they fail to explain. Sexual behaviour often proves more imaginative and varied than is recognized by these theories. Undoubtedly biology plays a part in human sexuality; reproductive capacities, in particular, are strikingly different for men and women. What is problematic is the attempt to explain all human behaviour on the basis of biology.

Sociologists provide a different framework for understanding sexuality, yet their arguments have similar flaws in that masculinity and femininity are seen in reductive terms, with social roles replacing biology as the essential root of sexual behaviour. Nurture and learned behaviour take over from biological explanations. In their case society rather than biology is seen as the predominant force. These are important influences on sexuality. The problem occurs when the attempt is made to explain all sexuality in these terms.

Psychoanalysis provides a more satisfactory range of theories of sexuality as it takes into account the meaning individuals give to their sexual activities. The role ascribed to the unconscious gives scope for fantasies, irrationality, contradictions and conflicts as the individual struggles to give meaning to psychic development. Neither gender identity nor sexual object choice (the gender of the desired sexual partner) are easily acquired, rather they are somewhat precariously attained through the resolution of developmental conflicts. There are many competing psychoanalytic theories of sexuality but Freud's work remains central (Freud, 1977). He saw human beings as all potentially bisexual, with gender identity and heterosexuality acquired through difficult developmental challenges through which the infant negotiates his or her way. The meaning each of us gives to sexual acts, to body parts and to relationships is far from straightforward and remains tenuous and provisional throughout our lives.

In psychoanalytic theory the roots of what is known as abnormal sexual behaviour are found in the infantile sexuality of all of us. Perverse solutions to developmental crises are available to everyone and heterosexuality is achieved only with difficulty. Within this framework it is possible to explain practices such as fetishism, and it is comprehensible that someone could be born biologically female, identify themselves as male and choose either gender or both as object choices.

However, there is a tension in Freud's work between his understanding of the complexity and fluidity of sexuality and his idea that there is a true adult sexuality. Homosexuality is regarded as a regression, as infantile, in opposition to heterosexuality which is described as 'mature object love'. His arguments were based on reproduction as the biological aim of sexuality. Because sexual acts *can* lead to procreation, it is argued, that is the purpose of sexuality. This is a basic premise of religious and biological views on sexuality upon which moral systems and scientific theories are founded. The problem is that, once again, human sexuality refuses to conform to this. It manifestly fails to explain the continuation of sexual desire after the menopause, when one partner is infertile, when contraception is being used and in homosexual relationships. The belief that sexual expression ought to be solely for procreation may produce guilt, shame or grief in individuals who are sexually active when not procreative, but it cannot explain the presence of sexual desire in these circumstances.

Also, Freud is less convincing about female sexuality, and his theory of penis envy, the claimed superiority of the vaginal orgasm and patriarchal view of women have been thoroughly critiqued by both psychoanalytic and feminist writers. By comparison, the work of Kinsey *et al.* (1953) and Masters and Johnson (1966) was refreshing. They debunked the myth of the superiority of the vaginal over the clitoral orgasm. They also emphasized the similarities of male and female sexual responses. Masters and Johnson were motivated by their beliefs in the equality of the sexes and their wish to promote good, satisfying sex as the foundation of marriage. However, their conclusions were influenced by this ideological position as much as the data. Consequently, although they emphasize similarities, their research shows that women and men have very different numbers of orgasms and their peak ages of sexual interest and activity are totally incompatible. Their work was funded to help marital happiness, yet, ironically, when orgasm is seen as central to sexual satisfaction the partner is relatively unimportant.

> With orgasm defined as the single, universal goal of what they call human sexual response, masturbation wins out every time as the most effective means of achieving it!
>
> (Segal, 1994)

Indeed, Masters and Johnson's work demonstrates that the penis has no great advantage over a hand, tongue or vibrator in bringing about orgasms; in fact, it rather suggests the reverse. If this is the case, and if orgasm is all important as a sexual goal, then heterosexuality has no inherent superiority over homosexuality.

Their work was conducted in a laboratory and they describe neat stages of responses and a linear progression of sexual excitement. Such descriptions are useful but many sexual encounters are experienced in more diverse ways that do not fit into their account.

These limitations to their theory should not detract from the importance of their contribution. Their work broke new ground and it has been used in combination with other approaches to form new sex therapies that are available to the benefit of many individuals and couples.

More recently, Michel Foucault's writing on sexuality has transformed the whole concept of sexuality, bringing about a radical examination of the concealed agendas in scientific, medical, psychological and sociological definitions of sexuality. His work usefully illuminates hidden assumptions, and brings into question how we think about power, diversity and identity in relation to sexuality (Foucault, 1987–88).

Finally, the feminist, gay and lesbian movements have fundamentally challenged traditional views of sexuality. Their campaigns and questions, in conjunction with the availability of birth control and safe terminations of pregnancy, have probably had more impact than anything else on women's sexuality and health. The availability of reliable contraception has profoundly affected the way women experience and think about their sexuality. It is possible, because of effective contraception, to separate sexuality from reproduction.

The advent of AIDS has also fundamentally affected how we think about sex. As a result of the AIDS epidemic, actual sexual practice has had to be examined more carefully and explicitly than ever before.

Models of sexual health that focus on rational, consciously held attitudes and beliefs have been shown to be seriously limited. Joffe (1997) argues that it would be more useful to focus on 'the interlinked issues of emotion, identity and identity enhancement'. Her discussion highlights how feelings of intimacy and love are more important than consciously known risks of becoming HIV positive. Willig (1997) also explores the role of trust in deciding to practise safer or unsafer sex. Research is becoming more sophisticated in the theories of sexuality on which it is based (Boulton, 1994) and the meaning, interactions between partners, and context of sexual encounters are seen as central. AIDS has made it more urgent than ever to understand sexual behaviour in all its complexities and to question prevailing theories of sexuality and the ways they obscure and illuminate our understanding.

Female sexual development

The first thing that everyone wants to know about a newborn baby is its biological sex. People are uncomfortable around infants when neither their name nor their attire indicates their gender. We respond differently in both subtle and obvious ways to boy and girl babies. Our behaviour shapes the child's responses into conforming to gender-appropriate behaviours even, at times, when we consciously intend to do otherwise. How we do this and what we regard as acceptable and unacceptable varies in different eras and in different places. It is also the result of our own personal histories, how we feel about our own mothers and fathers, brothers and sisters. Much of what we communicate will be unconscious and irrational and will contain contradictions and conflicts. Each child will actively construct his or her individual meaning as they attempt to make sense of all these messages.

The way in which girls experience their bodies is crucially different from the way boys experience theirs. Boys handle their penises as a matter of course every day; they are visible, external and the changes in them are instantly obvious. For girls, the exploration of their genitals is less frequently a part of their daily experience. This is not to say that their curiosity and satisfaction in playing with their genitals is less than that of boys, but their actual experience is different in significant respects. Many women have never looked at their own vulvas and indeed to do so is far from easy, given that it requires a mirror. Female genitals are often not accurately named. The vulva is often referred to as the vagina. In Webster's dictionary, earlier this century, there was no word for female genitals except the vagina.

> One might question how pride in femininity could flourish at a time when our language did not include a word for the part of the female anatomy most richly endowed with sensory nerve endings and with no function other than that of sexual pleasure.
>
> (Goldhor Lerner, 1988)

Vague information regarding sexuality and the nature of sexual differences can lead to anxiety, confusion and shame as the environment provides no language to help describe and understand sexual feelings. Gay and lesbian children face a similar challenge as little in the world around them reflects their experiences.

This sense of female bodies as mysterious and unknowable even to women themselves affects the expression of desire.

> The feminine sex organ is mysterious even to woman herself … Woman does not recognise herself in it and this explains in large part why she does not recognise its desires as hers.
>
> (De Beauvoir, 1953)

The infant does not experience her or himself as either gender. There is ample evidence to indicate that both sexes believe that they could become the other sex. For Freud and other psychoanalytic writers this is central to infantile sexuality. The fear of castration for the boy and the castration that has already taken place for the girl bring about different paths of development for girls and boys. Both sexes identify initially with the mother and the boy has to separate from her and learn to identify with his father, whereas the girl retains her identification with her mother but learns to desire her father. Whether this happens or not and how the crises are resolved by each individual child will provide the basis for their adult sexuality. The strength of this approach is that it accounts for the complexity of gender and sexual identity and demonstrates the role of fantasy and the unconscious.

Anyone who has contact with children knows that they have a rich and vivid fantasy life and that the distinction between reality and fantasy is only slowly and painfully learned. For the young baby there is no clear boundary between itself and the world. It is perhaps because of this that in all cultures the body is the boundary marker and many social and cultural rituals are organized around the body. In particular, the orifices are seen as central. Some anthropologists have suggested that the body is a metaphor for society and that therefore controlling what comes in and what goes out is crucial. Hence sexuality and its regulation is of public concern for any culture.

To the baby its body products are a source of pride and fascination. There is an erotic charge to sucking and defecating which is given up as controls are learned. These emerge again in foreplay and in many adult sexual activities. To the baby, all body parts and both sexes can be vested with sexual excitement. This is part of infantile sexuality and is given up slowly and with difficulty by the growing child. The roots of all 'abnormal' sexual behaviour can be found here. It reveals how sexuality can seek satisfaction in different ways, through any organ of the body and can be attached to any person we desire, regardless of their gender.

Because they have once been a source of intense pleasure and fascination, our body products can become a source of shame and disgust. Unconsciously we remember our earlier curiosity and feel a mixture of excitement and repulsion that can be hard to deal with. Nurses are constantly in touch with body products in a way that can cause discomfort for both them and their patients. Smell is important to sexual desire, and defecation and urination can be part of sexual activities. Yet the intimacy and potentially sexual nature of nursing tasks is not often thought about or spoken about. When sexuality is talked of, the body as a whole, touch, smell and the substances that issue from the body are ignored. Through examining infantile sexuality, it becomes evident that these are important foundations upon which our adult sexuality is formed.

As we mature, controls are developed but these can break down at critical points in our lives. Transitional maturational points (these are times of major social and biological change) are especially vulnerable times. Our infantile sexual conflicts can re-emerge in different ways at these times. This can add to the stresses experienced at puberty, marriage, pregnancy and at the menopause.

All of these transitions can bring up forgotten primitive anxieties that can shock women with their intensity. Ambivalent feelings and pressures to conform to impossibly conflicting expectations can make these times especially sensitive and demanding. Unlike the infant, adolescent and adult women are influenced by social and cultural values as well as by unconscious impulses and fantasies. This can produce feelings of shame and humiliation as adult controls seem less certain and irrational impulses are more demanding. Each woman will experience these transitions in her sexuality in unique ways. Assumptions we make during our work can inhibit patients from communicating distress they feel because they are not experiencing their pregnancy, for instance, as they think they ought to. Descriptions of puberty and the menopause can all too often become prescriptive as well as descriptive. Because of the values associated with good, natural sex it can be difficult to admit deviations from the hierarchy.

Bisexual and lesbian sexuality

From the picture drawn already about sexuality, lesbianism becomes more comprehensible as a choice all women could make. If we are to believe Freud, all of us are initially bisexual. Moreover, sexuality changes for many people throughout their lives.

Given the mutability of sexuality, it is easy to understand that someone can become lesbian after years of heterosexuality. Other women know they are attracted only to women from puberty and occasionally before. Still others have sexual encounters with women, but do not regard themselves as lesbians. Women may, therefore, identify themselves as lesbian, bisexual or hetero-sexual and the chosen identity may bear little relationship to the actual experiences of sex with other women. The choice of a lesbian or bisexual identity suggests an acceptance by these women of their sexuality. This is important for sexual health as self-esteem and self-acceptance greatly enhance sexual well-being.

Lesbians have become more visible in recent years but throughout history their existence has been ignored. Queen Victoria refused to believe lesbians existed (Ferris, 1993). This, at least, meant that there is no legislation against lesbians but it rendered them invisible. As female sexual-ity has been seen through male eyes it remains difficult for many men and women to under-stand how lesbians can have sex without a penis. Again we are confronted by how much sex con-tinues to be defined by penile penetration. Because lesbians are seen as 'other', their differ-ences from 'normal' heterosexuals are under-stood through frameworks that come from the dominant defining viewpoints. As a result, les-bians are understood in terms of 'butch' and 'femme' in an attempt to make sense of their practices to heterosexuals. Lesbians may indeed take on these roles, sometimes as a deliberate parody of heterosexual relationships and at other times because the women involved feel these roles to be appropriate. Any attempt to fit lesbian sexuality into these categories is made to render their sexuality less threatening. Lesbians are seen as outsiders. They may evoke strong feelings of excitement and danger, forbidden pleasures, disgust and abhorrence. That they may also be caring mothers, loving partners and may work as health care professionals cannot be contained in the usual construction of their sexuality.

Health care services have not taken into account the sexual health needs of lesbians. Services have been organized around contra-ception, disease control and fertility. Lesbians may require all of these services but there are many of their needs that are not catered for. Narrow definitions of sexuality, embodied in the health care services provided, fail to cater not just for lesbians but for any woman whose sexual needs fall outside of the present parameters.

Women who are disabled, ill, elderly or have learning difficulties similarly have to struggle to be seen as sexual and find services that cater for their sexual health needs.

Culture, ethnicity and religion

One of the fears most frequently expressed by health workers is of giving offence to women whose cultural and/or religious beliefs are dif-ferent from their own. In order to counter this fear, attempts are made to find out the attitudes to sexuality found in other religions and cultures (see also Chapter 6). This is a fascinating field of study but it is important that we are careful in how we use this information. Lists of cultural norms are of limited usefulness and can be applied in rigid and potentially racist ways (Montford and Skrine, 1993). Each woman's interpretation of her culture will be unique and the experiences of a second-generation Bengali woman, for instance, will differ from her mother's. There are as many differences within a culture as there are between them.

Also, attitudes and beliefs held publicly may bear little relation to practice. Roman Catholics who practise birth control and who have abortions despite their faith are a good example. This highlights how, for all of us, the beliefs that we hold and the values that we have may not be reflected in our behaviour. This can be a cause of shame and guilt and can be very detrimental to acknowledging our sexual health needs.

The complex relationship between different attitudes and values can also explain conflicting behaviour we observe in patients. For example, in some cultures menstruation is seen as an impor-tant regular cleansing for the body and is associ-ated with health (Caplan, 1987). Contraceptives that interfere with menstruation can consequently be rejected as unhealthy because of this. This reminds us once more that it is essential to explore the individual's own understanding of their health and sexuality in order to offer appropriate help.

One danger is that we will over-identify with people who have similar backgrounds to our own, and will assume that their experiences are the same as ours. As a result we fail to notice differences. On the other hand, it is equally possible to regard the experiences of people whose backgrounds differ from our own as totally foreign and strange. In this case we ignore common experiences. Stereotypes about race and sexuality can bring bizarre fantasies into play that can detrimentally affect health care. It is important to be as aware as we can be of the way these stereotypes can subtly influence us. It is impossible not to be affected by them, but it is crucial to attempt to be as non-judgemental as possible.

Conclusion

Most of us tend to see our own sex life as normal, understandable and natural while the sex life of 'others' may be frightening, bizarre or disgusting. The danger is that the sex lives of people regarded as 'different' are rarely seen in their terms and constantly they face ignorance and prejudice. This affects the elderly, the ill, people with learning difficulties and the disabled, as well as lesbians, prostitutes and cultural and ethnic minorities. The sexuality of all of these people is stereotyped in very different ways, but all of these stereotypes have a destructive effect on potential sexual health.

Nurses are dealing with their own feelings about sexuality whenever they enter the patient's private space. Taking cervical smears, touching, dealing with body products all involve intimacy that can be uncomfortable and disquieting. Yet how patients respond to routine procedures such as cervical smears can provide invaluable information about how they feel about their bodies which can be used by health professionals to promote sexual health.

We fear our own ignorance, feel embarrassed by the inadequate language available to talk about sexuality and worry that we will offend or open up histories of sexual abuse or rape that will overwhelm us. Yet the more we speak and learn the more our confidence grows. There is already a vast improvement from the ignorance prevalent a few generations ago.

How we think about sexuality is constantly changing as new variations on the theme of nature

versus nurture emerge. It is possible to think that these debates are irrelevant but in fact they affect health care profoundly. If a young girl of 13 comes in to discuss sexual health, how we think about sexual development will affect our response. Our values will be reflected in how we react if we find out her partner is a woman, 20 years older than her or that she is engaging in anal sex.

If we overemphasize biological differences in the sexual health care we offer we are in danger of ignoring women whose needs are not related to reproduction. On the other hand, if we emphasize similarities between women and men we may fail to cater for gender-specific needs. All aspects need to be reflected in the services we offer.

It may be that the appropriate concern of sexual health is mainly with safety and protection but unless sexuality is seen in much broader terms the care offered will be limited. Sexual health must connect with the experiences of the individual woman if it is to have relevance and meaning for her.

It is vital to remain open to the infinite variations in human sexuality and to acknowledge that sex is always going to be a highly charged and complex issue. To give good sexual health care we need to be curious about how each woman thinks of herself as a woman and a sexual being, and be alive to the fascination, excitement and challenge of sexuality.

Ideas for personal and professional development

- Compile a list of sexual health services available in your area. Possible suggestions for inclusion are: genitourinary medicine clinics, family planning services, young people's advisory agencies, HIV/AIDS services, psychosexual clinics, counselling, and rape and sexual assault services

- Liaise with as many of these services as you can: see if you can visit them and sit in with some of the staff

- Research the sexual health needs of specific groups of women in your area who do not use your services, to see if there are any ways in which you can improve the service you offer to meet their needs.

Further reading

COLMAN, J. and ROKER, D. (eds) (1998) *Teenage Sexuality. Health, Risk and Education.* Amsterdam: Harwood Academic.

HOLLAND, J., RAMAZANOGLU, C. and SCOTT, S. (1990) *Women Risk and AIDS Project Papers 1–8.* London: Tufnell Press.

HOLLAND, J., RAMANZANOGLU, C., SHARPE, S. and THOMPSON, R. (1998) *The Male in the Head. Young People, Heterosexuality and Power.* London: Tufnell Press.

LAWLOR, J. (1991) *Behind the Screens. Nursing, Somology and the Problem of the Body.* Edinburgh: Churchill Livingstone.

LINCOLN, R. (ed.) (1992) *Psychosexual Medicine.* London: Chapman and Hall.

MARTIN-SPERRY, C. (2003) *Couples and Sex.* Oxford: Radcliffe Medical Press.

MONTFORD, H. and SKRINE, R. (eds) (1993) *Contraceptive Care.* London: Chapman and Hall.

SAVAGE, J. (1987) *Nurses, Gender and Sexuality.* London: Heinemann Nursing.

SKRINE, R. (1997) *Blocks and Freedoms in Sexual Life.* Oxford: Radcliffe Medical Press.

TOLMAN, D.L. (2002) *Dilemmas of Desire.* London: Harvard University Press.

VAN OOIJEN, E. and CHARNOCK, A.J. (1993) *Sexuality and Patient Care: A Guide for Nurses and Teachers.* London: Chapman and Hall.

WEEKS, J. (2003) *Sexuality,* 2nd edn. London: Routledge.

WEEKS, J. and HOLLAND, J. (eds) (1996) *Sexual Cultures. Communities, Values and Intimacy.* London: Macmillan Press.

References

BEAUVOIR, S. DE (1953) *The Second Sex.* London: Jonathon Cape.

BOULTON, M. (1994) *Challenge and Innovation. Methodological Advances in Social Research on HIV/AIDS.* Southport: Taylor and Francis.

CAPLAN, P. (ed.) (1987) *The Cultural Construction of Sexuality.* London: Routledge.

DAVENPORT-HINES, R. (1990) *Sex, Death and Punishment.* London: Fontana.

FERRIS, P. (1993) *Sex and the British. A Twentieth Century History.* London: Michael Joseph.

FOUCAULT, M. (1987–88) *The History of Sexuality,* Vols 1, 2 and 3. Harmondsworth: Penguin.

FREUD, S. (1977) *On Sexuality.* Volume 7 of The Pelican Freud Library. Harmondsworth: Penguin.

GOLDHOR LERNER, H. (1988) *Women in Therapy.* New York: Harper and Row.

HOLLAND, J., RAMAZANOGLU, C. and SCOTT, S. (1990) *Women Risk and AIDS Project Papers 1–8.* London: Tufnell Press.

HOLLAND, J. and THOMSON, R. (1998) Sexual relationships, negotiation and decision making. In Colman, J. and Roker, D. (eds) *Teenage Sexuality. Health, Risk and Education.* Amsterdam: Harwood Academic.

JOFFE, H. (1997) Intimacy and love in late modern conditions. In: Ussher, J.M. (ed.) *Body Talk.* London: Routledge.

JOHNSON, M. and JOHNSTONE, F. (1993) *HIV Infection in Women.* Edinburgh: Churchill Livingstone.

KINSEY, A.C., POMEROY, W.B., MARTIN, C.E. and GEBHARD, P.H. (1953) *Sexual Behaviour in the Human Female.* Philadelphia and London: W.B. Saunders.

MASTERS, W.H. and JOHNSON, V.E. (1966) *Human Sexual Response.* London: Bantam Books.

MILLER, J.B. (1976) *Towards a New Psychology of Women,* 2nd edn. Boston: Beacon Press.

MONTFORD, H. and SKRINE, R. (eds) (1993) *Contraceptive Care.* London: Chapman and Hall.

PATTON, C. (1994) *Last Served? Gendering the HIV Pandemic.* London: Taylor and Francis.

SEGAL, L. (1994) *Straight Sex.* London: Virago Press.

TOLMAN, D.L. (2002) *Dilemmas of Desire.* London: Harvard University Press.

WEEKS, J. (2003) *Sexuality,* 2nd edn. London: Routledge.

WILLIG, C. (1997) Trust as risky practice. In Segal, L. (ed.) *New Sexual Agendas.* London: Macmillan Press.

2: Ethico-Legal Issues in Women's Health

Shirley R Jones

OBJECTIVES

This chapter should help you understand:

◆ The ethico-legal basis for the NMC documents provided for practitioners ◆

◆ Major ethical theories plus ethical and legal principles and their application to practice ◆

◆ Some ethico-legal aspects related to late termination of pregnancy ◆

◆ Some ethico-legal aspects related to sterilization of the younger woman ◆

◆ Some ethico-legal aspects related to antenatal testing for HIV ◆

◆ Some ethico-legal aspects related to domestic violence ◆

◆ Aspects of the practitioner's role as advocate and confidante ◆

◆ Some ethico-legal aspects of nurse prescribing. ◆

Introduction

Ethics and law, either together or as separate topics, are currently fundamental aspects of the education and training of nurses, midwives and health visitors. However, surprising as it may seem to the younger reader, these aspects only became overt topics in the various nursing/midwifery curricula from the late 1980s. Medical students who, until 1994, might have had an hour on ethics during their training, perhaps disguised within their psychology programme (verbally reported by a senior person in a medical school), also now have grounding in these areas (GMC, 1993). This educational provision is heartening. However, when we consider how many health care professionals currently in practice undertook their qualifying courses before the expected inclusion of ethics and law, it becomes clear that many practitioners missed such grounding.

Ongoing development is required by all health care professionals, as determined by their professional bodies. This development could be in order to change direction, for instance from general nursing to health visiting or practice nursing, or for academic enhancement or purely for professional updating. In most cases the practitioner will encounter something on ethics and law, whether it is a whole module or just a session in a study day. Some will even do complete degrees on the subjects. Whilst this may be reassuring in some ways, it does not guarantee that the individual will apply the new knowledge to practice; particularly if they only had a short exposure to the topic(s) compared with years of entrenched practice. The major point being made here is that while some practitioners have a good grounding in ethics and law, not only do they need to utilize it in their everyday practice, but they also need to be mindful of the fact that they may be working with practitioners who do not have that background knowledge or philosophy of practice.

Whilst those practitioners who have not studied ethics and law may not be familiar with the terminology used, they cannot plead total ignorance of the application to practice. The Nursing and Midwifery Council (NMC), as did the United Kingdom Central Council for Nursing, Midwifery and Health Visiting (UKCC) before it, provides ethico-legal direction and guidance in the form of documents sent free of charge to all its registrants. The *Code of Professional Conduct: Standards for conduct, performance and ethics* (NMC 2004a) and the *Practitioner–Client Relationships and the Prevention of Abuse* (UKCC, 1999) all provide clear ethical guidance to support all areas of practice. There are other similar documents that give guidance on specific aspects of practice, such as administration of medicines and record keeping (NMC, 2004b). Midwives have an extra document: *Midwives Rules and Standards* (NMC, 2004c), which indicates the legal and ethical aspects of their specific role. Other health care professionals have their own guidance documents, for instance doctors have the General Medical Council's code of conduct *Protecting Patients, Guiding Doctors* (GMC, 1993).

Having indicated a need for ethico-legal knowledge in health care, it would perhaps be useful to consider what ethics is and why it is so often linked with law.

> Ethics is the application of the processes and theories of moral philosophy to a real situation, concerned with the basic principles and concepts which guide human beings in thought and action, and which underlie their values.
>
> (Jones, 2000)

Ethics, then, implies more than just moral behaviour which is expected of everyone in a generally moral society. Moral behaviour, for most people, is greatly intuitive; an intuition developed through the various avenues of socialization and guided by conscience, perhaps exercised subconsciously at times. Ethical behaviour requires the conscious application of further knowledge of philosophical theory. It could be abstract, which the practitioner can leave to the mental posturing of academics, then access the end result by consulting textbooks and journal articles. It certainly needs to be practical, and knowledge of the basic theories and principles or concepts can be very useful, if only to help with thorough reflection after an event or incident.

Ethics can be related to any area of life. In this case it is health care and the legal link is obviously to health care law, which is generally dealt with in the civil courts through the law of torts, or civil wrongs, where compensation is being sought. There are some situations where criminal activity has occurred and this is dealt with through the criminal courts, where justice is sought; such as the well-publicized case of Dr Harold Shipman, convicted as a serial killer in January 2000. Some cases could appear in both courts. Civil law is underpinned by ethics and failure to uphold ethical practice can lead to claims of civil wrongs, hence practitioners need to be aware of the possible consequences of unethical practice.

This chapter considers briefly the major ethical theories in use. It includes a case study approach to discuss the application of ethico-legal principles to practice. While accepting that sound ethico-legal practice is essential to all areas of health care, the purpose of this chapter is to apply this knowledge to the care of women. Although it is acknowledged that there are many different health care professionals dealing with women's health issues, concentration is generally on nurses, midwives and health visitors. For ease of writing and rather than offend any particular group by use of the generic term 'nurse(s)', the term 'practitioner' and pronoun 'she' are used to denote the NMC professionals for the rest of the chapter.

Ethical theories

Ethical theories can be used to help resolve moral conflicts and dilemmas; a dilemma being where there is a choice of at least two courses of action, but neither option gives a perfect result. They can also be considered in retrospect, to try to understand the thinking behind someone's decision-making, particularly when that decision differs from the one we would make ourselves. Additionally, they can be used to aid reflection on events or incidents with inherent ethico-legal issues.

However, to do any of this, the theories must be known and understood by the practitioner. A brief overview of the major theories generally referred to is undertaken, but for more in-depth knowledge, it would be useful to access general texts as well as those where the authors have applied the ethics and law to the practitioners' areas of practice.

Duty-based theory

Deontology is the best known duty-based theory and there are three main schools of thought.

Rational monism (Kantian ethics) has a belief in one supreme driving force (hence the monism) – duty, based on good will (from God's will). Within this theory, proposed actions are judged according to the requirement for absolute observance of the principle of autonomy (which requires rationality) and their ability to be universalized. If a practitioner feels that she should undertake a specific course of action with one particular client, she would need to consider whether she is effectively observing that woman's autonomy and whether, if she took that action with all women in similar circumstances, it would still be seen as morally right. This does not mean that the action would *have* to be taken with all such women, just that it would not be wrong to do so; therefore, it is not as opposed to individualized care as it may initially seem.

There is a 'traditional' school within deontology, based on mainly Judeo-Christian beliefs, with the ten commandments as the code of conduct, each of which deals with a separate aspect of life and is, therefore, not liable to conflict. It is quite probable that any other religion which has a dutiful code of conduct, based on its scriptures, would also fit within this school.

The third school involves intuitionistic pluralism. This theory involves seven equal prima facie duties, determined by Ross (1930): fidelity, beneficence (doing good), non-maleficence (doing no harm), justice, reparation, gratitude and self-improvement. To reduce the amount of conflict possible in the application of these duties to any proposed action, a system of casuistry, case-based reasoning, can be used. This system allows prioritization of the duties according to the intuition of the individual. In the majority of health care situations, practitioners would be likely to consider beneficence, non-maleficence and justice as the priorities; however, conflict still commonly occurs between beneficence and non-maleficence.

Consequentialism

Utilitarianism is the best known consequentialist theory, where the anticipated consequences of an action are contemplated to determine the utility to be achieved. It was initially a hedonistic theory which sought pleasure from a person's actions; however, modern-day contemplation would probably seek benefit rather than pleasure. The intention is to achieve the greatest benefit for the greatest number of people. This theory has two schools of thought. The initial version, known as act-utilitarianism, considers every action with a view to achieving the aforementioned goal; it is therefore monist in outlook. This theory is objective, although benefit is not always measurable; it can also be harsh, as it is considered that 'the end justifies the means'. This maxim may result in the needs of the individual being overlooked to achieve benefit for the majority. A second school evolved with the intention of avoiding some of the difficulties, while still achieving utility. In this case, the possible outcome of an act is judged according to moral rules of conduct, similar to the universalization principle in Kantian theory.

To put this into context, consider the principle of truth-telling. For an act-utilitarian no principle is absolute, they are all negotiable, so if it is felt that the greatest benefit can be achieved by withholding the truth, or even telling a lie, this action would be acceptable. A rule-utilitarian, however, would consider that it is generally morally right to tell the truth, so he or she would choose to do so, while being mindful of the need to achieve utility.

In health care, it is possible to see both major theories in use. The professional codes and guidance for practitioners is deontological in nature, stressing the individual practitioner's duties to clients and patients, whereas the NHS itself is essentially utilitarian, aiming to create the greatest benefit for the greatest number of people. In practical terms, a practitioner undertaking a clinic session in contraception and sexual health can be deontological in her approach to every individual client. However, the manager responsible for keeping the whole service running has to be more utilitarian in approach. There are even times when a practitioner, whether she is aware of it or not, has to be a philosophical schizophrenic. One day she can be on duty on a ward where she is allocated a number of clients, in which case she can be deontological in approach. The next day she can be in charge of the whole ward and her approach will have to change to provide the best service possible for the total clientele and the staff.

Some people have a natural leaning toward one ideal or another, but for those who do not probably the way forward would be to adopt an eclectic approach, as has occurred with models of care – taking the best from each theory. There are elements of Kantian and pluralistic ethics that are suitable for client-centred care. At the same time, trying to achieve the greatest benefit for the greatest number of clients or patients, particularly within the NHS, is also a worthy cause. However, this latter point should not be achieved regardless of cost to individuals; the action cannot always be justified by the outcome (Jones, 2000).

Principlism

There are many ethical principles that the various theories can embrace, ignore or prioritize; however, this approach to resolution of conflict and dilemma relies on observance of just four main principles:

◆ Autonomy – where, unless proved otherwise, people are respected as self-determining and able to make rational decisions for themselves. This principle creates the obligation to provide information, obtain valid consent and maintain privacy and confidentiality (Beauchamp and Childress, 2001).

◆ Beneficence – one of two key principles in health care, requiring practitioners always to act for the good of the patient or client.

◆ Non-maleficence – the other key principle in health care, requiring practitioners to do no harm.

◆ Justice – requiring general fair play: equality in care given or in the expected endpoint; absence of any form of discrimination.

Virtue approach

This approach is based on the views of Aristotle. It relies on the development of attitudes and character through life experience. The virtues expected include honesty, courage, compassion, generosity, fidelity, integrity, fairness, self-control and prudence (Velasquez and Andre, 2003). These virtues should then be applied to decisions and actions towards the common good.

There are obviously criticisms of each of these approaches, but they will not be discussed here; further reading of texts listed and referenced will enable readers to develop critical thinking around the theories. In health care, it appears more usual to concentrate on deontology and utilitarianism when analysing cases.

Discussion

Abortion is the subject of great social and ethical debate. Those people who are opposed to abortion

 SCENARIO

Denise is 26 years old, she has one child aged 18 months and another of 10 months. The younger child was born at 24 weeks gestation and was left with long-term health problems which require a lot of care. Two weeks ago Denise had visited her doctor with some abdominal problems. She felt that she could not be pregnant as she had been experiencing fairly regular periods. However, a pregnancy test proved positive and she requested a termination of pregnancy (TOP) as she could not cope with another baby, in view of her existing difficulties.

Today, Denise arrived at a TOP clinic to follow through her request and she stated that she had experienced lower abdominal pain for the past few hours. On routine ultrasound scan it was discovered that Denise was at 23 weeks gestation and was in labour. She was transferred to the local maternity unit by ambulance, in well-established labour.

may have religious views which incorporate an absolute belief in the sanctity of life. Other objectors may have no religious belief, but object on moral grounds. Whatever the background, objections usually stem from the feeling that abortion is the destruction of a life. For some people the objection relates to abortion at any time, for others it would depend on the gestation. The difference of opinion usually relates to the views of the individual with regard to when life begins. Undoubtedly some people feel that life begins at conception, hence they may object to abortion at any stage. These people would usually be opposed to any method of contraception that does not prevent fertilization of the ovum, but prevents implantation of the blastocyst. For those people who believe that life does not begin until some later stage of development, such as presumed viability at 24 weeks, they may only be opposed to abortion from that particular point onwards.

Those people who support the woman's right to abortion are frequently supporters of the view that the woman's right to autonomy outweighs any moral rights that others may wish to bestow on the fetus. Legally, of course, the fetus has only one right, other than those contingent upon its being born alive, and that is the right not to be intentionally aborted except in accordance with the Abortion Act 1967 (as amended). This Act was amended by the Human Fertilization and Embryology Act 1990 and, while the upper gestational limit for most reasons for abortion was reduced to 24 weeks, there are three categories whereby there is no longer any upper limit (Morgan and Lee, 1991):

◆ To prevent grave permanent injury to the physical or mental health of the woman
◆ Where there is risk to the life of the woman
◆ Where there is substantial risk that the child would suffer from physical or mental abnormalities which would cause serious handicap.

In Denise's case, there is nothing to suggest that she will fit into either of the first two cases and, as she was not aware that she was pregnant until such a late gestation, she has had no opportunity for screening to determine any abnormality which

might come under the third category. She, therefore, would have been considered under the clauses relating to TOP prior to 24 weeks – with one week to go. There seems little doubt that both her own mental and physical health could suffer if she continued with the pregnancy, also her existing two children could suffer with the birth of another baby, thus satisfying clauses 2 and 3 of the Act. For these reasons, it would seem likely that she would have been successful in gaining the approval of the two medical practitioners necessary for the procedure to be undertaken.

Assuming that the documentation was completed, in view of the late gestation, the method of termination would most likely be the use of prostaglandins and an ensuing labour. The woman's condition would be monitored but not that of the fetus, as there would be no intention of taking any action to prevent the intended demise of the fetus. In fact, good practice would suggest that feticide should be carried out prior to the start of the process, to ensure that the baby is not born alive (RCOG, 1998). Although Callahan (1995, p. 271), in recognition of the antagonism of some people to this process, states that: 'a woman's right to terminate her pregnancy does not entail or include a right to death of her fetus'.

However, natural events appear to have overtaken Denise. Her pregnancy is coming to an end without interference. She feels unable to cope with another baby; therefore, as TOP was her wish, she will be hoping and possibly presuming that the fetus will die during labour. If the documentation has already been completed then the decision would probably be to treat the case as a TOP, thereby not monitoring the condition of the fetus during the labour. If the documentation has not been completed, the obstetricians and midwives in the maternity unit are now faced with a woman in established pre-term labour, where monitoring would be proposed. Denise, of course, is at liberty to refuse any offers of monitoring or intervention (St George's Healthcare NHS Trust v. S, 1998) during her labour.

All parties concerned could face difficulties on the birth of the baby should it be born showing signs of life, which is quite possible at this gestation. This labour may be viewed as an abortion, where the intention is 'to let the fetus suffer the labour to the point of its demise' (Jones, 2000), as it would be unsafe to consider an intra-cardiac injection of potassium chloride to the fetus during established labour. However, if it is born showing signs of life then it is a live birth and legally should be treated as such; this issue is covered by the Infanticide Act 1938 and the Human Rights Act 1998 (Article 2). If the condition of the baby at birth is poor, the paediatricians may choose not to undertake aggressive treatment, particularly in view of the circumstances. If, however, the condition is good, then they will have to deal with it in the same way that they would deal with any other very preterm baby, regardless of the circumstances. They cannot choose to leave it to die just because the mother's intention was for TOP. Now that it is a live birth it has the same legal rights as any other individual and the parents cannot determine that the child should die, unless the circumstances are such that 'treating to die' is in the best interests of the baby.

One of the problems for midwives in any late TOP where feticide has not been carried out is that paediatricians are often not keen to attend the delivery or to attend the live baby (Jones and Jenkins, 2004). This stance leaves the midwives in a dilemma. On the one hand the parent does not want the baby to live, but on the other hand the midwives are duty bound to treat a live birth as any live birth, particularly this close to the age of viability, therefore taking reasonable action until further instructions from a doctor on his/her arrival. The Infanticide Act 1938 states: 'anyone assisting in the commission of an act, or acquiescing in an omission resulting in the death of a child born alive, may be charged with murder'. It is perhaps important to note that even TOP clinics have to have neonatal resuscitation equipment available for such circumstances.

If this baby survives, the future could be very bleak for him or her and for the family. Denise has first-hand experience of the problems related to extreme prematurity and it could be suggested that, as this baby is one week younger in gestation than the previous one, it may have

greater problems. Added to the prematurity is the fact that Denise has had no antenatal care, therefore no advice and guidance with regard to her own health and well-being, which could have a detrimental effect on her fetus. Nor has she had any screening for fetal abnormality if this would have been her wish. Either of these last two points could even be the reason for the pre-term labour. The situation could arise where this baby 'would suffer from physical or mental abnormalities which would cause serious handicap' (Abortion Act 1967, as amended). However, where this would be grounds for the abortion of a fetus up to term, the law does not sanction active euthanasia of neonates with such abnormalities.

If this baby is born with a chromosomal or structural anomaly or develops a disability due to its prematurity, a deontological view would be that the best interests of the child, and only the child, should be taken into account. All practitioners having an impact on the care of the child have a duty to do the very best that they can, regardless of the consequences. This suggests that aggressive treatment should be undertaken with the aim of helping the child to survive. A utilitarian, however, would consider the consequences of various options to determine how to achieve the greatest benefit for as many of the concerned people as possible – the baby, Denise, her partner, the other two children. The consideration does not stop here. Providing ongoing care for such a pre-term baby has a resource implication, both in financial terms and the taking up of equipment and professional carers. It is possible, therefore, that a utilitarian would support the notion of 'treating to die' in these circumstances, especially if this was the wish of the parent(s). Peter Singer, an academic philosopher and well-known author in this field, is one such utilitarian, although he would go so far as to suggest that active steps should be taken to kill this baby, particularly if this is the preference of the parent(s); he sees little difference between killing a fetus in utero and helping him/her to die after birth (Toolis, 1999). Part of the reason for this is his view that neither a fetus nor a neonate is a person; neither possesses the rationality or self-consciousness necessary to be classified as such and therefore has no right to life. There are other commentators, such as Purdy and Tooley (1999), who consider a being's capacity to possess these personhood attributes. This consideration would include both the fetus and neonate as both have the capacity, or potential, to achieve these attributes – as long as they are not brain-damaged.

SCENARIO

Michelle is 21 years old and lives with her partner of 6 years, Kevin, in a two-bedroom council house. They receive some state benefit because Kevin is unskilled and a low-wage earner. They have four children: a boy of just 4 years old, a girl of 2 years and 9 months, another girl of 18 months and another son born 7 weeks ago. The first child was the result of not using contraception, whereas the other three followed failure of barrier and oral contraceptive methods; added to which, Michelle complained of headaches and fluid retention whilst taking the various contraceptive pills. Michelle is not a religious person but she does not like the idea of intrauterine contraceptive devices because of the way in which they work; in keeping with this view, she is also against abortion. She is a very loving mother but not very capable when it comes to keeping the house and the children clean. The children are fed well but that is because Kevin's parents live directly across the road and his mother brings their meals in for them. The baby is bottle fed but Michelle's technique for sterilization of equipment was of concern to the midwife; both the health visitor and social worker were informed.

Michelle brought the baby to the clinic to be weighed and to see the health visitor, Jenny, who knows Michelle and her family well. Jenny noticed that Michelle was unusually distracted and asked if she was alright. Michelle then explained that she had seen her GP the previous week, for her postnatal examination, and she had asked to be sterilized. He was not prepared to refer her for sterilization at the age of 21, so he discussed a variety of other contraceptive methods with her. He asked her to consider them and return the next week to discuss the matter further, but to remember that he would not support sterilization.

Discussion

This case could be debated from many points of view, but the issue to be focused on here is that of Michelle's wish to be sterilized and the GP's opposition to her request. If Michelle was 10–15 years older, even without her very difficult social circumstances, there would probably be no difficulty in persuading her GP that sterilization was a good option for her. While it has to be accepted that Michelle is very young to be considering such a permanent solution for control of her fertility, there certainly appear to be social reasons why this request might be considered more favourably.

The doctor's attitude in this case could be seen as medical paternalism – the doctor believes that he knows best what is right, or at least wrong, for Michelle. This attitude is historical, stemming from the view that women were not in control of their bodies, they were victims of their hormones, as demonstrated by menstruation, pregnancy and the climacteric (Rumbold, 1993); they were certainly not in control of their fertility. Some women today might say that little has changed, they are still victims of their hormones, but they would not believe that the male-dominated medical profession should be in control. Rather, its members should assist women to cope with any difficulties and, where it is possible, provide them with choice about the ways in which it can be done. Ethically, to be able to make choices one has to be autonomous which, according to Downie and Calman (1994), means possessing 'the ability to be able to choose for oneself or more extensively to be able to formulate and carry out one's own plans or policies.' This statement suggests a degree of rationality in the individual. It is generally accepted that most adults are rational, therefore autonomous, most of the time. In which case, they should be offered the opportunity to make informed choices, instead of well-meaning professionals making decisions for them.

It is generally considered that women today are in control of their fertility, partly because of the various methods of contraception available, but also because of their greater awareness of their anatomy and physiology. Undoubtedly, the availability of contraception has made a fundamental difference to the lives of women and often their families (Fredman, 1997). However, it could be argued that women are not always as 'in control' as we or they might think. How many women really choose their method of contraception?

A lot depends on the presentation of the information and the bias of the professional providing it. Anecdotal evidence and personal observation suggest that many women are persuaded to use hormonal methods, not just to satisfy the needs of the particular woman or couple, but to reduce the sequelae of unplanned or unwanted pregnancy from the resources point of view, in all its aspects. Such persuasion is often based on judgements made about the individual by the professional. For instance, where the practitioner does not trust the woman to remember to take her oral contraceptive pills regularly, she may persuade her that injection or implant would be better, instead of giving all the options and letting the woman assess her own reliability. Persuasion is really a more gentle form of coercion; therefore, persuasive practitioners are entering into the world of paternalism and control, attempting to override or reduce the autonomy of the individual. In some cases, the practitioners are not consciously aware of this effect of their behaviour, which suggests that there is little hope of changing practice through self-awareness, although true reflective practice could be effective.

Michelle is apparently a rational, autonomous being. She has thought about her current and possible future situation and made a decision about the course of action that she would like to take. It may well be that she has made her decision based on limited information; she may not be aware of all the possible consequences of undergoing sterilization, particularly so soon after the birth of her baby. The role of her doctor, in this situation, is surely to ensure that she has information about other effective methods of contraception. He should also consider the possible outcomes for Michelle and her family if she were to conceive more children in her remaining fertile years. Michelle has undoubtedly already considered this side of the argument, hence her decision. For Michelle, this is possibly a decision of last resort, in view of previous contraceptive failures. 'Last resort' may be the basis for legal rulings with regard to sterilization of mentally incompetent women (Cica, 1993); therefore, perhaps it should also be accepted as a valid reason in competent, autonomous women.

The doctor's current attitude is definitely paternalistic; he is limiting Michelle's options. It could be argued that he is also being ageist and therefore discriminatory. It is probable that he would be prepared to refer a woman of 35, perhaps with only one or two children, or even a younger woman where there is a history of genetic or congenital abnormality. This woman, who believes that she has completed her family by the age of 21, may feel that she is not being allowed the same freedom of choice as other women in her area. While it could be said that the principle of justice is being breached, the doctor probably feels, albeit paternalistically, that he is upholding the principles and duties of beneficence and non-maleficence. He would consider that he has upheld these principles by preventing Michelle from making a possible mistake. This mistake being to undergo a procedure that is intended to bring about a permanent end to her childbearing ability, when she has many fertile years ahead of her in which to change her mind. This is Michelle's point; she does have many fertile years ahead, in which she could find herself with many more children, particularly with her history of failed contraception. Her view may well be that her doctor has failed to uphold these principles and duties, by denying her the most reliable solution possible (Guillebaud, 1993), other than abstention from sexual intercourse. Legally, while Michelle would be able to give consent or refusal to any suggested health care treatment, she is not at liberty to demand that a procedure be undertaken if it is against the clinical judgement of the professional concerned (Dimond, 1999).

Jenny's role in this situation, as Michelle's health visitor, should involve counselling, advice and advocacy with regard to a vulnerable client (Rumbold, 1993). This is a fundamental part, or unwritten agreement (Husted and Husted, 1995), of the partnership between the practitioner and the client. She can discuss the various methods of contraception with Michelle, to determine her objections and to ensure that she has adequate knowledge on which to base her decision. She can then discuss the advantages and disadvantages of sterilization, to ensure that Michelle is making her decisions based on sound knowledge. If Michelle still wishes to be sterilized, Jenny can advise her that she could see another GP to try to gain a different opinion; she might even know whom to suggest. Also, as the original GP would not be undertaking the procedure himself, Jenny could suggest that Michelle asks to be referred to a gynaecologist to see what their view would be. She could also offer to speak to the GP to see if she can create a better picture of Michelle's situation. There would be no point in suggesting that Kevin, her partner, sought a vasectomy as his age would be against him too. Also, one of the GP's concerns would have been that Michelle's views might change if her current relationship broke down and she embarked on a new one. From Michelle's point of view, she may feel that, even in a new relationship, she would not want more children, therefore she would want to be the one to take the permanent step.

The private health care sector could, for some people, be an option when they wish to be sterilized and the NHS will not consider it (Evennett, 1996). Some nulliparous women, who choose to remain childless, request sterilization to remove the fear of pregnancy and the inconvenience of many years of less than perfect contraception. They also often have to resort to the private sector when the NHS will not support them (Campbell, 1999). Michelle, however, is highly unlikely to be able to access private health care to achieve her desire, as her financial situation is poor. The best that she can hope for is to convince this, or another, GP of her needs based on social grounds.

Discussion

When Hilary questioned the need for the Hep B and HIV screening, the midwife told her that she had no choice. Hilary, it would appear, gave implied consent by allowing a sample of her blood to be taken. It could be argued, however, that she was only giving consent to the other blood tests and that she felt coerced into allowing these additional two tests. The midwife apparently had the knowledge of a government directive enforcing testing, about which Hilary knew nothing. Knowledge creates power and power

SCENARIO

Hilary attended the booking clinic at the maternity hospital at 13 weeks of pregnancy. This was her third child, her previous two children being 8 and 6 years old. She had not planned this pregnancy but she, her husband and the children were very happy about it. When the time came for a blood sample to be taken, the student midwife listed the tests for which the blood was needed: these included syphilis, hepatitis B (Hep B) and human immunodeficiency virus (HIV). Hilary asked why these particular tests were being performed and the student explained as well as she could. Hilary stated that she really did not think that she needed a test for HIV. At this point the qualified midwife, who was overseeing the student, told Hilary that she had no choice. Her explanation was that the government had said that all pregnant women had to be tested, as HIV positive women could now be treated to prevent transmission of the disease to their babies, so it was in her baby's best interest. There was no further discussion and the blood was taken; the results of the tests in question were negative.

When Hilary was 36 weeks pregnant, a letter was received by the chief executive officer of the Trust, stating that Hilary and her husband were seeking to take legal action against the hospital for being wrongly advised with regard to the initial blood tests. Apparently, Hilary's family were planning to buy a bigger house to accommodate the increase in their family size. When it came to completing the application forms for the new mortgage, Hilary had answered 'yes' to the question asking whether a blood test for HIV had ever been taken. Their request for the mortgage was turned down. On further investigation, Hilary's husband had discovered that the refusal was related to the blood test, based on company health policy. He has also discovered that the test was optional, not compulsory.

can be used to control (Thompson *et al.*, 1994) and this was a perfect example. The situation was made worse by timing, as Hilary did not have time to consider what she had been told and then question further if necessary. The midwife was, of course, wrong on two counts.

First, Hilary should have had a choice both ethically, as an autonomous being, and legally. In 1985, in the Sidaway case, Lord Scarman stated: 'the existence of the patient's right to make his own decisions … may be seen as a basic human right protected by the common law.'

This was followed, in 1996, by Judge Wall's statement, that: 'A mentally competent patient has an absolute right to refuse consent to medical treatment for any reason, rational or irrational or for no reason at all, even where that decision will lead to his or her death.'

He then, effectively, defined competence as follows:

◆ Comprehending and retaining treatment information

◆ Believing such information

◆ Weighing such information in the balance to make a choice.

There is no reason to suppose that Hilary was not competent. She was just not given sufficient, or accurate, information; nor was she given time to think in order to exhibit her competence in this situation. The purist reader may consider that Judge Wall's statement only refers to treatment, not investigations. However, a later case in the Court of Appeal echoed Judge Wall's view but spoke of 'medical intervention' as opposed to treatment (Dyer, 1997). Investigation of a pregnant woman's blood with a view to treatment of the woman or treatment of the baby after birth is an intervention; in which case, Hilary should have been allowed to give her consent or refusal for these tests.

In 1986 Gillon gave a definition of consent which requires no alteration with the passage of time; it covers both ethical and legal aspects: 'a voluntary, uncoerced decision, made by a sufficiently competent or autonomous person on the basis of adequate information and deliberation, to accept rather than reject some proposed course of action that will affect him or her' (Gillon, 1986).

Hilary, although probably autonomous and competent, but not given the opportunity to prove it as she was not given adequate information, was coerced into the two tests in question. Her later innocence in completing a questionnaire, as she did not understand the implications, certainly affected her. This could have been foreseen and would have been included in any reasonable pre-test counselling. Lack of consent for HIV testing has already been the subject of concern to the General Medical Council, where a GP has been severely reprimanded for arranging HIV tests on patients without their knowledge (Dyer, 2000).

The second count on which the midwife was wrong was in the actual facts as she presented them. There is no government directive that states that all pregnant women must be tested for HIV, although it would appear so from an article by Harrison and Corbett (1999). There has been a policy in existence since 1994 (DoH) which encourages the offer of voluntary testing to all pregnant women in high-risk areas. Further consideration was given to the subject by the Intercollegiate Working Party on Antenatal HIV Testing (1998) and this body recommended that the provision, not the uptake, should be obligatory in London. The government, however, based on the further recommendations of an Expert Group, determined that the offer of HIV testing should be for all pregnant women nationwide (Report of an Expert Group, 1999; NHS Executive, 1999). All those reporting and determining on this subject have been in agreement that an underlying principle of informed consent is essential.

There are a number of possibilities as to how this situation occurred. First, the midwife could have misunderstood information given to her with regard to a new policy to offer HIV testing. In this case she is in breach of section 6 of the *Code of Professional Conduct: Standards for conduct, performance and ethics* (NMC, 2004a) and the *Midwives Rules and Standards* (NMC, 2004c) which require her to keep up to date and not take on duties for which she is not adequately prepared. In doing so she misrepresented the situation to Hilary.

Second, her failure to observe Hilary's right to autonomy and consent, by coercing her into apparently accepting the two blood tests in question, may have been based on lack of knowledge. Regardless of her responsibility to keep up to date, as previously stated, she should be familiar with such terms as autonomy and consent; they are commonly used and are explained in NMC literature with which she should be familiar (NMC, 2004a). In this case the actions of the midwife and student could be considered a trespass to the person and negligent; it is indefensible to plead lack of knowledge. Although the student was the person who actually took the blood, the midwife is accountable for the situation.

Third, and ethically the worst possibility, is that the midwife might have fully understood the situation but she chose not to give Hilary the choice, perhaps because she felt that she had the right to do so, or because adequate counselling would have been very time-consuming. In this case her actions could be viewed again in terms of trespass and negligence. In fact, the legal action referred to in a letter received by the Trust Officer would almost certainly be a lawsuit in the tort (civil wrong) of negligence. As the Trust would have to bear the vicarious liability for its staff, the action would be against the Trust, although the specific acts and omissions of the midwife and student would be in question.

To prove negligence and receive compensation, Hilary, through her legal representative(s), would have to prove that:

◆ A duty of care existed between the practitioners and Hilary

◆ The duty of care had been breached

◆ The breach had caused the harm being claimed.

The duty of care principle arose from the case of Donoghue v. Stevenson (1932) when Lord Atkin stated:

> You must take reasonable care to avoid acts and omissions which you can reasonably foresee would be likely to injure your neighbour … persons who are so closely and directly affected by my act that I ought to have them in my contemplation as being so affected when I am directing my mind to the acts and omissions which are called into question.

This particular midwife had taken responsibility for Hilary's care in the antenatal clinic on that occasion; therefore, there could be no question that her actions or omissions could affect Hilary. Hence a duty of care was owed. To determine whether this duty was breached, the actions of the midwife and student would be considered in line with the Bolam test, which has been in use since McNair J's ruling in 1957, and would be applied as follows:

> … the standard of the ordinary skilled [midwife] exercising and professing to have that special skill. A [midwife] need not possess the highest expert skill … it is sufficient that [she] exercises the skill of an ordinary competent [midwife] exercising that particular art.

The standard of this midwife's care, then, would be judged according to a body of midwifery opinion with regard to this case. That is, what would other midwives do in similar circumstances? Would they provide the opportunity for informed consent, or would they have taken the same action as this midwife? In determining appropriate standards of care since the inception of the Bolam test, various case rulings have clarified certain elements of the application of the test. For instance, someone's acts or omissions should be judged in accordance with the standards of the time in which they happened, not those of 3, 10 or 20 years later (Whitehouse v. Jordan and Another, 1981). It then became apparent that it was possible to have more than one standard of care by which the actions could be judged and deemed acceptable (Maynard v. West Midlands RHA, 1985). In 1997, however, it was deemed necessary to state that, while it was possible to have more than one body of opinion, each of those opinions should be reasonable, responsible and justifiable (Bolitho v. City & Hackney HA, 1997).

Having stated how the standards would be judged, it is now necessary to determine whether we think the midwife in this case acted according to current standards, as it was a recent case. Some of the problems related to HIV testing in general have been known and fairly well publicized in professional circles for a number of years. For instance, the issue of disclosure, by practitioners or by clients/patients, and the possible effects that it can have, such as difficulties with regard to new insurance policies and mortgages. This problem was foreseeable and Hilary should have been warned of the consequences of disclosure. This statement sounds as though we could be directing our clients to be deceitful when completing their application forms, but this is not the intention. Whether clients are totally honest, 'economical with the truth' or completely untruthful is a matter for their own consciences, but they do need to have the information in order to be prepared and make further autonomous decisions – about having the test and applications for policies and mortgages. It is highly unlikely that an expert witness would be prepared to support the actions of this midwife, whether they personally agreed with the idea of antenatal HIV testing or not. It is probable, therefore, that the actions and omissions in this case would be deemed to be negligent.

In order to be awarded compensation, however, causation must still be proved. It needs to be determined whether the harm being claimed, that is that they were turned down for a mortgage, was caused by the coerced HIV test (Bott, 2000). Hilary's husband has presumably been told that the company that he has approached has a policy not to agree to mortgages for people who have actual or potential serious health problems. Application forms usually require factual information, with no room for wordy explanations. Hilary, therefore, particularly as she has not been warned of the possible effects of disclosure, will have given a factual answer to the question of HIV testing, without any qualification that the reason for the test was because she was pregnant. Hilary will undoubtedly say that, had she been warned of the potential problems and known her rights, she would have refused the test. This is quite possible in view of the fact that she raised doubts about the need for it at the time. The company would probably presume that someone who has been tested has reason to believe themselves to be at risk of the disease and, therefore, is not a good insurance risk. On the balance of probabilities, it could be suggested that Hilary's harm was caused by the acts and omissions of the midwife and would be awarded compensation.

When consideration is being given to the future health of the nation, it is understandable that those people charged with creating or encouraging improvements consider the starting point – the baby. It is also reasonable that they should set their minds to the early development of that baby – in utero. However, in their search for improved beginnings, it is important that they do not trample on the 'ends'. The Kantian belief is that people, in this case women, are ends in themselves, not the means to someone else's ends (Palmer, 1999). Once a woman is pregnant she seems to be a physical and emotional captive within the health service. An antenatal clinic seems to be a ready source of material to determine all sorts of information and provide answers to all sorts of questions. Many invasions of body and privacy take place in the name of fetal well-being, or for the baby's sake. Most women, even those who spend their working lives challenging and questioning in one way or another, are prepared to suffer whatever comes their way if they think it is in the best interests of their baby. Practitioners are aware of this, they even take advantage of it. Women are often treated as a means to the fetus' end or, worse still, the professionals' end. Most procedures carried out on a pregnant woman are to determine something about the fetus, rather than for her own benefit. Some practitioners would argue that women want the frequent reassurance that all is well. They are probably correct, but it is the professionals who have created this dependence and insecurity over the years.

The position is unlikely to change. What should change, however, is the paternalistic attitude of many practitioners. If women were given more information, at the appropriate level for the individual, and encouraged to make decisions rather than being told what to do, then it would be possible to deal with the two ends (woman and fetus) in parallel, rather than by the subservience of the woman. In this way we would be adhering to deontological and utilitarian principles, therefore preventing moral sacrifice.

SCENARIO

Melanie attended for her appointment at the Assisted Conception Clinic for an ovarian scan. Janette, the nurse who had seen Melanie on a number of previous occasions, noticed a change in her behaviour. She was unusually withdrawn, avoiding eye contact and lacked her usual responsiveness to Janette's approach. When Melanie got onto the couch for her scan, she appeared to be moving awkwardly and, when asked to expose her abdomen, she appeared to be restricting access where previously she had exhibited no overt embarrassment.

As Melanie got up and moved her legs over the edge, the skirt of her dress dragged on the couch, exposing what appeared to be bruising on her back. Janette reached out and raised Melanie's skirt further, revealing extensive bruising from ilium to ribs. She asked the obvious question: 'What have you done?' Melanie started to cry, lowered her head and said: 'It's all my fault – the infertility. He's never done this before and I didn't want anyone to know.'

Discussion

This would appear to be a case of domestic violence. The intention here is not to discuss domestic violence itself, but the ethico-legal aspects for the practitioner. Janette must consider many ethical principles, not least those of beneficence, non-maleficence, justice, autonomy and confidentiality. She must do her best to help Melanie without making the situation worse. Dealing with victims of domestic violence is very difficult. It is understandable that some practitioners may pretend that it is not really happening, or none of their business, or they hide behind a screen of efficiency, taking control to set official wheels in motion. While this behaviour may be understandable, it is certainly not helpful to the woman, therefore it is unacceptable.

To be able to help Melanie at all, Janette must give her the opportunity to talk freely, perhaps with some direct questions to prompt, but mainly through active listening. Melanie is already exhibiting acceptance of guilt, so common in cases of domestic violence. She seems to be indicating that the infertility is all her fault and that this is what led to the violence, hence the violence is all her fault. Unwittingly, Janette may have emphasized this point in Melanie's mind by asking 'what have you done?' This question is almost routine when we see people with injuries of any sort, because the injury is usually related to an accident of some sort. In this case, however, Melanie may imagine the criticism that it is her fault. Perhaps a better question for practitioners

to ask is 'How did this happen?', or if they suspect abuse they could be more direct and ask 'Who did this to you?' One of the first steps to helping must be to acknowledge that abuse of any kind is unjust, and therefore wrong, and that it is the fault of the perpetrator, not the victim. At the same time it is not wise to be too condemnatory of the woman's partner as she probably loves him and wants to protect him, therefore, she might become antagonistic towards the practitioner. This could make matters worse, not least by closing the door to a potential source of help. Also, it is important to stress that infertility, while it may be attributed to a failure in the reproductive system in one partner, is nobody's fault. Blame is not attached to people who have a breakdown in other areas of their physiology, such as the development of diabetes mellitus or asthma.

In this case, if Melanie is to be believed, and it is important to show belief in the victim (Hunt and Martin, 2001), this is the first time that this has happened. Stress is often thought to be a root cause of domestic violence and both the acceptance and treatments of infertility are known to cause stress. Unfortunately, the extra physical and emotional stress of the abuse may create barriers to effective fertility treatment, thus a vicious circle could ensue. It is also possible that the partner has reached a point where he does not really want a child after all, but does not know how to tell Melanie, and it was this frustration that led him to be violent. It would seem that this couple might be helped with counselling (a service is provided by assisted conception clinics) before the situation becomes worse. As a nurse in this area of practice, Janette will be used to dealing with very sensitive, personal issues. She may be able to suggest counselling in such a way that Melanie feels in control and able to persuade her partner to attend with her.

If they continue with treatment, one potential problem to be considered for the future with this couple is the fact that they may be successful in achieving a pregnancy. It could be presumed that this would be a much-wanted pregnancy and would remove the stress that had caused the violence. However, Hunt and Martin (2001) suggest that domestic violence may be triggered by pregnancy for a number of reasons, not least the stress created by this life event. If this can happen for the first time in pregnancy, then possibly a woman who has been a victim prior to pregnancy might be at even greater risk. It is important that Janette keeps adequate records, particularly as there is the potential for them to be needed as evidence in the future. Domestic violence is a criminal offence and, should Melanie's situation continue, she may wish to take legal action, for which these records would be essential. At this stage Melanie may believe that she will not be abused again, and she might be right, so she may not be very willing to have records kept. She has already stated that she does not want anyone to know about the incident. Janette, however, would have to explain that legally she must keep professional records about issues of client safety (NMC, 2004b).

Confidentiality (including privacy) is one of the least upheld of the ethical principles in professional practice, as evidenced by many overheard conversations in nurses' stations, coffee-rooms, dining rooms or on public transport (Jones, 2000). Sadly, many practitioners are unaware that they have breached such principles; however, when faced with any case of actual or possible abuse all practitioners should be alert to the need for confidentiality. In planned counselling sessions it would be common practice to set ground rules regarding what the practitioner would feel they had to take further. However, in unplanned situations such as this one, it can be more difficult. Ground rules were not established before Janette saw the bruising and Melanie indicated the cause. Once she had indicated the cause, Janette could explain that there might be some matters upon which she would feel the need to seek further advice, but this could frighten Melanie, preventing her from saying any more, thus preventing her from getting any help.

Janette faces a dilemma. Either she sets the ground rules, as suggested, or she must agree to maintain confidentiality completely, in order to get Melanie to talk, thus providing a potential source of support and advice. As child abuse is not in question, Janette is not legally obliged to report the situation (Bridge *et al.*, 1990), and

therefore she is more at liberty to maintain confidentiality (NMC, 2002). If she chooses the confidential route then she will find herself alone in trying to support Melanie, although she could seek advice from others in a hypothetical way, for instance: 'If you had a case where ...?' It is possible that Melanie might feel more able to speak to others once she learns to trust Janette.

An additional aspect within Janette's dilemma is that, although there are no children involved in the case, there is the potential for children to be involved. All professionals working within the area of assisted conception are bound by the Human Fertilization and Embryology Authority's *Code of Conduct* (HFEA, 2003). This code requires nursing staff to be on the active NMC Professional Register, therefore subject to their rules and codes also. The code reiterates that one of the licensing conditions stated in the HFE Act (1990) relates to consideration of the welfare of the child:

> ... a woman shall not be provided with treatment services unless account has been taken of the welfare of any child who may be born as a result of the treatment (including the need of that child for a father) ...
>
> (HFEA, 2003)

Presumably, when Melanie and her partner were accepted initially for treatment, there were no apparent problems of this nature. However, the code later states:

> Centres should take note in their procedures of the importance of a stable and supportive environment for any child produced as a result of treatment.
>
> ... bear in mind ... any risk of harm to the child or children who may be born, including the risk of ... neglect or abuse ...
>
> (HFEA, 2003)

While it may seem unfair to Melanie, the victim in this situation, to contemplate reconsideration of the couple's suitability for treatment, it must be considered that future children could be at risk, if not of violence itself, then from the sequelae of violence in the home.

If Janette takes a deontological route to solving her dilemma, she will support Melanie's autonomy.

She will maintain confidentiality but keep a separate factual record, the contents of which Melanie will be aware of, which will not be available to others at this stage. According to Hunt and Martin (2001) this record should include Melanie's description of the incident of abuse, a detailed description of the injury and a description of her psychological state. They also suggest that visually identifiable, labelled photographs should be kept in the confidential record. However, it is probable, in this particular case, that Melanie would not consent to photographs at this time. Janette should also offer help in the form of counselling, plus provision of local support group details and the Women's Aid telephone number if Melanie would like them.

If Janette takes a utilitarian route to solution of the dilemma, she will seek the action that will achieve the greatest benefit for the greatest number of people. In this case, the people concerned are Melanie and her partner. To rush in and take aggressive action at this stage could be detrimental to both parties. Therefore, the utilitarian approach would probably be similar to that of the deontologist. Even if a utilitarian were also to consider the future child(ren), it is probable that they would take no different action at this stage. Whichever way forward Janette and Melanie choose to go, there will not be an overnight solution. Also, plans may have to change according to progress made, or lack of it.

Nurse prescribing

In addition to the issues that arise in normal practice, some of which were indicated in the cases above, practitioners face additional areas of responsibility and accountability generated by national initiatives. One such initiative related to prescribing of medicines and treatments by non-medical professionals. Midwives already had exemption from certain requirements of the Misuse of Drugs Act 1971 with authority for the prescription of a list of drugs stated in the Prescription Only Medicines (Human Use) Order 1997, SI 1997 No. 1830. This initiative created limited prescribing rights for a number of health care professionals but, within the NMC professions, it has become known as 'nurse prescribing'.

The initiative for nurse prescribing came from the recommendations in the Report on the Review of Prescribing, Supply and Administration of Medicines (Crown Report), which was finalised in March 1999. There was a need to balance improvements in services, by the best use of skills, against cost-effectiveness. Therefore, as there were concerns about potential cost increase by giving nurses the power to prescribe, it was determined that the extension of legal authority would be limited. In fact, that was the major criticism of the initiative – that it was too limited, in both the nurses who would meet the preconditions for training and the formulary from which they could prescribe. However, despite the criticisms, it was generally felt to be a positive move in primary care, by professional groups and patients.

In 2003 the Department of Health agreed to extend the prescribing rights and an 'Extended Formulary' was created for those who successfully undertake the appropriate, extended course. There are two categories of prescriber, initially known as independent and dependent prescribers but, along with the recent extension, the titles have changed to independent and supplementary prescribers.

Independent prescribers are community-based nurses and health visitors who have successfully undertaken specialist practitioner programmes, with prescriber training either incorporated into the programme or undertaken subsequently. The independent prescriber is responsible for the initial patient assessment, diagnosis and development of a written clinical management plan. The supplementary prescriber, also appropriately trained, works to the management plan by monitoring progress, prescribing within the stated limits and referring to the independent prescriber as required (DoH, 2003).

From a legal standpoint, nurses must be appropriately trained, as indicated above, through NMC-approved programmes. Having been successful in that training, a nurse for whom independent or supplementary prescribing is part of her stated professional duty is covered through vicarious liability by her employer. She will have a duty of care for all the patients for whom she prescribes and she must work within the standards of the day, which included abiding by the *Code of Professional Conduct: Standards for conduct, performance and ethics* (NMC, 2004a).

Ethically, nurses must ensure that the change in role does not affect the manner with which they deal with their patients or clients. Although they have increased professional autonomy, it should not lead to paternalistic behaviour and, therefore, a reduction in the autonomy of the patients. The nurse prescriber must ensure that sufficient information is given to the patient, with an opportunity to discuss any issues and consider the consequences of any options before making a decision. Basic principles of beneficence, non-maleficence, justice and truth-telling are all important, possibly prioritized according to the basic ethical theory underpinning the actions of the individual nurse.

Conclusion

This principle of accountability is often considered by practitioners to be of legal origin as their first thought is with regard to litigation. Undoubtedly there is a legal side to it but it has a basis in ethics too; it encompasses liability and duty and indicates that we are both responsible and answerable for our actions. In each of the scenarios used in this chapter, and in nurse prescribing, the practitioners are accountable for their decisions, their actions and omissions. Although in some aspects of care there is the potential for delegating responsibility, as to a student, there is no possibility of delegating accountability. We cannot plead that we took a certain action or omitted a certain action because someone else told us to do so. Once we decide to act, or not to act, we have agreed that this was the correct action or inaction. If we felt that it was wrong, then we would have no defence in saying '(s)he told me to'. As practitioners we owe a duty of care, both ethically and legally, to all our clients/patients, but never more so than to those who are most vulnerable; sadly, this commonly refers to women.

Ideas for personal and professional development

- Regularly access the NMC website (www.nmc-uk.org) to keep abreast of current professional issues, literature and consultations
- Attend an NMC Conduct and Competence hearing to gain greater knowledge of the issues and processes related to allegations of professional misconduct or incompetence
- Access further literature on ethics and law in your professional field, to ensure good grounding and assistance with application to practice
- Access the Formularies in use for nurse prescribing, to see which products can be prescribed by appropriately trained nurses and midwives
- Consider your professional role and whether it would be appropriate to undertake a nurse prescribing course.

Patient education points

- Facilitate patients' knowledge of their health care rights and the exercise of their autonomy
- Ensure that all patients have access to information about all aspects of domestic violence and how to get help.

Further reading

BEQUAERT HOLMES, H. and PURDY, L.M. (eds) (1992) *Feminist Perspectives in Medical Ethics*. Bloomington, USA: Indiana University Press.

BOWDEN, P. (1997) *Caring. Gender-Sensitive Ethics*. London: Routledge.

HAWS, J.M., BUTTA, P. and GIRVIN, S. (1997) A comprehensive and efficient process for counseling patients desiring sterilization. *The Nurse Practitioner* **22**(6):52–9.

HUMPHRIES, J. and GREEN, J. (eds) (2002) *Nurse Prescribing*, 2nd edn. Hampshire: Palgrave.

MONTGOMERY, J. (2003) *Health Care Law*, 2nd edn. Oxford: Oxford University Press.

ROSSER, J. (1999) Editorial: The force of the law (re HIV and breastfeeding). *The Practising Midwife*, **2**(9):4–5.

SEEDHOUSE, D. (1998) *Ethics. The Heart of Health Care*, 2nd edn. Chichester: John Wiley.

WAITE, M. (2004). *Nurse Prescribing Programme*. Oxford: Radcliffe Medical Press.

WARNOCK, M. (1999) *The Intelligent Person's Guide to Ethics*. London: Gerald Duckworth.

WEDGWOOD, F. (2000) HIV screening choices (a mother's story). *The Practising Midwife*, **3**(2):18–19.

References

ABORTION ACT (as amended) (1967) London: HMSO.

BEAUCHAMP T.L. and CHILDRESS J.F. (2001) *Principles of Biomedical Ethics*, 5th edn. New York: Oxford University Press.

BOLAM v. FRIERN HMC (1957) 2 All ER 118.

BOLITHO v. CITY & HACKNEY HA (1997) 4 Med LR 381.

BOTT, J. (2000) HIV screening issue for midwives. *British Journal of Midwifery* **8**(2):72–8.

BRIDGE, J., BRIDGE, S. and LUKE, S. (1990) *Blackstone's Guide to the Children Act 1989*. London: Blackstone Press, p. 28.

CALLAHAN, J.C. (1995) Ensuring a stillborn: The ethics of lethal injection in late abortion. Introduction to Part III. In Callahan, J.C. (ed.) *Reproduction, Ethics, and the Law. Feminist Perspectives*. USA: Indiana University Press, p. 271.

CAMPBELL, A. (1999) *Child Free and Sterilized: Women's Decisions and Medical Responses*. London: Cassell, p. xiv.

CICA, N. (1993) Sterilising the intellectually disabled: The approach of the High Court of Australia in Department of Health v. JWB and SMB. In Kennedy, I. and Grubb, A. (eds) *Medical Law Review* **1**(2):186–231.

DIMOND, B. (1999) Is there a legal right to choose a caesarean? *British Journal of Midwifery*, **7**(8):515–18.

DoH (Department of Health) (1994) *Guidelines for Offering Voluntary Named HIV Antibody Testing to Women Receiving Antenatal Care*. London: DoH.

DoH (1999) *Report on the Review of Prescribing, Supply and Administration of Medicines* (Crown Report). London: The Stationery Office.

DoH (2003) *Supplementary Prescribing by Nurses and Pharmacists Within the NHS in England*. London: DoH.

DONOGHUE v. STEVENSON (1932) AC 562 (HL).

DOWNIE, R.S. and CALMAN, K.C. (1994) *Healthy Respect*. Oxford: Oxford Medical Publications, p. 52.

DYER, C. (1997) Court of Appeal decision. *British Medical Journal*, **314**:993.

DYER, C. (2000) GP reprimanded for testing patients for HIV without consent. *British Medical Journal*, **320**:135.

EVENNETT, K. (1996) *Women's Health: An Essential Guide for the Modern Woman*. London: Ward Lock, Chapter 3, p. 42.

FREDMAN, S. (1997) *Women and the Law*. Oxford: Clarendon Press, p. 130.

GENERAL MEDICAL COUNCIL (1993) *Protecting Patients, Guiding Doctors*. London: GMC.

GILLON, R. (1986) *Philosophical Medical Ethics*. Chichester: John Wiley, p. 113.

GUILLEBAUD, J. (1993) Contraception. In McPherson, A. (ed.) *Women's Problems in General Practice*, 3rd edn. Oxford: Oxford University Press, Chapter 3, p. 109.

HARRISON, R. and CORBETT, K. (1999) Screening of pregnant women for HIV: the case against. *The Practising Midwife*, **2**(7):24–9.

HFEA (Human Fertilization and Embryology Authority) (2003) *Code of Conduct*, 6th edn. London: HFEA, pp. 17(3.12, 3.14), 18(3.17h).

HUMAN FERTILIZATION and EMBRYOLOGY ACT (1990) London: HMSO.

HUMAN RIGHTS ACT (1998) London: The Stationery Office.

HUNT, S.C. and MARTIN, A. (2001) *Pregnant Women, Violent Men. What Midwives Need to Know*. Oxford: Butterworth-Heinemann, Chapters 5 and 6.

HUSTED, G.L. and HUSTED, J.H. (1995) *Ethical Decision Making in Nursing*, 2nd edn. St Louis, USA: Mosby, Chapter 4, p. 43.

INFANTICIDE ACT (1938) London: HMSO.

INTERCOLLEGIATE WORKING PARTY FOR ENHANCING VOLUNTARY CONFIDENTIAL HIV TESTING IN PREGNANCY (1998) *Reducing Mother to Child Transmission of HIV Infection in the United Kingdom, Executive Summary and Recommendations*. London: Royal College of Paediatrics and Child Health.

JONES, S.R. (2000) *Ethics in Midwifery*, 2nd edn. London: Mosby, Chapters 1, 5 and 8.

JONES, S.R. and JENKINS, R. (2004) *The Law and the Midwife*, 2nd edn. Oxford: Blackwell.

MAYNARD v. WEST MIDLANDS RHA (1985) 1 All ER 635.

MORGAN, D. and LEE, R.G. (1991) *Blackstone's Guide to the Human Fertilization and Embryology Act 1990*. London: Blackstone Press, p. 28.

NHS EXECUTIVE (1999) *Reducing Mother to Baby Transmission of HIV. HSC 1999/183*. London: NHSE.

NMC (Nursing and Midwifery Council) (2004a) *Code of Professional Conduct: Standards for conduct, performance and ethics*. London: NMC.

NMC (2004b) *Guidelines for Records and Record-Keeping*, paras 9, 11, 13, 14. London: NMC.

NMC (2004c) *Midwives Rules and Standards*. London: NMC.

PALMER, M. (1999) *Moral Problems in Medicine*. Cambridge: Lutterworth Press, p. 113.

PURDY, L. and TOOLEY, M. (1999) Is abortion murder? In Palmer, M. *Moral Problems in Medicine*. Cambridge: Lutterworth Press, p. 45.

REPORT OF AN EXPERT GROUP (1999) *Targets Aimed at Reducing the Number of Children Born With HIV*. London: UK Health Departments.

ROSS W.D. (1930) *The Right and the Good*. Oxford: Clarendon Press.

ROYAL COLLEGE OF OBSTETRICIANS and GYNAECOLOGISTS (1998) *A Consideration of the Law and Ethics in Relation to Late Termination of Pregnancy for Fetal Abnormality*. London: RCOG, p. 11.

RUMBOLD, G. (1993) *Ethics in Nursing Practice*, 2nd edn. London: Baillière Tindall, pp. 212–13.

SIDAWAY v. BETHLEHEM RHG (1985) 1 All ER 643.

ST GEORGE'S HEALTHCARE NHS TRUST v. S (1998) 3 All ER 673.

THOMPSON, I.E., MELIA, K.M. and BOYD, K.M. (1994) *Nursing Ethics*, 3rd edn. Edinburgh: Churchill Livingstone, p. 80.

TOOLIS, K. (1999) The most dangerous man in the world. *The Guardian Weekend*, November 6, pp. 52–5.

UKCC (1999) *Practitioner–Client Relationships and the Prevention of Abuse*. London: UKCC.

VELASQUEZ, M. and ANDRE, C. (2003) A Framework for Moral Decision Making. www.scu.edu/ethics/practicing/decision.

WALL, JUDGE (1996) *Tameside and Glossop Acute Services Trust v. CH* (1996) 1 FCR.

WHITEHOUSE v. JORDAN and ANOTHER (1981) 1 All ER 267.

3: Promoting a Healthy Lifestyle

Liz Illman and Catrina Donegan

OBJECTIVES

This chapter should help you understand:

◆ What is meant by good health ◆

◆ The dimensions of health ◆

◆ Health promotion – before the cradle to the grave ◆

◆ Saving lives: working in partnership to tackle poor health ◆

◆ The targets: tackling causes of premature death ◆

◆ How to help clients make healthy choices about diet, exercise, smoking, alcohol and drugs ◆

◆ Planning, delivery and evaluation of health promotion. ◆

Introduction

Before thinking about health promotion one needs to consider what we mean by 'health'. There is no universally accepted definition. Similarly, there is a lack of consensus about the best approach to promote health. The following health definitions reflect the range of thought.

> The state of being bodily and mentally vigorous and free from disease.
>
> (Collins Dictionary)

> A process of adaptation. It is not the result of instinct, but of an autonomous yet culturally shaped reaction to socially created reality. It designates the ability to adapt to changing environments, to growing up and to ageing, to healing when damaged, to suffering and to the peaceful expectation of death. Health embraces the future as well, and therefore includes anguish and the inner resources to live with it.
>
> (Illich, 1977)

Health is holistic and includes different dimensions which each need to be considered.

> (Aggleton and Homans, 1987; Ewles and Simnett, 1992)

> A state of complete physical, mental and social well-being and not merely the absence of disease and infirmity.
>
> (World Health Organization, 1946)

Naidoo and Wills (1998) state that health promotion should be based on sound theoretical underpinnings and adhere to certain core principles, whilst remembering to reflect on what we are doing and what we are trying to promote.

Since health means different things to different people, your client may not share your personal or professional ideas about, for example, the benefits of stopping smoking, eating more fruit and vegetables, or taking exercise. She may regard herself as 'healthy' so long as she feels in control or able to go to work and cope with everyday routine. She may regard doctors and nurses as people to see only when she is ill.

33

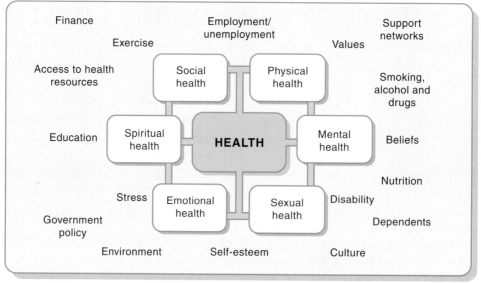

Figure 3.1 Dimensions of health: a holistic view.

Figure 3.1 illustrates how the various dimensions of health interact and are influenced by a range of factors. Some of these are fixed; for example, genetic inheritance and gender. Others can be influenced by environmental, social and lifestyle factors; and quality of and access to health care services.

 SCENARIO

Jenny is 24 and has three children. She and her partner have a two-bedroom flat on a rundown estate. He has been unemployed for two years. Jenny feels constantly tired and stressed. She is overweight and smokes 20 cigarettes a day which, she says, she cannot afford. She knows they are bad for her, but feels unable to do anything about it.

Jenny's story underlines the need for health care practitioners to have a flexible approach to health promotion, which takes account of lifestyle and environmental factors and pressures, which can make it difficult for women like Jenny to change their habits. Jenny needs support with childcare, housing and financial help before she has the strength to tackle the issues such as smoking that are important for her own health.

The political perspective

Government plans for health promotion emerged in the White Paper *The New NHS: Modern, Dependable* (DoH, 1997a). Primary Care Trusts, together with other agencies, were given responsibility for promoting the health of the local population.

A further White Paper, *Saving Lives: Our Healthier Nation* (DoH, 1999a), describes the Government's action plan to tackle poor health and health inequality – the UK has one of the worst records in Western Europe for coronary heart disease (CHD), breast cancer and teenage pregnancy. Delivery of the strategy relies on partnerships between government, local organizations and individuals. It sets targets for 2010 focusing on the principal causes of premature death and avoidable ill health in the country. The four priority areas are:

◆ Cancer

◆ CHD and stroke

◆ Accidents

◆ Mental illness.

Other key issues include alcohol, drugs, food safety, communicable diseases and sexual health.

Health promotion

Defining health promotion

The World Health Organization (1984) states that health promotion is a process which enables people to increase control over, and to improve their health. Health promotion is generally regarded as an umbrella term encompassing a range of activities. Naidoo and Wills (1998) identify four elements:

- Disease prevention – activities focusing on individuals or groups, e.g. screening and immunization
- Health education and information – activities aimed at preventing disease and enhancing health through education giving, e.g. nurse–client consultations and media campaigns
- Public health promotion – activities that promote health through social and environmental measures, e.g. improving access to services, housing, smoking bans
- Community development – activities that enable individuals to develop personal skills, knowledge and social networks, e.g. women's health groups, exercise classes for older people.

Promoting health is a major part of the nurse's role. Nurses are increasingly influential in planning and implementing local initiatives through representation on Primary Care Trusts. Funding arrangements may determine which health promotion activities take a higher priority. However, these activities may be compromised by heavy workloads or time constraints.

Debate continues over the best ways to promote health. Traditional health education was designed to change the behaviour of the individual towards healthier lifestyles by making people fit the environment. However, this did not make the environment a healthier place to live in and has resulted in 'victims' being blamed for their own ill health. This traditional approach had a further limitation: it was based on the conviction that the expert (usually the doctor) knew best. Ewles and Simnett (1992) point out:

> There is a danger of imposing alien values on a client. Frequently this is an imposition of white, middle-class values on working-class people. For example, a doctor may perceive that the most important thing for a patient is losing weight and lowering blood pressure, but drinking beer in the pub with friends may be far more important to the overweight, middle-aged, unemployed patient. Who is to say which set of values is right? Whose life is it anyway?

The client-centred approach involves working with clients on their own terms and helping them to make decisions and choices. Clients are valued as equals. The key is self-empowerment evolving from increasing self-awareness and self-esteem. This is in stark contrast to the traditional paternalistic model.

Planning health promotion

Much health promotion is opportunistic – done during a busy clinic or over the phone. A few minutes may be all that is available, or necessary. Issues needing more time can be followed up when it is more convenient – by an individual appointment or a group session. Remember that the best plan can go wrong: your colleague is ill; the video breaks down; your client is more concerned about last night's TV programme on breast cancer than her smoking habits. Be flexible and prepared to depart from your plan.

When constructing a programme it will help to:

- Assess your client's needs
- Decide on your aims
- Set objectives, i.e. goals to be achieved
- Select which methods/strategies to use
- Ensure support from your manager and colleagues
- Check that everyone involved has the appropriate knowledge and skills
- Contact your local health promotion department for advice and resources
- Find out what services your local agencies provide – can clients self-refer?
- Compile a list of national and local organizations, helplines and support groups – ask for promotional materials
- Devise an evaluation strategy for clients, e.g. a questionnaire

◆ Allow time for staff debrief/feedback – clinical supervision may provide a supportive environment for developing ideas

◆ Audit helps future planning and to monitor quality standards.

Changing health behaviour

Achieving changes in health-related behaviour forms an element of many of the National Service Frameworks.

◆ Helping patients make healthy choices is a challenge for all nurses.

◆ Individuals have freedom of choice and some patients may choose to continue with unhealthy behaviour (such as smoking) because they believe the benefits outweigh the risks.

◆ Changing health-related behaviour is a complex process involving psychological, social and environmental issues.

Stages of change

Research has demonstrated that a behaviour change model is effective in changing a variety of health-related behaviours such as drug abuse and weight control (Ewles and Simnett, 1999). Prochaska and DiClimente (1984) identified stages in the process of behaviour change. Using this model you can help your patients to make changes by focusing on moving them one step further around the cycle.

◆ Pre-contemplation stage. At this point the patient has no awareness of a need to change. Health education and advice can be used at this stage to raise awareness of the unhealthy behaviour. Questions, delivered in a non-judgemental way such as 'how do you feel about smoking?' may prompt consideration of the health-related behaviour.

◆ Contemplation stage. This is where the change starts. Patients in this stage are sufficiently motivated to begin to think about making a change. Patient self-empowerment is key to moving through this stage of the cycle.

◆ Commitment stage. Patients in this stage are making a serious decision to change an aspect of their health-related behaviour. In this stage you can help to turn a decision into action by developing an action plan, coping strategies and identifying sources of support. A date to change behaviour and to review progress can be set.

◆ Action stage. Patients in this stage are changing their health-related behaviour. Support during this phase can be given through continued sessions with a health professional, as part of a support group, from friends and family, via telephone help lines or a combination of some or all of these.

◆ Maintenance stage. This is the stage where patients are endeavouring to maintain the behaviour change they have made. Using the coping strategies identified during the commitment stage will improve maintenance. Continuing to gain support is also vital and satisfaction is gained from maintaining the behavioural change. Remember most patients are not successful at maintaining their health behaviour at their first attempt.

◆ Relapse stage. In this stage they have relapsed back into their old behaviour. You can help patients identify this relapse as a stage on the way to making their change, and move them on to the comtemplation stage again. On average, smokers take three cycles of the change model to successfully quit smoking.

◆ Exit stage. This is the stage where a health-related change has been successfully made and can be maintained.

Remember that practical problems may limit change. A woman may see no need to alter her lifestyle. She may lack the self-esteem and confidence to cope with big changes. She may be unable to change because she lacks control over her life at home or at work, maybe due to financial problems or insufficient support. In addition, you may not have the necessary time she needs in order to help her.

All these pressures highlight the need to strike a balance between meeting government targets, respecting your client's wishes and being realistic about what is achievable for both you and your client.

Preconception care and early pregnancy

Preconception care has two aims:

◆ To give the baby the best possible start to life by minimizing risks associated with lifestyle, heredity, medical history and maternal age

◆ To promote the health of the mother.

A woman wishing to conceive can be given advice about timing intercourse during the most fertile phase of the menstrual cycle, i.e. 14 days before the expected start of the next period (see also page 287).

In theory, a contraception, sexual health or well-woman consultation provides an ideal opportunity to discuss plans for planning a pregnancy, to check your client's general health and to arrange appropriate screening. In practice, however, you may not see your client until she presents for a pregnancy test. A negative result will determine if she needs either contraception or preconception counselling. A positive result will enable you to discuss other issues covered in this section or the possibility of counselling for termination of the pregnancy.

The first four weeks of a pregnancy are the most critical in a baby's development – the time of maximum velocity in cell division, when the heart, brain, spine and other major organs begin to develop. This is why it is so important to give health promotion advice before conception, rather than after pregnancy is confirmed. Nevertheless, even if the client does not present for several weeks, you can still emphasize that it is never too late to make healthy lifestyle changes.

A report for the British Dietetic Association (Doyle, 1994) says that women with a high risk of poor pregnancy outcome (Box 3.1) should be targeted for nutrition counselling. Their needs may extend beyond diet and call for a more holistic approach.

Preconception and early pregnancy care should include:

◆ A review of medical and family histories

◆ Advice on smoking, alcohol and other drugs

Box 3.1 Risk factors for poor pregnancy outcome
◆ Poor obstetric history, e.g. previous low-birth-weight baby or congenital abnormality
◆ Smoking, heavy drinking or abuse of other drugs
◆ Adolescence
◆ Pre-existing medical conditions, e.g. diabetes, hypertension and malabsorption states
◆ Low socio-economic group and poor housing
◆ Close birth spacing and large families
◆ Very under- or overweight
◆ An inadequate diet, e.g. some vegans with a limited nutritional intake or families with poor cooking facilities
◆ Eating disorders, e.g. anorexia or bulimia.
(Doyle, 1994)

◆ Nutritional advice

◆ Advice on exercise, lifestyle and occupational hazards for both partners

◆ Information about stopping contraception.

A woman who becomes pregnant whilst taking hormonal contraception should be advised to stop immediately, but be reassured that studies do not show any detectable increased risk of fetal abnormality (Guillebaud, 1999).

Medical history

A review of general medical history should include illness, previous surgery and any medication. Gynaecological and obstetric history should cover previous pregnancies: deliveries, miscarriages, abortions, stillbirth and intra-uterine death, toxaemia, fertility investigations, sexually transmitted infections, hepatitis and HIV status, if known. Ask about previous cervical smears, rubella status and sickle cell and thalassaemia trait.

Take a family history for both partners, if possible, and offer screening for inherited disorders. Women who have had recurrent miscarriages, and couples with a family history of inherited disorders may be referred for genetic counselling. Screening in specialist centres is available for conditions such as cystic fibrosis, muscular dystrophy and fragile X syndrome.

Nutrition advice

The importance of a healthy diet before and during pregnancy cannot be overemphasized. With the exception of folic acid, there are no proven benefits associated with taking vitamin or mineral supplements unless the diet is inadequate or very restricted, e.g. vegan. 'Fortified' breads and breakfast cereals are a good source of extra vitamins and minerals. Zinc deficiency reduces sperm count and is believed to be associated with poor pregnancy outcome. Zinc is lost when alcohol intake increases. Calcium is important for adequate mineralization of fetal bone, particularly in the third trimester. Adequate iron intake is required throughout pregnancy to prevent anaemia and for normal fetal brain development, and iodine plays a role in cognitive functioning of the baby. Maternal intake of vitamins A and D influence development of visual and skeletal systems, and long-chain fatty acids from fish oils promote neural development (HEA, 1998a).

Weight control

Women who are overweight should be advised to cut down high calorie foods; but to avoid restricting their diet if they are actively trying to become pregnant. Ideally, they should aim to lose weight well in advance of conception to let their weight and metabolism stabilize. An underweight woman or one who is over-exercising may have difficulty conceiving. Being underweight also increases the risk of having a small baby. Chronic long-term dieters should try to eat three good meals a day to ensure the baby is adequately nourished in those important first few weeks of pregnancy (Doyle, 1994).

Folic acid

Folic acid supplements can reduce the incidence of neural tube defects, such as spina bifida. The Department of Health advises women planning pregnancy to take 400 μg of folic acid daily, in addition to dietary intake, until the 12th week of pregnancy. If there is a family history of spina bifida the woman is advised to take a higher daily supplement of folic acid (5 mg). The DoH (1992a) recommended that this daily dose should be reduced to 4 mg if a licensed preparation became available. There is still no 4 mg licensed preparation available to date, so women should continue to take 5 mg.

Vitamin A

An excessively high intake of retinol or animal forms of vitamin A is associated with birth defects. The plant form (beta-carotene) is safe. Pregnant women are advised to avoid cod liver oil and vitamin A supplements in excess of 700 μg or foods known to be high in vitamin A, such as liver or liver products.

Food-related infection

Immunity is reduced in pregnancy and some women may fall prey to illnesses more easily.

Listeriosis is a bacterial infection common in animals, including cattle, pigs and poultry. It may also affect humans. Maternal infection can result in miscarriage, stillbirth, brain damage or severe illness in a newborn baby. Foods to avoid in pregnancy include ripened soft cheeses, e.g. Brie, Camembert and blue-veined cheeses. Unpasteurized milk and unpasturized milk products and pâté may contain high levels of listeria. Cooked-chilled meals and ready-to-eat poultry should be avoided unless they are thoroughly reheated.

Raw or partially cooked eggs or foods containing raw egg (e.g. mousses and mayonnaise) and undercooked chicken can cause salmonella poisoning and should be avoided.

Remind your client about food hygiene. Emphasize the importance of hand washing before and after handling food, especially raw meat, eggs, etc.; and the need for separate chopping boards and knives for raw and cooked foods (DoH, 1997b).

Exercise, lifestyle and occupational hazards

Advice on exercise is given on page 41. Adequate sleep and relaxation is also important. Both partners should avoid occupational hazards, e.g. exposure to chemicals and radiation. Ask your client to encourage her partner to eat healthily, reduce alcohol consumption and to cut down or stop smoking. The mutual support that a partner can give by adopting a healthy lifestyle is a positive factor and lays the foundations for bringing up children with a similar approach.

Ask your client if she has any pets. Toxoplasmosis is an infection caused by a parasite found in cat's faeces, raw and partially cooked meat and unpasteurized goat's milk and cheese. Exposure in early pregnancy can cause miscarriage and fetal damage, which may lead to mental retardation and blindness. Pregnant women should avoid changing cat litter; but if this is essential, they should wear rubber gloves. They should be especially careful to wash their hands thoroughly after handling animals, cat litter, earth or raw meat; avoid eating rare meat; wash salads thoroughly and wear gloves for gardening. On farms, pregnant women should avoid lambing.

Women and nutrition

It is generally accepted that nutrition plays a significant part in leading causes of morbidity and mortality in women, e.g. CHD, stroke, osteoporosis, diabetes and some cancers. Risk factors for these diseases could be reduced by adopting a healthier way of eating. In addition, a healthy diet has been linked to the onset of menarche and bone development. The relationship between nutrition and menstrual disorders such as amenorrhoea and PMS has also been studied. The main focus of research for women of childbearing age has been the association between nutrition and reproduction. Good nutrition is important to the mother herself who needs to maintain her health as well as providing for a growing fetus (HEA, 1998a).

Deciding what to eat

Women play a key role in buying and preparing food and in educating the family about healthy eating. However, dietary preferences of the family at large help to determine what appears on the table. Employment trends and food technology also affect the family menu. Convenience foods appeal to women juggling the conflicting demands of home and outside jobs. A healthy diet can cost more in terms of shopping, preparation and cooking. Local street markets offer cheaper produce and reflect the dietary preferences of the local ethnic community.

Self-image also affects what women buy and eat. Up to 70% of women diet at some time in their lives. Many pursue an elusive ideal figure of the kind promoted by glossy magazines, and the burgeoning dieting industry. Obsessive dieting associated with a distortion of body image can lead to eating disorders.

What makes a healthy diet?

A good diet provides all of the nutrients essential to sustain life and to maintain adequate health. In defining a healthy diet the British Dietetic Association states that two objectives should be fulfilled:

◆ It must provide sufficient energy and nutrients to maintain normal physiological functions and permit growth and replacement of body tissues

◆ It must offer the best protection against the risk of disease.

In an attempt to improve the health of the nation, the Government defined numerical targets for the intakes of specific nutrients. The Balance of Good Health produced by the former Health Education Authority (HEA, 1996b) translates these targets into a form that is more easily understood. The principal messages conveyed are that it is important to consume a variety of foods, and that 'starchy' foods, along with fruits and vegetables, should form the greatest proportion of energy intakes.

Benefits of and implementing a healthy diet

Evidence for the benefits of a good diet comes from a variety of sources. Epidemiological and prospective studies indicate that those with lower intakes of animal products and higher intakes of fruit and vegetables have a lower prevalence of cardiovascular disease, hypertension and certain cancers. Fruit and vegetables are thought to protect health through their supply of vitamins, minerals, dietary fibres and other bioactive compounds.

The Balance of Good Health model provides a framework for more in-depth dietary advice. Most people should be encouraged to eat at least five portions of fruit and vegetables a day and to opt for unsaturated sources of fat. Those with anaemia can be encouraged to eat red meat and individuals with osteoporosis can be encouraged to include calcium-rich foods from the 'milk and dairy' group. Older housebound people are advised to take a supplement of vitamin D (10 mg) each day.

Diet and fertility

What a mother eats before and during pregnancy may influence her child's subsequent health. Research has shown a significant association between retarded growth *in utero* and increased rates of coronary heart disease, hypertension and non-insulin-dependent diabetes later in adult life. Low-birthweight babies are at increased risk from these problems in later life. They have been linked to fetal undernutrition at different stages of gestation (Barker, 1993).

Women of childbearing age need to know what to eat, particularly if they take risks with contraception. A woman may not realize she is pregnant until she has missed a period, several weeks after conception. Therefore they need encouragement to eat a well-balanced diet and cut down on bad habits, such as smoking and drinking, that can affect them and their baby's health, before and during the pregnancy.

Pregnancy and breastfeeding

Emphasize the benefits of a healthy, varied diet and the hazards of overeating. Specific points to include are:

◆ Appetite is the best guide to energy needs. Think of 'eating for two' not as twice as much, but as getting the nutrients that both she and her baby need

◆ Most pregnant women build up a store of 2–4kg of body fat to support energy requirements for breastfeeding

◆ Increased quantities of a varied diet will provide all the energy and nutrients most breastfeeding women require

◆ Some women need to drink more when breastfeeding, especially while lactation becomes established

◆ Calcium requirements during breastfeeding rise from 700 to 1250 mg/day. This represents, on average, two extra servings of calcium-rich food – a total of five a day (e.g. a glass of milk, a pot of yoghurt, 30 g of cheddar cheese, two canned sardines).

Research indicates that increased calcium intake is not required in pregnancy as the body adapts to allow it to absorb more calcium from food (DoH, 1998d). However, pregnant women, particularly teenagers, need to ensure adequate calcium intake especially if they eat little dairy produce.

Adolescence

Teenagers are inclined towards erratic eating habits: missed breakfasts, junk food snacks, irregular meals and crash diets. Growth and development are rapid during the teenage years, and the demand for energy and most nutrients is relatively high. In both sexes, an average of 23 cm is added to height and 20–26 kg to weight. Before adolescence, both girls and boys have an average of 15% body fat. During adolescence this increases to about 20% in girls and decreases to about 10% in boys. The rapid increase in bone mass means that they require more calcium than adults. Girls should aim for 800 mg/day – 3 to 4 servings of calcium-rich food. Pregnant teenagers need extra care, but can be a difficult group to reach: they may not present until late in pregnancy and may disregard nutritional advice.

One way to obtain sufficient energy is by consumption of frequent snacks as well as meals. However, some adolescents eat more than they need and may become overweight, particularly if they are inactive. In the past ten years levels of obesity have trebled among 15-year-olds, and are continuing to rise. This situation has been described as 'a health time bomb' by the chief medical officer for England in his 2002 Annual Report (DoH, 2002a).

It is better to try to prevent obesity than to encourage strict dieting in this age group. The best way to manage overweight young people is to encourage regular exercise and healthy eating – increasing starchy foods for energy and reducing fatty and sugary foods. This should check weight gain whilst not inhibiting growth. Encouraging leisure pursuits (including exercise) should provide a distraction from eating. Good habits practised now will be likely to benefit their health for the rest of their lives. Parents may need education and support to encourage their children towards healthier eating. The school nurse may be a good source of help and monitor of progress.

There is an increasing tendency for teenagers, particularly girls, to control their weight by unsuitable methods such as smoking or by adopting very low-energy diets. Restriction of many food items can lead to nutrient deficiencies and health problems in later life. During adolescence iron requirements are increased in order to help growth and muscle development. After menstruation begins, girls need more iron to replace menstrual losses. The National Diet and Nutrition Survey (DoH, 2000a) found that 9% of girls aged 15–18 had a haemaglobin level lower than the limit for women. The survey also found that teenage girls between 15 and 18 years had intakes of iron below the lower reference nutrient intake.

Bread flour is fortified with iron by law and iron is also added to most breakfast cereals. This makes breakfast an important means of acquiring iron. However many adolescents skip breakfast, so these foods should be encouraged as snacks, together with food or drinks containing vitamin C, e.g. fruit juice. Adolescents should not be put on reducing diets. These can restrict growth and may precipitate anorexia nervosa which affects about 1% of young women (see also page 161). Bulimia nervosa also affects this age group. An obese or underweight teenager may need referral to a

---

Box 3.2 Body mass index (BMI)

BMI is calculated by applying the formula:

$$BMI = \frac{Weight\ (kg)}{Height\ (m)^2}$$

BMI grades

Less than 20 = Underweight

20–24 = Acceptable

25–29 = Overweight (some health risk)

30–40 = Obese (moderate health risk)

Over 40 = Severely obese (high health risk)

---

dietitian or for psychological assessment. See Box 3.2 for body mass index (BMI) measurements.

Diet, PMS and the menopause

Eating regular, well-balanced meals throughout the menstrual cycle and avoiding foods high in salt, sugar and caffeine premenstrually can help women with premenstrual syndrome (see page 435).

A healthy diet and regular weight-bearing exercise will help women prepare for the menopause and guard against osteoporosis.

The food standards agency

This agency was set up in the wake of the scares over BSE, *E. coli* and salmonella and is responsible for formulating policy and legislation; advising government on all aspects of food safety and standards and on certain aspects of nutrition. The Agency's role is described in the White Paper *A Force For Change* (DoH, 1998a).

Health and physical activity

◆ Seven out of ten women between 16 and 74 years of age do not do enough physical activity to benefit their health

◆ Only a third of young women (16–24 years of age) achieve recommended levels of exercise

◆ Women of all ages are less active than men, increasingly as they grow older.

(Hansbro, 1997)

Physical activity can:

◆ Reduce the risk of heart disease and stroke

◆ Promote psychological well-being

◆ Relieve the symptoms of anxiety and depression

◆ Help to promote self-image and a sense of well-being

◆ Encourage women to make time for and feel good about themselves

◆ Be fun and affordable

◆ Help to reduce social isolation and promote integration – encouraging a sense of community and a social focus for families and young people.

You can play an important role by emphasizing the benefits of exercise and how to make it enjoyable. There is evidence that a lack of physical activity plays a major role in the deterioration of bone quality that accompanies osteoporosis (DoH, 1998d). Weight-bearing exercise such as walking, jogging, dancing and tennis protect against osteoporosis. Pelvic floor exercise helps to promote continence and can increase sexual enjoyment (see page 495). Moderate weight-bearing and non-weight-bearing exercise (e.g. swimming) can improve the course of pregnancy. Physical activity stimulates metabolism and plays a role in controlling weight and managing obesity.

Despite all these benefits, women are still not getting the message. The greatest health benefits will be gained by encouraging people who are currently sedentary to get involved in some physical activity. It is also important to encourage those who are already active to remain active and possibly to increase their activity levels, in terms of time spent, frequency and intensity.

Getting fit

In 1996 the HEA launched the *Active For Life* campaign (HEA, 1996a) to encourage people to lead more active lives, particularly those who do not enjoy exercise or sport. The campaign gives comprehensive guidance for people of all ages and all ethnic groups. (Black and minority ethnic groups have disproportionately high rates of certain diseases, e.g. CHD and diabetes.) The campaign also recognizes the specific needs of disabled people.

The current recommendation is to incorporate activity into everyday routine, building up to 30 minutes of 'moderate intensity' activity on 5 or more days a week. The idea is to encourage activity which results in breathing slightly harder; a slightly raised heart rate, but not out of breath or sweating profusely.

This can be achieved by walking to school or getting off the bus a couple of stops early or climbing the stairs rather than taking the lift. Recreational activities do not need to be expensive – brisk walking, rollerblading, dancing, swimming, golf and gardening. Suggest your client chooses activities she can do with a friend or joins a class at a centre with a crèche.

People who are already fit may benefit from increasing the intensity and length of their workout or choosing a new activity to exercise a different range of muscles. They may need advice from a qualified instructor. How vigorous should activity be? Advise clients that they should feel their heart beating faster, but not racing, be able to continue talking whilst exercising, and to feel in control.

Activity and stamina should be built up gradually. Advise clients with medical problems to consult you or their doctor before embarking on a new or more vigorous routine. To reduce risk of injury, remind clients to 'warm-up' and do some gentle stretching before vigorous exercise and end with a 'cool-down' period and further stretching.

The menstrual cycle

Research suggests that exercise triggers the body to produce endorphins, natural opiates that promote a sense of well-being in addition to relieving pain. Anecdotal evidence suggests that moderate exercise can help dysmenorrhoea perhaps by distracting attention from pain, producing a feeling of relaxation, and reducing stress. Similarly, exercise may relieve some of the symptoms of PMS. Yoga and relaxation techniques are recommended for PMS and dysmenorrhoea.

Sexual activity and orgasm are also said to help dysmenorrhoea.

Excessive exercise, especially in competitive athletes, can lead to irregular periods, anovulatory cycles and amenorrhoea. An inadequate diet or anorexia nervosa can compound such problems, leading to subfertility and long-term risk of osteoporosis. Periods usually revert to normal and fertility to its previous level with restoration of a healthy BMI through an appropriate diet and reduction in exercise.

Pregnancy and well-being

Studies have shown elevated stress and depressed mood during pregnancy, but few have examined exercise in relation to psychosocial outcomes during pregnancy. Da Costa *et al.* (2003) examined associations between leisure-time physical activity (LTPA) patterns during pregnancy, and psychological well-being. Data collected for pregnant women who exercised were compared with those women who did not exercise. Women who exercised reported significantly less depressed mood, stress, anxiety and daily worries in the first and second trimester. Women who exercised in the third trimester reported less anxiety compared to non-exercisers. These results suggest that there is an association between enhanced psychological well-being, as measured by a variety of psychosocial inventories and LTPA participation, particularly during the first and second trimesters of pregnancy. In healthy pregnant women, even low-intensity regular exercise may be a potentially effective low-cost method of enhancing psychological well-being.

Pregnant women can continue to exercise so long as there are no complications (e.g. vaginal bleeding or hypertension). They should consult their midwife or GP if in doubt. Exercise in moderation reduces risk of miscarriage and premature birth. Beneficial activities include walking, swimming, stationary cycling and yoga. A gradual transition to non-weight-bearing exercises is recommended as pregnancy progresses and weight increases. Vigorous physical activity is best avoided for 6–8 weeks after delivery, but women should be encouraged to do postnatal and pelvic floor exercises during this time.

The middle years and beyond

Bone mass should be maintained (thus minimizing the risk of osteoporosis) through diet and weight-bearing exercise such as brisk walking, dancing, cycling, racquet sports, weight training and gardening. Hormone replacement therapy will also protect against bone loss as oestrogen levels decline. Swimming, although good for the cardiovascular system, is non-weight-bearing and does not protect against bone loss. Exercise has the additional advantage of increasing agility and dexterity, thereby preventing falls and associated fractures.

Encourage women to keep active after the menopause, with modifications to type and intensity as the years go by. Women disabled by degenerative or neurological disease may need your advice about suitable options. Many community centres run exercise classes for older people and provide transport for the housebound.

Women and drugs

> We are surrounded by drugs ... the cups of coffee and tea, the glasses of beer, wine and whisky, the cigarettes, the snorts of cocaine, the joints, the tablets of acid, the fixes of heroin and the ubiquitous tranquillisers and sleeping pills ... So long as there are drug takers, there will be drug casualties ...drug taking is here to stay and one way or another, we must all learn to live with drugs.
>
> (Gossop, 1993)

Drug use has risen disproportionately among women, according to the Institute for the Study of Drug Dependence (ISDD, 1999a). National figures suggest that women account for one in four users presenting to drug services; over 90% are of childbearing age (DoH, 1999b; SCODA, 1997). However, as a high proportion of these women conceal their drug use and do not seek treatment, these figures must be a significant underestimate (Mounteney, 1999).

Female drug use does not conform to the image of women as carers, mothers and partners. Public prejudice may result in marginalization of drug-using women from mainstream society. They may be discouraged from attending women and children's services for fear of being viewed negatively. A common concern is that their children may be taken into 'care' (Mounteney, 1999).

Drug use is often blamed for family breakdown, legal or financial difficulties, but these factors may be a precipitating cause of drug problems. Adult drug users often report poverty, violence, child abuse and family dysfunction (Mounteney, 1999).

As with smoking and alcohol, the biggest focus of concern is young people: 16- to 19-year-olds have the highest prevalence, with almost a third taking drugs on a regular basis. Homeless young people are especially at risk – nine out of ten are estimated to be taking illicit drugs. Almost all 'clubbers' are reported to have tried a drug; ecstasy, cannabis and amphetamines being the most common. Increasing availability and cheaper prices have led to an increase in cocaine use, often in combination with alcohol (ISDD, 1999b).

'Tackling drugs'

In 1998 the government published a 10-year anti-drugs strategy: *Tackling Drugs To Build A Better Britain* (DoH, 1998c). Collaboration between government and the statutory, private and voluntary sectors was promoted as the key element in this new approach. These bodies continue to work closely with local partnerships set up by Drug Action Teams to facilitate a coordinated approach to local drug issues.

Drug Misuse and Dependence. Guidelines on Clinical Management (DoH, 1999c) was published to help practitioners working in primary care and stressed the importance of multi-professional shared care.

Self-image and drugs

It is common for female drug users to have poor self-image and low self-esteem. You should take care not to add to these negative feelings. It is important to create an atmosphere of trust and support by adopting an open and accepting attitude, and avoiding judgemental terms such as 'abuse' and 'addiction'. At the same time, you must be clear about policy governing breach of confidentiality in the event of a child protection concern. The child's welfare is paramount.

Psychoactive drugs

This section discusses the effects of psychoactive drugs, both legal and illicit, therapeutic and recreational. Further information about physical and psychological effects and the legal status of individual drugs is described in the 7th edition of the ISDD's *Drug Abuse Briefing* (1999a). Alcohol and tobacco are discussed in more detail later. In essence, however, all drugs are used for similar reasons: to feel good, to relax, to alleviate stress, to block out reality, to calm anxiety or to stimulate mind and/or body.

Drugs, the menstrual cycle and fertility

Disruption of the menstrual cycle is common among women using drugs like ecstasy, amphetamines, opiates and anabolic steroids. Periods may become irregular, lighter or heavier; and there can be intermenstrual bleeding. Ecstasy, amphetamines and heroin can reduce appetite leading to weight loss and amenorrhoea as a result of suppression of ovulation. Poor nutrition, a common problem with heavy drug users, and long-term amenorrhoea are risk factors for osteoporosis. Amenorrhoea may lull women into a false sense of security that they will not become pregnant and risks may then be taken with contraception.

Anabolic steroids can affect fertility and sexuality. They are associated with menstrual disturbance, increased sex drive, decrease in breast size and irreversible development of virilizing effects. These may affect a female fetus if drug use continues during pregnancy.

Alcohol and cannabis are sometimes used to 'treat' dysmenorrhoea and premenstrual syndrome, but they may exacerbate PMS symptoms rather than alleviate them.

Drugs, sex and contraception

Ecstasy has been called the 'love drug' and the 'hug drug'. Other drugs reported to promote feelings of closeness and sexual pleasure include cannabis, alkyl nitrites ('poppers'), LSD and amphetamines. However, ecstasy and amphetamines may inhibit orgasm. Antidepressants may also cause sexual dysfunction. Mixing drugs and sex can make it difficult to stay in control, to use effective contraception and to practise safer sex. Sharing injecting equipment or having unprotected sex increases the risk of hepatitis, sexually transmitted infections (STIs) and HIV.

Oral contraception may be unsuitable for heavy drug users. They may forget to take it regularly. The combined pill is contraindicated for women with a history of deep vein thrombosis or liver damage: common complications of intravenous drug use. Oral contraceptive users need to know that drug interaction may occur with antibiotics, some anti-HIV treatments, e.g. protease inhibitors, antiepileptics, barbiturates, tranquillizers and hypnotics (see page 268). The combined pill may also alter the effects of other drugs, including chlordiazepoxide, diazepam, imipramine and amitriptyline.

A progestogen injectable or implant are better options: they are highly effective and non-intercourse-related. In addition, reduced menstrual loss benefits women with anaemia and HIV infection. Other reliable methods, depending on medical history and sexual lifestyle, are the intrauterine device (IUD) and the levonorgestrel intrauterine system (IUS). The IUS has the advantage of reducing menstrual loss and possibly the risk of pelvic infection.

Condoms, used carefully, provide protection against STIs and HIV. Female condoms may give women more personal control. Diaphragms and caps are less reliable and do not protect against STIs. Rapid weight loss can occur with drug use, necessitating a change in diaphragm size. All clients using barrier contraception should be reminded about emergency contraception.

Drugs mixed with other substances could cause interactions. Cocaine, amphetamines and ecstasy can increase blood pressure.

Drugs and pregnancy

Lifestyle associated with heavy drug use may put mother and baby at risk through self-neglect and poor nutrition. Drugs also directly affect the baby. The small risk of drug-related malformations is at its greatest in the first trimester.

Many heavy drug users have healthy babies, but heavy drug use (including alcohol and smoking) in pregnancy is associated with miscarriage, premature labour, low birthweight, fetal abnormality and stillbirth. Risk to babies whose mothers are taking benzodiazepines is believed to be low. However, studies have shown a link with cleft palate when taken in the first trimester. Babies born to heavy, long-term users of tranquillizers, opiates and barbiturates may show signs of withdrawal.

Methadone maintenance can improve pregnancy outcome among opiate users. Barbiturates, opiates or tranquillizers should not be withdrawn suddenly. Women wanting to reduce or stop drugs should aim to do so slowly during the second trimester, with support and medical supervision. The timing of reduction or withdrawal is important to minimize the risk of miscarriage or premature labour. Inpatient treatment is recommended for barbiturate withdrawal because of the risk of fits.

Pregnant women and those planning a baby should, if possible, avoid all drugs. Clients taking prescription medicines need to consult their doctor/midwife to discuss continuation and any associated risks to a developing fetus. Women continuing to use opiates or benzodiazepines may require extra care during pregnancy and labour. Their babies may be at risk from fetal distress; and, after birth, from respiratory depression and neonatal drug withdrawal problems. Fear of hostile attitudes by staff or pressure to have an abortion may discourage disclosure of drug use, resulting in late booking for antenatal care – or none at all. A well-coordinated multi-agency approach is vital in the care of a woman with a high-risk pregnancy and her new baby.

Tranquillizers and hypnotics

Withdrawal from tranquillizers can take weeks or months (Box 3.3). During this time, women may be vulnerable not only to re-emergence of the old problems which led to them starting medication, but also to new ones related to withdrawal. The National Association for Mental Health (MIND) has details of local support groups and helplines (see Resources). Many women successfully come off tranquillizers without medical help, whilst others need support

from a community drugs team or residential care. Very few residential units accommodate children and there are even fewer mother and baby units.

Sources of help

Drugs have an impact on all of us, our lives, worries and aspirates, so it would be useful to compile a list of local services that can help clients, their partners and families including:

◆ GPs
◆ Street agencies
◆ Community drug teams
◆ Drug dependency/treatment units.

Services provide a wide range of help, including advice on harm minimization, safer injecting techniques, needle exchange, safer sex, counselling, legal and housing help. Some agencies work with GPs to provide a prescribing programme. Ask for their promotional materials and perhaps arrange to visit them.

Women and smoking

Smoking, the UK's largest single cause of preventable death and disability, accounts for more than 120,000 deaths a year, 30,000 of which are women and costs the NHS in England about £1.7 billion each year (DoH, 2002b; Callum, 1998). We smoke more cigarettes per person than the European average and more deaths are caused by smoking in the UK than in other countries. The problem could be getting worse. The long downward trend in smoking since the 1960s may now be levelling out. Increasing numbers of young people are starting to smoke. Smoking hits poorer people harder, widening inequalities in health among social groups (DoH, 2002b). Around 10 million people in Britain (about 1000 a day, on average) have stopped smoking in the last 15 years; and 70% of the remaining 13 million cigarette smokers are reported to want to do so; however, approximately 26% of women and 10% of 11- to 15-year-old girls continue the smoking habit (DoH, 1998b).

Box 3.3   Coming off tranquillizers

The Council for Involuntary Tranquillizer Addiction (CITA) gives the following advice to people wanting to withdraw from benzodiazepines:

◆ Ensure you have support from family/friends (perhaps your practice nurse or drug agency can help too)

◆ Do not stop suddenly – this may cause severe withdrawal symptoms

◆ Enlist your GP's support

◆ Ask to change to diazepam; it is long-acting and available in different strength doses

◆ Divide the dose so that it is taken 3 times a day – morning, noon and night – with a larger dose at night

◆ Stabilize for 2 weeks on this dose before starting to reduce

◆ Decrease dose **gradually** – no more than 1 mg/fortnight initially. (Younger people may be able to reduce by 2 mg/fortnight.) Follow this by a 0.5 mg reduction when you feel ready

◆ Take it at your own pace. Stay at the same dose for longer if you are finding it too difficult

◆ Talk to a supportive friend, ex-user or helpline

◆ Read the leaflets/books (see Resources)

◆ Do not start counselling or therapy until withdrawal is complete – it is too much to cope with

◆ Aim for the winning post. Remember many others have made it already.

The White Paper on tobacco *Smoking Kills* (DoH, 1998b) sets three targets for England to be achieved by 2010. These are to reduce smoking among:

◆ Children age 11–15 years: from 13% to 9%, with a fall to 11% by 2005

◆ Adults: from 28% to 24%, or less by 2010, with a fall to 28% by 2005

◆ Pregnant women: from 23% to 15%, with a fall to 18% by 2005.

This was supported by the NHS Plan (DoH, 2000b) with the aim to reduce the number of smokers by 1.5 million by 2010, a fall of 125,000 smokers per year. Measures taken have included the NHS cessation programme in designated areas, the availability of nicotine replacement therapies on prescription and the development of the NHS Stop Smoking Helpline.

In 1999 the government launched England's first evidence-based guidelines: Smoking Cessation Guidelines for Health Professionals published in Thorax (Raw et al., 1998), with Guidance for Commissioners on the Cost Effectiveness of Smoking Cessation (Parrott et al., 1998). The government is setting tough targets to improve the health of the people of this country, including cancer and heart disease. We can only succeed in meeting these targets if we tackle smoking now, through a determined, concerted and strategic effort. While overall smoking rates have fallen for decades, they have barely changed among the least disadvantaged.

Why do women smoke?

Women's ambivalent relationship with tobacco seems to have been strongly established in the 1920s when consumption rose rapidly alongside the fight for sexual equality (Graham, 1993). Cigarette smoking became identified as a symbol of emancipation. It was a fashion accessory for the affluent, upwardly mobile woman: an image that is often perpetuated by today's media (Ernest, 1985). The image of smoking as 'liberating' is ironic, as the link between smoking and social disadvantage is well established (Graham, 1993).

Oakley (1994) linked women's smoking to social deprivation, stress and disadvantage.

Research has shown that there are pronounced socio-economic differences in women's smoking and it is more prevalent in semi- and unskilled groups than in professional classes (see Figure 3.2). Women experiencing depression and those with psychosocial difficulties, such as difficulties in daily domestic roles, have high rates of persistent smoking (Pritchard, 1994). Single mothers living in poverty may smoke as a way of taking a few moments for themselves and making the stress of daily life tolerable (Blackburn and Graham, 1994).

Women are less likely to give up smoking than men and not just because of self-image and fear of gaining weight. Research suggests women are more likely to smoke under emotional pressure, while men prefer more relaxed circumstances. Women are also said to rely more on cigarettes to cope when feeling angry and frustrated. Studies show that quitting smoking depends upon the interaction of at least three crucial factors:

◆ Perception of stress

◆ Self-confidence

◆ Dependence on cigarettes.

Not only do women feel less confident and more dependent on cigarettes than men, but they also

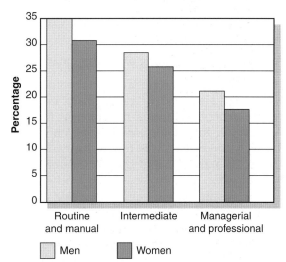

Figure 3.2 Prevalence of cigarette smoking by sex and socio-economic classification based on the current or last job of the household reference person (ONS, 2002).

see themselves as being under more stress – which in turn boosts their dependence on cigarettes (Jacobson, 1986).

Tomorrow's smokers

About 82% of smokers start as teenagers (ONS, 1998). The main influences are the smoking status and attitudes of parents, older siblings and peer pressure (HEA, 1995). Children from households where one parent smokes are twice as likely to become regular smokers than those from non-smoking homes. Other factors include low self-esteem, problem behaviour and poor school performance. Teenagers are especially susceptible to the addictive nature of nicotine. They soon experience cravings, become irritable and suffer sleep disturbances (Bellow and Ramsay, 1991).

In 1996 only 4% of 12-year-old girls were regular smokers. By the age of 14 this increased to 24% and at 15 years 33% were regular smokers (ONS, 1997). If current smoking rates continue, around one million of today's UK teenagers and children will die by middle age (Doll *et al.*, 1994).

The government believes that a range of strategies will help protect young people by making it less likely that they will begin to smoke and also by helping them to stop. Such strategies include:

◆ Minimal tobacco advertising in shops

◆ Tough enforcement on under-age sales

◆ Proof of age cards

◆ Strong rules on siting of vending machines.

A change in the law outlawing tobacco advertising marks the end of a long, hard battle by campaigners, including the British Medical Association and Action for Smoking on Health. Tobacco advertising was finally banned in the UK in 2003 and tobacco sponsorship of sports banned after 2005. However, some advertising will be possible at the point of the sale of cigarettes (Eaton, 2003).

The tobacco industry needs to recruit about 330 smokers a day to replace those killed by smoking related diseases. Young people are a prime target. Smoking is still associated with 'looking cool', being mature and staying slim.

Adult role models – musicians, models, actors, sports celebrities, etc. – seen smoking may encourage young people to experiment, possibly leading to lifelong addiction.

Smoking and fertility

A substantial body of literature suggests that smoking reduces a couple's chances of a successful pregnancy, not to mention having adverse health effects on children. It is estimated that around one in six couples in the UK experience problems in conceiving at some time. A large study (Klonoff-Cohen *et al.*, 2001) demonstrated double the risk of childlessness five years after discontinuing contraception in smoking couples compared to non-smoking couples.

Infertility is usually defined as not having conceived after 12 months of unprotected sex. The fertility problems observed in smokers may result (at least in part) from alterations in sex hormone metabolism. Substances present in cigarette smoke have been found to be toxic to the testes and ovaries. Women who smoke are twice as likely to be infertile as non-smokers (US DHHS, 2001).

Studies that have assessed the risks of different types of infertility have found some evidence that smokers are at particular risk of tubal infertility, in which the underlying problem is thought to involve the function of the fallopian tubes (Phipps *et al.*, 1987). Daling *et al.* (1987) found that women with primary tubal infertility were almost three times as likely to be smokers as were fertile women. The effect of smoking on fertility appears to be reversible: most studies show that women who have stopped smoking take no longer to become pregnant than women who have never smoked.

Smoking is associated with abnormal menstrual patterns, premature ageing (including skin wrinkling), earlier menopause by 2 or 3 years, and an increased risk of osteoporosis. Twenty cigarettes a day throughout adulthood may reduce bone density in women by 5–10% (Hopper and Seeman, 1994). Smoking also alters the normal physiological levels of reproductive hormones, reduces the chances of embryo implantation and increases the risk of pelvic inflammatory disease by altering the immune function.

Smoking and pregnancy

Smoking during pregnancy is an important cause of ill health for both mother and her developing fetus. As well as increasing the mother's risk for potentially serious complications, smoking during pregnancy is the largest preventable cause of fetal and infant ill health and death (RCP, 2000). Smoking is associated with an increased risk of ectopic pregnancy (Poswillo and Alberman, 1992) even after adjustment for other predisposing factors, such as STIs and pelvic inflammatory disease.

Studies have shown that the risk of ectopic pregnancy is increased 1.5–2.5 times in women who smoke (RCP, 1992; Saraiya *et al.*, 1998).

It is estimated that about one-third of all perinatal deaths in the UK are caused by smoking. Smokers are more likely to lose their baby through stillbirth.

Women who smoke during pregnancy are three times more likely to have a low-birthweight baby (RCP, 1992): on average, 200–250 g lighter than those of non-smokers. The greater the number of cigarettes smoked during pregnancy, the less well the fetus grows and develops. Smoking is a more important determinant of birthweight and growth of the fetus than the mother's height, weight, number of previous pregnancies and their outcomes, or the sex of the baby (Windsor, 2001).

Stopping smoking reduces the risk of many of the adverse effects of smoking on pregnancy. Studies show that women who quit during the first trimester reduce the impact of smoking on birthweight. Smoking fewer cigarettes has no beneficial effect.

Smoking and cervical abnormalities

Epidemiological evidence strongly links smoking with squamous cell cervical cancer and high-grade CIN (see Chapter 13). Studies among women who are infected with HPV have found that women who smoke are at higher risk of developing preinvasive and invasive cervical cancer. Typically, smoking increases the risk of invasive cervical cancer some two- to threefold (Catellsague *et al.*, 2001). Nicotine and tobacco-specific carcinogens have been detected in the cervical mucus of smokers (Prokopczyk *et al.*, 1997). Cigarette condensate increases the frequency of malignant transformation in cultured cervical cell infected with HPV (Yang *et al.*, 1996). There is also some evidence that smoking may result in a reduced immune response to the cervix (Poppe *et al.*, 1995). Other research suggests that smoking cessation could have a beneficial effect on early cervical abnormalities, reducing the size of some lesions (Szarewski *et al.*, 1996).

Smoking and breast cancer

A recent US study suggests women who smoke are 30% more likely to develop breast cancer (Reynolds *et al.*, 2004).

Passive smoking

Passive smoking kills hundreds every year and causes misery for many. Tobacco smoke is estimated to contain more than 4000 chemicals including over 40 carcinogens. Passive smoking or exposure to environmental tobacco smoke is recognized as a cause of cancer and CHD. It is also known to aggravate respiratory conditions and allergies. It is thought to cause several hundred deaths from lung cancer every year in the UK (DoH, 2002b). The hazards were highlighted by the entertainer Roy Castle, a non-smoker, who died after spending much of his working life in smoky nightclubs. Non-smokers inhale both 'mainstream' smoke inhaled/exhaled by the smoker and 'sidestream' smoke from the burning end of cigarettes. Only 15% of smoke is inhaled by the smoker. Non-smokers exposed to tobacco smoke over long periods have an estimated 15% increased risk of lung cancer (Copas and Shi, 2000). Most vulnerable are babies and children who are at increased risk from asthma and other respiratory and ENT conditions.

A national enquiry into stillbirths and infant death provided strong evidence linking sudden infant death syndrome to smoking. The risk was twofold: first, from the mother smoking during pregnancy; and second, from those exposing the pregnant mother or infant to passive smoking. The study estimated that the number of cot deaths could fall by almost two-thirds if parents did not smoke (Blair *et al.*, 1996).

Why do women want to quit?

Reasons include:

◆ Social pressure
◆ Pregnancy
◆ To increase self-respect
◆ To feel in control
◆ To improve health
◆ To save money
◆ To set an example to children and safeguard their health
◆ To look, feel and smell better.

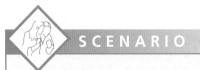

SCENARIO

Karen, aged 24, tried to stop smoking several times. She finally succeeded when her 5-year-old asked her not to kiss him good night because she smelt so horrible. She said: 'I felt so guilty'.

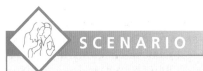

SCENARIO

Sarah started smoking when out with her friends – but never at home. After leaving for university, she began to smoke whilst studying – more before exams. Soon she was getting through a pack of 10 a day, sometimes more. When she renewed her Pill prescription, the nurse pointed out that she was spending £20 a week on cigarettes. Shocked to realise how much of her loan was going on smoking (£1040 a year), she set a quit date after her exams and persuaded her boyfriend to give up with her.

What stops women quitting?

Knowing the risks of smoking does not necessarily help. Women often fail to stop because of the following factors:

◆ Withdrawal symptoms
◆ Possible weight gain
◆ Fear of losing control
◆ Anticipation of increased stress
◆ Enjoyment of smoking
◆ Lack of support
◆ Lack of confidence and low self-esteem.

Helping smokers to quit

The smoking cessation guidelines recommend an integrated approach by all health professionals to assess the smoking status of individuals at every opportunity. Guidelines should be incorporated into health improvement programmes, in collaboration with local Primary Care Trusts. Smoking cessation services should be specified within clinical governance arrangements (Raw *et al.*, 1998). Initially, Health Action Zones were the first areas to benefit from government funding.

Whilst smoking cessation advice should be directed at all clients, priority groups include women who are pregnant or trying to conceive; have young children; are young themselves; are taking the combined contraceptive pill; have health problems, e.g. diabetes, cardiovascular or respiratory disease; and those on a low income.

Assess what updating, or new skills you need. Check training available at your local health promotion unit. Assemble a starter pack of information/leaflets for clients. Advertise what services you offer and where more intensive help is available. Follow the '4As' for brief intervention: ask, advise, assist and arrange.

Ask

Assess and document smoking status. Use open-ended questions to explore your client's attitude to smoking – both positive and negative. For example, would you like to give up smoking if you could do it easily? The next question might be: What stops you? or What do you like/dislike about smoking? These questions may provide valuable insight into her motivation to stop.

You also need to assess her dependence on nicotine. Ask how soon after waking she has her first cigarette and what is the longest time she goes without one. How many does she smoke? How old was she when she started smoking? Has she stopped before? What degree of support does she think she will need? A carbon monoxide monitor can be a powerful motivator before and after quitting – it is also a means of verifying reports of abstinence.

Advise

Stress the benefits of quitting (Table 3.1) and the dangers of continuing. Be positive and discuss the real potential of nicotine replacement therapy

(NRT) and professional support – including helplines and specialist services. Plan possible strategies to reduce the 'triggers' she may associate with smoking.

Assist

Try to establish with her what level of assistance is required. Her individual needs will be determined by nicotine dependence, previous attempts to quit; and other factors such as pregnancy, lack of support and financial difficulties. Set the quit date. Both of you should write it down. Draw up an action plan – you could base a quit programme on information contained in *Stopping Smoking Made Easier* (HEA, 1998b) or *Smoking: Don't Give Up Giving Up* (DoH, 1999d). Ask her to try and anticipate problems. Why did previous attempts fail? What did she learn from them? Will any non-smoking friends/colleagues support her through the initial critical period?

Help her to select and use an NRT product. Clients who have tried NRT before may need a different delivery system or a higher/more frequent dose over a longer period. Some areas are operating a one-week free treatment voucher scheme for clients entitled to free prescriptions – the money that would have been spent on cigarettes pays for the next week's NRT. Be aware of local arrangements and promote community pharmacists as a reliable source of information. Discuss alternative anti-smoking aids, especially if NRT is contraindicated. These could include hypnotherapy, acupuncture, relaxation therapy, sugar-free gum, counselling and helplines.

Provide her with reinforcing literature. Websites may prove to be an effective source of help for many smokers. They are confidential and easily accessible (see Resources).

Arrange

Make a follow-up appointment 2–4 weeks after the quit date. Offer to see her earlier if she needs extra support and promote the quitlines. A smoker who has made repeated attempts or has experienced severe withdrawal symptoms should be offered a specialist programme, if available, in your area.

Table 3.1	Cessation of smoking: the benefits
Time since quitting	**Benefits**
20 MINUTES	Blood pressure and pulse return to normal. Circulation improves
8 HOURS	O_2 blood levels return to normal. Nicotine and CO levels reduced by 50%
24 HOURS	CO eliminated from the body. Lungs start to clear out mucous and other smoking debris
48 HOURS	Nicotine is no longer detected in the body. Taste and smell are improved
72 HOURS	Breathing becomes easier as bronchial tubes relax. Energy levels increase
2-12 WEEKS	Circulation improves, making walking easier
3-9 MONTHS	Cough, wheezing and shortness of breath improve. Lung function increased by 5-10%
5 YEARS	Risk of heart attack falls to about half that of a smoker
10 YEARS	Risk of lung cancer falls to about half that of smoker. Risk of heart attack falls to about the same as lifelong non-smoker

Source: The Health Benefits of Smoking Cessation. A Report of the Surgeon General 1990 (US Department of Health and Human Services) and QUIT (1996).

Brief advice

Quit rates of 5% may be achievable with the help of brief advice. This may not sound much, but given the multitude of smokers nationally it translates into large absolute numbers. However, health professionals often fear that people will resent being advised to quit. Perhaps the first step is to select the patient with care. Advice on quitting is incongruous for someone who consults about a laceration to his or her finger. However a presentation with a related condition such as a cough, or shortness of breath is a golden opportunity. One strategy for a brief advice is 'the 30-second approach' outlined in Box 3.4.

Withdrawal effects: symptoms of recovery

Between 50% and 70% of people attempting to stop after smoking more than 10 cigarettes a day experience withdrawal symptoms meeting diagnostic criteria for nicotine withdrawal syndrome. Explaining why these symptoms occur may help your client overcome them and understand the value of NRT. Tell her the symptoms are a positive sign that her body is recovering from the effects of tobacco.

Nicotine withdrawal syndrome is defined as the emergence of four or more of the following symptoms within 24 hours of abrupt cessation or reduction of nicotine use:

◆ Cravings

◆ Dysphoric or depressed mood

◆ Insomnia

◆ Irritability, frustration or anger

◆ Anxiety/tension

◆ Poor concentration or loss of concentration

◆ Restlessness

◆ Decreased heart rate

◆ Increased appetite or weight gain.

(Hughes *et al.*, 1991; Hughes, 1992)

Associated symptoms include:

Cough. Reactivation of the cilia, slowing down of mucus production and increased viscosity of sputum may make coughing more difficult for a few weeks.

Constipation. May result from reliance of the bowel on the laxative action of tobacco.

Dizziness. May be due to improved blood supply to the brain as carboxy-haemoglobin is eliminated and red blood cells carrying a greater concentration of oxygen.

Mouth ulcers and sore tongue. May be due to changes in bacterial flora.

Sleep disturbances. May include nocturnal tobacco craving. Insomnia may be related to a temporary fall in electro-cortical activity when smoking stops.

Tingling sensations. May occur with improved circulation. Elimination of nicotine from the body restores normal arterial tone, lowering heart rate and blood pressure.

Smoking cessation aids

Nicotine replacement therapy (NRT)

Inhalation through cigarettes is the most addictive form of nicotine delivery, providing a 'fix' within 20 seconds. NRT helps quitting by providing nicotine at a slower rate, in a safer form and without the harmful constituents of tobacco smoke. Products include transdermal patches, chewing gum, nasal spray, inhalator, sub-lingual tablets and a lozenge. Using NRT in primary care can double cessation rates from about 5% to 10%;

> **Box 3.4** The 30-second approach to brief smoking cessation intervention
>
> ◆ Do you smoke?
>
>   Yes/No → Record in patient notes
>
>   ↓
>
> ◆ Would you like to stop?
>
>   Yes/No → Provide the patient with a leaflet and emphasize that when they do want to stop, you and your team will be available to help
>
> ◆ There are treatments available – would you like our help?
>
>   Yes/No → Reinforce the idea that you and your team can help
>
> ◆ Encourage the patient to arrange a double appointment with the GP, nurse or smoking cessation counsellor. Provide a leaflet.

and in intensive settings, from about 10% to 20%. All NRT methods have similar success rates (Raw *et al.*, 1998). Smoking cessation therapies are now available on an NHS prescription.

Encourage NRT use – without creating unrealistic expectations. Clients need accurate information about the various delivery systems and how to use them. Under-dosing or stopping NRT too soon is a common reason for relapse. NRT is not a miracle cure, nor is it meant to feel the same as smoking, but it reduces cravings and withdrawal symptoms. Reassure clients it is much safer and less addictive than cigarettes and that they cannot overdose on it. It is the tar, carbon monoxide and other poisonous chemicals that cause disease. Moreover, NRT costs no more than 20 cigarettes a day (around £32–34 a week) with the prospect of long-term financial gains. Data sheets warn that smokers should stop completely while using NRT.

NRT is, as yet, contraindicated in pregnancy because of lack of data, even though nicotine without tar and carbon monoxide may be safer for the fetus. What about young people? It seems ironic that 16-year-olds can legally buy and smoke cigarettes, yet data sheets guidelines restrict NRT use (with the exception of chewing gum) to those over 18. An assessment may need to balance the increasing risk of addiction against any risks associated with NRT.

Bupropion hydrochloride SR (Zyban)

Bupropion, the first non-nicotine pharmacological smoking cessation aid, is now available on prescription. Originally developed as an antidepressant, bupropion has been shown to be highly effective in helping motivated, nicotine-dependent smokers to quit when used in combination with counselling and support. It reduces craving and withdrawal symptoms by altering two neurotransmitters involved in nicotine addiction: dopamine and noradrenaline (Jorenby *et al.*, 1999; Covey *et al.*, 2000).

Smokers wishing to use bupropion need medical assessment. Pregnant or breastfeeding women should not use it, nor is it recommended for people under 18. It is contraindicated in smokers with certain pre-existing conditions

including epilepsy, eating disorders and severe liver disease.

Guidance from the National Institute for Clinical Excellence (2002) now recommends NRT and bupropion (Zyban) for smokers who want to stop. In fact these therapies are presented as being among the most cost-effective of all healthcare interventions.

Helping relapsers

Many smokers go round the cycle several times before quitting for good (Figure 3.3). Help clients explore what happened last time and find a better way for the future. Feelings of failure and guilt are common and may put them off trying again. You may also feel demoralized if clients fail and wonder whether you are giving them the right advice; but remember the quit rate is no more than 20% even with intensive support.

Your continuing support and non-judgemental approach may spur clients on to have another go. You can suggest:

◆ Checking on reasons for quitting. Does she *really* want to stop? Is she committed?

◆ Trying NRT (perhaps a different type)

◆ Seeking more support from a specialist cessation service

◆ Working out the best time to try again

◆ Having a break until she is really ready to quit.

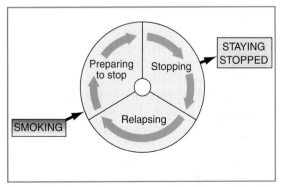

Figure 3.3 Preparing to stop smoking. *Source: Stopping Smoking Made Easier*, HEA, 1992. The diagram is like a revolving door. Many smokers go round several times before leaving it.

Note: Smoking is still a major problem among nurses. Some people may question whether they are in a position to encourage others to give up. Nurses who smoke need to address their own personal issues, but should continue to advise, support and encourage their clients. See Box 3.5 for top tips for self-help.

Women and alcohol

Alcohol, the most popular drug in Western society, is associated with good times: celebrations, weddings, social occasions and family gatherings – when many young people experience their first drink. It is also a means of 'drowning our sorrows'. Until recently, problem drinking was predominantly associated with men, but the move to sexual equality is believed to have encouraged women to drink more. Alcohol Concern in 2000 stated that the proportion of women drinking in excess of 14 units a week had increased from 10% in 1988 to 15% in 1998, an increase of 50% over a ten-year period.

The Health of the Nation (DoH, 1992b) set a target to reduce the proportion of women drinking more than 14 units a week to 7% by 2005. Alcohol Concern says that if current trends continue this is extremely unlikely. The Alcohol Harm Reduction Strategy for England (DoH, 2004) whilst acknowledging that women benefit from drinking small amounts aims to:

◆ Tackle alcohol-related disorder

◆ Improve treatment and support

◆ Clamp down on irresponsible promotion

◆ Provide better information to consumers about the dangers of alcohol misuse.

Due to the contributing factors causing alcohol consumption amongst women and the health risks involved, it is evident that a coherent strategy is needed to combat harmful drinking among women. High-profile health promotion is needed, which informs women about guidelines on sensible drinking. There needs to be a clear focus on the benefits of alcohol as well as the health risks, as currently there appears to be conflicting and confusing information.

The DoH advises that men should not drink more than 3–4 units per day of alcohol and women should only drink 2–3 units daily, due to lower body weight, smaller livers, less body fluid and less alcohol dehydrogenase (which breaks down alcohol). These daily benchmarks apply whether you drink every day, once or twice a week, or occasionally. A unit of alcohol is 10 ml of pure alcohol. Counting units of alcohol can help us to keep track of the amount we are drinking (see Table 3.2).

According to surveys in 1996, women were drinking on average about 5.4 units a week. Men, in comparison, were drinking 15.4 units a week. But both these amounts may have been an underestimate (BLRA, 1996). The proportion of men drinking more than recommended levels has remained fairly constant at 27% since 1984. In contrast, the proportion of women drinking at such levels had risen steadily from 9% to 14% over the same period (ONS, 1998).

Alcohol advertising and promotion is frequently directed at women and young people, with images of women who drink as glamorous and successful. Attempts to raise concern among teenagers about alcohol misuse are difficult when advertising equates adult success and

Table 3.2 Number of units of alcohol in common drinks

Drink	No. of units
A pint of ordinary strength lager (Heineken, Carling Black Label, Fosters)	2
A pint of strong lager (Stella Artois, Kronenbourg 1664)	3
A pint of bitter (John Smith's, Boddingtons)	2
A pint of ordinary strength cider (Dry Blackthorn, Strongbow)	2
A 175 ml glass of red or white wine	Approx. 2
A pub measure of spirits	1
An alcopop (e.g. Smirnoff Ice, Bacardi Breezer, WKD)	Approx. 1.5

attractiveness with drinking. In reality, women often drink excessively because they are lonely, unhappy, stressed and lack confidence and support. Recent research has shown that women at the top of their profession are more likely to have a drink problem than their male colleagues. The stress of competing in a male-dominated environment is blamed for driving one in seven high-flying females to alcohol (Eaton, 2004).

According to Alcohol Concern, the executive or professional full-time employee, without dependent children, in her mid-20s or early 30s, is probably most at risk. Also at risk are single women under 25. Women in professional households are almost twice as likely to exceed recommended limits than those in semi-skilled or unskilled households. This appears to be the reverse of trends seen in smoking, where the least well-off women in unskilled manual jobs make up the highest rate of smokers.

Current concern about drinking trends is centred on young adults who are the heaviest drinking section of the population and have the highest rate for signs of dependence on alcohol. Research shows that:

◆ Almost a fifth of 16- to 24-year-old women drink above the recommended limits (ONS, 1998)

◆ Average alcohol consumption among 11- to 15-year-olds in England more than doubled in the 1990s (Goddard, 1997)

◆ Nearly 12% of young men and 7% of young women (16–19 years) showed signs of alcohol dependence (Melzer *et al.*, 1995).

Young people are heavily influenced by their parents' attitude and use of alcohol. In a multiracial study of 9- to 15-year-olds, African-Caribbean and white children were most likely to have tried alcohol (71% and 65% respectively). Only 19% of Asian children were reported to have done so. For a significant proportion of 15- to 16-year-olds, drinking is an established habit rather than an occasional treat (HEA, 1991).

The impact of 'alcopops' is still being assessed. Alcohol Concern says that teenagers describe alcopops as 'trendy, fresh-tasting and suitable for girls'. In contrast, beer is a 'drink for the lads' (HEA, 1997). But anecdotal evidence suggests that alcopops may not be as popular as originally anticipated: they do not project a 'mature' image. Alcohol content is around 5% – stronger than normal-strength beers.

Where do women seek help?

Social taboos still make it generally unacceptable for women to drink heavily, especially those with children. Thus, women at risk are more inclined to consult people not specifically associated with alcohol abuse. GPs and primary care nurses are readily accessible: there is no stigma attached to consulting them. They can reach many women with alcohol problems who might otherwise be neglected.

Young people may not use primary care services or see themselves at risk, are more difficult to reach and may regard any discussion about their drinking habits as none of your business. Health promotion opportunities can therefore be difficult to create. Building an atmosphere of trust and confidentiality during any consultation may allow you to introduce drinking into the discussion.

Why do women drink?

Women drink alcohol for many reasons, including:

◆ To socialize

◆ To boost confidence

◆ To relax and to promote sleep

- ◆ To cope with work, domestic and financial pressure
- ◆ To 'treat' sexual problems
- ◆ To relieve stress, boredom and loneliness
- ◆ To help cope with major life events (e.g. bereavement, job loss, abuse)
- ◆ To switch off.

Anxiety, depression, shame, guilt, grief can all trigger and be exacerbated by drinking. Depression in women may be more marked premenstrually, postnatally and at the menopause. Drink can cause a vicious circle in which depression triggers drinking, which in turn results in low self-esteem and lack of confidence which, in turn, aggravates depression.

Women play a central role in the family, often putting others' needs before their own. Women in general, and problem drinkers in particular, often feel guilty about taking time for themselves and may perceive themselves to be 'bad mothers' or 'bad partners'. They need to learn how to meet their own needs (Plant, 1993). Another potential problem – 'the empty nest syndrome' – may develop when children leave home, and can be a trigger in increasing alcohol intake.

Less well known is the susceptibility of lesbian women: a third are reported to have alcohol problems. Lesbians are between three and five times more likely to have a drink problem than heterosexuals. Most at risk are isolated adolescents in conflict with their sexuality. They may use alcohol as a means of escaping their feelings about being different. Alcohol and drugs are an integral part of gay culture.

Problems identified by lesbians include attitudes of health care workers who 'assume everyone is heterosexual' and lack understanding about the effects of homophobia. Other problem areas include mental health, substance misuse and sexual health (Lesbian Information Service, 1998). Women with a history of sexual, physical or emotional abuse, or of problem drinkers in the family, are also at increased risk.

Women and the effects of alcohol

Women are more vulnerable to the effects of alcohol than men as they have a higher proportion of fat to water. This results in higher blood alcohol concentrations after drinking the same quantity of alcohol. Drinking the same amount of alcohol at different phases of the menstrual cycle is reported to produce varying blood alcohol levels. The peak is said to occur during ovulation and premenstrually. Oral contraception slows down metabolism of alcohol, meaning that it takes longer for blood alcohol levels to revert to zero. (Alcohol is normally metabolized at the rate of a unit per hour.) Alcohol is a central nervous system depressant and potentiates the action of sedative drugs. The combination of alcohol with tranquillizers, antidepressants, 'recreational drugs' and narcotics is potentially dangerous and sometimes lethal. Prolonged heavy use of alcohol causes increased metabolism of some drugs, including antiepileptics, hypoglycaemic agents and metronidazole.

Fatty deposits in the liver from heavy alcohol exposure will resolve if drinking stops and the liver is given a rest. Prolonged heavy drinking leads to scarring and cirrhosis and possibly to cancer. Women, on average, develop cirrhosis within 13 years, 9 years earlier than men (Plant, 1993). A government report in 2001 suggested that 'cirrhosis of the liver kills more women now than cervical cancer' (DoH, 2001).

Alcohol, sex and contraception

Drink-related sexual problems are associated with loss of libido, dyspareunia and vaginismus. Affected women may resort to alcohol to 'treat' themselves, reinforcing the popular myth that it enhances sexual pleasure. They may even perceive it to be an aphrodisiac, perhaps because of its disinhibiting effect. But as Shakespeare observed: 'It provokes the desire, but takes away the performance'. It is not only performance that may be lost: the relaxing effect of alcohol discourages effective contraception. Alcohol Concern (2000) stated 1 in 6 women (16%) admit to having unsafe sex after drinking too much. Hird (2003) suggests this percentage is higher – even as high as 41%. These findings are alarming, given the current climate in which we live, where HIV and sexually transmitted infections are on the increase.

Alcohol and the menstrual cycle

Women who drink heavily are susceptible to menstrual disturbances and reduced fertility, whilst heavy-drinking men may experience temporary impotence after a drinking binge. Five units a day can reduce sperm counts.

PMS is more common in women with alcohol-related problems. Many sufferers are reported to 'self-medicate' with alcohol in the hope of relieving symptoms. Alcohol can trigger hot flushes at the menopause, and heavy consumption is a risk factor for osteoporosis, especially in smokers. Excess drinking puts women at increased risk of falls and fractures.

Alcohol and pregnancy

Alcohol freely crosses the placenta, so the concentration of alcohol in the developing baby will be the same as that in the mother. A baby's liver is less efficient at eliminating alcohol.

The UK Department of Health and the Royal Society of Obstetricians and Gynaecologists say there is no ill effect of light alcohol consumption – that is 10 g of alcohol a day – on the fetus. The UK government guidelines suggest that consumption should be limited to one or two units (8 g) once or twice a week. Women who are trying to conceive are advised to follow the same guidelines (in addition to reducing caffeine and smoking), to improve fertility. In practice it is not always possible to give preconception advice, as so many pregnancies are unplanned, leaving women unaware that they are pregnant until several weeks after conception. Thus, all sexually active women should be aware that alcohol consumption may:

◆ Increase the risk of spontaneous abortion

◆ Retard intrauterine growth

◆ Cause damage to the developing fetus ranging from minor problems to full-blown fetal alcohol syndrome.

Breastfed babies may also be affected by alcohol passing into the breast milk in small quantities, disturbing their feeding, sleeping and bowel habits. Breastfeeding mothers should follow the same advice as given in pregnancy.

Alcohol and breast cancer

Recent research has focused on a possible relationship between moderate alcohol consumption and development of breast cancer. The National Cancer Institute study in 1998 illustrated a decrease of risk of breast cancer up to a limit of 14 units a week, but a sharp increase of risk at above 30 g of alcohol intake a day (that is just under four units or three glasses of wine daily). So if government guidelines are adhered to it is believed that women are at no increased risk by drinking sensibly (Smith-Warner *et al.*, 1998).

Sensible drinking

The Department of Health's *Sensible Drinking* report (1995) recognizes the variability in individual responses to alcohol; and suggests a daily benchmark of between two and three units for women and between three and four units for men. Consistently drinking more carries an increasing health risk. The report says that one or two units a day can provide some protection against coronary heart disease in postmenopausal women and men aged 40 and over. This effect may be negated by other predisposing factors such as smoking. The beneficial effect of alcohol lasts for 24 hours, hence the message is to drink moderately and regularly.

It is important to emphasize the risks of intoxication and binge drinking, to which young people are especially vulnerable. You may need to explain the importance of avoiding alcohol for 48 hours after heavy drinking to allow the body time to recover.

How can you help?

Nurses are often thought of as more approachable and as having more time than doctors. But what about the nurses themselves? Many feel they lack the skills to handle the complex underlying causes of alcohol problems, particularly if they drink heavily themselves. Before helping others, they may need to address their personal situation.

Developing counselling skills helps to build up confidence and expertise to raise the subject, encouraging clients to discuss their drinking habits in an open and honest way. Many local alcohol services or health promotion units now offer training/education sessions in alcohol awareness.

A client may present with anxiety, depression, panic attacks, general malaise or an injury, and may not recognize or admit that her problem is alcohol-related. Regular visits to the surgery with such problems may indicate a serious underlying problem she has not yet voiced.

Taking a drink history

Asking about alcohol consumption in a routine health check can encourage discussion without causing offence. Questions must be open and non-judgemental. A client may ask if she is drinking too much. An effective response may be to ask how drink is affecting her life (Box 3.6). Keeping a drink diary for a week or two may help her to establish if she is at risk. A diary can also pinpoint situations when she feels vulnerable and in need of a drink. Emphasize that if the diary is to be useful, it must be a true record. Tell your client that she does not have to show it to anyone unless she wishes, which should encourage honesty.

Check that she understands about units of alcohol and the different strengths of alcoholic drink. A pub measure of spirits in England and Wales (25 ml) contains one unit; a drink poured at home may contain much more. She may not know, for example, that extra-strong lager contains almost three times as much alcohol as ordinary lager. A 440 ml can of extra-strong lager contains four units (see Table 3.2). For more information on this and how to record a drink diary see *Say When ... How Much is Too Much* (HEA and Alcohol Concern, 1997).

Avoid pressurizing your client to stop drinking: women who drink heavily use alcohol as a coping mechanism. Physically dependent drinkers should not stop suddenly or without medical supervision.

Use the initial assessment to find out what your client wants to do. You can help her to explore her options: to continue drinking at current levels, to cut down (Box 3.7) or to stop. Many women can cut down successfully, but a dependent heavy drinker may need to stop completely, recognizing that abstinence is her only hope. Acceptance that alcohol is – or could be – a problem marks a major step forward.

Box 3.6   Warning signs of harmful drinking

- Needing alcohol close at hand
- Making drink the number one priority
- Drinking faster than others in social situations
- Needing to increase the amount or type of drink to maintain the effect, i.e. developing a tolerance to alcohol
- Feeling angry/irritated when others talk about your drinking habits
- Feeling tired/lethargic, sick
- Hangovers, 'the shakes' or sweats
- Sleep problems
- Disruption of relationships and friendships
- Drink-related accidents or injuries
- Difficulty maintaining normal routine at home and work.

Some problem drinkers may show only one of these signs; others may show several.

Box 3.7   The following tips may be useful when discussing how to moderate alcohol consumption with a client

- Set yourself a limit for the day/week/or a special occasion, e.g. a party
- Enjoy the taste. Make it last. Take smaller sips and put the glass down in between
- Avoid rounds. Do not feel obliged to keep up with other people
- Dilute spirits with low-calorie mixers to make a long drink
- Pace your drinks with non-alcoholic 'spacers'
- Eat a meal before or while drinking
- Avoid cocktails and 'strong' lagers. They contain several units of alcohol
- Find other ways to relax and unwind. Take a walk, have a long bath, try a new hobby or evening class and make friends outside your drinking circle
- Give yourself a treat with the money you have saved.

Your client may need further information, referral to a GP or specialist alcohol service, and support from a social worker or health visitor. Encourage her to play an active role in planning her own recovery.

Stress

Stress has been defined in a variety of ways and means different things to different people and is a normal part of everyday life. However, it is important to remember that 'stress' is almost always assumed to be negative and harmful. Whilst there is little doubt that stress (however defined) can have quite devastating effects on individuals, it can also be seen in a positive light in some circumstances. Short-term stress can have a constructive effect, making us take stock of difficult situations, or alerting us to potential threats or hazards. In contrast, long-term, unresolved stress is potentially destructive.

Long-term stress in modern life can result in a state of over-alertness and prolonged anxiety, which prevents the body from winding down. Coping with a job or unemployment while trying to bring up a family can cause prolonged stress. The breakdown of the traditional extended family has compounded stress in family life by leaving many women unsupported. Doctors estimate that emotional stress plays an important role in more than half of all medical problems, e.g. ulcers, hypertension and heart disease. If people learn new ways of coping, these can remain with them for the rest of their lives.

Stress in women is variable. A source of stimulus for one person may reduce another to a state of nervous exhaustion. Stress in women may be caused by many factors including:

◆ Raising a family – young children, teenagers, lone parenting, a low income, poor housing
◆ Employment/unemployment problems
◆ Ill health
◆ Caring for an elderly or sick relative
◆ Racism
◆ Sexual discrimination and sexual orientation

◆ Living in a violent relationship
◆ Bereavement

Many of the chapters in this book deal with potentially stressful issues, such as infertility, pregnancy, abortion, abnormal smears, PMS, rape and urinary incontinence. Stress associated with issues like these may be exacerbated by lack of information and understanding and by fixed, inaccurate ideas of the 'my mother told me' variety.

Counselling skills can help you to help clients. However, it is important to recognize your limitations and be able to refer those who may need more specialist counselling.

Dealing with stress

The harmful effects of stress do not depend exclusively on the characteristics of stressful events. Sarafino (1998) describes coping as the process by which people try to manage the perceived discrepancy between the demands placed on them and the resources available to deal with a stressful situation. Being aware of what causes stress, how a person reacts and how much they can cope with, can help them to take control. Accepting that no one is perfect and an ability to see the funny side of things may help to defuse stressful situations.

Relaxation techniques can be effective, easy to teach, and used in many different situations: alone or in groups; or with an audio cassette. A simple routine that you can recommend is outlined in Box 3.8.

Nurses under stress
Nurses themselves are not immune from stress and may need support. Cooper and Baglioni (1988)

Box 3.8 A simple relaxation routine

◆ Sit right back in a chair and uncross your legs. Rest your hands in your lap
◆ Put your feet flat on the floor
◆ Close your eyes and breathe easily and normally
◆ Tense and relax the main groups of muscles starting with the toes and ending with the face. Notice the difference in the sensations
◆ When you feel ready, open your eyes. You should feel renewed and refreshed.

found nursing to be one of the most stressful jobs in a review of more than 100 occupations. Personal problems may be intensified by professional ones in a health service that is increasingly beset by pressure to reach targets, lack of resources, low pay and increased public expectation. There is little research about why nurses smoke, drink and use other drugs to alleviate stress in their professional or personal lives. This seems ironic in a profession dedicated to health care. An article in the *Nursing Times*, 'Nursing makes you sick' (Wing, 1999), suggests that a culture of absenteeism pervades the NHS. With nurses facing huge workloads and low morale, the article concludes that this is hardly surprising.

The Nuffield Trust report (Williams *et al.*, 1998) *Improving the Health of the NHS Workforce* highlighted the cost of stress-related sickness, estimating that a 1% reduction in sickness absenteeism rates would save £140 million a year. Failure to deal with stress-induced problems is identified as a cause of rapid staff turnover, which can impact on nursing standards.

Effective clinical supervision allows nurses to examine their practice in a safe, supportive environment. Encouraging staff to share experiences may help them to develop insight into their own difficulties, resolve problems and find ways of coping with work pressures. Reflective practice and self-assessment are a means of identifying areas needing further development. These processes reinforce strengths, and build up confidence, self-esteem and a sense of professional identity. Empowerment may have an insulating effect against stress.

The RCN Counselling Service offers free counselling to members for personal or work-related issues and there are some excellent books dealing with stress management and staff support for health professionals (see Resources).

Conclusion

Nurses, midwives and health visitors play a key role in health promotion by encouraging women to take care of themselves and their families. Try to empower your client to make her own decisions about health and lifestyle, but respect her final decision – even if it runs contrary to your own view. Her upbringing, culture, and values, and social and financial circumstances will influence what she does.

It is beyond the scope of this chapter to present a fully comprehensive view of health promotion, but we hope it will stimulate further exploration and learning and give you ideas for your own clinical practice and local needs.

Ideas for personal and professional development

- Investigate smoking cessation services and courses and visit any local services. What are the opening times? Is an appointment needed or are they 'drop in' sessions? Can patients self-refer?
- Investigate alcohol services and visit any local services. Ask the above questions
- Investigate drug abuse services and visit any local services. Ask the above questions
- Compile a resource directory of all the services including alternative therapists and charges. Include opening times, addresses, telephone numbers, websites, etc., for clients and other health professionals to use
- Design a poster for the waiting area encouraging women to ask for help if they have any of the above problems.

Patient education points

Clients should be aware of:

- The importance of a healthy diet
- Implications on health caused by smoking and the benefits to be gained by giving up smoking
- Implications on health caused by drug and alcohol abuse
- Preconceptual information if considering pregnancy.

Resources

Health promotion

Department of Health (DoH)
Richmond House, 79 Whitehall,
London SW1A 2NS
Tel: 020 7210 4850 (enquiry desk)
www.doh.gov.uk

FPA Direct
PO Box 1078, East Oxford DO,
Oxon OX4 5JE
Tel: 01865 719413 Fax: 01865 748746
www.fpa.org.uk
Family Planning Association bookshop
and mail order service.

Health Development Agency
Holborn Gate, 220 High Holborn,
London WC1V 7BA
Tel: 020 7430 0850
For publications
PO Box 90, Wetherby, Yorkshire,
LS23 7EX
Tel: 0870 121 4194
www.hda.nhs.uk
www.hda-online.org.uk

Health Education Board for Scotland
Woodburn House, Canaan Lane,
Edinburgh EH10 4SG
Tel: 0131 536 5500
www.hebs.scot.nhs.uk

**Health Promotion Agency for
Northern Ireland**
18 Ormeau Avenue, Belfast BT2 8HF
Tel: 01232 311611
www.healthpromotionagency.org.uk

Health Promotion England
50 Eastbourne Terrace, London W2 3QR
Tel: 020 7725 2880 Fax: 020 7725 2881
www.hpe.org.uk

Health Promotion Wales
Ffynnonlas, Tyglas Avenue, Llanishen,
Cardiff CF14 5EZ
Tel: 01222 752222
www.hbw.wales.gov.uk

NHS Careers
PO Box 376, Bristol BS99 3EY
Tel: 0845 6060655 Fax: 0117 921 9562
www.nhs.uk/careers
Provides information and advice on continuing
professional education.

Wired for Health
www.wiredforhealth.gov.uk
Addresses all aspects of health for young
people.

Women's Health
52 Featherstone Street, London EC1Y 8RT
Tel: 020 7251 6580
www.womenshealthlondon.org.uk
Provides a wide range of information and
leaflets. Send a stamped addressed envelope
for a publications list.

Preconception, early pregnancy care and nutrition

GIG – Genetic Interest Group
Unit 4D, Leroy House, 436 Essex Road,
London N1 3QP
Helpline: 020 7704 3141
www.gig.org.uk
A resource for families and health professionals.
Information on regional genetics centres and
self-help groups.

Maternity Alliance
45 Beech Street, London EC2P 2LZ
Tel: 020 7588 8583; 020 7588 8582 (24-hour
information line)
Publishes books, reports and leaflets for
parents-to-be and professionals on
preconception advice, pregnancy and
the first year of life.

WellBeing
27 Sussex Place, Regent's Park, London NW1 4SP
Tel: 020 7262 5337 Fax: 020 7724 7725
www.wellbeing.org.uk
Sainsbury's/WellBeing eating for pregnancy
helpline: 0114 242 4084
A health research charity for women
and babies.

www.foodstandards.gov.uk

www.nutrition.org.uk

www.diabetes.org.uk

Health and physical activity

Active for Life Campaign
www.active.org.uk
www.Nrgize.co.uk (aimed at 11- to
 15-year-olds).

British Heart Foundation
14 Fitzhardinge Street, London
 W1H 4DH
Tel: 020 7935 0185
www.bhf.org.uk
Advice from the Medical Information
 Department. Video and publications list
 available.

Women and drugs

ADFAM National
Waterbridge House, 32–36 Loman Street,
 London SE1 0EE
Tel: 020 7928 8898
Helpline: 02079288900 (Monday–Friday
 10 am–5 pm)
A resource for families and friends of
 drug users.

Blenheim Project – 'Changing Gear'
Tel: 020 8960 5599
For women using drugs.

**Council for Involuntary Tranquilliser
 Addiction (CITA)**
Cavendish House, Brighton Road, Waterloo,
 Liverpool L22 5NG
Tel: 0151 474 9626 Helpline: 0151 949 0102
www.liv.ac.uk/~csunit/community/cita.htm
Provides support for people withdrawing from
 tranquillizers.

Drugs in School
Helpline: 0808 8000 800 (office hours).

DrugScope
Waterbridge House, 32–36 Loman Street,
 London SE1 0EE
Tel: 020 7928 1211
www.drugscope.org.uk

The UK's leading centre of expertise on drugs.
 DrugScope conducts research, gives advice on
 policy and practice and all aspects of drug
 use. It is the national coordinating body for
 drug agencies and organizations.

**MIND (The National Association for
 Mental Health)**
Granta House, 15–19 Broadway, London E15 4BQ
Tel: 020 8519 2122
Information line: 020 8522 1728
www.mind.org.uk

National Drugs Helpline
Tel: 0800 776600
For 24-hour advice, counselling and
 information about local agencies. Advice
 in other languages is available on request.

Northern Ireland Council for Voluntary Action
127 Ormeau Road, Belfast BT7 1SH
Tel: 01232 321224
www.nicva.org

Release
Tel: 020 7729 9904
A national advice line offering drug and legal
 advice and support from 10 am to 6 pm
 Monday to Friday.
Emergency 24-hour helpline: 020 7603 8654.

Scottish Drugs Forum
Shaftsbury House, 5 Waterloo Street,
 Glasgow G2 6AY
Tel: 0141 221 1175
www.sdf.org.uk

UK Psychiatric Group
Tel: 020 7919 2999
Based at the Maudsley Hospital. Helpline for
 the public, staffed by pharmacists, for queries
 on drugs.

Welsh Drugs and Alcohol Unit
4th Floor, St Davids House, Wood Street,
 Cardiff CF10 1ER
Tel: 02920 667766.

Women and smoking

Action on Smoking and Health (ASH)
102 Clifton Street, London EC2A 4HW

Tel: 020 7739 5902
www.ash.org.uk

QUIT
Victory House, 170 Tottenham Court Road,
    London W1P 0HA
Quitline: 0800 002200
Tel: 020 7251 1551
www.quit.org.uk
E-mail counselling: stopsmoking@quit.org.uk

NHS Smoking Helpline and Tobacco
    Information Campaign
Tel: 0800 169 0169
www.givingupsmoking.co.uk

Quitline and Pregnancy Quitline
Tel: 0800 00 22 00
Offers advice, support and a Quitpack to
    smokers trying to stop. Also Asian
    languages helpline.

Alternative therapies
British Acupuncture Council
34 Alderney Street, London
    SW1V 4EU
Tel: 020 8964 0222

British Hypnotherapy Association
1 Wythburn Place, London, W1H 5WL
Tel: 020 7723 4443.

Women and alcohol

Al-Anon Family Groups and UK and
    Eire (AFG) and Alateen
61 Great Dover Street,
    London SE1 4YF
Tel: 020 7403 0888
www.hexnet.co.uk/alanon
Supports families and friends of
    problem drinkers.

Alcohol Concern
Waterbridge House, 32–36 Loman Street,
    London SE1 0EE
Tel: 020 7928 7377
Drinkline: 0800 917 8282
www.alcoholconcern.org.uk
Publishes research (including regular
    bulletins) and provides information

and resources for professionals and
    the public.

Alcohol in Moderation
PO Box 2282, Bath BA1 2QY
Tel: 01225 471444
www.drinkingandyou.com

Alcohol Recovery Programme
Women's Alcohol Centre, 66a Drayton Park,
    London N5 1ND
Tel: 020 7226 4581
Free counselling. Black and lesbian counsellors
    available. Child care, day and residential care
    available.

Aquarius Action Project
6th Floor, 111 New Street,
    Birmingham B2 4EU
Tel: 0121 6324727
Offers information and advice to women living
    in the Midlands, with or affected by alcohol
    problems.

Lesbian and Alcohol Project
PO Box 9, Todmorton, Lancashire OL14 5TZ
Tel: 01706 817235.

Northern Ireland Community Alcohol
    Service
Tel: 01232 66 44 34.

Scottish Council on Alcohol
Tel: 0141 333 9677.

Stress

National Association for Staff
    Support (NASS)
9 Caradon Close, Woking,
    Surrey GU21 3DU
Tel: 01483 771599
http://ourworld.compuserve.com/
    homepages/nassupport
A charitable association providing a network
    and resource service to help professionals
    promote good staff support practices.

Personal support for nurses
Nurseline
Tel: 020 8681 4030 Email: nurseline@rcn.org.uk

An independent, confidential advice and information service for *all* nurses, midwives and health visitors, including students and retired nurses. Provides support and advice on personal matters, careers, housing and finance.

RCN Counselling Service

20 Cavendish Square, London W1G 0RN
Tel: 020 7647 3464 RCN Members' Line:
08457 697064
E-mail: counselling@rcn.org.uk
Free confidential counselling, either by phone or at RCN offices throughout the UK. The service is a member of the British Association for Counselling and Psychotherapy (BACP).

RCN Work-Injured Nurses Group (WING)

Tel: 020 8649 9536 E-mail: WING@rcn.org.uk
Offers help to members with work-related injury, mental or physical illness or disabilities.

Further reading

ALCOHOL CONCERN (2001) 'Women and Alcohol the Facts': A pilot evaluation of a self-help resource. London: Alcohol Concern.

ARMSTRONG, P. (1992) *Back to Life*. The Print Organization. Available from CITA (see Resources).

BRYANT-JEFFERIES, R. (2003). *Counselling a Recovering Drug User*. Oxford: Radcliffe Medical Press.

CHAMBERS, R., HAWKSLEY, B. and TEERANLALL, R. (1999) *Survival Skills for Nurses*. Oxford: Radcliffe Medical Press.

CHAMBERS, R., SCHWARTZ, A. and BOATH, E. *Beating Stress in the NHS*. Oxford: Radcliffe Medical Press.

DoH (1999) *Smoking: Don't Give Up Giving Up*. London: The Stationery Office. Campaign pack for health professionals. NHS Smoking Helpline 0800 169 0169, or Smoking Pregnancy Helpline 0800 169 9169; website: www.giving-upsmoking.co.uk.

DoH (2003) NHS: The Pregnancy book. Your complete guide to a healthy pregnancy.

HARDMAN, A. and STENSEL, D. (2003) *Physical Activity and Health: The Evidence Explained*. London and New York: Routledge.

HEA (1996) *Promoting Physical Activity in Primary Health Care: Guidance for the Primary Health Care Team*. London: HEA.

HEA (1999) *Physical Activity and Inequalities*. A briefing paper. London: HEA.

HEA (2000) *Helping Smokers Stop: A New Approach for Health Professionals*. London: HEA.

McDONALD, M. (1994) *Gender, Drink and Drugs*. Oxford: Berg.

MIND (1998) *Making Sense of Treatments and Drugs: Minor Tranquillizers, 1998*. London. Available from MIND (see Resources).

NAIDOO, J. and WILLS, J. (2000) *Health Promotion, Foundations for Practice*. London: Baillière Tindall.

OGDEN, J. (2002) *Health Psychology*. Open University Press.

PRIME MINISTER'S STRATEGY UNIT (2004) *Alcohol Harm Reduction Strategy For England*. www.strategy.gov.uk.

SCAPE (Smoking Cessation Action in Primary Care) (2002) Smoking cessation consultations – simple solutions for general practice.

SHAIKH, Z. and NAZ, F. (2000) *A Cultural Cocktail. Asian Women and Alcohol Misuse*. London: Alcohol Concern.

STOTTER, D.J. (1997) *Staff Support in Health Care*. Bodmin: Blackwell Science.

THOM, B. (1997) *Women and Alcohol: Issues for Prevention*. London: HEA.

TREVELYAN, J. and BOOTH, B. (1994) *Complementary Medicines for Nurses, Midwives and Health Visitors*. London: Macmillan.

WELLS, R. with TSCHUDIN, V. (eds) (1994) *Wells' Supportive Therapies in Health Care*. London: Baillière Tindall.

References

AGGLETON, P. and HOMANS, H. (1987) *Educating About AIDS*. NHS Training Authority.

ALCOHOL CONCERN (2000) Women and alcohol – a cause for concern? Autumn, No. 27, pp. 1–7.

BARKER, J.P. (1993) Fetal nutrition and cardiovascular disease in adult life. *Lancet* 341:938–41.

BELLOW, B. and RAMSAY, I. (1991) *Towards a Smoke Free Generation*. London: HEA and DoH.

BLACKBURN, C. and GRAHAM, H. (1994) Smoking among Working Class Mothers: Information Pack. Department of Applied Social Science, University of Warwick.

BLAIR, P.S., FLEMING, P.J., BENSLEY, D. et al. (1996) Smoking and sudden death syndrome: Results from 1993–95. Case study for confidential inquiry into stillbirth and deaths in infancy. *British Medical Journal* 313:195–8.

CALLUM, C. (1998) *The Smoking Epidemic*. London: HEA.

CATELLSAGUE, X., BOSCH F.X., and MUNOZ, N. (2001) Environmental co-factors in HPV carcinogenesis. *Virus Research* 89:191–9.

COOPER, C.L. and BAGLIONI, A.J. (1988) A structural model approach toward the development of a theory of the link between stress and mental health. *British Journal of Medical Psychology* 61:87–102.

COPAS, J. and SHI, J. (2000) Reanalysis of epidemiological evidence on lung cancer and passive smoking. *British Medical Journal* 320:417–18.

COVEY, L.S., SULLIVAN, M.A., JOHNSTON, J.A. et al. (2000) Advances in non-nicotine pharmacotherapy for smoking cessation. *Drugs* 59:17–31.

DA COSTA. D, RIPPEN, N. et al. (2003) Self-reported leisure-time physical activity during pregnancy and relationship to psychological well-being. *Journal of Psychosomatic Obstetrics & Gynaecology* 24(2):111–19.

DoH (Department of Health) (1992a) *Folic Acid and the Prevention of Neural Tube Defects. Report from an Expert Advisory Group*. London: The Stationery Office.

DoH (1992b) *The Health of the Nation. A Strategy for Health*. London: The Stationery Office.

DoH (1995) *Sensible Drinking. Report of an Interdepartmental Working Group*. London: The Stationery Office.

DoH (1997a) *The New NHS: Modern, Dependable.* London: The Stationery Office.

DoH (1997b) *While You Are Pregnant: Safe Eating and How to Avoid Infection from Food and Animals.* London: The Stationery Office.

DoH (1998a) *The Foods Standards Agency: A Force for Change.* London: The Stationery Office.

DoH (1998b) *Smoking Kills: A White Paper on Tobacco.* London: The Stationery Office.

DoH (1998c) *Tackling Drugs to Build a Better Britain: The Government's Ten-Year Strategy for Tackling Drug Misuse.* London: The Stationery Office.

DoH (1998d) *Report on Health and Social Subjects No 49: Nutrition and Bone Health.* London: The Stationery Office.

DoH (1999a) *Saving Lives: Our Healthier Nation.* London: The Stationery Office.

DoH (1999b) *Statistical Bulletin: Statistics from the Regional Drug Misuse Databases for Six Months Ending March 1998.* London: The Stationery Office.

DoH (1999c) *Drug Misuse and Dependence. Guidelines on Clinical Management.* London: The Stationery Office.

DoH (1999d) *Smoking: Don't Give Up Giving Up.* London: The Stationery Office.

DoH (2000a) *Report of the National Diet and Nutrition Survey,* Vol 1. London: The Stationery Office.

DoH (2000b) *NHS Plan: A Plan for Investment. A Plan for Reform.* London: The Stationery Office.

DoH (2001) *Annual Report of the Chief Medical Officer.* London: The Stationery Office.

DoH (2002a) *Annual Report of the Chief Medical Officer. Check On the State of the Public Health.* London: The Stationery Office.

DoH (2002b) *Statistics on Smoking. Cessation Services in England, April 2001 to March 2002,* London: DoH.

DoH (2004) *The Alcohol Harm Reduction Strategy for England,* London: DoH.

DOLL, R., PETO, R., WHEATLEY, K., GRAY, R. and SUTHERLAND, I. (1994) Mortality in relation to smoking: 40 years observations on male British doctors. *British Medical Journal* **309**:901–11.

DOYLE, W. (1994) *Teach Yourself Healthy Eating.* London: Hodder and Stoughton.

EATON, L. (2003) United Kingdom finally bans tobacco advertising. *British Medical Journal* **326**:351.

EATON, L. (2004) UK government announces plan to tackle alcohol. *British Medical Journal* **328**:659.

ERNEST, V. (1985) Mixed messages for women: a social history of cigarette smoking and advertising. *New York State Journal of Medicine* July:335–40.

EWLES, L. and SIMNETT, I. (1992) *Promoting Health. A Practical Guide.* London: Scutari Press.

EWLES, L. and SIMNETT, I. (1999) *Promoting Health. A Practical Guide.* London: Baillière Tindall.

GODDARD, E. (1997) *Young Teenagers and Alcohol in 1996; vol 1 England.* London: The Stationery Office.

GOSSOP, M. (1993) *Living With Drugs,* 3rd edn. Aldershot: Ashgate.

GRAHAM, H. (1993) *When Life's a Drag: Women, Smoking and Disadvantage.* London: HMSO.

GUILLEBAUD, J. (1999) *Contraception: Your Questions Answered,* 3rd edn. Edinburgh: Churchill Livingstone.

HANSBRO, J. (1997) *Health in England 1996.* London: The Stationery Office.

HEA (Health Education Authority) (1991) *Factfile: Young People and Drink. Drinkwise Campaign.* London: HEA.

HEA (1992) *Stopping Smoking Made Easier.* London: HEA.

HEA (1995) *Tracking Teenage Smoking, track 7.* Carried out by MORI for the HEA. London: HEA.

HEA (1996a) *Active for Life Campaign.* London: HEA.

HEA (1996b) *The Balance of Good Health: Information for Educators and Communicators.* London: HEA.

HEA (1997) *Young People and Alcohol: A Survey of Attitudes and Behaviour Towards New Types of Alcoholic Drinks in England.* London: HEA.

HEA (1998a) *Effectiveness of Interventions to Promote Healthy Eating in Pregnant Women and Women of Childbearing Age.* London: HEA.

HEA (1998b) *Stopping Smoking Made Easier.* London: HEA.

HEA and ALCOHOL CONCERN (1997) *Say When … How Much is Too Much?* London: HEA.

HIRD, L. (2003) Drink and be merry. *The Guardian,* 16 November, pp. 1–3.

HOPPER, J.L. and SEEMAN, E. (1994) The bone density of female twins discordant for tobacco use. *New England Journal of Medicine* Feb:387–92.

HUGHES, J.R. (1992) Tobacco withdrawal in self-quitters. *Journal of Consulting and Clinical Psychology* **60**:689–97.

HUGHES, J.R., GUST, S.W., SKOOG, K. *et al.* (1991) Symptoms of tobacco withdrawal: a replication and extension. *Archives of General Psychiatry* **48**:52–9.

ILLICH, I. (1977) *Limits to Medicine – Medical Nemesis: The Exploration of Health.* London: Pelican Books.

ISDD (Institute for the Study of Drug Dependence) (1999a) *Drug Abuse Briefing,* 7th edn. London: ISDD.

ISDD (1999b) *UK Drugs Situation: 1999.* London: ISDD.

JACOBSON, B. (1986) *Beating The Ladykillers: Women and Smoking.* London: Pluto Press.

JORENBY, D.E., LEISCHOW, S.J., NIDES, M.A. *et al.* (1999) A controlled trial of sustained-release bupropion, a nicotine patch, or both for smoking cessation. *New England Journal of Medicine* **340**:685–91.

KLONOFF-COHEN, H. *et al.* (2001) Effects of female and male smoking on success rates of IVF and gamete intra-fallopian transfer. *Human Reproduction* **16**:1382–90.

LESBIAN INFORMATION SERVICE (1998) *Lesbians and Alcohol Misuse: A Guide for Alcohol Workers.* London: LIS.

MELZER, H., GILL, B., PETTICREW, M. *et al.* (1995) *OPCS Surveys of Psychiatric Morbidity in Britain: the Prevalence of Psychiatric Morbidity Among Adults Living in Private Households.* London: The Stationery Office.

MOUNTENEY, J. (1999) *Drugs, Pregnancy and Childcare. A Guide for Professionals.* London: ISDD.

NAIDOO, J. and WILLS, J. (1998) *Practising Health Promotion: Dilemmas and Challenges.* London: Baillière Tindall.

NATIONAL INSTITUTE FOR CLINICAL EXCELLENCE (2002) Guidance on nicotine replacement therapy (NRT) and bupropion (technology appraisal 39). London: NICE.

OAKLEY, A. (1994) Who cares for health? Social relations, gender and the public health. *Journal of Epidemiological Community Health* **48**:427–34.

ONS (Office for National Statistics) (1997) *Smoking Among Secondary School Children in England in 1996.* London: The Stationery Office.

ONS (1998) *Living in Britain: Results from the 1996 General Household Survey.* London: The Stationery Office.

ONS (2000) *Living in Britain: Results from the 1998 General Household Survey.* London: The Stationery Office.

ONS (2002) *Living in Britain: 2001 Results from the General Household Survey.* London: The Stationery Office.

PARROTT, S., GODFREY, C., RAW, M. *et al.* (1998) Guidance for commissioners on the cost of smoking cessation interventions. *Thorax* **53**(Suppl 5, Part 1).

PHIPPS, W.R. *et al.* (1997) The association between smoking and female infertility as influenced by the cause of the infertility. *Fertility and Sterility* **48**:377–82.

PLANT, M. (1993) Drink problems. In McPherson, A. (ed.) *Women's Problems in General Practice.* Oxford: Oxford University Press.

POPPE. W.A. *et al.* (1995) Tobacco smoking impairs the local immunosurveillance in the uterine cervix. An immunohistochemical study. *Gynaecol. Obstet. Invest.* **39**:4–8.

POSWILLO, D. and ALBERMAN, E. (1992) *Effects of Smoking on the Fetus, Neonate, and Child.* Oxford: Oxford University Press.

PRIME MINISTER'S STRATEGY UNIT (2004) Alcohol Harm Reduction Strategy For England.

PRITCHARD, C.W. (1994) Depression and smoking in pregnancy in Scotland. *Journal of Epidemiological Community Health* **48**:377–82.

PROCHASKA, J.O. and DICLEMENTE, C.C. (1984) *The Transtheoretical Approach: Crossing Traditional Boundaries of Therapy.* Homewood, IL: Dow Jones-Irwin.

PROKOPCZYK, B. *et al.* (1997) Identification of tobacco-specific carcinogen in the cervical mucus of smokers and non-smokers. *Journal of the National Cancer Institute* **89**(12):868–73.

QUIT (1996) *Helping Smokers to Quit* (1994, updated 1996). London: QUIT.

RAW, M., McNEIL, A. and WEST, R. (1998) Smoking cessation guidelines for health professionals. A guide to effective smoking cessation interventions for the health care system. *Thorax* **53**(Suppl 5, Part 1).

REYNOLDS, P., HURLEY, S., GOLDBERG, D.E. *et al.* (2004) Active smoking, household passive smoking, and breast cancer: evidence from the California teachers study. *Journal of the National Cancer Institute* **96**(1):29–37.

ROYAL COLLEGE OF NURSING (2002) *Clearing the Air 2.* London: Royal College of Nursing.

ROYAL COLLEGE OF PHYSICIANS (1992) *Smoking and the Young.* London: Royal College of Physicians.

ROYAL COLLEGE OF PHYSICIANS (2000) *Nicotine Addiction In Britain.* London: Royal College of Physicians.

SARAFINO, E.P. (1998) *Health Psychology: Biopsychosocial Interactions.* New York: Widen.

SARAIYA, M. *et al.* (1998) Cigarette smoking as a risk factor for ectopic pregnancy. *American Journal of Obstetrics and Gynecology* **178**:493–8.

SCODA (Standing Conference on Drug Abuse) (1997) *Drug-using Parents: Policy Guidelines for Inter-Agency Working.* London: LDGF.

SMITH-WARNER, S.A., SPIEGELMAN, D., SHIAW-SHYUAN, Y. *et al.* (1998) Alcohol and breast cancer in women: a pool analysis of cohort studies. *Journal of the American Medical Association* **279**(7):535–40.

SZAREWSKI, A., JARVIS, M.J., SASIENI, P. *et al.* (1996) Effect of smoking cessation on cervical lesion size. *Lancet* **347**:941–3.

THOMAS B. (ed.) (2001) *Manual of Dietetic Practice*, 3rd edn. Oxford: Blackwell Science.

THOMAS, M., WALKER, A., WILMOT, A. *et al.* (1996) *Living in Britain: Results from the 1996 General Household Survey ONS.* London: The Stationery Office.

US DHHS (Department of Health and Human Services) (1990) *The Health Benefits of Smoking Cessation: A Report of the Surgeon General.* Atlanta: Public Health Service Centers for Disease Control.

US DHHS (2001) *Smoking and Women's Health. A Report of the Surgeon General.* Rockville: USDHHS.

WILLIAMS, S., MICHIE, S., PATTANI, S. *et al.* (1998) *The Nuffield Report: Improving the Health of the NHS Workforce.* London: Nuffield Trust.

WINDSOR, R.A. (2001) Smoking, cessation and pregnancy. In *WHO Women and Tobacco Epidemic: Challenges for the 21st Century.* WHO/NMH/TFI?01.1.

WING, M. (1999) Nursing makes you sick. *Nursing Times* **95**:24–5.

WORLD HEALTH ORGANIZATION (1946) *Constitution.* Geneva: WHO.

WORLD HEALTH ORGANIZATION (1984) Health promotion: a WHO discussion document on the concepts and principles. Reprinted in *Journal of the Institute of Health Education* **23**(1):1985.

YANG, X. *et al.* (1996) Malignant transformation of HPV-16 immortalised human endocervical cells by cigarette smoke condensate and characterisation of multistage carcinogenesis. *International Journal of Cancer* **65**:338–44.

4: Using Complementary Therapies to Aid Women's Sexual Health

Denise Tiran ◆

OBJECTIVES

This chapter should help you understand:

◆ The basic principles of a range of the most common complementary therapies used in Britain today ◆

◆ How aspects of complementary and alternative medicine can be used to enhance and improve women's sexual health ◆

◆ The limitations of your own professional role when advising women on aspects of complementary therapies. ◆

Introduction

Most women accept as normal the physiological changes which occur throughout their lives, but for those who find times such as menarche, pregnancy, the premenstrual and perimenopausal phases difficult, there is a whole range of strategies to help them cope. Some are highly technological, such as contemporary infertility treatments; some, whilst controversial, are considered almost routine, for example hormone treatment for the menopause; and others cover a wide variety of self-help treatments.

This self-management of health is facilitated by the plethora of natural remedies available in health food stores, but these are not necessarily universally acceptable, proven or safe. Whilst health professionals would encourage partnerships in care to empower women to achieve optimum health, consumers need to appreciate that self-administering natural remedies is not always wise. No complications should occur from sensible use of self-help strategies for minor health problems, but it is possible that herbal or other remedies may mask more serious problems, or indeed produce side effects or interfere with current pharmacological treatments.

If women with sexual health problems choose not to consult conventional health care professionals, they may seek advice from a practitioner of complementary medicine. However, for maternity care it is illegal for anyone, other than a midwife or doctor, or one in training, to be the sole provider of care, except in an emergency, and therefore any therapies used must be complementary rather than alternative to other care provided.

Complementary and integrative medicine

Complementary and integrative medicine (CIM) encompasses all those strategies or systems of diagnosis and treatment that currently fall outside the sphere of conventional health care (see Box 4.1). The term 'alternative' medicine continues to be applied when the therapies are used *instead* of orthodox care, but increasingly the therapies are being used to *complement* conventional care.

Box 4.1 Classification of complementary therapies

Professions supplementary to medicine
  Osteopathy
  Chiropractic

Therapies often practised by GPs and some nurses
  Homeopathy
  Acupuncture
  Herbal medicine

Therapies incorporated relatively easily into nursing, midwifery and health visiting practice
  Aromatherapy
  Massage
  Reflexology
  Hypnotherapy
  Shiatsu/acupressure

Additional therapies that can be used as self-help strategies by women
  Tai ch'i
  Yoga
  Bach flower remedies
  Alexander technique
  Relaxation techniques.

Indeed, the gradual *integration* of many of the commonly used therapies has more recently led to the coining of the phrase 'integrative medicine' (see Figure 4.1).

One in three people in Britain, two-thirds of them women, have used one or more forms of complementary therapy; and although NHS provision is increasing, people are prepared to spend considerable amounts of money accessing private CIM (Thomas *et al.*, 2001). Their main reasons for seeking complementary medicine appear to be a generalized dissatisfaction with the orthodox health care system and a desire for a more person-centred, holistic and empowering approach to care. There is, however, a misconceived belief that, because many therapies are

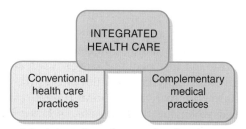

Figure 4.1 Integration of conventional and complementary therapies (Tiran, 1999).

natural, they must also be safe, but unfortunately this is not so. Also, people fear their doctor's disapproval and often fail to inform them of their use of CIM, which increases the risk of problems such as potentiation or inhibition of, or interaction with, conventional medical treatments (Crock *et al.*, 1999).

Professional accountability of nurses, midwives and health visitors in relation to complementary therapies

It is important to acknowledge the benefits *and* limitations of CIM in helping women to achieve optimum sexual health. Nurses and midwives should engender an open facilitative attitude about complementary therapies to avoid confrontation, implicitly giving 'permission' to ask questions so that patients can obtain sufficient detail to make informed choices within the boundaries of effectiveness and safety. The Nursing and Midwifery Council (NMC) stresses the right of individuals to self-administer alternatives or to consult practitioners outside the conventional system but suggests that they may require assistance to identify the most appropriate therapy or therapist (NMC, 2000a). As with conventional care it is essential that complementary therapies are based, where possible, on comprehensive contemporary evidence on safety and efficacy. NMC registrants wishing to advise on or utilize therapies must recognize their own personal professional boundaries. If they are in any doubt about a particular form of CIM or their own personal knowledge-base they must refrain from attempting to offer advice which may be incorrect, not so much through error, but rather through omission, and should seek guidance from a relevant expert (NMC, 2000b).

Just because many remedies are easily accessible to women in the high street, health professionals should not assume that they are automatically safe or that they have been quality tested, particularly essential oils, herbal remedies, Chinese herbs and homeopathy. Similarly, it is vital that nurses appreciate the widely varying standards of complementary practitioners, as a result of differing levels of education and subsequent experience.

Under English common law it is still possible for anyone to set up in practice with little or no training, although this situation is likely to change as a result of demands from Europe and from concerned health care professionals across the whole spectrum.

The NMC exists primarily to protect the public by statutorily regulating the work of its registrants, and can only issue directives related to CIM when applied to nursing, midwifery or health visiting practice. Individual practitioners are responsible for ensuring that, if they wish to use or advise on CIM, they are adequately and appropriately educated, fulfil their requirements for professional updating for both aspects of their practice and act always in a way to safeguard the interests of their patients and clients (NMC, 2000b). These issues are summarized in Box 4.2.

Nurses, midwives and health visitors may be in a position to advise on self-help remedies, or make suggestions regarding therapies to which women could refer themselves or, following appropriate training, may incorporate some of the therapies into their own work. It is therefore important to have an appreciation of how the commonly used therapies may help, but this chapter will not equip readers to utilize the therapies in their own practice without further reading and/or training.

The main complementary therapies in use in Britain today

There are over 200 therapies classified as 'non-conventional' but a core of approximately 20 therapies are commonly accepted, classified into two main groups (House of Lords, 2000). Group 1 includes osteopathy, chiropractic, acupuncture, homeopathy and herbal medicine, which are considered to be complete, discrete systems of health care with formalized, nationally regulated education programmes and an expanding research base. Group 2 is the 'supportive therapies' which complement other forms of care, have a less well regulated education system and limited research evidence. Supportive therapies are often practised by nurses and midwives and include massage, aromatherapy, reflexology, hypnotherapy, nutrition, yoga, stress management, Alexander

---

Box 4.2 Professional accountability issues for nurses, midwives and health visitors wishing to implement complementary therapies into their practice

- ◆ Adequate and appropriate training with continuing professional updating
- ◆ Act as the woman's advocate wherever possible
- ◆ Acknowledge limitations of the therapy within the constraints of conventional practice
- ◆ Evidence-based practice where contemporary research available
- ◆ Ensure safe and effective practice of the therapy
- ◆ Communication and collaboration with colleagues
- ◆ Consent; acknowledge the woman's right to refuse the therapy
- ◆ Policies and guidelines to set parameters for practice of the therapy
- ◆ Record keeping
- ◆ Evaluation and audit of individual care and of the service.

---

technique, shiatsu, counselling, reiki and Bach flower remedies. Most other therapies, which are less well recognized and may be considered 'fringe' therapies are classified in group 3 which is sub-divided into traditional systems of health care such as Chinese and Indian Ayurvedic medicine and diagnostic techniques, for example, iridology and kinesiology (see Box 4.3). Group 3 therapies are not dealt with in this chapter.

Osteopathy and chiropractic

Osteopathy and chiropractic are related therapies based on the realignment of the musculoskeletal system by a series of specialist movements, often used in conjunction with massage and soft tissue manipulation, on the principle that all conditions arise as a result of postural misalignment. Neither osteopathy nor chiropractic are without potential dangers or side effects, although the lengthy education and stringent regulations regarding practice and continuing professional development will certainly eliminate the poorly qualified or over-enthusiastic novice from treating patients without supervision. They are statutorily regulated by the General Osteopathic Council and General Chiropractic Council respectively.

Box 4.3 Classification of complementary and alternative therapies

Group 1
    Osteopathy
    Chiropractic
    Homeopathy
    Herbal medicine
    Acupuncture

Group 2
    Massage
    Shiatsu
    Reflexology
    Aromatherapy
    Nutritional therapy
    Yoga
    Stress management
    Bach flower remedies
    Hypnotherapy
    Alexander technique
    Counselling
    Healing, reiki

Group 3
    Traditional systems of medicine, e.g. Chinese,
        Tibetan, Ayurvedic
    Other alternative therapies, e.g. kinesiology,
        radionics, crystal healing, dowsing

Acupuncture and shiatsu

Acupuncture is part of traditional Chinese medicine (TCM) based on the principle that the body has energy lines, called meridians, flowing from top to toe through major areas of the body. When the body, mind and spirit are in optimum health the energy ('Chi') flows along the meridians unimpeded, but when physiological stressors or pathological conditions arise, blockages occur along the meridians at specific points. Application of needles (acupuncture) or thumb pressure (acupressure) to these points releases the blockages and realigns the body's energy flow. Shiatsu is a more contemporary Japanese therapy similar to acupressure, also based on the correction of energy flow ('Ki' in Japanese). Acupuncture is self-regulated by the British Acupuncture Council, but shiatsu is not currently regulated at a national level, with several organizations in existence.

Homeopathy and Bach flower remedies

Homeopathy is a form of energy medicine in which minute amounts of substances are used, which in larger doses would actually cause the symptoms being treated. Although the remedies are usually in tablet form, homeopathy does not work pharmacologically or chemically. It can be simplistically likened to the principle of 'like cures like' but is an extremely complex system of medicine in which all aspects of the client's health, lifestyle, personality and the complete symptom picture are significant. Care must be taken when self-prescribing as inappropriate use of the incorrect remedy can cause a 'reverse proving' in which the symptom picture intended to be treated by the (wrong) remedy can be precipitated by its use without treating the existing symptom picture. Symptoms may worsen before improving but this is part of the body's innate healing reaction. Long-term, chronic pathological conditions should always be treated by a qualified homeopath. Homeopaths who are also medically qualified doctors, dentists or veterinary surgeons are members of the Faculty of Homeopathy based at the Royal London Homeopathic Hospital, and lay homeopaths belong to the Society of Homeopaths.

Medical herbalism and aromatherapy

Medical herbalism is the precursor of modern pharmaceuticals, but herbal remedies differ from drugs in that generally the whole plant is used so that the required active ingredient is balanced by other constituents in the plant. This contrasts directly with the manufacture of drugs in which the active ingredient is isolated and then produced synthetically so that the product can be patented, but which increases the likelihood of side effects from the chemicals in the drug. Aromatherapy is the use of highly concentrated essential oils extracted from plants and administered through massage, inhalation, in baths, compresses, via the mucous membranes as pessaries or suppositories and occasionally neat or by mouth. Although the aroma plays a significant role in affecting mood, chemicals within essential oils act pharmacologically, the action being enhanced by the method of administration, particularly massage. It is important to understand that essential oils should be considered as drugs which may act therapeutically but which also have the potential, if misused or abused, to do harm. Health professionals should not prescribe essential oils unless they understand fully the uses, contraindications, precautions, side effects and potential interactions with other medications. Most herbalists are members of the National Institute of Medical Herbalists and most aromatherapists register with the International Society of Professional Aromatherapists.

Reflexology

Reflexology is based on the principle that the feet (and hands) represent a map of the rest of the body, so that by working on the feet, other parts of the body can be treated. Reflexology is *not* just a relaxing foot massage, but involves very precise movements over the entire surface of the feet in order to elicit areas that may indicate significant physiological or pathological changes and can be harmful if abused. Reflexology is especially effective for the prevention and treatment of stress-related conditions such as generalized anxiety, hypertension and as an adjunct to other relaxation therapies following physical or psychological stressors, but it is also beneficial for physiopathological conditions not necessarily exacerbated by stress. Although it is not intended as a diagnostic technique, it is possible to identify, from the feet, previous, current or impending health conditions, as well as changing physiology such as stages of the menstrual cycle. Although the profession is attempting to regulate itself under the Association of Reflexologists, there remain several registering bodies for reflexology.

Massage

Massage is the applied use of touch to relax or stimulate physiological and psychological well-being, either with or without essential oils. There are many different forms of massage such as Swedish (involving the traditional cupping and hacking movements), lymphatic drainage, shiatsu massage and others. Many nurses and midwives use massage and touch informally in their work, perhaps even subconsciously. It can be administered as a therapeutic intervention, for example to relax women prior to investigations or surgery, or to stimulate excretion, for example lymphatic drainage following mastectomy or peristalsis after abdominal operations. Massage is known to reduce pain, alleviate stress, anxiety and depression, and to stimulate the immune function (Field, 1998).

Hypnotherapy

Hypnotherapy is the medical use of hypnosis, or the applied use of deep relaxation techniques, mainly to treat problems of psychological origin, such as reducing pain perception, or changing behaviour, for example drug addiction, smoking, weight loss and enuresis. Practitioners utilize sophisticated counselling skills and may induce the hypnotic state in clients or may teach them how to self-induce.

Using complementary therapies for women's sexual health

Pre-menstrual syndrome

The herbal remedy Vitex agnus castus has become popular in recent years for the treatment of pre-menstrual syndrome (PMS). A study that compared a commercial preparation containing agnus castus with pyridoxine (vitamin B6) demonstrated greater alleviation of complaints such as breast tenderness, depression and stress, headache, constipation and oedema in the herbal group, although some minor side effects were observed (Lauritzen *et al.*, 1997). Betz (1998) questions the validity of this study in which there was no control group and a relatively small number of participants ($n = 175$), but a larger study ($n = 1634$) (Loch *et al.*, 2000) showed an 81% rate of overall improvement in pre-menstrual symptoms. Agnus castus appears to be particularly effective in relieving pre-menstrual mastalgia as a result of prolactin suppression by dopaminergic compounds in the plant (Wuttke *et al.*, 2003) and compares favourably with the serotonin reuptake inhibitor Fluoxetine (Atmaca *et al.*, 2003). Other herbal remedies, including gingko biloba and St John's wort, have been investigated although further work needs to be undertaken and nurses should not advise these remedies unless they understand fully their potential side effects or interactions with drugs (see Harkness and Bratman, 2003; McKenna *et al.*, 2003).

Homeopathic medicines for PMS have also been explored in two double-blind placebo-controlled studies. One study had an extremely small sample due to stringent exclusion criteria ($n = 10$) (Chapman *et al.*, 1994), but a later trial showed reduced use of medication for pain relief or depression and fewer days off work than a placebo group (Yakir *et al.*, 2000). Acupuncture has been found to be beneficial for pre-menstrual symptoms such as breast tenderness, insomnia and gastrointestinal disturbance compared to placebo, due to its effects on the serotoninergic and opioidergic neurotransmission that modulates various psychosomatic functions (Habek *et al.*, 2002).

Headaches and migraines may respond to massage, which relieves pain by intercepting pain impulses, eases stress and enhances well-being through a reduction in cortisol and an increase in serotonin (Hernandez Reif *et al.*, 1998). A later specific study of pre-menstrual women showed improvements in physical but not mood-related symptoms after massage (Hernandez-Reif *et al.*, 2000). Oleson and Flocco (1993) used a combination of foot, hand and ear reflexology and produced statistically significant symptom improvements in a large group of women, although treatment was long term and the positive results may have been due to the accumulative effects of relaxation. Yoga and meditation may improve manual dexterity through an improvement in concentration levels which is relevant during the premenstrual phase for some women (Manjunath and Telles, 1999; Raghuraj and Telles, 1997). Osteopathy or chiropractic may also be of value (Walsh and Polus, 1999).

The peri-menopausal phase

Homeopathy may offer an effective alternative to long-term use of hormone replacement therapy for some women (Thompson *et al.*, 2002). It would, however, be difficult for nurses without some training in homeopathy to advise precise remedies as they must be prescribed for each individual's precise symptoms, but they could certainly suggest that homeopathy can have a part to play in relieving menopausal symptoms. Work by Polish researchers (Warenik-Szymakiewicz *et al.*, 1997) investigated the use of a homeopathic preparation, Feminon N, in 20 post-menopausal women and found significantly lower levels of follicle stimulating hormone and menopausal symptoms in the trial group but did not identify significant changes in oestradiol levels after 6 months of the treatment. Clover and Ratsey (2002) also found improvement in peri-menopausal symptoms using homeopathic medicines in a pilot study. However, this study was undertaken without the use of a control group and highlights the difficulties in randomizing a standard remedy to a non-standard group of individuals with different symptom pictures which impacts on the validity of homeopathy research, despite the fact that much of the British work has been undertaken by medically qualified homeopaths.

Commonly used phytoestrogens (oestrogen-like compounds found in plants) for treatment of menopausal symptoms, as an alternative to HRT, include red clover, chasteberry (*Vitex agnus-castus*), hops, Asian ginseng, dong quai (*Angelica sinensis*), licorice and black cohosh (*Cimicifuga racemosa*) (Liu *et al.*, 2001). *Agnus castus* in essential oil form may also be of use (Chopin Lucks, 2003). Certain foods such as soybean, green and mung beans and alfalfa sprout also contain the active isoflavones which have been shown to have a beneficial cardiovascular effect (Garcia-Martinz *et al.*, 2003; Steinberg *et al.*, 2003; Teede *et al.*, 2003), improve bone density, memory loss and cognitive functioning (Setchell and Lydeking-Olsen, 2003). Black cohosh and red clover may be useful for symptoms such as hot flushes (Kronenberg and Fugh Berman, 2002; van de Weijer and Barentsen, 2002), although the beneficial effects of black cohosh may be central rather than hormonal (Borrelli *et al.*, 2003; Mahady 2003). Red clover also appears to have an anti-prolferative effect on the endometrium (Hale *et al.*, 2001), although Murray *et al.* (2003) dispute this. In a 6-month study Balk *et al.* (2002) found a maximum 35% risk of stimulation of the endometrium from phytoestrogen use in the form of soybean, and a significant reduction in night sweats, hot flushes and vaginal dryness, although the incidence of insomnia was greater in the trial group than the control. However, Mahady *et al.* (2003) express concern about the high incidence of self-administration of herbal remedies and dietary supplements without medical knowledge, which presents the possibility of potentiation, while Abebe (2002) focuses on the risk of interaction with analgesic drugs such as aspirin. Conversely, in a systematic review of herbal medicinal products for menopausal symptoms, Huntley and Ernst (2003) suggest that there is insufficient evidence to support their use, although they acknowledge promising results on the value of black cohosh and red clover.

Concern has been expressed about the potential of phytoestrogens to predispose women to breast cancer due to their structural similarity to physiological oestrogens although the incidence of breast cancer is lowest in nations whose consumption of phytoestrogens is highest (Barnes, 1998). However, Nikander *et al.* (2003) found that isoflavones from phytoestrogens did not relieve subjective menopausal symptoms in a group of women with a history of breast cancer and Kurzer (2003) suggests that isoflavones should not be recommended to women at high risk of breast cancer until more safety data are available.

St John's wort (*Hypericum perforatum*) is a herbal anti-depressant which appears to work through the action of hyperforin which elevates sodium ions to inhibit reuptake of serotonin and nor-adrenaline and dopamine (Nathan, 1999; Singer *et al.*, 1999), although it is probably most effective for treatment of mild to moderate, rather than severe, chronic depression (Deltito and Beyer, 1998). In 2000 the Committee on Safety of Medicines reviewed new evidence about important interactions between St John's wort preparations and certain prescribed medicines leading to a loss of therapeutic effect of the prescribed medicine. These medications include MAOIs, HIV protease inhibitors, warfarin, anticonvulvsants, digoxin, theophylline and oral contraceptives. The latter is obviously very important for women of reproductive age, as potentially St John's wort could increase the risk of an unplanned pregnancy (Committee on Safety of Medicines, 2000). The remedy is also

contraindicated during the preconception period and pregnancy as it may damage oocytes (as may also ginkgo biloba and echinacea at high concentrations) (Ondrizek *et al.*, 1999a) and inhibit sperm motility (Ondrizek *et al.*, 1999b).

Acupuncture appears to be useful for reducing vasomotor symptoms but has little effect on libido (Dong *et al.*, 2001; Porzio *et al.*, 2002), nor does it lower blood pressure in hypertensive menopausal women (Kraft and Coulon, 1999), while animal studies suggest that it may improve memory through the stimulation of norepinephrine and dopamine transmission from the brain (Toriizuka *et al.*, 1999). Electro-acupuncture is thought to be more effective and more long lasting than superficial needle insertion for elevating mood (Sandberg *et al.*, 2002). Reflexology may be relaxing but has not been shown to be superior to generalized foot massage in reducing psychological symptoms (Williamson *et al.*, 2002). Tai Ch'i and other gentle forms of relaxation and exercise may help in preventing falls, lessen the risks of osteoporosis and aid maintenance of general health and fitness (Henderson *et al.*, 1998; Lane and Nydick, 1999).

Gynaecological in-patient care

Women admitted to hospital for gynaecological investigations or surgery may wish to use complementary therapies as an adjunct to their care, for relaxation or pain relief. Bach flower rescue remedy, an anti-stress remedy, may be useful prior to surgery, although research regarding its effectiveness is inconclusive and it may simply act as a placebo (Walach *et al.*, 2000). Hypnotherapy and biofeedback offer other alternatives for treating anxiety and problems such as needle phobia (Pinnell and Covino, 2000). Homeopathic arnica is advocated for bruising, shock and trauma, although, again, trial results have been variable (Hart *et al.*, 1997; Vickers *et al.*, 1998) and systematic reviews have reached the conclusion that its value is as a placebo (Ernst and Pittler, 1998; Linde *et al.*, 1997).

Pain has been shown to be significantly reduced by massage, in a randomized controlled trial of women who had laparoscopic sterilization as day case patients, while another small study suggests that it may assist women in coming to terms with altered body image following mastectomy (Bredin, 1999). Several studies have explored the physiopsychological effects of back massage in hospitalized (and therefore stressed) patients and demonstrate increased relaxation and well-being (Gauthier, 1999; Smith *et al.*, 1999). However, the results specifically for reflexology are less clear: a German trial (Kesselring, 1999) found that reflexology after gynaecological surgery actually increased abdominal pain rather than relieved it, although an earlier trial by Kesselring *et al.* (1998) demonstrated the positive effects of reflexology on postoperative micturition.

Acupuncture is thought to be analgesic due to the stimulation of beta-endorphins and neuropeptides and increase in interleukin-2 cells and natural killer cells (Bin, 1994). Post-operative nausea and vomiting can be relieved with acupuncture or acupressure, and is one of the most well-researched of complementary therapy techniques, through stimulation of the Pericardium 6 (P6) or Neiguan point on the inner wrist (Pearl *et al.*, 1999). However, although the incidence and severity of nausea and vomiting in women receiving chemotherapy for breast cancer improved slightly, the results of a study by Dibble *et al.* (2000) were inconclusive. Hypnotherapy is also useful for nausea and vomiting associated with chemotherapy, particularly anticipatory symptoms (Marchioro *et al.*, 2000; Montgomery *et al.*, 2002). The value of hypnotherapy in reducing anxiety and pain perception in cancer patients has also been considered (Curtis, 2001).

Massage and aromatherapy can be invaluable in aiding relaxation, easing pain and discomfort, reducing blood pressure, stimulating peristalsis and preventing infection. A well-researched essential oil is Australian tea tree, renowned for its strong anti-infective actions against bacteria, viruses and fungi, including vaginal thrush, and Methicillin-resistant *Staphylococcus aureus* (MRSA) (Chan and Loudon, 1998; Concha *et al.*, 1998; Hammer *et al.*, 1999; Harkenthal *et al.*, 1999) although skin sensitivity and anaphylactic shock to essential oils has been reported (Giordinano-Labadie *et al.*, 2000; Reider *et al.*, 2000; Southwell *et al.*, 1997).

Infertility

The herbal remedy vitex agnus castus may be appropriate for infertility due to secondary amenorrhoea or luteal insufficiency although a case of multiple follicular development following self-administration was reported by Cahill *et al.* (1994) and a homeopathic dilution may be safer (Bergmann *et al.*, 2000). Nutritional supplementation may be effective for some women, although care should be taken to caution against excessive use, as this may be counter-productive – high levels of chromium, for example, may exacerbate sterility and trigger mutations (Hepburn *et al.*, 2003). Sperm motility in men may also respond to dietary isoflavones or supplementation with selenium and vitamins E and C (Sierens *et al.*, 2002; Rolf *et al.*, 1999), although studies on the use of magnesium have proved inconclusive (Zavaczki *et al.*, 2003). Acupuncture is thought to affect the hypothalamic–pituitary–ovarian axis (Chang *et al.*, 2002; Chen, 1997) and, in men, has been shown to improve sperm density and quality (Zhang *et al.*, 2002; Siterman *et al.*, 2000). Relaxation therapies such as hypnotherapy or yoga may have an impact on conception rates when included as part of preconception and *in vitro* fertilization treatment (Khalsa, 2003; Poehl *et al.*, 1999).

Pregnancy and childbirth

Nausea and vomiting in pregnancy may respond to herbal medicines although it should be recognized that ginger is *not* a universal solution and in some women can be harmful (see Tiran, 2003). Acupuncture or acupressure wristbands are used by many women with variable success but this may be due to positioning or failure to stimulate the relevant acupressure point at intervals (Steele *et al.*, 2001; Werntoft and Dykes, 2001). Hypnotherapy may be useful if hyperemesis gravidarum develops (Torem, 1994); studies on women in labour also indicate a value in using hypnotherapy to relieve pain (Brann, 1995; Jenkins and Pritchard, 1993).

SCENARIO

Maria was a student midwife who consulted the complementary therapy midwife initially for pre-conception advice as she had been trying to conceive for over 18 months. Although she had three other children this was to be the first with her new partner. After two treatments with reflexology Maria conceived and had a largely unremarkable pregnancy. However, at 35 weeks' gestation the fetal presentation was found to be breech. Maria was desperate to avoid caesarean section or the potential complications of a vaginal breech delivery and she returned to the complementary therapy midwife requesting moxibustion. She was shown how to administer the treatment at home. Her family was very sceptical about the use of a smoking herb stick to turn the fetus but on the third day whilst performing the fifth treatment they were amazed actually to witness, from the movement of Maria's abdomen, the baby appearing to writhe around under the surface! The next day Maria had a booked ultrasound scan and was delighted to see that the fetus had indeed turned to a cephalic presentation, which progressed to a normal vaginal delivery four weeks later.

Moxibustion, an aspect of Chinese medicine, is increasingly being used to turn breech presentations to cephalic. Moxa sticks, containing compressed dried mugwort, a herb, are used as a heat source above the Bladder 67 acupuncture points on the little toes, for 15 minutes twice a day for 5 days at between 32 weeks' gestation and term. Research appears to indicate that, even allowing for the incidence of spontaneous cephalic versions in control groups, the number of spontaneous cephalic vaginal deliveries at term is greater in the moxibustion group than in groups matched for control or the more conventional external cephalic version treatment (Cardini and Weixin, 1998; Kanakura *et al.*, 2001). It is thought that the moxa heat affects the relevant acupuncture point and the Chi flowing along the meridian, to increase myometrial contractility and sensitivity and also stimulate fetal movement to encourage the fetus to turn itself.

Labrecque *et al.* (1999) found that daily 10-minute perineal massage from 34 weeks' gestation was effective in reducing the risk of perineal trauma at delivery in women having their first vaginal delivery but not in those who had had previous vaginal births. Twice-weekly massage during pregnancy has been found to improve sleep, reduce anxiety and alleviate backache (Field *et al.*, 1999). Pain relief in labour may be achieved through the careful use of aromatherapy or reflexology (Burns *et al.*, 2000; Motha and McGrath, 1993).

Conclusion

The philosophy of complementary medicine is one of holism, the interdependence of body, mind and spirit, with an appreciation of the impact of each element upon the individual. Truly holistic practitioners would question the reductionist approach to orthodox health care and challenge the isolation of specific strategies from different complementary therapies as a means of treating a range of symptoms, although it is through this symptoms-based approach that conventional health care professionals can begin to appreciate the value of complementary medicine.

Nurses, midwives and health visitors can develop an understanding of the place of complementary and alternative medicine, although they may not always be in a position to use it in their own practice. Care is about endeavouring to find the most appropriate means of helping

Ideas for personal and professional development

● Compile a list of issues to consider when recommending complementary therapies/therapists to women for help with their reproductive health

● Identify situations when it might be inappropriate for women to resort to complementary medicine

● Collate the questions which women have asked you about the use of complementary medicine and identify areas for further learning

● Discuss with your colleagues how you may best facilitate women's use of complementary therapies and natural remedies effectively *and* safely.

Patient education points

- 'Natural' does not always mean 'safe' or without side effects: always check with your doctor or nurse before using natural remedies which might interfere with any drugs you may be taking

- Therapists providing complementary therapies for women with specific reproductive health issues should have a thorough working knowledge of the relevant pathophysiology and the conventional treatments

- Herbal remedies for the relief of menopausal symptoms may not give protection against complications which occur later (e.g. osteoporosis) and often cost more than prescriptions of hormone replacement

- During pregnancy any complementary therapies must be used in conjunction with normal maternity care from a midwife or doctor.

patients and clients, whilst acknowledging the importance of safety and evidence-based practice. Complementary therapies can offer an expanded range of strategies with which to assist the women in our care, and should be seen truly as a beneficial adjunct to the conventional management of women's sexual health. Collaborative, communicative and facilitative relationships between patients/clients and all their caregivers will lead to satisfaction and success for all; complementary and alternative medicine may go some way towards achieving that.

Patient education points

Resources

Association of Reflexologists
www.aor.org.uk

British Acupuncture Council
63 Jeddo Road, London W12 9HQ
Tel: 020 8735 0400 Fax: 020 8735 0404
E-mail: info@acupuncture.org.uk

Complementary Maternity Forum
c/o Denise Tiran, Chair, by e-mail:
   www.expectancy.co.uk

Forum website: www.c-m-f.co.uk (password for the Noticeboard is 'childbirth')

General Chiropractic Council
www.gcc-uk.org

General Council of Osteopaths
www.osteopathy.org.uk

International Federation of Professional Aromatherapists
www.ifparoma.org

National Institute of Medical Herbalists
www.nimh.org.uk

Prince of Wales' Foundation for Integrated Health
12 Chillingworth Road, London N7 8QJ
www.fihealth.org.uk

Research Council for Complementary Medicine
27a Devonshire Street, London W1G 6PN
Tel: 020-7935-7499
info@rccm.org.uk

Royal College of Nursing – Complementary Therapies Forum
RCN, 13 Cavendish Square, London W1M 0AB

Society of Homeopaths
www.homeopathy-soh.org

Further reading

ERNST, E., PITTLER, M.H., STEVINSON, C. and WHITE, A. (2001) *The Desktop Guide to Complementary and Alternative Medicine*. Edinburgh: Mosby.

MACKERETH, P. and TIRAN, D. (2002) *Clinical Reflexology: A Guide for Health Professionals*. London: Elsevier Science.

TIRAN, D. (2003) *Nausea and Vomiting in Pregnancy: An Integrated Approach to Care*. London: Elsevier Science.

TIRAN, D. (2001) *Clinical Aromatherapy in Pregnancy and Childbirth*, 2nd edn. London: Churchill Livingstone.

TIRAN, D. and MACK, S. (eds) (2000) *Complementary Therapies for Pregnancy and Childbirth*, 2nd edn. London: Baillière Tindall.

References

ABEBE, W. (2002) Herbal medication: potential for adverse interactions with analgesic drugs. *Journal of Clinical Pharmacology & Therapeutics* **27**(6):391–401.

ATMACA, M., KUMRU, S. and TEZCAN, E. (2003) Fluoxetine versus vitex agnus castus extract in the treatment of premenstrual dysphoric disorder. *Human Psychopharmacology* 18(3):191–5.

BALK, J.L., WHITESIDE, D.A., NAUS, G., DE FERRARI, E. and ROBERTS, J.M. (2002) A pilot study of the effects of phytoestrogen supplementation on postmenopausal endometrium. *Journal of the Society of Gynecological Investigations* 9(4):238–42.

BARNES, S. (1998) Phytoestrogens and breast cancer. *Baillière's Clinical Endocrinology and Metabolism* 12(4):559–79.

BERGMANN. J., LUFT, B., BOEHMANN, S., RUN-NEBAUM, B. and GERHARD, I. (2000) The efficacy of the complex medication Phyto-Hypophyson L in female hormone-related sterility. A randomised placebo-controlled clinical double-blind study. *Forsch Komplementarmed Klass Naturheilkd* 7(4):190–9.

BETZ. W. (1998) Commentary – William Betz, Brussels *Forschende Komplementarmedizin* (Basel) 5:146–7.

BIN, W. (1995) Effect of acupuncture on the regulation of cell medicated immunity in patients with malignant tumours. *Chen Tzu Yen Chiu* 20(3):67, cited in Spencer, J.W. and Jacobs, J.J. (1999) *Complementary/Alternative Medicine: An Evidence-based Approach*. St Louis: Mosby, p. 138.

BIN, W., ZHOU, R.X. and ZHOU, M.S. (1994) Effect of acupuncture on interleukin-2 level and NK cell immunoactivity of peripheral blood of malignant tumour patients. *Chung Kuo His I Chieh Ho Tsa Chih* 14(9):537, cited in Spencer, J.W. and Jacobs, J.J. (1999) *Complementary/Alternative Medicine; An Evidence-based Approach*. St Louis: Mosby, p. 138.

BORRELLI, F., IZZO, A.A. and ERNST, E. (2003) Pharmacological effects of Cimicifuga racemosa. *Life Science* 73(10):1215–29.

BRANN, L. (1995) The role of hypnosis in obstetrics. *The Diplomate* 2(2):95.

BREDIN, M. (1999) Mastectomy, body image and therapeutic massage: a qualitative study of women's experience. *Journal of Advanced Nursing* 29(5):1113–20.

BURNS, E., BLAMEY, C., ERSSER, S., LLOYD, A.J. and BARNETSON, L. (1999) The use of aromatherapy in intrapartum midwifery practice: an observational study. *OCHRAD* Oxford.

CAHILL, D.J., FOX, R., WARDLE, P.G. and HARLOW, C.R. (1994) Multiple follicular development associated with herbal medicine. *Human Reproduction* 9(8):1469–70.

CARDINI, F. and WEIXIN, H. (1998) Moxibustion for correction of breech presentation. A randomized controlled trial. *Journal of the American Medical Association* 280(18):1580–4.

CHAN, C.H. and LOUDON, K.W. (1998) Activity of tea tree oil on Methicillin-resistant *Staphylococcus aureus* (MRSA). *Journal of Hospital Infection* 39(3):244–5.

CHANG, R., CHUNG, P.H. and ROSENWAKS, Z. (2002) Role of acupuncture in the treatment of female infertility. *Fertility and Sterility* 78(6):1149–53.

CHAPMAN, E.H., ANGELICA, J., SPITALNY, G. and STRAUSS, M. (1994) Results of a study of the homeopathic treatment of PMS. *Journal of the American Institute of Homeopathy* 87:14–21.

CHEN, B.Y. (1997) Acupuncture normalizes dysfunction of hypothalamic-pituitary-ovarian axis. *Acupuncture and Electrotherapy Research* 22(2):97–108.

CHOPIN LUCKS, B. (2003) Vitex agnus castus essential oil and menopausal balance: a research update. *Complementary Therapies in Nursing & Midwifery* 9(3):157–60.

CLOVER, A. and RATSEY, D. (2002) Homeopathic treatment of hot flushes: a pilot study. *Homeopathy* 91(2):75–9.

COMMITTEE ON SAFETY OF MEDICINES (2000) Important interactions between St John's wort (*Hypericum perforatum*) preparations and prescribed medicines. Open letter to doctors and pharmacists.

CONCHA, J.M., MOORE, L.S. and HOLLOWAY, W.J. (1998) Antifungal activity of Melaleuca alternifolia (tea tree) against various pathogenic organisms. *Journal of American Podiatric Medical Association* 88(10):489–92.

CROCK, R.D., JARJOURA, D., POLEN, A. and RUTCHEKI, G.W. (1999) Confronting the communication gap between conventional and alternative medicine: a survey of physicians' attitudes. *Journal of Alternative Therapies in Health and Medicine* 5(2):61–6.

CURTIS, C. (2001) Hypnotherapy in a specialist palliative care unit: evaluation of a pilot service *International Journal of Palliative Care Nursing* 7(12):604–5.

DELTITO, J. and BEYER, D. (1998) The scientific, quasi-scientific and popular literature on the use of St John's wort in the treatment of depression. *Journal of Affective Disorders* 51(3):345–51.

DIBBLE, S.L., CHAPMAN, J., MACK, K.A. and SHIH, A.S. (2000) Acupressure for nausea: results of a pilot study. *Oncology Nurses Forum* 27(1):41–7.

DONG, H., LUDICKE, F., COMTE, I., CAMPANA, A., GRAFF, P. and BISCHOF, P. (2001) An exploratory pilot study of acupuncture on the quality of life and reproductive hormone secretion in menopausal women. *Journal of Alternative & Complementary Medicine* 7(6):651–8.

ERNST, E. and PITTLER, M.H. (1998) Efficacy of homoeopathic arnica – a systematic review of placebo-controlled trials. *Archives of Surgery* 133(11):1187–90.

FIELD, T. (1998) Massage therapy effects. *American Psychologist* 53(12):1270–81.

FIELD, T., HERNANDEZ REIF, M., HART, S., THEAKSTON, H., SCHANBERG.S. and KUHN, C. (1999) Pregnant women benefit from massage therapy. *Journal of Psychosomatic Obstetrics and Gynecology* 20(1):31–8.

GARCIA-MARTINEZ, M.C., HERMENIGILDO, C., TARIN, J.J. and CANO, A. (2003) Phytoestrogens increase the capacity of serum to stimulate prostacyclin release in human endothelial cells. *Acta Obstetrics and Gynecology Scandinavia* 82(8):705–10.

GAUTHIER, D.M. (1999) The healing potential of back massage. *Online Journal of Knowledge Synthesis for Nursing* 6(5):U1–U6.

GIORDANO-LABARDIE, F., SCHWARZE, H.P. and BAZEX, J. (2000) Allergic contact dermatitis from camomile used in phytotherapy. *Contact Dermatitis* 42(4):247.

HABEK, D., HABEK, J.C. and BARBIR, A. (2002) Using acupuncture to treat premenstrual syndrome. *Archives of Gynecology and Obstetrics* 267(1):23–6.

HALE, G.E., HUGHES, C.L., ROBBOY, S.J., AGARWAL, S.K. and BIEVRE, M. (2001) A double-blind randomized study on the effects of red clover isoflavones on the endometrium. *Menopause* 8(5):338–46.

HAMMER, K.A., CARSON, C.F. and RILEY, T.V. (1999) Antimicrobial activity of essential oils and other plant extracts. *Journal of Applied Microbiology* 86(6):985–90.

HARKENTHAL, M., REICHLING, J., GEISS, H.K. and SALLER, R. (1999) Comparative study on the *in vitro* anti-bacterial activity of Australian tea tree oil, cajuput oil, niaouli oil, manuka oil, kanuka oil and eucalyptus oil. *Pharmazie* **54**(6):460–3.

HARKNESS, R. and BRATMAN, S. (2003) *Handbook of Drug–Herb and Drug–Supplement Interactions*. St Louis: Mosby.

HART, O., MULLEE, M.A., LEWITH, G. and MILLER, J. (1997) Double-blind placebo-controlled randomized clinical trial of homoeopathic arnica 30C for pain and infection after total abdominal hysterectomy. *Journal of the Royal Society of Medicine* **90**(2):73–8.

HENDERSON, N.K., WHITE, C.P. and EISMAN, J.A. (1998) The roles of exercise and fall risk reduction in the prevention of osteoporosis. *Endocrinology and Metabolism Clinics of North America* **27**(2):369–87.

HEPBURN, D.D., XIAO, J., BINDOM, S., VINCENT, J.B. and O'DONNELL, J. (2003) Nutritional supplement chromium picolinate causes sterility and lethal mutations in Drosophila melanogaster. *Proceedings of the National Academy of Sciences USA* **100**(7):3766–71.

HERNANDEZ REIF, M., DIETER, J., FIELD, T., SWERD-LOW, B. and DIEGO, M. (1998) Migraine headaches are reduced by massage therapy. *International Journal of Neuroscience* **96**(1–2):1–11.

HERNANDEZ REIF, M., MARTINEX, A., FIELD, T., QUINTERO, O., HART, S. and BURMAN, I. (2000) Premenstrual symptoms are relieved by massage therapy. *Journal of Psychosomatic Obstetrics and Gynecology* **21**:9–15.

HOUSE OF LORDS SELECT COMMITTEE ON SCIENCE AND TECHNOLOGY (2000) *Sixth Report on Complementary and Alternative Medicine*. Norwich: The Stationery Office.

HUNTLEY, A.L. and ERNST, E. (2003) A systematic review of herbal medicinal products for treatment of menopausal symptoms *Menopause* **10**(5):465–76.

JENKINS, M. and PRITCHARD, M. (1993) Hypnosis: practical applications and theoretical considerations in normal labour. *British Journal of Obstetrics and Gynaecology* **100**:221.

KANAKURA, Y., KMETANI, K., NAGATA, T., NIWA, K., KAMATSUKI, H., SHINZATO, Y. and TOKUNAGA, Y. (2001) Moxibustion treatment of breech presentation. *American Journal of Chinese Medicine* **29**(1):37–45.

KESSELRING, A. (1999) Foot reflexology massage – a clinical study. *Forschende Komplementarmedizin* **6**(Suppl 1):38–40, cited in *MEDLINE* ® ISSN 1021-7096.

KESSELRING, A., SPICHIGER, E. and MULLER, M. (1998) Foot reflexology: an intervention study. *Pflege* **11**(4):213–18, cited in *CINAHL* ® Database 1997–1999/07.

KHALSA, H.K. (2003) Yoga: an adjunct to infertility treatment. *Fertility and Sterility* **80**(Suppl 4):46–51.

KRAFT, K. and COULON, S. (1999) Effect of a standardized acupuncture treatment on complaints, blood pressure and serum lipids of hypertensive, postmenopausal women. A randomized, controlled clinical study. *Forsch Komplementarmed* **6**(2):74–9.

KRONENBERG, F. and FUGH-BERMAN, A. (2002) Complementary and alternative medicine for menopausal symptoms: a review of randomized, controlled trials. *Annals of Intern Medicine* **137**(10):805–13.

KURZER, M.S. (2003) Phytoestrogen supplement use by women. *Nutrition* **133**(6):1983S–1986S.

LABRECQUE, M., EASON, E., MARCOUX, S. *et al.* (1999) Randomised controlled trial of prevention of perineal trauma by perineal massage during pregnancy. *American Journal of Obstetrics and Gynecology* **180**(3), Pt 1:593–600.

LANE, J.M. and NYDICK, M. (1999) Osteoporosis: current modes of prevention and treatment. *Journal of the American Academy of Orthopaedic Surgeons* **7**(1):19–31.

LAURITZEN, C., REUTER, H.D., REPGES, R., BOHNERT, K.J. and SCHMIDT, U. (1997) Treatment of premenstrual tension syndrome with vitex agnus castus – controlled double-blind study versus pyridoxine. *Phytomedicine* **4**(3):183–9.

LINDE, K., CLAUSIUS, N., RAMIREZ, G. *et al.* (1997) Are the clinical effects of homoeopathy placebo effects? A meta-analysis of placebo-controlled trials. *Lancet* **350**(9081):834–43.

LIU, J., BURDETTE, J.E., XU, H., GU, C., VAN BREEMEN, R.B. *et al.* (2001) Evaluation of estrogenic activity of plant extracts for the potential treatment of menopausal symptoms. *Journal Agriculture and Food Chemistry* **49**(5):2472–9.

LOCH, E.G., SELLE, H. and BOBLITZ, N. (2000) Treatment of premenstrual syndrome with a phytopharmaceutical formulation containing vitex agnus castus. *Journal of Women's Health & Gender-based Medicine* **9**:315–20.

MAHADY, G.B. (2003) Is black cohosh estrogenic? *Nutrition Review* **61**(5Pt1):183–6.

MAHADY, G.B., PARROT, J., LEE, C., YUN, G.S. and DAN, A. (2003) Botanical dietary supplement use in peri- and post-menopausal women. *Menopause* **10**(1):65–72.

MANJUNATH, N.K. and TELLES, S. (1999) Factors influencing changes in tweezer dexterity scores following yoga training. *Indian Journal of Physiology and Pharmacology* **43**(2):225–9.

MARCHIORO, G., AZZARELLO, G., VIVIFANI, F., BARBATO, F., PAVANETTTO, M., ROSETTI, F., PAPPAGALLO, G.L. and VINANTE, O. (2000) Hypnosis in the treatment of anticipatory nausea and vomiting in patients receiving cancer chemotherapy. *Oncology* **59**(2):100–4.

MCKENNA, D.J., JONES, K. and HUGHES, K. (2003) *Botanical Medicines: The Desk Reference for Major Herbal Supplements*, 2nd edn. New York: Haworth Herbal Press.

MONTGOMERY, G.H., WELTZ, C.R., SELTZ, M. and BOVBJER, D.H. (2002) Brief presurgery hypnosis reduces distress and pain in excisional breast biopsy patients. *International Journal of Clinical and Experimental Hypnosis* **50**(1):17–32.

MOTHA, G. and McGRATH, J. (1993) The effects of reflexology on labour outcomes. *Reflexions: Journal of the Association of Reflexologists* November:2–4.

MURRAY, M.J., MEYER, W.R., LESSEY, B.A., OI, R.H., DeWIRE, R.E. and FRITZ, M.A. (2003) Soy protein isolate with isoflavones does not prevent estradiol-induced endometrial hyperplasia in postmenopausal women: a pilot trial. *Menopause* **10**(5):456–64.

NATHAN, P.J. (1999) The experimental and clinical pharmacology of St John's wort (Hypericum perforatum L.). *Molecular Psychiatry* **4**(4):333–8.

NIKANDER, E., KILKKINEN, A., METSA-HEIKKILA, M., ADLERCREUTZ, H., PIETENEN, P., TIITENEN, A. and YLIKORKALA, O. (2003) A randomized placebo-controlled crossover trial with phytoestrogens in treatment of menopause in breast cancer patients. *Obstetrics and Gynecology* **101**(6):1213–20.

NURSING & MIDWIFERY COUNCIL (2000a) *Standards for the Administration of Medicines*. London: NMC.

NURSING & MIDWIFERY COUNCIL (2000b) *Guidelines for Professional Practice*. London: NMC.

OLESON, T. and FLOCCO, W. (1993) Randomized controlled study of premenstrual symptoms treated with ear, hand and foot reflexology. *Obstetrics and Gynecology* **82**(6):906–11.

ONDRIZEK, R.R., CHAN, P.J., PATTON, W.C. and KING, A. (1999a) An alternative medicine study of herbal effects on the penetration of zone-free hamster oocytes and the integrity of sperm deoxyribonucleic acid. *Fertility and Sterility* **71**(3):517–22.

ONDRIZEK, R.R., CHAN, P.J., PATTON, W.C. and KING, A. (1999b) Inhibition of human sperm motility by specific herbs used in alternative medicine. *Journal of Assisted Reproduction and Genetics* **16**(2):87–91.

PEARL, M.L., FISCHER, M., McCAULEY, D.L., VALEA, F.A. and CHALAS, E. (1999) Transcutaneous electrical nerve stimulation as an adjunct for controlling chemotherapy-induced nausea and vomiting in gynecologic oncology patients. *Cancer Nursing* **22**(4):307–11.

PINNELL, C.M. and COVINO, N.A. (2000) Empirical findings on the use of hypnosis in medicine: a critical review. *International Journal of Clinical & Experimental Hypnosis* **48**:170–94.

POEHL, M., BICHLER, K., WICKE, V., DORNER, V. and FEICHTINGER, W. (1999) Psychotherapeutic counseling and pregnancy rates in *in vitro* fertilization. *Journal of Assisted Reproduction and Genetics* **16**(6):302–5.

PORZIO, G., TRAPASSO. T., MARTELI, S. *et al.* (2002). Acupuncture in the treatment of menopause-related symptoms in women taking tamoxifen. *Tumori* **88**(2):128–30.

RAGHURAJ, P. and TELLES, S. (1997) Muscle power, dexterity skill and visual perception in community home girls trained in yoga or sports and in regular schoolgirls. *Indian Journal of Physiology and Pharmacology* **41**(4):409–15.

REIDER, N., SEPP, N., FRITSCH, P., WEINLICH, G. and JENSEN-JAROLIM, E. (2000) Anaphylaxis to camomile: clinical features and allergen cross-reactivity. *Clinical and Experimental Allergy* **30**(10):1436–43.

ROLF, C., COOPER, T.G., YEUNG, C.H. and NIESCHLAG, E. (1999) Antioxidant treatment of patients with astheno-zoospermia or moderate oligoasthenozoospermia with high-dose vitamin C and vitamin E: a randomized, placebo-controlled, double-blind study. *Human Reproduction* **14**(4):1028–33.

SANDBERG, M., WIJMA, K., WYON, Y., NEDSTRAND, E. and HAMMAR, M. (2002) Effects of electro-acupuncture on psychological distress in postmenopausal women. *Complementary Therapies in Medicine* **10**(3):161–9.

SETCHELL, K.D. and LYDEKING-OLSEN, E. (2003) Dietary phytoestrogens and their effect on bone: evidence from in vitro and in vivo, human observational, and dietary intervention studies. *American Journal of Clinical Nutrition* **78**(3 Suppl):593S–609S.

SIERENS, J., HARTLEY, J.A., CAMPBELL, M.J., LEATHAM, A.J., and WOODSIDE, J.V. (2002) In vitro isoflavone supplementation reduces hydrogen peroxide-induced DNA damage in sperm. *Teratogens, Carcinogens, and Mutagens* **22**(3):227–34.

SINGER, A., WONNEMANN, M. and MULLER, W.E. (1999) Hyperforin, a major antidepressant constituent of St John's wort, inhibits serotonin uptake by elevating free intracellular Na^+. *Journal of Pharmacology and Experimental Therapeutics* **290**(3):1363–8.

SITERMAN. S., ELTES, F., WOLFSON, V., LEDERMAN, H. and BARTOOV, B. (2000) Does acupuncture treatment affect sperm density in males with very low sperm count? A pilot study. *Andrologia* **32**(1):31–9.

SMITH, M.C., STALLINGS, M.A., MARINER, S. and BURRALL, M. (1999) Benefits of massage therapy for hospitalised patients: a descriptive and qualitative evaluation. *Alternative Therapies in Health and Medicine* **5**(4):64–71.

SOUTHWELL, I.A., MARKHAM, C. and MANN, C. (1997) Skin irritancy of tea tree oil. *Journal of Essential Oil Research* **9**:47–52.

STEELE, N.M. FRENCH, J., GATHERER-BOYLES, J., NEWMAN, S. and LECLAIRE, S. (2001) Effect of acupressure by Sea Bands on nausea and vomiting of pregnancy. *Journal of Obstetric, Gynecological and Neonatal Nursing* **30**(1):61–70.

STEINBERG, F.M., GUTHRIE, N.L., VILLABLANCA, A.C., KUMAR, K. and MURRAY, M.J. (2003) Soy protein with isoflavones has favorable effects on endothelial function that are independent of lipid and antioxidant effects in healthy postmenopausal women *American Journal of Clinical Nutrition* **78**(1):123–30.

TEEDE, H.J., McGRATH, B.P., DeSILVA, L., CEHUN, M., FASSOULAKIS, A. and NESTEL, P.J. (2003) Isoflavones reduce arterial stiffness: a placebo-controlled study in men and postmenopausal women. *Arteriosclerosis, Thrombosis, and Vascular Biology* **23**(6):1066–71.

THOMAS, K.J., NICHOLL, J.P. and COLEMAN, P. (2001) Use and expenditure on complementary medicine in England: a population based survey. *Complementary Therapies in Medicine* **9**(1):2–11.

THOMPSON, E.A., TICE, J.A., ETTINGER, B., ENSRUD, K., WALLACE, R., BLACKWELL, T. and CUMMINGS, S.R. (2002) Homeopathy and the menopause. *Journal of the British Menopause Society* **8**(4):151–4.

TIRAN, D. (2003) *Nausea and Vomiting in Pregnancy: An Integrated Approach to Care*. London: Elsevier Science.

TOREM, M. (1994) Hypnotherapeutic techniques in the treatment of hyperemesis gravidarum. *American Journal of Clinical Hypnosis* **37**(1):1.

TORIIZUKA, K., OKUMARA, M., IIJIMA, K., HARUYAMA, K. and CYONG, J.C. (1999) Acupuncture inhibits the decrease in brain catecholamine contents and the impairment of passive avoidance task in ovariectomized mice. *Acupuncture and Electrotherapy Research* **24**(1):45–57.

VAN de WEIJER, P.H. and BARENTSEN, R. (2002) Isoflavones from red clover (Promensil) significantly reduce menopausal hot flush symptoms compared with placebo. *Maturitas* **42**(3):187–93.

VICKERS, A.J., FISHER, P., SMITH, C., WYLLIE, S.E. and REES, R. (1998) Homeopathic arnica 30X is ineffective for muscle soreness after long-distance running: a randomized double-blind placebo-controlled trial. *Clinical Journal of Pain* **14**(3):227–31.

WALACH, H., RILLING, C. and ENGELKE, U. (2000) Bach flower remedies are ineffective for test anxiety: results of a blinded, placebo-controlled randomized trial. *Forsch Komplementarmed Klass Naturheilkd* **7**:55.

WALSH, M.J. and POLUS, B.I. (1999) A randomised placebo-controlled clinical trial on the efficacy of chiropractic therapy on premenstrual syndrome. *Journal of Manipulation and Physiological Therapeutics* **22**:582–5.

WARENIK-SZYMANKIEWICZ, A., MECZEKALSKI, B. and OBREBOWSKA, A. (1997) Feminon N in the treatment of menopausal symptoms. *Ginekol – Pol.* **68**(2)89–93, cited in *MEDLINE* http://libweb.gre.ac.uk/scripts/webspirs.cmd 10/5/98.

WERNTOFT, E. and DYKES, A.K. (2001) Effect of acupressure on nausea and vomiting during pregnancy. A randomised placebo-controlled pilot study. *Journal of Reproductive Medicine* **46**(9):835–9.

WILLIAMSON. J., WHITE, A., HART, A., and ERNST, E. (2002) Randomised controlled trial of reflexology for menopausal symptoms. *British Journal of Obstetrics and Gynecology* **109**(9):1050–5.

WUTTKE, W., JARRY, H., CHRISTOFFEL, V., SPENGLER, B. and SEIDLOVA-WUTTKE, D. (2003) Chaste tree (Vitex agnus-castus) – pharmacology and clinical indications. *Phytomedicine* **10**(4):348–57.

YAKIR, M., KREITLER, S., BZIZINSKY, A., BENTWICH, Z. and VITHOULKAS. G. (2000) Homeopathic treatment of premenstrual syndrome – repeated study. *Proceedings of the Annual Conference of the International Homeopathic League.* Budapest, Hungary.

ZAVACZKI, Z., SZOLLOSI, J., KISS, S.A., KOLOSZAR, S., FEJES, I., KOVACS, L. and PAL, A. (2003) Magnesium-orotate supplementation for idiopathic infertile male patients: a randomized, placebo-controlled clinical pilot study. *Magnesium Research* **16**(2):131–6.

ZHANG, M., HUANG, G., LU, F., PAULUS, W.E. and STERZIK, K. (2002) Influence of acupuncture on idio-pathic male infertility in assisted reproductive technology. *Journal of Huazhong University of Science and Technology (Medical Sciences)* **22**(3):228–30.

5: Psychosexual and Emotional Care

Jane Selby ◆

OBJECTIVES

This chapter should help you understand:

◆ That it is appropriate for nurses to enquire about a woman's sexual life as part of holistic care ◆

◆ How to observe, listen to, reflect and respond to a woman's sexual anxieties ◆

◆ That nurses wishing to advise on psychosexual issues should recognize their professional boundaries and seek appropriate training ◆

◆ The long-term impact that childhood sexual abuse and post-traumatic stress disorder can have on well-being ◆

◆ That depression, grief and bereavement affect people in a variety of ways ◆

◆ That there are other types of loss apart from death. ◆

Psychosexual nursing

This section describes how the sexuality of patients can be addressed as part of normal clinical practice. Psychosexual nursing as discussed in this chapter is a mind/body approach. This approach, whichever field of nursing you work in, can be used for the care of your patients. The sexual lives of your patients are an important part of holistic care but sadly it is still often neglected in our everyday clinical practice. This approach is a change from 'unfeeling' clinical nursing to one where there is a consideration of 'building emotional bridges' between the practitioner and the patient, and can offer an opportunity for you and your patient to talk more freely about feelings associated with sexuality and life events (Clifford, 2000).

Most women whom you meet professionally do not have deep-seated psychological causes for their worries and anxieties. Women may use any consultation with you to ask about sexual matters, sexual development and anxieties. They see you as not being personally involved with their life, and welcome the opportunity of a consultation with a concerned and sensitive nurse. The aim of this chapter is to encourage you to use and increase the skills that you already possess but which often lie dormant and unrecognized. Sometimes it may take just as much courage for you to overcome your inhibitions with patients as it does for them to be brave and raise sexual matters with you.

Nurses are human beings, and you share the same gifts, faults and failures as your patients. You have emotional experiences and personal events which can be drawn upon when talking to women, but you should remember that these belong to you alone and should never be personalized in a consultation. An additional problem is that we like some patients and some patients like us more than others, i.e. we feel we 'work well' and relate with them, but we may have negative attitudes towards others. Some feel that nurses should not react in this way, but all human

81

beings have these prejudicial emotions. The ability to recognize and share emotions with patients and colleagues can be revealing and is often enough to relieve anxiety. In itself, this can be a significant help to the patient. Sexuality is still seen to be private even with today's more liberal attitudes and thinking. Therefore the patient's behaviour can be noted and her wishes respected.

When patients make enquiries to you about sexual matters, you 'hear' but are often fearful of the outcome and fail to respond appropriately because you think 'I might be seen to be prying' or 'I might get out of my depth' and go on to think 'I don't know how to solve the problem'. In psychosexual nursing the most important thing is to listen and learn that you do not have to solve the patient's problems. It is the patient who has to do that, with your help.

A knowledge of emotional development is helpful in order to acknowledge sexual maturation. This can be done by looking at everyday behaviour around you, reading novels and magazines, watching television as well as by professional study. You can practise your new learning by observing, reflecting and studying how you relate to each patient as well as how the patient behaves towards you. Ideally, this should be with some supervised training to enable you to develop professional confidence. You will then be able to notice when normal steps in sexual growth seem to have been missed out, or events have happened that cause or leave damage and trauma, which appear to affect a woman's sexual health. An enquiry can then be made and interpreted with her. We all learn from our patients and John Bowlby (1986) dedicates his book on *Loss, Sadness and Depression* to 'My patients who have worked hard to educate me'.

Psychosexual nursing is often painful and frightening for both you and your patient. The temptation is not to stay with these uncomfortable emotions but to go down the safer route of clinical illness: the familiar route where the patient may feel more comfortable and you feel more skilled.

It should be your responsibility to listen, understand and share these ordinary everyday fears and worries, and enable your patient to explore her problems with you and then lead her to an understanding of them. You will then discover that you have skills, often hidden and not used, that allow you to make a move forward in offering psychosexual care. This can give satisfaction not only to your patient but also to yourself.

Scenarios are included throughout this chapter to illustrate how problems can be presented to you, and to show that the presenting problem may well cover deep unspoken sexual anxieties. Recognition of this fact alongside sensitive questioning can mean that a small amount of help from you may be all that is needed to prevent minor anxieties becoming major psychosexual problems.

Presentation of sexual anxieties

Sexual anxieties are presented in a variety of ways and you need the knowledge and skills to be alert to these in order to communicate effectively. Nurses who work in women's health have a valuable opportunity to ask about sexuality as part of their holistic care. Sadly such enquiries do not always take place, and if they do they may well come from the patient herself rather than from the nurse.

The overt presentation

Anxiety may be openly presented by your client in various forms:

◆ A client may just ask you a direct question about sexuality or sexual life. This usually comes as a surprise and you may feel taken aback initially, sometimes even bordering on panic, for instance during a consultation when sexual abuse is revealed

◆ The patient may feel she wants to 'test you out'. In spite of feeling you have been asking relevant questions in your consultation which might have allowed her to voice an anxiety, nothing has actually been revealed. It is only when she feels she can trust you and your attitude, that she can say something

◆ Sometimes the patient waits to the very end of the consultation until she asks the question.

It may be that she has had to screw up her courage to raise her anxiety. This can create a reciprocal anxiety for you because time is running out and other patients are waiting. It then becomes difficult to deal with the problem satisfactorily. Offer another appointment to discuss the anxiety further. But to avoid this problem it is advisable to try and raise any sexuality issues early in the clinical consultation.

Tears represent a variety of emotions (Box 5.1). Some people cry easily and will then apologize afterwards. Others remain dry-eyed even whilst telling harrowing stories when you feel they should be crying. Absence of tears does not necessarily indicate a lack of feeling. You need to recognize and interpret with the patient the feelings that lie behind the need to cry.

> **Box 5.1 Types of tears**
>
> ◆ *Happy tears* of excitement and joy are perhaps the easiest to cope with. They may represent relief from anxiety as well as joy, e.g. childbirth, or on hearing that a breast lump is not malignant
>
> ◆ *Tears of anger* that 'come in bucketfuls' may be a result of a feeling of frustration with a problem at home, or perhaps with medical care; a treatment may not be working or an old complaint may be recurring; in women's health, cystitis and vaginal discharge are common causes for anger as these not only affect general health but are also closely tied up with sexual life. The anger is not only with the initial complaint, but also with themselves and their partner
>
> ◆ *Tears of sadness* that well out of the eyes and roll down the cheeks, despite the woman's attempts to control them, may make the nurse feel she has provoked sadness by an innocent enquiry. Loss is often the clue in such a situation. It may not be a recent event; the emotional pain may have been controlled not just for days or weeks but sometimes many years, e.g. the termination of an earlier pregnancy
>
> ◆ *Sobbing tears* where the whole body seems to be involved can occur in acute stress situations, e.g. divorce. The woman has felt perhaps for some considerable time that she must stay in control and when she meets someone who appears empathetic, it is then that she breaks down.

SCENARIO

Sandra, a young woman of 23, married for just two months, had come to see the nurse in the surgery. She was the last patient of a late clinic. When she was called in she shot through the door, sat down and burst into tears. The nurse held her hand and waited – not easy when time was short. Sandra blurted out that she didn't love her husband and nearly didn't marry him, but felt too frightened to say no. The nurse felt taken aback. Sandra then said she thought she might be pregnant. Her husband wanted a baby and they had not used contraception, but she didn't want a baby yet. The nurse thought he sounded most uncaring. The pregnancy test was indeed positive and Sandra revealed that her husband was in the waiting room. The nurse went to fetch him, and found a young man who appeared very concerned and quite different from her assumptions. She left them to talk together. The husband walked out as the nurse returned, and Sandra appeared calmer and said she wasn't going to have a termination. She and her husband then went in to see the doctor and on returning to the waiting room she flung her arms round the nurse saying 'thank you'.

For Sandra, the emotional upheaval of marriage and a quick pregnancy was just like receiving an electric shock: frightening and overwhelming. The nurse shared these emotions, she waited and used the skill of touch, a professional privilege, to 'stay' with Sandra throughout this encounter. The way Sandra said goodbye to the nurse was important, as she showed relief and grateful appreciation of her help and concern.

The covert presentation

Hidden and often unspoken anxieties will require all your skills of observation and listening, if you are to uncover the real problem.

Nurses are well trained in clinical observation, which is one of the early skills learnt in basic training, but psychosexual nursing observations are about the patient's feelings and emotional life; these require very perceptive antennae. Nurses sometimes feel that it is unprofessional and not part of the job to pry into women's sexual lives. This can be overcome with training and recognized as one of the defences we use to avoid the issue. A sensitive nurse should offer an opening for any patient to talk about her sexual health during a consultation.

The setting and first observations

This could be the surgery, the clinic, the outpatient department, the ward, the waiting room and even the corridor. The way she walks into the room and greets you can be an important clue. Who accompanies her? A child, children, her boyfriend, partner, husband or friend? How does she behave with them? What does she bring with her? Does she bring lots of bags? This may be only the shopping, but note how she organizes the bags; she may need support even from them. If she comes on her own, does she seem to be in control but not very confident? Could this be hiding some painful emotional feelings?

Appearance

Is she dressed appropriately for her age group? Does she dress up or down? Observe her make-up and appearance of her nails; if they are bitten it will often indicate anxiety. Hair, particularly for the young is an excellent curtain to hide behind. If you see someone regularly, note any changes from one visit to the next. You do not always have to verbalize your thoughts to the patient but appearances indicate mood and emotional changes as well as life changes. It may be useful to make a comment and acknowledge these changes.

Smell

This can be unpleasant and embarrassing both for the patient and for you. Is it the smell of a dirty body, unwashed or dirty clothes? Is it the smell of urine? If so, you could raise a question about her continence as she may suffer from stress incontinence which she has never felt able to discuss before. As all continence advisers will tell us, it is a common problem which affects all age groups and once the question has been raised and incontinence acknowledged, help is often gratefully received (see Chapter 17).

Alcohol on the breath may well be a sign of a problem, especially if the time of day appears to be inappropriate. Alcohol and drugs are widely used to help both short-term anxieties and long-term emotional problems, but they also can cause havoc with people's sexual lives.

SCENARIO

Sally was a professional woman aged 36 and held a responsible administrative job. She appeared tired and overweight. She had come for a repeat pill prescription. The nurse noticed a smell of alcohol on her breath although it was mid-morning. Sally said that although she and her partner both worked for the same organization they hardly ever saw each other. On enquiry from the nurse, she also admitted there was hardly any sexual life. She was worried about her recent increase of weight and admitted that her eating habits were erratic as she was always home late and her partner was even later. She was a non-smoker which then led to the nurse enquiring about her drinking habits. She had to entertain at lunchtime – often with wine – and had a drink again when she got home in the evening. On discussing this she was shocked to realize that over the last 6 months she had started with one glass of wine in the evening but now quite frequently finished the bottle by herself. Her health and sexual life were in jeopardy, and the small clue to this unhappiness was the faint whiff of alcohol mid-morning that the nurse had noticed and sensitively enquired about.

Facial expressions

The eyes often give the clue – sad, flashing, defiant, or unable to look at you. Look at the face as you talk to your patient and obtain information from her. Note any change in facial expressions – all the emotions can be expressed, ranging from excitement to sadness. The nose that wrinkles, as in a family planning consultation, where the nurse learnt from the young girl that they were using condoms as she had a new boyfriend. She knew that the nurse was expecting to hear that they were practising safer sex, but the nurse noted the nose twitch and the brief downward look. On commenting 'You don't look very happy about that' she learnt the true story where the condom was not always used and a gamble was consequently taking place for both infection and contraception. One small sign gave the observant nurse the opportunity to discuss other methods of contraception and the importance of safer sex.

Common sexual anxieties and problems

Women come to you to seek and receive professional help, information and advice, often with the added pressure of expecting you to find a solution for them. In psychosexual nursing the patient has to find the solution for herself, but you can help her. Women frequently present with problems that seem irrelevant and this can confuse both of you. You should try to sift out and clarify what is relevant to your nursing role. The importance of identifying the real anxiety becomes your primary task, whether it is physical, emotional or a combination of both. Nichols (2003) suggests 'this is the task of making oneself aware of the patient's psychological state' and he goes on to look at the reality of the situation and comments 'it is more an issue of attitudes, value and style'.

The feelings that adversely affect a woman's sexuality are summarized in Box 5.2.

The encounter can be uncomfortable for both of you and patience may be required as usually nothing significant will be revealed if the woman is feeling hassled. Silence may hide the distress of a woman struggling with her inner feelings which she feels are unspeakable. Try not to be afraid of this silence, bear with it and more often than not you will be rewarded with a response.

Many events and changes in women's lives only cause temporary sexual anxieties and not long-lasting problems. They are certainly more likely to be temporary if they are discussed early on rather than later or not at all.

Sexual anxieties and problems are often classified as being *primary* or *secondary*. Primary problems have been present since the start of sexual activity whereas secondary problems develop after a period of satisfactory sexual function. Common forms of sexual anxiety and dysfunction are listed in Table 5.1.

Loss of libido

Loss of libido is defined as absence of interest and lack of sexual arousal. It is sometimes referred to as 'feeling frigid'. This is a common complaint and many women have a feeling of failure both for themselves and their partners.

Primary lack of sexual libido may be the result of difficulty during early sexual maturation, e.g. child sexual abuse or rape.

Box 5.2 Feelings that adversely affect a woman's sexuality

Misunderstanding about sex
- Ignorance about sex
- Not knowing what to expect
- Not knowing how to behave
- Expectations too high.

Bad feelings about sex
- Fear of being caught
- Fear of making too much noise and being overheard
- Fear of being interrupted
- Fear of failing to perform 'normally'
- Fear of being undignified or incontinent
- Guilty, believing that sexual intercourse or sexual acts are wrong
- Disgust that sex is dirty and messy.

Problems in the relationship
- Feeling angry, even rage and violence
- Feeling resentful and bitter
- Feeling contempt for a partner
- Feeling insecure
- Fear of being physically hurt
- Fear of partner leaving
- Fear of the future.

Bad feelings from women
- Depression
- Worthlessness
- Low self-esteem
- Unattractive
- Unhappy with her body image.

Circumstances which cause lack of sexual feelings
- Too tired
- Worried
- Preoccupied with other things
- Babies and children of all ages
- Lack of warmth and comfort
- Losses and bereavement
- No privacy.

Table 5.1 Sexual anxiety and dysfunction	
DYSFUNCTION	**CAUSE**
Loss of libido	Emotional
Dyspareunia	Physical and emotional
Vaginismus	Physical and emotional
Dry vagina	Physical and emotional
Orgasmic dysfunction	Emotional

Secondary lack of libido presents more frequently, and is likely to be associated with either current life events or a past emotional or physical event. Women may also feel generally depressed with their current situation. Such situations could include:

◆ Difficulties in a relationship with poor communication between the couple

◆ Infertility problems

◆ Pregnancy, birth and postnatal problems

◆ Redundancy, job failure or career changes

◆ Retirement and ageing

◆ Bereavement

◆ Losses, e.g. leaving home, selling and moving house

◆ Anxieties over medical problems and ill-health

◆ Gynaecological problems including cervical cell changes and the effects of colposcopy.

It is often the anger, frustration and resentment at the above situations which leads to a withdrawal of feelings to have a sexual relationship. Gentle enquiries such as 'I wonder how *you* felt about that situation?' are often gratefully accepted and can clarify the problem for you and your patient. Remember it is your patient's feelings that are often transferred to you, and you should stay 'alongside' her and understand her feelings rather than try to reassure her (Clifford, 2000).

Dyspareunia

Dyspareunia is pain during or after sexual intercourse. This can occur for pathological reasons and a clinical cause such as infection should be

SCENARIO

Carol came to the surgery to have a cut finger dressed. She was well known to the nurse and asked if she remembered telling her last time that 'she felt nothing when making love'. The nurse did not remember the remark but she did this time!

Carol was now 6 months postnatal after her third child and commented 'I never felt like this after the other two'. The nurse offered to examine Carol and noticed that the episiotomy had healed well with no pain but Carol then said her vagina felt 'numb'. The nurse felt baffled, just as Carol felt, so suggested she should return for some counselling. It was then that Carol said very angrily that would be impossible as she was having to move across the country because of her husband's job. The nurse recognized and identified with her this feeling of anger, which led on to Carol saying she did not want to leave this happy neighbourhood and all her friends, but had to move as the house was now sold. The discussion that followed made her realize she was also angry with her husband, leaving her no desire to make love as well as having a 'numb' vagina.

The nurse's skill during this encounter was to work with the angry feelings of Carol which were only revealed when the nurse examined her. A relatively minor complaint may cover and disguise a far larger problem and may only be revealed when the woman has found a sympathetic listener.

investigated first. You should find out the type of pain:

◆ Superficial pain at the introitus

◆ On penetration of the penis into the vagina

◆ On deep penetration

◆ Marked tenderness of the cervix to movement of the penis in the vagina

◆ Chronic illness – particularly back pain.

Dyspareunia can also be an expression of emotional pain causing muscle tension. If digital vaginal examination shows there is no evidence or expression of pain from the woman, then further enquiries may reveal the true anxiety. Factors leading to dyspareunia can include:

◆ Parental influence

◆ Past sexual experiences

◆ Termination of pregnancy

Diane, a 22-year-old, came to the nurse complaining of pain on intercourse for the last 9 months. She was in a loving relationship but now 'dreaded' having intercourse. The nurse asked when they last had sex and was told that it was over a month ago and it had been very infrequent since she had a colposcopy 9 months previously. The nurse wondered if that had been the problem, as Diane described the experience of colposcopy as 'quite a shock as it was so painful'. The nurse shared this experience with her and explained the necessity for colposcopy treatment. Diane described the pain as 'being outside and very sore as he entered'. She was examined by the doctor who identified some slight soreness of the fourchette and prescribed salt baths and a short treatment of oestrogen cream to aid healing. The nurse then went on to discuss with Diane her fear of sex and of her boyfriend hurting her, and why she had waited so long to discuss this. An appointment was made to return in 2 weeks to see the nurse. When she returned the pain had gone and Diane described having sexual intercourse as 'great again'.

Here the problem was identified by the patient but she needed both prescriptive help and emotional help from the nurse. To make a brief follow-up appointment to share the outcome is always a good idea as it will encourage you in future consultations with patients with similar problems. If the problem had not been resolved then more skilled psychosexual counselling and help should be made available.

◆ Childbirth

◆ Previous gynaecological disease

◆ Fear of cancer

◆ Ill health

◆ Feeling inadequate as a sexual partner.

Vaginismus

Vaginismus occurs when there is an involuntary spasm of the muscle surrounding the lower third of the vagina, making penetration difficult or impossible. It is often described as 'a blockage' and experienced as pain, representing an unconscious expression about a woman's vagina.

Primary vaginismus indicates there has been no penetration of the vagina by the woman herself or the penis. Non-consummation is no penetration

of the vagina in a sexual partnership. The sexual response of the woman in all other ways may be normal; she can be orgasmic and makes use of other sexual expressions to satisfy her sexual needs, e.g. masturbation and oral sex. This can leave her partner feeling impotent and may also lead to some erectile dysfunction. A woman may often disclose this problem after some years in a partnership when there is a wish to start a family, or in starting a new relationship where a previous relationship has not been consummated. A lot of courage may have been required for a woman to disclose this failure in her sexual relationship. Specialist psychosexual counselling should always be offered and an appropriate referral made if you meet this problem.

Secondary vaginismus may take place after sexual or emotional trauma, including sexual abuse, rape or a traumatic gynaecological experience or examination. Other causes include:

◆ Infertility investigations and the demands of treatments

◆ Discharges and vaginal infections – the vagina is felt to be dirty

◆ Fantasies of thinking the vagina is too small or the penis will damage the inside

◆ Ante- and postnatal anxieties

◆ After hysterectomy or bladder surgery

◆ Anxiety about contraception.

You should try to explore the feelings surrounding vaginismus and the anxiety it poses for the individual woman. It can be helpful for her to explore or re-explore her vagina with your help as described on page 93.

Dry vagina

If the natural vaginal secretions are reduced for any reason then penetration can be uncomfortable and painful. The emotional reasons stated under dyspareunia will also cause a feeling of dryness. Sexual stimulation may be unsatisfactory and foreplay may be either too slow or too quick and the woman not sufficiently sexually aroused. For peri- and post-menopausal women the physical complaint of the vagina becoming dry and tight is due to a fall in oestrogen levels and can be treated by local or systemic oestrogen. Water-based jellies and lubricants are an alternative treatment for some women. There may also be other changes going on in their lives which will require emotional care and support.

Orgasmic dysfunction

Orgasmic dysfunction means difficulty in having an orgasm despite a normal sexual responsiveness, and only becomes a problem when the woman regards it as such. Orgasm can occur through stimulation by a partner or from self-masturbation and is a unique experience which makes it difficult to define and where a loss of control will take place.

Sometimes a woman may enquire what an orgasm is or how she can become orgasmic. You can discuss with her that you cannot make her orgasmic: this often leads to laughter and a release of tension. You can also enquire about what else is happening in her life (both past and present) and start to uncover her anxieties and listen to any contributory factors that she may express such as:

◆ She has high expectations aroused by the media, but in real life orgasm seems ordinary

◆ Orgasm does not happen as frequently as she wishes

◆ She never has vaginal orgasm but comes before or after penetration

◆ They do not 'come together'

◆ Their sexual technique is poor or inadequate

◆ She has a real fear of losing control and 'letting go'

◆ She feels she is abnormal and simulates orgasm to protect her self-esteem.

Postnatal lack of orgasm is common, and is hardly surprising with the many changes that have taken place: tiredness, breastfeeding, physical discomfort, as well as the birth itself which may not have been as she wished (see Chapter 8). Anorgasmia is a disappointment and the woman may feel she is failing her partner.

SCENARIO

Pat had recently registered at the surgery, so was unknown to the nurse. She called Pat in to her room where she sat very upright with her hands clasped, her face quite expressionless apart from the occasional wry smile. The nurse felt uncomfortable but asked how she could help. Pat said 'I want help with my sex life'. Pat then told her she was 39 years old and had a previous relationship of 8 years, but she now had a new boyfriend and she had never had an orgasm. She then sat back and waited. The nurse wondered where to start. She asked some questions but all Pat replied was 'I don't know'. The nurse felt quite irritated by this behaviour and felt that her enquiries and the negative responses were getting nowhere. She suggested she should make an appointment to see the counsellor in the surgery which was accepted by Pat. The nurse, reflecting on the encounter later on, realized that this degree of control by Pat and denial of any feelings was going to make it very difficult for her to become orgasmic. Perhaps deep down there was some hidden pain which never allowed her to 'let go'.

Defence mechanisms for nurses and patients

When working in the field of women's sexual health, both nurses and patients put up barriers. These act as a means of defence against working with emotional feelings and any pain involved in the consultation. These barriers protect you and your patient from discomfort. It is often difficult at the time of the consultation to identify what is happening and why the encounter may not be going too well, but a clue can often be found in the ebb and flow of communication which takes place during the consultation. Nichols (2003) urges health care practitioners 'to make sure that some exploratory initiatives have been taken to give "permission" for sexual issues to be included on the agenda'. The interest that you and your patient show in each other can range from boredom to being over-anxious. It is therefore important that you, the nurse, recognize these defences and how they affect verbal and non-verbal communication. They should be treated with respect and not dismissed as a sign of failure. This then allows you to make changes in your nursing practice, to accept and work with defensive as well as positive feelings.

You arrive at work with the same variety of emotions as patients have when they come to see you. Sometimes you feel well and on top form, and other days you arrive feeling strained and stressed. You may have left ill children, the child-minder has arrived late, there are financial anxieties, a row with your partner, bereavement or any other event that upsets the routine. Your professional training enables you to continue to work with people when you feel like this, but such training is aimed at giving information, advice and using well-practised skills and techniques to give treatment. Talking about sexual health is different as this is about exploring and discovering reality with your patient. The demands that come from your patient may be overwhelming for you, and you can experience a feeling of helplessness and uselessness and not wanting to be involved. Then what do you do? Frequently you may try to make things better by talking too much or asking lots of closed questions, desperately hoping to find a solution. The responses often reveal irrelevant information and you and your patient may feel you are getting nowhere. A referral may be made which can be equally unhelpful and the moment for helping your patient is lost and her anxiety has not been explored. The patient feels let down, and often dissatisfied. It is these defences that you may use that you need to recognize in your day-to-day work with your patients.

Reassurance

How often do you read the word 'reassured' in medical notes? What does it mean? What has been offered to the patient? Reassurance implies that the patient requires comfort, and therefore there is some worry, anxiety or even anger. The facts behind this anxiety may be unknown or felt too awful to communicate. Inevitably this can increase anxiety and not allay it. Physiological and pathological questions can be answered by clinical knowledge; but with sexuality, where the emotional pain and anxieties are often hidden,

'reassurance' is easier to record. If you see this in your patient's notes, refer back to the initial consultation and make another enquiry. The problem may not be so acute but often it has not been fully resolved or understood by the patient or the professional.

Lack of time

Lack of time is another major defence that nurses tend to use. Even a brief amount of time if carefully planned can be used effectively for your patient. It is the quality of time given and not the quantity that is important (Balint and Norell, 1973). The excuse of 'lack of time' is frequently used to avoid listening and hearing the spoken or unspoken cry for help from your patient. Of course it is not only nurses who have this excuse; patients may often use the same defence – pleading that they are in a hurry rather than verbalize a problem. They may also appear to want to have a social chat, rather than asking for your professional help. You should remember that your patients are often busy as well and may have waited to see you, and to use the consultation time for 'social chat' may be an 'avoiding technique' for you both. The disciplined use of time by using appropriate and professional remarks at the introduction as well as during the consultation and at its conclusion can be very effective. It is easy to find an excuse not to have time for your patient when you have a waiting room full of people, or are working on a busy ward.

You may feel that talking about sexuality will take even more time. Why does it feel like that? It seems easier for nurses to ask women about their last menstrual period or when their bowels were open, details that are just as intimate for the patient concerned, than to ask about their sexual life. Because sexual maturation has often not been recognized as an integral part of health care, then 'lack of time' will continue to be used as an excuse not to discuss the matter. When you are able routinely to include sexuality in your care, it is seen to be time well spent for both you and your patient. The importance of being punctual and keeping to the boundaries is as important for your patient as it is for you. The sharing of limited time becomes disciplined and the offer to continue the discussion later will always be appropriate. You may be disappointed if your patient fails to return, but it may not necessarily be for negative reasons; your patient could have had time to think, reflect and feel positive about her initial consultation with you.

Lack of confidence

Sexuality is frequently not raised as an issue because you fear you will be 'out of your depth', 'make the situation worse' or you feel that you 'cannot offer a solution'. This lack of confidence can make you think and feel that only 'experts' talk about sexuality. This is not true as women choose the place and 'the face' where they feel comfortable and able to discuss everyday emotions about their sexuality and feelings. They will not usually talk about sexual dysfunction and rarely about sexual deviation, but will often wish to share the emotional feelings surrounding sexuality. During a vaginal examination, how often do you hear colleagues say 'just relax'? Try to do the same when discussing sexuality with a patient – relax and be yourself, and realize there is no need to feel out of depth or to produce a solution. Women generally respond very positively when they meet a nurse who is uninhibited, sensitive and flexible in approach. It is rewarding to try.

Lack of privacy

Lack of privacy can act as another excuse not to open or even respond to a question about sexual health. Sexuality is a private area and Dr Margaret Gill comments in her chapter 'Defences in the patient': 'The private parts are not so called for nothing' (Gill, 1989). There are degrees of privacy for everyone, depending on our upbringing and circumstances. As nurses we perform daily tasks which are very intimate, such as: washing a patient, cleaning the incontinent, passing a catheter, dressing a surgical wound such as a mastectomy or colostomy, vaginal examination, passing a speculum and treatment of sexually transmitted infections. The midwife has similar tasks: examination and delivery of a baby followed by postnatal care of the perineum and breasts. Sometimes these tasks

are performed with only curtains as a barrier but the patient may still choose such a moment to confide in you. This can sometimes be identified as 'a moment of truth' when she is enabled to talk about her inner feelings, where intimacy and touch by you are the releasing factors. Some women do not feel the need to wait and find privacy; they can accost nurses in the corridor, the waiting room or even in the supermarket. It is usually only *your* feelings of embarrassment and intrusion that get in the way. It is the woman's choice when to talk about an anxiety and acknowledgement of this is always appropriate, but it must be your professional judgement that decides about future consultations. Your offer of finding privacy may be brushed aside with a comment such as 'I just wanted to ask you now', and once again the moment may be lost for the patient.

Finding a solution

The need to find a solution for your patient's anxieties could mean that you start advising on techniques in sexual nursing for which you have not been trained. The works of Masters and Johnson (1970) and their techniques (a behaviourist therapy) are frequently quoted and offered by nurses to their patients because it is seen to be constructive and therefore better than nothing. This is not good practice, as all recognized therapies require training, practice and supervision before they are offered to patients. The important factor that enables you to move forward in psychosexual nursing is to realize that you do not need to find a solution for your patient and the anxiety should always belong to the patient and not to you. Be available to listen, share and reflect on what you hear but remember your role is to facilitate your patient finding her own solution.

Referral

It is well recognized that some doctors use the prescription pad as a defence mechanism when they are running late or do not know the answer to a patient's problems. This excuse is not generally available to nurses, so instead of prescribing nurses may suggest to the patient that they should see the doctor to ask their discomforting questions. Some doctors have training in psychosexual skills just as some nurses are trained, but many have no more skills than nurses and their perception and experience of patients are the same. Again, you should ask yourself 'Why did the patient choose me?' Do you have skills you fail or choose not to recognize? Do you fear that colleagues will mark you out as 'the nurse who always deals with sex problems'? You may feel the need for additional training to increase your skills (see page 97). In psychosexual nursing it is always worth trying 'to stay' with the woman rather than referring her, but be aware of the defences from you both that may hinder or stop your work. It is never easy, often painful but immensely satisfying and rewarding for both you and your patient.

Approaches to vaginal examination

Throughout women's lives the vaginal examination is one of the most frequent and intimate examinations by the medical and nursing profession. It should never become routine but, as is discussed here, should be observed and thoughtful each time it is undertaken. Vaginal examination is a skill for all nurses and midwives to learn, practise and revise when necessary and it can then become a basis for psychosexual nursing. It has been well documented that a vaginal examination can often offer 'the moment of truth' for women who have troubled sexuality (Tunnadine, 1970, 1992).

In medical practice, vaginal examination is usually done to exclude pelvic pathology or to assess progress during labour. In nursing it is possible to use a vaginal examination as an extension of your psychosexual nursing skills. In such cases it becomes therapeutic and can help both you and your patient towards a better understanding of a problem and for some women the revealing of a hidden difficulty. The examination does not necessarily have to be a bimanual examination but can be a digital examination or the passing of a speculum or only the examination of the external genitalia. You may notice a degree of vaginismus. Nurses and midwives may need to involve the doctor in order to make a clinical diagnosis and if a woman requests a doctor then her wish must be respected. More often than not women are only too pleased to have continuity of care from the nurse to whom they initially revealed their anxiety.

Occasionally women will ask for a vaginal examination when it is not appropriate. Some reasons for this are listed in Box 5.3. Clearly, a valid indication for a vaginal examination should be established before the procedure is started.

Observations

It is relevant to notice the woman's reaction to the suggestion of a vaginal examination and the defences she may put up to avoid it such as:

◆ Menstruation at repeated visits
◆ 'I haven't washed'
◆ 'I'm in a hurry today'
◆ Arriving late for an appointment
◆ Keeping her pants on as she gets on the couch.

All of these can be observed and an appropriate comment made which can allow the woman to voice an anxiety. It is not always possible to predict how a woman will react to a vaginal examination. Women who you think could be difficult to examine may lie back, appear relaxed and 'behave' perfectly.

Box 5.3 Some reasons why women come for examination where it may not be appropriate

◆ Some women want to be examined to be told they are normal
◆ Some women feel they *should* be examined. Are they missing out? What have they lost? Perhaps the loss of never having had sexual intercourse?
◆ They receive a request to have a cervical smear. Compliance seems to be important for them although there is no clinical indication for a smear as no vaginal intercourse has ever taken place.

On the other hand, it may only be when an examination is attempted on an outwardly relaxed woman that you realize she may have difficulties. There is no guarantee that if previous examinations caused no problems that the woman's behaviour will be 'perfect' on a subsequent examination. All nurses, whether they are observing, chaperoning or performing examinations, should be alert and observe any distress signs at each particular occasion.

There is acceptable and unacceptable behaviour during an examination. A very detached, uncaring attitude from your patient where there appears to be no modesty, may indicate that she really does not value her sexuality or her vagina. She almost 'throws it away' and can make you feel uncomfortable at the lack of some degree of modesty. Too much modesty, on the other hand, may be indicated by vaginismus, abductor spasms, moving up the couch as you approach, the lifting of buttocks and arching the back off the couch, as well as a verbal expectation of pain. All these reactions arouse different feelings in you, which may include sympathy, impatience, annoyance and occasionally anger. If you are sensitive and have gained insight and understanding then you can share and enquire about these feelings with her rather than being tempted to ask a barrage of questions and ignore your patient's verbal and non-verbal signs. The examination can then have a positive outcome for your patient. Her attitude at the time may indeed also be a clue to the way she affects her partner, or vice versa, and more may be gained if this issue is discussed during the examination rather than waiting until later.

Preparation for examinations

Your patient should be adequately prepared for an examination by a clear explanation of the procedure as well as by discussing any fears and anxieties she may have. There are many myths, even nowadays, about vaginal examinations and it is relevant to discuss her attitude to menstruation and her experience of sexual intercourse. Never make an assumption that your patient is or has been sexually active but ask

SCENARIO

Maria was complaining to the nurse of soreness and feeling dry during intercourse. The nurse noted a history of recent thrush and genital warts which had been treated and Maria had been given the 'all-clear'. During the discussion Maria said quite angrily 'He gave it to me'. The nurse offered to look again but Maria was reluctant and said 'I've been examined so much'. The nurse encouraged her to have another examination and the vulva and vagina showed no indication of soreness or dryness. The nurse wondered 'what was going on here' and remembered the anger in Maria's answers. She enquired how Maria felt about her partner and learnt that she was very angry with him for 'infecting her' as she said. A short discussion followed where they felt it could be the emotional anger with him which was making intercourse uncomfortable and Maria acknowledged that the nurse's examination did not hurt. The anger and fury (soreness and dryness) really got in the way of her sexual life and the nurse was able to make this interpretation with Maria.

'Have you ever had sexual intercourse?' If the reply is 'no' then the reason for coming for an examination can be discussed. Vaginal examination in a woman who is sexually active and sexually mature is usually achieved with few problems.

Preparation can also include:

◆ Showing the woman a speculum if she wishes, and explaining that it is smaller than a penis

◆ Warming the speculum

◆ Using a hand mirror to look at the genitalia or the cervix when the speculum is in position

◆ Allowing the woman to insert the speculum herself.

The flexibility of your approach is the secret of success. Sadly, insensitive examinations all too frequently take place, leaving women with anxieties about vaginal examination that are never forgotten. It can be similar to an experience of violent intercourse and the mental and physical pain will always be remembered.

During the examination

Women must be asked to lie in a comfortable position. The dorsal position is the most common, with the shoulders off the pillow and easy access to a light. It is also easier for you to observe the non-verbal communication of your patient. Some gynaecologists use the left lateral position and in some instances this position is necessary for clinical reasons. It may be helpful to insert a finger before insertion of the speculum so that the size of the introitus can be assessed and the position of the cervix identified before taking a cervical smear.

At this point it may be useful to assess the woman's attitude towards her vagina by asking a few careful questions (Box 5.4). You may suggest that it is quite acceptable and normal for a woman to explore her vagina and that she can try it now or in private at home if she wishes. She might need a simple anatomy lesson first and is often grateful for this as she feels she should know more about herself but is frightened to reveal her own ignorance. A simple diagram can be helpful as well as describing the best position to feel inside, e.g. by putting one foot on a chair or by squatting on her heels and inserting one or two fingers into the vagina in a downward direction towards the floor.

There is no right or wrong way for self-examination but you should aim to make it acceptable and achievable for your patient. Sadly for some, self-examination remains abhorrent despite referral and skilled help.

During a vaginal examination you can talk to the woman and ask her to perform simple tasks to help you. Perhaps you could ask her to:

◆ Put her hands underneath her buttocks to tilt her pelvis if the cervix is difficult to visualize

◆ Contract and relax the vaginal muscles and introitus

◆ Bear down to aid removal of the speculum

◆ Cough to expose the cervix.

Women often express hidden feelings by asking questions or making comments:

◆ 'How big is the vagina?'

◆ 'My vagina seems too small' (or too big)

◆ 'My vagina is dry'

◆ 'My partner seems to be very big'

◆ 'It starts to sting and hurt as he goes in'

◆ 'It always seems so messy'

◆ 'I don't like using contraception'

◆ 'I wish he would use a condom'

◆ 'I never seem to "come"'

◆ 'I often think of other things when *he* makes love'.

If a woman complains of dyspareunia, this should always be explored by asking:

◆ At what stage of intercourse does she feel the pain (e.g. penetration or with deep movement)?

◆ Can she describe the pain?

◆ Is the pain worse in some positions than others?

Clinical problems

Pathology must be excluded and this might require examination by a doctor. If tests and investigations are necessary, these in themselves

---

Box 5.4 Questions you could use that may reveal a woman's attitude towards her vagina

◆ *'Do you use tampons with an applicator?'* The use of these indicates that she feels able to insert something into her vagina and feels no blockage. However, there is a cardboard tube and therefore no need to actually feel inside the vagina

◆ *'Do you use tampons without an applicator?'* With these there will be finger contact with the introitus and vagina. Some women will say they have tried without success and 'it hurt'. If they want to try again a simple explanation, usually of the direction to push the tampon, is all that is required

◆ *'Have you ever felt inside your vagina?'* The answer may be 'no' and implies that the woman may think that part of her is private and not your business, or she may feel unsure of your reaction if she says 'yes'. She may think she should not feel inside or you may think her 'dirty'.

often give rise to further anxiety. If there is no clinical reason for dyspareunia it is helpful to find out what might be getting in the way.

Vaginal fantasies

Many women have fantasies about their vagina, which can get in the way both of sexual intercourse and vaginal examination. These fantasies are not controlled by factual knowledge and although she may know her anatomy, she feels that *her* vagina is different.

Women may ask questions which can offer a clue to these fantasies, such as 'Where does it go to?' 'Is it really very small?' or 'Are the walls rigid?' She may describe her vagina as dark, dirty, disgusting, messy or red and raw – all bad feelings. The good feelings of the vagina like 'velvet', 'soft and comfortable' or 'soft and crinkly' and 'it feels surprisingly familiar just like the inside of the mouth' are also sometimes expressed.

Perhaps a woman thinks her vagina is remote and does not belong to her, so how does she give or offer it to anyone else? She may feel she needs to be given permission to use her vagina. Does marriage give permission? Sometimes being a virgin before marriage is important for religious or cultural reasons. Others may have tried to have sexual intercourse before marriage and failed, but hope that when they get married everything will be different. Sadly, this is often not the case. The woman feels a failure and finds it difficult to seek help. You may be tempted to 'take over' and can give inappropriate instructions in a desperate attempt to improve the situation. Logical thought and explanations are really not effective against illogical, inexpressible fears and fantasies about the vagina. You should refer these women to a skilled psychosexual counsellor for help.

Disclosure of sexual abuse by women in adulthood

Violence against women and children is also discussed in Chapters 6 and 8. Although it has become more common for nurses to hear about sexual abuse, both physical and verbal, it still remains a shock when a woman discloses this.

Media publicity has made it less of a taboo subject, but that does not mean that women find it easy to make a disclosure of sexual abuse. Their secrets are often deeply buried and have been hidden for many years in their emotional minds. It may seem easier not to expose themselves to the pain that will have to be revealed if the experience is shared with someone else. Some women, however, have been able to have the strength to talk about their experiences and draw attention to the crime of child abuse.

Women who have been sexually abused are all victims: how they cope with the trauma of abuse varies. Some may feel the need to protect themselves by dressing and behaving in a sexually provocative manner, but in subsequent relationships find they are unable to be a sexual person for fear of arousing memories of their previous experiences. The disclosure of abuse may come through the presentation of a psychosexual anxiety or problem. They may have made many appointments and tried to drop hints about their emotional distress but these have not been 'picked up'. You may suspect a problem and it may be appropriate to enquire gently whether they have been abused in the past.

A change in a woman's life or a crisis may become a trigger point that enables her to talk. Your attitude and sensitivity could enable her to say something that may indicate her secret. A disclosure cannot be ignored, and your client may have expectations that as a health professional you have expert knowledge and the ability to help her. It is much more likely, however, that you will be working from ignorance and the disclosure of childhood sexual abuse leaves you feeling shocked and confused as to how you can best help her. It is important to keep these normal feelings of shock, distress, anger and condemnation to yourself as her story is heard.

Childhood abuse can be physical or verbal and the abuser often implicitly or explicitly threatens the child to ensure secrecy. Discussion with a caring professional can enable the woman to sort out what she remembers and whether it was physical abuse, mental torture or a combination of both. It is then that she can decide how to proceed and if she requires ongoing help.

Some women, when disclosing their violation, may find some excitement and arousal from recounting their experiences. Afterwards they may feel guilty, helpless and ashamed, causing them to become defensive of their situation. The health practitioner will also produce her own defences against these feelings. Initially, the emotions may seem to be overwhelming, making it difficult to listen to the story and think clearly. But, if these feelings are acknowledged by the professional, they can then be shared with the woman and recognized as a normal sexual response, despite being in an abusive situation.

Each woman has to find her own way back to remember the feelings of being abused: this will then allow her some healing and resolution of her distress and guilt. Most victims will have some remaining emotional pain and unpleasant memories, but are relieved in having shared the pain they have lived with for many years. The emotions may include:

◆ Helplessness
◆ Powerlessness
◆ Violation
◆ Betrayal
◆ Guilt
◆ Excitement – sexual feelings
◆ Inability to blame the abuser.

Wakeley (1991) says: 'It would be wrong to conclude that everybody who has had these experiences suffers to the same degree or has the same long term problems'. Briere (1984) suggests that some suffer the long-term effects of sexual abuse or 'a post sexual abuse syndrome'. These women can be demanding and require considerable support, but this may also increase the powerlessness of the individual and their dependency on the professionals: it is important to make some clear boundaries to prevent this happening.

Doyle (1994) says: 'People are born with different characteristics and have varying degrees of resilience' and continues: 'sexual abuse is not the only childhood experience that can cause difficulty as they mature'. Other traumas experienced, such as the loss of mother or father, ill-health or the experience of war, may be easier to talk about more freely without the embarrassment of talking about sexual matters.

The effects of post-traumatic stress disorder, discussed later in this chapter, may also apply to those suffering from childhood sexual abuse. Any treatment will require the professional to understand the importance of concentrating and listening to the history of the woman's unique relationships and sexual life.

Helpful suggestions that could be offered to victims of childhood sexual abuse include:

◆ Talking with a health professional
◆ Referral to a specialist therapist or counsellor
◆ Joining a group of survivors
◆ Books or tapes which they can use in their own time
◆ Doctor's appointment for advice on a prescription of antidepressants
◆ Relaxation and stress-relieving techniques.

As a professional, you may also wish to have the chance to talk through this experience in a supervision session. This would support you and become a learning experience for others.

Psychosexual referrals

The reason for referral to a psychosexual counsellor must be established between you and your patient before referral is made and the woman must be willing to see someone else. She should be encouraged to make her own appointment as this gives her some control and then she is more likely to keep this appointment. Waiting lists for psychosexual counselling are often long, and in some cases this is due to women who are unwilling or not yet ready for counselling. Some women may have previously sought advice or had counselling, often over a period of years, and it is important to find out why this was not satisfactory before making another referral. Some women 'do the rounds', which is not necessarily their fault as previous referrals for help may have been inappropriate. When women become desperate for help they may self-refer to an agency or therapist, often at great expense to themselves. In vain, women try to seek help from various people; some of these will be skilled but others may be unskilled and offer dubious therapy, with a poor outcome.

Psychosexual help within the National Health Service is very patchy and there will often be long waiting lists. Some GPs, family planning and hospital doctors have undertaken seminar training, a psychodynamic approach under the Institute of Psychosexual Medicine, but the counselling offered is not intended to be an extended therapy. Such sessions are held in GP surgeries, family planning clinics and in some hospitals. Nurses may also have the opportunity to work alongside doctors as independent psychosexual nurse counsellors in some areas.

Counsellors or social workers in primary care, community or hospital clinics may only offer general counselling and do not necessarily work with their patient's sexuality, although some community psychiatric nurses may offer sexual counselling. Before referring any woman to a counsellor it is important that you establish how the counsellor works and whether they are capable of working with sexual anxieties.

Some women are unfortunately referred to busy gynaecological departments, where staff change frequently and clinical problems are examined and discussed, but the emotional anxieties associated with the complaint are rarely addressed. In hospital, with the high turnover of inpatients and busy outpatient departments, you may observe and hear of sexual anxieties, but these will usually have a low priority over other more pressing problems.

Although you wish to make a referral you may feel restricted because of a lack of knowledge and contacts in your district. Where troubled sexuality is identified, communication must be made between professionals. Where you know of no counselling facilities, you can alert the GP, district nurse, health visitor or community midwife by letter or by a personal telephone call rather than leaving the problem and hoping that someone else will 'pick up the pieces'! Nurse specialists with counselling skills play a very important role, particularly the breast counsellor, continence adviser, stoma adviser, infertility counsellor and

family planning nurse specialists. The conditions presented to these advisers can have an impact on all aspects of sexuality.

Outside the NHS there are many counsellors with a wide variety of training and experience. Again, before referring it is important to check what they offer as many may only give general counselling and do not necessarily work with sexual anxieties. Find out how they work and whether they would be suitable for a particular woman's problem. There will be fees to pay so it is important that you have up-to-date information.

Relate has trained psychosexual counsellors offering a behaviourist therapy. All clients are assessed before being accepted for a course of therapy and it is normal practice to be seen as a couple. They also have marital and reconciliation counselling where they will see single people. Some Relate offices are able to offer an assessment in a crisis situation. Donations or fees are required for their services.

To summarize, it is helpful to keep a list of counsellors, agencies and services available for appropriate help in your locality. Use the checklist in Box 5.5 to obtain relevant information.

Finally, if it is possible, arrange to meet those offering the service, and see where they work. Then you can give first-hand information to your patient and be sure that you are sending her to the right place. With the difficulty of finding

---

Box 5.5 Questions to ask of counsellors, agencies and services

1. Who is available?
2. Where are they?
3. When do they work – days and times?
4. How long is the waiting list?
5. What sort of therapy or treatment do they offer?
6. What type of training have the counsellors received?
7. Do they offer short- or long-term therapy?
8. How do you refer a woman?
9. Do they make an assessment first and then decide to offer therapy?
10. What payment is required, or is it free?

skilled help, it is even more necessary nowadays for you to know what is available and if it is appropriate for the individual woman or couple.

Training in psychosexual nursing

In order to be effective, training in psychosexual nursing has to be tailored to your role as a nurse. The skills learned must be relevant and possible to use in your day-to-day clinical practice. Expectations that training will give you answers and make you an expert must be dispelled. A knowledge of emotional development and an understanding of sexual maturation (see Chapter 1) is important, just as the knowledge of anatomy and physiology is essential for clinical nursing. Skill is needed to communicate effectively with all women about sexual matters whether they are well or unwell, and you will need continuing opportunities where the individual nurse/patient relationships can be studied to assess and develop these skills. There is very little training in psychosexual nursing in the UK, so it is a bonus when sexual care is well integrated into pre- and post-registration courses. Training is expensive and nurses often have to find the finances themselves. Sadly, nurses who wish to gain psychosexual skills have to 'fight' to be heard by their managers and educators. Holistic care is difficult to measure and unfortunately 'value for money' is frequently measured in terms of quantity of patients and not quality of care.

It is necessary to recognize that in psychosexual nursing your role is not the same as the doctor, the social worker or the counsellor. But like doctors, you have the privilege and ability to touch, examine and treat women intimately. Female patients perceive you to be a 'carer' and will trust and confide in you. This can provide you with the opportunity to make positive use of your professional role to share women's fantasies, fears and joys. The encounters with women who have sexual anxieties are often brief with little opportunity for follow-up. This brief encounter can be just as important to the patient as a longer consultation.

Reasons for psychosexual training

There are many reasons why you might want to have further training in psychosexual skills, ranging from a genuine desire to help to 'collecting another certificate'. These reasons could include the following:

Women are asking you questions about their sexuality and sexual health. You feel inadequate and feel you require further skills:

◆ You want to know about psychosexual problems and how best to help

◆ You have been on lots of training days and none of them have answered your needs, so you continue searching

◆ You have your own personal problems and difficulties which are unresolved. In this case, personal therapy would be more appropriate before undertaking psychosexual training.

Choosing suitable training

Training needs to be at a convenient location as travelling is both time-consuming and expensive and requires a positive commitment. Questions that you should consider include:

◆ What training is on offer?

◆ What work do they require of you?

◆ How much time do you have available?

◆ What approach does the course have?

◆ Who will be the tutors – what are their skills and experience?

◆ How long is the course?

◆ Is further training offered if required?

◆ Is there a recognized qualification?

Post-registration courses

Post-registration courses offer an ideal opportunity to extend skills in psychosexual training, particularly for those who work in women's health. Your own individual life experiences have increased as well as your nursing skills, and you have started to recognize any difficulties you may have in discussing patients' sexuality.

You are also beginning to expand your own role, taking on more responsibilities and specializing with growing confidence, often training other nurses and setting standards for a pattern of care. Sexuality must be integrated throughout a post-registration course from the beginning if it is to be of value, and not offered as a 'one-off' or 'token' lecture at the end of a course. The discussion of sexuality and the opportunities to practise communication skills can take place and clinical encounters from your daily work can be reflected on during the course. You should be encouraged to get away from thinking there is a right and wrong way to work with sexuality and not to make assumptions because you feel uncomfortable discussing feelings. You may then feel able to offer help without a fear of saying the wrong thing.

The need for further training is an individual matter, but an enormous amount of job satisfaction can be gained when you can offer your patients a more holistic approach by integrating the theory of sexuality with increased counselling skills.

Counselling and communication courses

There are numerous courses offered by a variety of organizations and agencies. Some are specialized, such as abortion or bereavement counselling, but many are more general and only offer basic counselling skills. Some nurses feel very disappointed with the outcome of the course they attended: thus emphasizing the need to find out beforehand what the course offers and that it will be helpful and relevant for your work.

Courses on sexuality

Courses on sexuality are often multidisciplinary and offer a theoretical knowledge, with the expectation that you will be prepared to discuss your own anxieties about sexuality during training. With such a course you will need to think carefully about whether you are able to share your private feelings and experiences and whether it will be relevant to your patient care. Role play and problem-solving exercises are often offered as the method of study, and your day-to-day work may not be explored. Some courses may require

you to undergo personal therapy yourself before or during training.

The Association of Psychosexual Nursing organizes a one-year, part-time course of Psychosexual Awareness for Registered Health Care Practitioners. This is credit rated by Greenwich University at Level 3 and 30 credits. The seminar training in this course offers the opportunity for reflection, supervision and action research of patients' sexual anxieties that are met in everyday practice.

Balint-style seminar training

Balint-style seminar training occurs when a group of nurses meet together with a leader for experiential learning and present clinical encounters from their daily work. The aim of such seminars is to increase skills by honest discussion and reflection where counselling is seen as an integral part of clinical care. The focus of the work is on the interaction between the nurse and the patient and the feelings invoked, offering participants the opportunity to listen, think and discuss not only their own work with patients' sexual anxieties but also those of others in the group. The training is similar to a pattern of training developed by the Institute of Psychosexual Medicine. For seminar training to be effective nurses must be working in clinical practice, so that changes they make in their practice can be self-assessed and evaluated within the group. It is therefore not suitable for short training but it has been recognized that six seminars at monthly intervals does allow new thinking and some exploration and discovery of skills with patients (Bell *et al.*, 1997). A more permanent change can take place after 20–30 seminars of 2 hours each held weekly or fortnightly (Clifford, 1998).

Clinical supervision is recognized as important for continuing professional development whilst a Balint-style seminar offers the required focus, training and supervision for psychosexual nursing (Selby, 2000).

Workshops

Workshops may take place over one or more days and can be very valuable as you will normally work in groups. However, some nurses find it threatening to participate in a group, particularly when there is a fear of having to put their own feelings about sexuality forward. The skill of the facilitator is paramount in establishing an atmosphere where feelings about sexuality can be discussed freely, and the focus must be on the patients, the nurses' clinical practice and the relationship between them. Many sensitive nurses feel they work in total isolation with their patients' sexuality, as colleagues do not always take this subject seriously and seem unsupportive when concerns are raised. Signs of amusement and laughter will often cover other people's embarrassment. In a workshop you are given the chance to meet other nurses who are committed to a holistic approach and this allows you to acknowledge skills and feelings that you may have hidden from your colleagues.

Lectures

Lectures are generally 'one-off' events where you listen, take notes and there are no demands to get involved. Lectures usually represent a non-threatening form of education. Theoretical knowledge and information is given and you may gain some insight into sexual problems and anxieties by listening to new ideas and different communication skills. You may then come away fired with enthusiasm to try them in your own clinical practice. Often, unfortunately, it is easier to revert to old ways of practice and fail to address your patients' sexual care. On the other hand, the information learnt may be very positive and inspire you to seek further training.

Support groups

In support groups nurses can meet for discussion of cases and for mutual support. Unfortunately, there is often no aim or structure to these groups or even a designated facilitator. The tendency is then for the group to become a 'social' group of professionals where training and therefore learning is minimal. Properly organized clinical supervision, however, can be very supportive.

Conclusions

All women go through life with sexual feelings, fears and fantasies which may persist into old age and can include sexual experience of masturbation, heterosexuality or homosexuality. Many changes take place during their sexual maturation, both physical and emotional. For some women their sexual lives are fulfilled and they feel happy, supported and loved, whilst others feel their lives are in a turmoil and they feel depressed, angry, confused and lonely.

It is important for all nurses to realize that you can help by developing your observing and listening skills when you meet women in your everyday clinical practice where their sexuality, sexual health care and sexual lives can be nursed with the same respect and equality as the other care that you offer and give.

If a woman hints at or verbalizes a problem it is vital that you respond appropriately at the first mention so that the issue can be more fully explored, and that you should be able to offer her relevant skills or else refer her for the holistic care she needs.

Depression

Depression not only affects the sufferer but also can have a debilitating effect on family and friends. It can occur in all age groups from childhood to old age and is more common in women than men. Rutter (1992) writes: 'Depression becomes more prevalent in adolescence and shows a marked female preponderance only at and after adolescence'. Research in Scotland by Shajahan and Cavanagh (1998) indicates there has been a change in the balance between men and women, and that depression in men is increasing. In the mid-nineteenth century depression began to be medicalized and came under the growing discipline of psychiatry, thus becoming part of 'mental illness', although symptoms are often presented as a physical illness. Treatments such as electroconvulsive treatment and antidepressant drugs began to be used. More recently, psychiatry has looked at early events in the life of the patient, which can manifest as depression later in life. The importance of these previous psychological effects is increasingly being recognized as a factor in the diagnosis and treatment of depression.

The use of the word 'depressed' is common-place and is frequently used when people are feeling 'low'. A woman said after a severe bout of influenza: 'One day I felt so low. I am on my own now, having been widowed a year ago but a good friend came and talked me through this feeling and that was a great help'. She was lucky, but many people have to overcome this feeling on their own. The difficulty for professionals is to sort out the degree and severity of the problem when the word is used. Stuttaford (1999) suggests that all people have a standard mood with swings of elevation or depression: 'the intensity will vary and come and go'. He comments: 'Left untreated, the majority, but not all, will in time improve but, even so, over 50% of people who have a major depressive episode will suffer a recurrence'.

As health professionals we should try not to make assumptions and jump to the incorrect conclusion, but to elicit why a woman is feeling depressed. Depression can often present with a physical problem and many women do not connect their mind to their body symptoms. They are sometimes interwoven. Women may visit you over a number of years with various physical complaints (see Box 5.6) but leave after each appointment without having had a chance to say anything that concerns their feelings. A gentle probing question, a listening ear and a non-judgemental response can save many future visits and hours of professional time.

Conversely, many genuine health problems cause a feeling of depression. These range from minor self-limiting illnesses such as flu to chronic conditions such as multiple sclerosis. Women who experience loss, either from bereavement or in a physical sense (loss of a breast, womb or a limb), may also be depressed.

For some women depression may occur as the result of childhood events and deprivation. Every woman's interpretation of 'depression' is unique, and the use of the word will need to be analysed with each patient. Nichols (2003) suggests you need to focus 'on sensing' the feelings of each patient: the skill for the health professional remains an ability to listen and interpret individual stories. It is always helpful to know if there is a family history of depression, particularly where children are involved: it may then be possible to modify the effects on other children in order to prevent a cycle of depression. Parents lay down the genetics of their children, but their upbringing is influenced by the emotional care they are given. (Postnatal depression is discussed in Chapter 8.)

Internal or external factors in the home, such as marital problems or financial worries, can trigger a feeling of depression. For some women it may be a 'one-off' depressive episode but for others it may be the beginning of a recurring cycle of depression. Depression can bring periods of blackness and misery, with a tendency towards isolation and withdrawal. Even everyday tasks seem too difficult to undertake; concentration is lost and a woman may appear apathetic with confused ideas and thoughts. Other women may be agitated or restless and have abnormal sleep patterns with insomnia. The feelings of hopelessness, failure and despair are common with severe depression and sometimes you will hear women expressing the thought that it does not seem worth continuing with life, indicating suicidal tendencies. They may then require urgent help and referral. It will usually be the role of the doctor to prescribe treatment either by psychotherapy, counselling or drugs. Antidepressant drug treatment has greatly improved with the advent

---

Box 5.6 Feelings and symptoms that may be observed when depression is mentioned

- Isolation
- Withdrawal
- Apathy
- Poor memory
- Poor appetite
- Lack of concentration
- Weight loss
- Alcohol intake
- Drug use
- Disturbed sleep patterns/insomnia
- Anorexia/bulimia
- Agitation and restlessness.

of selective serotonin reuptake inhibitors such as fluoxetine.

Nurses are in an ideal position to follow up the woman's care, and to monitor compliance with therapy as well as to evaluate the effects of treatment. The therapy may be given over weeks, months or in some cases years. Monitoring must be vigilant as changing circumstances, even over a short time, may alter a women's perception of her depression and her compliance with treatment.

In elderly women it is common to overlook underlying depression and to make an assumption that the symptoms are the onset of senile dementia or Alzheimer's disease. If there is any suspicion that this is the case they can be referred for a psycho-geriatric assessment and their treatment modified accordingly.

The UK has seen many changes in social life and cultural practices over the past few decades, but there continues to be widespread hardship in many communities. Work roles have changed as well as family life. These changes have been accompanied by increasing rates of alcoholism, drug abuse and suicide. Violence both emotional and physical has also increased but this is often hidden within the home situation. All these factors inevitably contribute to how women will cope in their own situation.

Sadness is a normal response to any misfortune including loss of status. It is important not to equate sadness and unhappiness with depression. Occasionally, normal reactions to human problems might be mistaken for clinical depression and an inappropriate or unnecessary drug regime started. All a woman may need is the empathetic ear of a health professional to realize that her unhappiness is a natural emotional response to an event. Once this is shared there is often an understanding that brings relief.

Bowlby (1986) suggests that: 'It is characteristic of the mentally healthy person that he can bear with this phase of depression and disorganisation, and emerge from it after not too long a time with behaviour, thought and feeling beginning to be reorganised for interactions of a new sort' and comments 'his sense of competence and personal worth remains intact'. The message can therefore be one of hope for many women despite the disruption of their psychosocial life.

Post-traumatic stress disorder

Post-traumatic stress disorder (PTSD) is the result of a major traumatic event that results in the personal threat of death or serious injury or a threat to the physical integrity of self or others. At the event the person will have felt intense fear, helplessness or horror (Rogers and Liness, 2000). The reactions can be experienced by adults, young people, children and families. The formal psychiatric definition is clearly given in the diagnostic statistical manual *Coping with Loss* (Parkes and Black, 1998).

Background to PTSD

The concept of human distress caused by a major traumatic event was not recognized until the end of World War I when troops, apparently traumatized with 'shell shock', were given treatment by a few army doctors interested in psychiatry. During World War II the need for treating those with this condition was again recognized and treatment was offered. After the war a group of psychiatrists and psychoanalysts continued to study and develop therapies for those suffering from their war experiences. It was realized that this human distress required skilled people who could listen to the experience of the traumatic event and were able to focus and make appropriate observations on the emotional experiences. The study of treating those who had been traumatized concentrated on the whole human experience which enabled a breakthrough in the treatment and recovery (Main, 1989).

In the UK this work escalated after the fire on the underground at King's Cross station in 1987 when a large number of people were affected by the tragedy. Nowadays traumatic experiences are identified not only with fires but also with violent crime, murder, bombings, shootings, rape, car crashes, torture, sexual abuse and many other life-threatening events. Close relatives, although they may not have experienced the actual incident, also suffer and may require treatment.

Children can also suffer acute trauma as the result of family violence, accidents, disasters and traumatic bereavements.

The theory developed that counselling should be offered as soon as possible to everyone following a major stressful event, the idea being that stress and strain are usually seen as undesirable and should therefore be managed and removed.

After any painful event it is normal to experience strong feelings. Emotional trauma is an individual event: everyone reacts differently and help may not always be required in the immediate aftermath of a stressful episode. During a clinical encounter you may meet a woman or family who have experienced a major traumatic event: an enquiry as to how they feel now will often be appropriate, even if it is some weeks or months since the traumatic episode. If their reactions appear to be prolonged or severe (see Box 5.7) then it is important to direct them towards appropriate treatment.

Skilled help can come from a multi-professional group including clinical psychologists, psychotherapists, psychiatrists and family therapists, and is available in traumatic stress clinics and hospitals. These experienced professionals will often give an initial assessment before treatment is offered. There is an opportunity for the patient to talk about what has happened and the

way their life has been affected. The stress can then become recognized and understanding is more likely within their psychosocial context. There is no definitive treatment for PTSD sufferers but the most effective comes from cognitive behavioural therapy using exposure and cognitive techniques. Such treatments generally require from 8 to 16 sessions (Marks *et al.*, 1998).

The results of seven randomized controlled trials were recently analysed and showed no evidence that debriefing helped victims in the long term, and even suggested that it might have harmed them (Rick and Briner, 2000). The debriefing offered was a highly structured one-off counselling session lasting several hours. Rick commented: 'At best its efficacy is neutral and at worst it can be damaging' and she went on to say 'that, with 75% of all victims overcoming post-traumatic stress disorder without debriefing, organizations such as banks and shops need to assess whether it was necessary'.

More recently attitudes to PTSD vary and new initiatives are now being tested with UK combat soldiers. Some psychiatrists are concerned that the diagnosis of PTSD may be abandoned in the UK and Gillian Mezey, a forensic psychiatrist at St George's Hospital Medical School, says 'dismissing PTSD as a diagnosis denies the sufferings of people exposed to severe and life-threatening trauma (Feinmann, 2003).

When you are caring for women, mothers will sometimes comment about their children's behaviour and reaction to an event. You should be alert to these remarks as they can be an indication of emotional trauma that could have taken place in the past or be taking place now. This can be particularly relevant when child abuse and family violence has occurred. Children's reactions to stress can be very similar to adult reactions but may also include a return to younger behaviour, bedwetting, over-activity and a fear of being left alone.

Box 5.7 Reactions that can occur long after an event of PTSD

◆ Flashbacks
◆ Sleep disturbance
◆ Anxiety about death
◆ Disturbed concentration
◆ Inability to make decisions
◆ Persistent anxiety
◆ Heart palpitations
◆ Nightmares
◆ Clinical depression
◆ Numb feeling
◆ Memory loss
◆ Feeling irritable and short tempered
◆ Sweating.

Bereavement

All of us will experience death and bereavement at some stage in our lives. Nurses may find their first close experience of death is not until after they have started their training. How you will cope with bereavement is an entirely individual and personal reaction and will not be known until the event itself. The feeling of being out of control is strong and can be frightening. We can read about the effects of bereavement and the processes of mourning that take place in preparation for ourselves, and to help us to work with our patients, but it is often bewildering and puzzling how individual people react to loss, and it may be very different from the behaviour expected both of ourselves and our patients. The actual process of grief is little understood and there is no right or wrong way to grieve. It does not mean that people are coping when they do not show their grief like everyone else. Patients need to be allowed to feel and behave as they are – individuals.

The study of grieving and loss is crucial for all nurses, as there is a profound effect on the psychosocial and psychosexual lives of those concerned. Nurses not only meet loss that is current, but also loss from the past, where grieving, for whatever reason, has not taken place. Where this has not been expressed, emotional trauma can remain hidden, leaving damage for the patient you are seeing as well as for partners, husbands, family and friends. An illustration of this sometimes occurs when a midwife takes an obstetric history from a pregnant woman. Routine questions about previous pregnancies are asked but the midwife may not stop to ask how the woman is feeling now about a previous termination of pregnancy, miscarriage, stillbirth or death of a child. All these questions may provoke memories of a loss that has not been resolved and can then cause emotional anxiety. The midwife can observe the response of the woman, which may be obvious, such as welling tears or she may appear quite dismissive of the loss. This is often a clue that the grief is hidden and there is still unexplored psychological pain. If the midwife can then share the woman's feeling of dismissal and of not wanting to talk about past events, then the woman may feel able to say something like 'I feel so silly and anyhow it was a long time ago'. Work can then start to allow some resolution of her loss before the birth of the next baby.

Many of us, whether nurses, midwives or health visitors, underestimate our skills and the very fact that the loss has been raised, acknowledged and discussed is frequently enough for self-healing to take place. If the emotional pain is too great then referral to a bereavement counsellor or an organization such as Cruse may be an appropriate solution (see Resources).

The period of mourning should normally be completed within two years. This does not mean forgetting, but a fading of feelings which allows emotional healing to take place, and the opportunity to start to build a new, separate life. The grief process describes the common reactions and feelings that are normal and appropriate. Most people who experience bereavement are not ill themselves, and if they are treated as being unwell they may retreat into helplessness, i.e. withdrawing from what is going on around them to get away from the pain, rather than allowing themselves to experience the necessary stages of emotional pain to stop grieving. Grief has been studied in depth by Colin Murray Parkes, and his book *Bereavement* (Parkes, 1996) is a highly informative and useful book for all health professionals.

It is important for you as a nurse to relate the identified stages of grief and feelings to your everyday clinical practice, with the knowledge that anyone you meet may be experiencing loss in a variety of forms (Parkes and Black, 1998). This may not necessarily be the death of a loved person, but could also be the loss of a job, divorce, financial loss or burglary, as well as loss experienced through surgery and illness. Loss not only involves the patient you meet but their family as well; whether in hospital, general practice, the community or the home, they all may need your support and care.

When you are nursing a child or adult with a chronic illness you will have noticed how much has to be sacrificed by the carers, the family and the patient. There are many losses, one of which can be a sexual life for the carers as well as for the adult patient. You can sometimes wonder in these circumstances as to who is the 'real' patient. Is it the carer or the sufferer? It is also important to recognize that all those who are involved have their own emotional needs that may require your help at different times.

In Western culture, bereavement is still seen as private and not to be publicly displayed. In other cultures, particularly Asian, there is often a set period of mourning with open tears and acceptance of rituals and behaviour which helps all those involved to come to terms with their loss.

The stages of grief

Shock

This phase usually lasts for a short while. It will be particularly pronounced when death is sudden and unexpected, leaving a state of confusion where reactions will vary, from feeling completely numb or apathetic to being over-reactive. As Lily Pincus in *Death and the Family* says, 'for physical shock, rest and warmth are the recognized methods of treatment' (Pincus, 1997). The same treatment applies equally to emotional shock and it should be remembered that to 'keep going' is not necessarily a good cure for emotional pain. The need for tender loving care will be important particularly when the main feeling is of being left alone and abandoned. The return of the bereaved to the family home, after leaving hospital following a death where perhaps only a short time previously everything had been normal, gives rise to feelings of disbelief, which can rapidly turn to extreme distress bordering on hysteria. Feelings of being out of control, not able to cope, fear, the inability to relax and restlessness are all common. Sleep patterns are disturbed and it could be you who might encourage the bereaved to take medication at this stage.

Nowadays people live much more in isolation, with relations and family often living far away and neighbours and friends out at work during the day. In fact neighbours may only be known by sight and not by name. Thus the feeling of loneliness can be intensified.

When the death has been expected, and some preparation for mourning has already started, the immediate reaction may be one of relief rather than shock. This reaction will vary with the individual situation and the temperament of the bereaved, but it does not mean to say the emotions will be any less intense.

During this stage of grief arrangements have to be made, the funeral organized and the bereaved will be supported by relatives and friends. It is important for you to remember, whatever your work setting, that many other people will be mourners and may be grieving as well as the immediate relatives. This is particularly relevant for those in a close community.

Nurses must also mourn. Where nursing care has been given, often over a long period of time, either on a one-to-one basis or with a team approach, nurses can become very close to both the dying and their relatives, so it is only to be expected that they should experience a similar reaction. In hospital the turnover in bed occupancy is so rapid that there may be no time for adjustment to a new patient in a bed where a death has recently occurred. The bed is remade and clean and it becomes hard to remember the recent death and nurses might even have a feeling of guilt that this can happen so quickly. Time should be made on a ward or in general practice for discussion of individual deaths and acknowledgements of the feelings that other nurses and professional colleagues have. Other patients may also need support; they have watched the comings and goings and wonder what has happened. They know when a death has taken place and their enquiries must be answered truthfully. Even though other patients' deaths may not be imminent, there is always the individual knowledge that they will die at some time in the future. This can be frightening. The death of someone else will often evoke painful memories of a previous experience of death.

In home nursing, the contact between the nurse and patient is much more intense. The acceptance of care comes from the patient and those living in the home, and a close relationship often develops. Even then the role of the nurse has to be non-intrusive, especially at the time of dying. Nevertheless, for the nurse to be present and available is usually seen to be important to the family; to be on call in the event of change in the patient's condition is reassuring for everyone. The nurse who is unable to be present at the end may have feelings of 'letting the family down' and of leaving the task incomplete both for her and the relatives. Contact with the bereaved is much more likely to continue after a home death, particularly where the nurse may be known and seen in the neighbourhood. This is often a real benefit in the healing process for both the nurse and those who are bereaved.

Searching

After the initial shock response, relatives and friends leave and a feeling of isolation takes over. The bereaved may start looking for the lost person, with the inability to accept this loss. Pining is a noticeable wish for the lost person. The adult may see this as irrational behaviour, but that does not mean they are out of control. Their behaviour may be restless and tense with lots of repetitive talking and recalling past events. The bereaved may give vivid descriptions of 'seeing' the dead person or feeling their presence. This is a common phenomenon and can be a comfort to them and is not necessarily upsetting. These symptoms will decrease as the reality of the loss is accepted.

Some people may experience feelings that are new to them of anger and aggression, even over trivial events. Nurses may be aware of hostile feelings often directed towards them and other medical staff as the bereaved feel the need to express blame. Depression, not necessarily pathological, and despair are common; these may not be prolonged but have acute phases and then disappear. The feeling of guilt about what might have been said or not said, or regrets that they should have done something can leave a feeling of unfinished business. For the bereaved, there is sometimes a loss of interest in their personal appearance as there is no one to make an effort for and no one to compliment them.

Concentration, whether at home or at work is always difficult. Many women have jobs, either full- or part-time, and usually only a brief leave of absence is given or taken. It may be therapeutic to return to work as the activity keeps them occupied, but it can also leave feelings of not being able to cope and being less efficient, resulting in a lack of confidence.

The home becomes difficult to organize and the family may feel neglected, especially if there are young children, who may find it difficult to understand why routines are upset and they are not receiving the same attention as before. Children need just as much support and understanding during a bereavement as adults. The mother can then feel guilty as she is not able to be the provider and organizer for her children whilst she is trying to cope with her own grief.

Possessions may become very important. Sometimes there is the temptation to get rid of everything too early but it is important to allow some time before making final decisions as regrets are then less, and specific possessions will remain as reminders of happy times. Other people get rid of nothing or may leave a room untouched. The possessions then seem to remain a 'living' memorial. Memories and recollections are particularly painful throughout this time but happier memories will replace them as the pain starts to fade. When death was sudden and there was no time for farewell, the bereaved may feel that they never had a chance to say 'goodbye' which makes the task of mourning even harder, and longer.

Acceptance and adaptation

During this phase the emotional pain of bereavement lessens and acceptance of the loss becomes a reality. Changes take place and a new identity is established with the environment where the deceased lived or the loss took place. Relationships that may have suffered within the family may need to be renewed, even if the idea seems totally alien to other members of the family. It then starts to become possible to reinvest emotional feelings in new relationships. Family affairs have to be reorganized and where the bereaved has never dealt with financial matters these have to be understood and new skills learnt.

If the wife and mother becomes the provider, family administrator and planner she is often surprised at how well she can cope. Support and encouragement will continue, but it is important to stop grieving otherwise the new identity will not develop. Parkes (1996) describes 'turning points; that is events associated with a major revision of their feelings, attitude and behaviour'. He goes on to point out that 'the timing of such turning points is important'. They can be an anniversary, a holiday or a memorial service and should not go unnoticed by those around. It is at such 'turning points' that problems can be discussed and arrangements for the future made which will continue to allow further adaptation to the new situation.

Pathological grief

The signs that all is not well are when physical symptoms persist with no pathology: there may be excessive guilt or anger or an anxiety state with uncontrollable tears and depression. Maybe the grieving is being avoided or the problem as in chronic grief is how and when to stop this process. You need to be able to identify that there is a problem and offer suitable support and perhaps onward referral. This can then lead to an acceptance of the bereavement.

Other types of loss

Other types of loss take place frequently throughout life and cover a wide range of issues (Box 5.8). The feelings of grief are exactly the same. Some losses pass quickly, fade equally quickly and leave little or no trauma. But for others, because it is not necessarily a death of a person, it is difficult to understand why the feelings of grief should be there at all. Nurses feel the same and wonder why a loss that appears remote or happened a long time ago should have a bearing on the current situation. Even if we are told of a 'loss event' the interpretation of this may be difficult, and we fail to 'hear' the patient's emotional pain and continue to concentrate on the physical symptoms. The temptation to ignore a recent loss is common as you may feel the event is 'too close' and be afraid of upsetting the patient and provoking sadness and tears. Women themselves have the same fear that 'I should be getting over it now' and will often apologize for crying.

You may also find that your own personal experiences of loss and bereavement may not have been adequately resolved and consequently

---

Box 5.8 Losses that can affect women's sexual health

Most of these losses take place in a normal lifecycle and many of them are mentioned elsewhere in this book but it was felt important to group them together in this section on bereavement. You will encounter many different types of loss in your daily clinical work:

- Loss of parental control: children rejecting parents, teenage trauma, truancy from school, running away from home, drugs, alcohol and eating disorders
- Children leaving home for school, college, university, a new job or to live with a partner
- Loss of virginity – particularly traumatic following sexual abuse and rape
- Loss of confidence and self-esteem
- Getting engaged and married
- Loss of husband or partner through separation, divorce or death. Partners separated by work
- Loss of parents and close relatives
- Never having had the opportunity to have children
- Pregnancy: unable to have a normal delivery; unable to breastfeed
- Loss of employment, redundancy, financial loss, early retirement as well as retirement at the standard age
- Buying and selling a house, moving neighbourhood, moving to a new country
- Menopause with loss of periods and loss of fertility
- Death of a pet
- Burglary.

Physical loss
- Medical illness which can be short or long term, acute or chronic, or progressive and incurable, e.g. diabetes, asthma, stroke
- Changes in personality, memory loss, senility
- Loss of function in any part of the body by accident or illness
- Paraplegia
- Incontinence of bladder and rectum
- Infertility.

Surgical loss
- Loss of limb
- Hysterectomy, vulvectomy
- Mastectomy
- Miscarriage, ectopic pregnancy, stillbirth
- Termination of pregnancy.

get in the way of working with your patients over their own experiences of loss.

The positive message for you as a nurse involved in women's health is that you must be open and willing to listen to the psychosocial events that surround women's lives, and then make enquiries. You will gain information on loss whilst taking a medical history, in conversation with a patient during a consultation, from a concerned professional colleague with or without referral and even from the 'grapevine'. You must aim to acknowledge this loss, to pause and then allow the patient to share her feelings with you. It need only be very brief but it is important to resist the temptation to ignore or pass over the loss. You need to observe how the woman responds to your acknowledgement of her loss. It may be so painful that it is dismissed with 'I'm alright'. Experience tells you they are seldom 'alright'. You can then ask a pertinent question, such as 'Tell me what you mean by alright.' This allows the patient to hear that you are listening and empathetic. Then her true feelings may be revealed, which you can identify and share with her as being a normal reaction to her loss. This is often a relief and a revelation, especially where the loss has been hidden. At this stage of talking about loss you are not offering counselling and therapy, but acting as a concerned nurse alongside the woman. It will be your observations and clinical experience that will determine with the woman the need for more time and counselling in the future.

As we have seen already, the value to the woman of being allowed to recognize her feelings over the loss is often therapy itself. When working in women's health we should constantly remember that we are not only caring for a woman's physical needs, but also her psychosexual and psychosocial well-being. Remember that the loss can be exciting and pleasurable, such as loss of virginity, and therefore not always one of trauma and sadness.

Summary of help you can offer the bereaved

◆ Your help should be an enabling process where you endeavour to help the bereaved cope for themselves. You should avoid telling them what to do.

◆ A consultation with you can be very short or more prolonged, just as in the grieving process itself

◆ One of the crucial skills you require is to be able to listen to really painful events and information without becoming emotionally swamped yourself

◆ Let your genuine concern and care show, but be able to stand back and think about your responses

◆ Allow the bereaved to express how they are feeling in the 'here and now'; listen and hear what they want to share with you. When the subject is too painful it is only too easy to try and change the subject which can then allow both of you to run away from the pain. Try to stay with the current situation

◆ If you are asking questions, make them open ended. 'How are you feeling now?' elicits a fuller reply than 'Are you feeling a bit better now?', when the answer is often 'Yes', even if they are not! Questions that start with 'how', 'what', 'when' and 'why' will give your patient more time to express herself fully

◆ Encourage women to be patient and not to expect too much of themselves too quickly

◆ Encourage the family to talk about their individual feelings. Communication in families is often poor and remote, but distress if shared can be a positive benefit

◆ The friends and family you meet will also want to know how they can help. They can be encouraged to just listen, even if it may be repetitive

◆ The bereaved must have the true facts about the death which may relieve their individual feelings of guilt and blame. This is especially important in accidents and in instances of sudden death

◆ Allow them to understand that the reactions and feelings they have are 'normal' and experienced by others in similar situations.

Difficulties you might experience when offering help

◆ You may feel so helpless yourself that you imagine you will be of no use. Patients are your educators and you can learn by listening to them. If you have experienced a loss or bereavement yourself and you feel you have come to terms with it, you will have much to offer to others. Never be tempted to personalize from your own experiences

◆ You may be tempted to avoid talking about emotions and painful events because you want to try and make patients feel better. Do not try to change the subject to make it more comfortable for you and run away from the pain that the woman is feeling

◆ Empathize rather than sympathize. You must avoid saying 'I know how you must be feeling'. You may like to think you know, but everyone's grief pattern is different and individual to them. It is important not to belittle or devalue their feelings and not to make assumptions

◆ Avoid the temptation to tell patients how they should be feeling now and how they will feel in the future and what they should do

◆ Try not to feel sorry for the patient. This can then lead to a feeling of pity or even contempt, which will stop your care for the bereaved. This should not be confused with the sadness that is appropriate when dealing with your patient's loss.

Conclusion

Bereavement and grief are commonplace and cover many types of loss apart from death. If you as a nurse can acknowledge your patient's sadness and participate in helping her through the grief process then the care you can offer your patients will be truly holistic.

Ideas for personal and professional development

● Did you ask your patients about their sexual life or psychosexual needs during an encounter this week? How did you address this? Reflect in writing how and why you did this, and whether the outcome was positive or negative

● Make a list of the personal difficulties and defences that you experience when discussing a patient's sexuality

● Keep a brief reflective diary of the patients you meet and their sexual anxieties for a week. Make an opportunity to discuss this clinical material with one or two colleagues

● Compile a list of counsellors, their charges, how they work with clients (either singly or as a couple) and what they specialize in

● Consider attending a workshop or enrolling for a series of seminar training.

Patient education points

● Many events and changes in women's lives can lead to sexual anxieties

● Early discussion with a health professional may prevent a temporary anxiety from becoming a permanent problem

● A current crisis or recent change may become a trigger point that enables discussion about the past

● Encourage women to ascertain, before seeing a counsellor, that the councellor would be suitable for dealing with their specific problem.

Resources

Psychosexual issues

Association of Psychosexual Nursing
PO Box No 2762, London W1A 5HQ
Can advise on psychosexual nurse training, seminars or workshops.

British Association of Sexual and Relationship Therapy
PO Box 13686, London SW20 9ZH

Tel: 020 8543 2707
www.basrt.org.uk

British Association of Counselling and Psychotherapy
BACP House, 35-37 Albert Street, Rugby, Warwickshire, CV21 2SG
Tel: 0870 443 5252
www.bacp.co.uk

British Society of Psychosomatic Obstetrics, Gynaecology and Andrology
11 Hagholm Road, Cleghorn, Lanark ML11 7SG
www.bspoga.org

Institute of Psychiatry
De Crespigny Park, London SE5 8AF
Tel: 020 7703 5411
www.iop.kcl.ac.uk

Institute of Psychosexual Medicine
11 Chandos Street, London W1G 9DR
Tel: 020 7580 0631
www.ipm.org.uk

Relate Central Office
Herbert Gray College, Little Church Street, Rugby CV21 3AP
Tel: 01788 573241
www.relate.org.uk

Tavistock Centre
120 Belsize Lane, London NW3 5BA
Tel: 020 7435 7111
www.tavi-port.org

The Tavistock Institute
30 Tabernacle Street, London EC2A 4UE
Tel: 020 7417 0407
www.tavinstitute.org

Traumatic stress

Traumatic Stress
73 Charlotte Street, London W1P 1LB
Tel: 020 7530 3666
www.traumaclinic.org.uk

Bereavement

ARC (Antenatal Results and Choices)
73–75 Charlotte Street, London W1P 4PN
Tel: 020 7631 0280

Helpline: 020 7631 0285
www.arc-uk.org

Child Bereavement Trust
Aston House, West Wycombe, High Wycombe, Bucks HP14 3AG
Tel: 01494 446648
www.childbereavement.org.uk

Compassionate Friends
53 North Street, Bristol BS3 1EN
Tel: 0117 966 5202 Helpline: 08451 232304
www.tcf.org.uk

Cruse Bereavement Care
126 Sheen Road, Richmond, Surrey TW9 1UR
Tel: 020 8939 9530
Helpline: 0870 167 1677
www.crusebereavementcare.org.uk

Foundation for the Study of Infant Deaths
Artillery House, 11-19 Artillery Row, London SW1P 1RT
Tel: 0870 787 0885
Helpline: 0870 787 0554
www.sids.org.uk/fsid

Hospice Information Service
St Christopher's Hospice, 51–59 Lawrie Park Road, London SE26 6DZ
Tel: 020 8768 4500
www.stchristophers.org.uk
A national referral and training centre for adults, children and families.

Rape Crisis Federation
Unit 7, Provident Works, Newdigate Street, Nottingham NG7 4FD
Tel: 0115 900 3560
www.rapecrisis.co.uk

Road Peace
PO Box 2579, London NW10 3PW
Tel: 020 8838 5102 Helpline: 0845 4500 355
www.roadpeace.org
Support for those bereaved by road accidents.

SAMM (Support after Murder and Manslaughter)
Cranmer House, 39 Brixton Road, London SW9 6DZ

Tel: 020 7735 3838
www.samm.org.uk

SANDS (Stillbirth and Neonatal Death Society)
28 Portland Place, London W1B 1LY
Tel: 020 7436 7940 Helpline: 020 7436 5881
www.uk-sands.org

Further reading

BALINT, M. (1957) *The Doctor, His Patient and the Illness*. London: Pitman.

BANCROFT, J. (1989) *Human Sexuality and its Problems*, 2nd edn. Edinburgh: Churchill Livingstone.

BURNARD, P. (1999) *Counselling Skills for Health Professionals*, 3rd edn. Cheltenham: Stanley Thomas.

CASEMENT, P. (1985) *On Learning from the Patient*. London: Tavistock.

HALL, L. and LLOYD, S. (1993) *Surviving Child Sexual Abuse*. London: Falmer Press.

HEATH, H. and WHITE, I. (eds) (2002) *The Challenge of Sexuality in Health Care*. Oxford: Blackwell Science.

IRWIN, F. (1998) Nursing an adult survivor of childhood sexual abuse. In Barnes, E., Griffiths, P., Ord, J. and Wells, D. (eds) *Face to Face with Distress*. Oxford: Butterworth Heinemann, Chapter 6, p. 83.

KLUGER-BELL, K. (1998) *Unspeakable Losses*. Harmondsworth: Penguin.

KUPERFERMANN, J. (1992) *When the Crying's Done*. London: Robson Books.

MATSOUKIS, A. (1996) *I Can't Get Over It*, 2nd edn. California: New Harbinger.

NICHOLS, K. (2003) *Psychological Care For Ill and Injured People: A Clinical Guide*. Philadelphia: OUP Maidenhead.

ORBACH, S. (1994) *What's Really Going on Here?* London: Virago.

PARKES, C. and MARKUS, A. (eds) (1998) *Coping With Loss*. London: BMJ Books.

ROWE, D. (1988) *Choosing Not Losing. The Experience of Depression*. Oxford: Radcliffe Medical Press.

SACKS, O. (1991) *A Leg to Stand On*. London: Picador.

SAVAGE, J. (2003) Emotions in practice. A study of Balint seminar training as experiential learning for qualified nurses. RCN Institute.

SKRINE, R. (1997) *Blocks and Freedoms in Sexual Life*. Oxford: Radcliffe Medical Press.

SKRINE, R. and MONTFORD, H. (2001) *Psychosexual Medicines: An Introduction*, 2nd edn. London: Arnold.

SKYNNER, R. and CLEESE, J. (1984) *Families and How to Survive Them*. London: Methuen.

SMITH, P. (1992) *The Emotional Labour of Nursing*. London: Macmillan Press.

THOMAS, J. (1993) *Supporting Parents when a Baby Dies Before or Soon after Birth*. Available from Child Bereavement Trust, Brindley House, 4 Burkiss Road, Beaconsfield, Bucks HP9 1PB.

THOMAS, J. and KOHNER, N. (1993) *Grief After the Death of Your Baby*. Available from Child Bereavement Trust, Brindley House, 4 Burkiss Road, Beaconsfield, Bucks HP9 1PB.

VALINS, L. (1992) *When a Woman's Body Says No to Sex*. Harmondsworth: Penguin.

Van OOJEN, E. and CHARNOCK, A. (1994) *Sexuality and Patient Care*. London: Chapman and Hall.

WELLS, D. (ed.) (2000) *Caring for Sexuality in Health and Illness*. Edinburgh: Churchill Livingstone.

WORDEN, J. (1991) *Grief Counselling and Grief Therapy*, 2nd edn. London: Routledge.

ZILBERGELD, B. (1999) *The New Male Sexuality*. London: Bantam.

References

BALINT, E. and NORELL, J.S. (1973) *Six Minutes For the Patient*. London: Tavistock.

BELL, J., RUTTER, M., SELBY, J. and WARD, M. (1997) Nurse-led family planning. *Practice Nurse* **14**(4):265–7.

BOWLBY, J. (1986) *Loss, Sadness and Depression*, Vol 3. London: Pelican.

BRIERE, J. (1984) *The Effects of Childhood Sexual Abuse on Later Psychological Functioning: Defining a Post Sexual Abuse Syndrome*. Paper presented at the 3rd National Conference on Sexual Victimisation of Children, Children's Hospital National Medical Center, Washington DC.

CLIFFORD, D. (1998) Psychosexual nursing seminars. In Barnes, E., Griffiths, P., Ord, J. and Wells, D. (eds) *Face to Face with Distress*. Oxford: Butterworth Heinemann.

CLIFFORD, D. (2000) In Wells, D. (ed.) *Caring for Sexuality in Health and Illness*. Edinburgh: Churchill Livingstone.

DOYLE, C. (1994) *Child Sexual Abuse. A Guide for Health Professionals*. London: Nelson Thornes.

FEINMANN, J. (2003) Have they got it all wrong? *The Times*, 29 October 2003.

GILL, M. (1989) Defences in the patient. In Skrine, R. (ed.) *Introduction to Psychosexual Medicine*. London: Chapman and Hall.

MAIN, T. (1989) Clinical problems of repatriates. In John, J. (ed.) *The Ailment and Other Psychoanalytic Essays*. London: Freedom Press.

MARKS, I. *et al.* (1998) Treatment of post-traumatic stress disorder by exposure and/or cognitive restructuring: a controlled study. *Archives of General Psychiatry* **55**:317–25.

MASTERS, W.H. and JOHNSON, V.E. (1970) *Human Sexual Inadequacy*. Edinburgh: Churchill Livingstone.

NICHOLS, K. (2003) *Psychological Care For Ill and Injured People: A Clinical Guide*. Philadelphia: OUP Maidenhead.

PARKES, C.M. (1996) *Bereavement: Studies of Grief in Adult Life*, 3rd edn. Harmondsworth: Pelican.

PARKES, C.M. and BLACK, D. (1998) Disasters. In Parkes, C.M. and Markus, A. (eds) *Coping with Loss*. London: BMJ Books.

PINCUS, L. (1997) *Death and the Family*. London: Faber and Faber.

RICK, J. and BRINER, R. (2000) *Trauma Management Versus Stress Debriefing: What Should Responsible Organisations Do?* Paper presented to the British Psychological Society, Occupational Psychology Conference, January 2000.

ROGERS, P. and LINESS, S. (2000) Post-traumatic stress disorder. *Nursing Standard* **14**(22):47–52.

RUTTER, M. and RUTTER, M. (1992) *Developing Minds*. London: Penguin.

SELBY, J. (2000) Coaching for psychosexual awareness. In Wells, D. (ed.) *Caring for Sexuality in Health and Illness*. Edinburgh: Churchill Livingstone.

SHAJAHAN, P.M. and CAVANAGH, J.T.O. (1998) Admission for depression among men in Scotland. 1980–95: a retrospective study. *British Medical Journal* **316**:1496–7.

STUTTAFORD, T. (1999) *In Your Right Mind*. London: Faber and Faber.

TUNNADINE, P. (1970) *Contraception and Sexual Life*. London: Tavistock (out of print).

TUNNADINE, P. (1992) *Insights into Troubled Sexuality. A Case Profile Anthology*. London: Chapman and Hall.

WAKELEY, G. (1991) *Sexual Abuse and the Primary Care Doctor*. London: Chapman and Hall.

6: Women with Special Needs and Concerns

Marjorie Hickerton

OBJECTIVES

This chapter should help you understand:

- How the outreach family planning service works and who can benefit from such a service
- The importance of sensitivity in dealing with people with learning disabilities
- The impact of sexual abuse and rape on women
- How different cultures and religions influence female sexuality.

Introduction

The title of this chapter 'Women with special needs and concerns' could cover a wide range of women with very different needs, concerns and problems and easily become a complete book in its own right. It is not within the scope of this chapter to cover the subject in such depth but it is hoped that by concentrating on a few specific areas you will be able to understand and be aware of the sexual health and contraceptive needs of different groups of people in society. Women with special needs are often confused, their problems are complex and you will need time, patience and the ability to enlist the help of counsellors, social workers and others in order to help them.

Domiciliary family planning

Domiciliary family planning is a specialized service visiting women at home to give advice on contraception and sexual health. The service has also been described as: 'preventative community services which should bridge the gap between medical and social services' (Christopher, 1980). This is in line with the *Health of the Nation* document (DoH, 1992), which states that 'family planning services should be appropriate, accessible and comprehensive to meet the needs of those who use or may wish to use them' (Box 6.1).

Box 6.1 Domiciliary services available

All the following services can be carried out in a domiciliary capacity:

- Information and advice on all methods of contraception
- Abortion counselling and referral
- HIV and AIDS counselling and referral
- Cervical screening/breast awareness
- Menopause counselling and referral
- Post-termination counselling
- Preconceptual advice
- Pregnancy testing
- Premenstrual syndrome counselling and advice
- Psychosexual counselling
- Referral to genitourinary medicine clinics
- Sterilization/vasectomy counselling and referral
- Health promotion.

The provision of domiciliary family planning was established in the late 1950s, when pilot studies were set up in Newcastle, York and Southampton. The aim of the service was to establish and maintain contact with those women who were in need of the service and defined as 'hard to reach' and could not or would not go to family planning clinics.

In 1972 the Secretary of State recommended that the service should be available within the National Health Service and about this time 140–150 domiciliary family planning services were started up throughout the country (Leathard, 1985). These services were mostly situated in the larger cities and in their surrounding areas. Today this service is often referred to as 'outreach'.

The domiciliary service can be run by nurses with a doctor, or by nurses alone. If it is run solely by nurses, then clients who are unable to attend clinics can be taken to a clinic to be seen by a doctor. This is necessary for clients who choose prescribable methods of contraception for the first time, i.e. the pill or injection, and for insertion of intrauterine devices. The increasing use of patient group directions or protocols in reissuing hormonal contraception has given nurses greater autonomy. Protocols, however, as Jones (1998) reminds us, must be regularly reviewed so that they comply with the review by June Crown (NHSE, 1998). With the increase in nurse prescribing, suitably qualified nurses will be able to take over more of this role in the future.

Staff working in the domiciliary service need considerable training and experience in all aspects of sexual health and in working within the community. Courses specializing in women's health needs, with particular emphasis on contraception and sexual health, are desirable, thus enabling the nurse to function autonomously at an advanced level within a multidisciplinary context and a rapidly changing health environment. Close liaison between social services and the domiciliary service may be required in order to provide access to additional support.

Many of the women seen by the domiciliary service have low self-esteem, poor education and limited skills. This can lead to a lack of finances and poor housing which in turn compounds

SCENARIO

Mary, a 15-year-old single girl, was referred to the service having just had her first baby. Her pregnancy was unplanned. She said that as she had not got pregnant after her first experience of unprotected sexual intercourse she was sure she was infertile. Her partner was the same age as her and they both seemed immature for their age.

They eventually married but were divorced within three years, leaving Mary with a second child. Both children were boys and they would have posed a handful to raise even for a more mature couple with no additional problems. The boys seemed beyond parental control by the time the first was 5 years old. The elder boy had spent short periods of time in care and on one occasion had even set the house on fire.

The boys refused to go to school and their teacher told Mary that when they were there they behaved so badly that it was not acceptable to put them with the other children. There were constant complaints from neighbours about their behaviour and Mary and her family became more and more isolated. She existed between periods of deep depression, sometimes bordering on suicide, and periods of just managing to cope. Mary herself had spent part of her own childhood in children's homes and desperately did not want the same to happen to her own children.

Originally Mary was on the combined oral contraceptive pill but was an unreliable pill-taker and required emergency contraception on a number of occasions. This failed on one occasion and Mary had a termination. It was about this time that Mary's husband left her. After the termination she needed regular counselling and support. It was decided that a more reliable method of contraception requiring easy compliance was necessary and from the choices offered Mary chose the injectable method.

This proved successful and she remained with this method for the next 6 years. During this time her elder child had to be placed in care and was eventually fostered. She regularly called the GP to her remaining son and neglected her own health. She smoked heavily and had a very poor diet. Regular check-ups were given and Mary also received advice on a more healthy lifestyle. After a routine cervical smear test Mary required a colposcopy. She became very anxious and failed to attend numerous colposcopy appointments so eventually the domiciliary family planning nurse accompanied her to the clinic. Mary felt guilty and over-anxious that the necessity for a colposcopy might have been due to her number of sexual partners and was eventually referred for psychosexual counselling.

Her problems resolved after a number of sessions, and her lifestyle and self-esteem improved. Last year she met a new partner who has accepted her and her child and she is pregnant again. This time it is a planned pregnancy and she hopes for a more stable future.

the problem. Under these circumstances contraception becomes a very low priority and this in turn leads to even more hardship. If help and advice are given at an early stage then many of the pitfalls that clients experience could be avoided.

Referral system

Outreach services are provided around large cities and areas of social deprivation. Clients are referred to this service from many sources. Any health care worker who recognizes a woman in need may refer, having first obtained permission from the client. Referrals can be made verbally by telephone or on the appropriate form. It is the intention of the service that each new client is seen either by a doctor or a nurse within 48 hours of professional contact.

A relatively new outreach initiative at St George's Hospital in south London has been established where midwives refer young mothers of 18 years and under to the service. The nurse ensures that all new referrals are seen within three weeks after delivery, and most are followed up for at least one year. This service is proving very successful in preventing further unplanned pregnancies.

Reasons for referral are often complex and multifactorial reflecting the crises and difficulties experienced by this client group. Current trends in health care provision are recognizing the value of outreach services in targeting special needs groups such as those listed in Box 6.2.

Staff working in domiciliary family planning need to have considerable training in all aspects of health care and a wide variety of experience is required as, on most occasions, nurses will make decisions on their own. Detailed protocols should be in place to give health care professionals guidance and support. The Royal College of Nursing has also produced guidelines for domiciliary family planning services and this document assumes familiarity with, and an acceptance of, the RCN *Nursing Standards of Care for Family Planning Nurses* (RCN, 1991a) and the RCN *Family Planning Manual for Nurses* (RCN, 1991b).

There have been those who complain that the outreach service is expensive, even though it is, in fact, only marginally more expensive than

---

Box 6.2 Women who would benefit from domiciliary services

- Young people in care
- Those who have opted out of mainstream education
- Teenage mothers
- Single mothers with several young children
- Those with learning disabilities or mental illness
- Those with physical disabilities
- Some women who have religious or cultural limitations
- Those who are lacking in motivation to seek advice
- Women who are suspicious of conventional facilities.

---

a visit to the doctor. Success of the service, however, cannot be measured by cost alone. Because the women catered for are often poorly motivated and, by nature, intermittent contraceptive users, unplanned pregnancies will still occur, adding to the already difficult situation these women are in, but these pregnancies will be more widely spaced than they would be without the outreach service. The benefits to the client in allowing her to take control of her sexuality and lifestyle cannot be measured in terms of cost or client satisfaction.

The service is needed more than ever today in our multicultural society. Many clients come from countries where sex education and contraception are either forbidden or non-existent. They find attending clinics or GP centres intimidating and feel isolated and insecure in strange and often very formal surroundings. They feel more confident having a home visit with their families around them. Family planning services are inexpensive in terms of total NHS expenditure. For every £1 spent on family planning there is a saving of £11 to the taxpayer (McGuire and Hughes, 1995).

Many people involved in domiciliary family planning believe that it is a much under-funded service. Its value and potential need to be recognized by health care workers and especially by GPs, some of whom are completely unaware of the services available and how their patients who are needy and at risk could benefit. It can cost £1000 per week to keep a child in care, depending on the child's needs. This is money that could easily be directed at expanding the domiciliary service and preventing unplanned pregnancies in those women who find it difficult to attend the usual clinics.

More information about local outreach family planning services can be obtained from your PCTs and health care trusts that provide family planning services.

Women with learning disabilities

When defining learning disability it was once thought that intelligence was the 'gold standard'. However, intelligence cannot be defined in a precise way; it is made up of a number of components, including cognition, language, motor skills and social abilities (Sims and Owens, 1993). In the past, and in ICD-10 (a WHO classification of mental and behavioural disorders), an IQ score of 70 or below has been regarded as indicative of a learning disability, but the definition is by no means as simple as this.

A survey at one psychiatric hospital showed that of the people admitted, more than half had IQs above 70, a quarter recorded scores above 80, and 7% had scores between 90 and 100. There are, most certainly, genetically and environmentally caused medical disorders which may have a profound effect on physical and mental development. Such conditions include Down's syndrome (a chromosomal abnormality), tuberose sclerosis (a single gene error), cytomegalovirus (due to infection) and fetal alcohol syndrome (resulting from prenatal environment). A good account of these and many other disorders may be found in Craft and Craft (1985).

People with learning disabilities have the same rights as other individuals within the community and are encouraged to live as independent a life as possible. Over the past two decades there have been moves towards greater care at local levels, away from large institutions and into small residential units within the community. Here there are greater opportunities for

SCENARIO

Terrie, aged 21 years, suffers from Smith-Lemli-Opitz syndrome, a hereditary syndrome transmitted as an autosomal recessive trait and characterized by microcephaly, mental retardation, hypotonia, a short nose with anteverted nostrils and syndactyly of the second and third toes. She is slim, blonde, of average height and attractive. Her verbal capacity and understanding are limited and her facial movements are minimally distorted. At times she becomes aggressive and will then throw anything within her reach at anyone present at the time.

Terrie lived in residential care but went home to see her parents on a regular basis. She attended a day centre for people with learning difficulties and the staff became aware and concerned that she was becoming sexually active. Terrie had not considered the possible outcomes of sexual intercourse and was not using any form of contraception. A domiciliary family planning nurse was asked to visit the day centre to discuss the matter with her.

On the first contact Terrie was very withdrawn and non-committal and the nurse used this session to assess her level of understanding and the language she used to refer to her own sexuality. Terrie had a limited understanding but recognized her sexual feelings. On the second visit her boyfriend, who also attended the day centre, was present with her. He had a greater understanding of sexual matters and in his presence Terrie was much more communicative.

They discussed with the nurse their relationship and their hopes and plans for the future. They both stated that they wanted a home and a family but realized they would need support to achieve this. The couple set up home together, and with supervision they managed to cope. Terrie was advised on methods of contraception but it soon became obvious that she was unreliable with any method that involved self-compliance.

Terrie eventually became pregnant and when the baby was born the care that was given was limited. Eventually both parents and their baby moved into residential care where greater supervision was available. The baby, a little girl, appeared to be quite normal and the couple were loving and caring parents. Terrie realized that she could not cope with another child and requested a reliable method of contraception that required minimal compliance on behalf of either partner. After discussion of all the methods Terrie eventually chose to have the contraceptive injection.

Terrie and her partner manage, with considerable help, to bring up one child but have realized that more children would put considerable stress on their relationship. Their understanding of sexual matters, contraception and sexuality has increased dramatically since Terrie was referred to the domiciliary service and the involvement of her partner at the outset was of considerable help to her.

education and training and many have found worthwhile jobs whilst living in supervised housing. The majority are unaffected by physical handicap and generally have no problems with sexual functioning.

Attitudes towards people with learning disabilities have gradually changed as the general public have become more aware of the needs of this group. There is a growing acceptance that they are as entitled as the rest of the population to lead as normal a life as is possible. However, this requires understanding on the issues relating to their sexuality. Problems can arise if these issues are not dealt with sensitively. An individual's sexuality is intimately connected with her mental health, and disruption of one can have a serious effect on the other.

It would appear that the old-fashioned argument concerning people with a mental handicap still often applies, 'if we don't talk about it, we won't put ideas into their heads and they will not show any interest in sex'. This is nonsense as all humans have sexual needs and drives and although these may vary from individual to individual they still exist and need to be acknowledged by health professionals.

No human being is asexual. Sex education and health education are vitally important but should not take place in isolation and should include discussion about relationships and social interactions. Many of these young people will not have the ability to select the appropriate reading materials for themselves or possess the capacity to absorb and interpret their meanings. Most young people learn a significant amount about their sexuality from peer group discussion but this invariably is not the case with young people with learning disabilities.

Schools that cater for children up to the age of 16 years with learning disabilities are increasingly featuring sex education (Craft, 1990) in the curriculum and many have discussion groups about matters surrounding adolescent sexuality at which parents are encouraged to attend. Anxieties can be shared and parents realize that many of the issues they worry about are common problems which can be discussed together, e.g. 'My son aged 14 regularly gets an erection in

class, this upsets some of the other pupils who look at him and want to touch him'.

Another common problem is that of masturbation by females, particularly when this is done in public. It is important to acknowledge and recognize the sexual pleasure that is obtained but young women should be told that this is best done in private. Contraceptive advice should always be accompanied by advice and counselling in sexual behaviour and personal relationships. Methods of contraception that require minimal or no compliance are often the most suitable. The use of simple charts and diagrams and plenty of time are necessary to facilitate understanding. There is a fear amongst those who are not used to dealing with people with learning disabilities, that by educating these young people in matters of sex and sexuality they may be encouraged to explore further with each other.

Parents in general find it difficult to talk to their children about sexuality and this is even more so with young people with learning disabilities who are often more sheltered as their parents or guardians believe that sexual activity is not an option for them. It is unfortunately the case that the carers have become used to making all the decisions for those in their care. Although this is completely understandable it may leave the individual with the disability less likely to think for his or herself and they may then lack the confidence to make future decisions for themselves.

Carers of the disabled should be helped and guided by other health care professionals, e.g. the mental handicap and social workers, to provide the maximum support in this delicate area of learning. Those working with clients with learning difficulties need to be sensitive when teaching sexual awareness.

It is important to be constantly aware of how vulnerable these groups are to the possibility of exploitation and abuse, both mental and physical, without being able to take any action for themselves. This abuse can start at an early age, regardless of the degree of learning disability (McCarthy, 1993).

Obviously a great deal will depend upon the severity of the disability. Those with severe problems, who are unable to take any meaningful

SCENARIO

Jane, aged 35 years, with a history of mental illness was visited by a family planning nurse. She could not read or write and had two children by previous partners. Both children had been taken into care. The nurse noticed on the first visit that Jane was very withdrawn and that her present partner never left her alone. Her partner was a few years older than her and was physically disabled with no use of his left arm.

After a few visits Jane managed to speak to the nurse on her own. She then told her that her partner beat her and never gave her any money. She was never allowed out on her own and was kept locked in the flat most of the time. This was reported to the appropriate authority and action was taken. Jane's partner was asked to leave the flat and was bound over by the local magistrates' court.

part in society, will need full-time residential care. Others have a good quality of life living at home and receiving day care. Some are able to work and to take part in the community with limited assistance and supervision but all have their sexual wants and needs and these must be addressed by the carers in society.

Concern also needs to be shown for the families of the disabled; their lives can be taken over completely by the person with the disability.

McCarthy (1993) also provided evidence of a high prevalence of smoking among women with learning disabilities. We now know there is a strong association between cigarette smoking and cytological abnormalities of the cervix

SCENARIO

The Brown family had a daughter with a severe learning disability. There were two older teenage boys in the family but virtually all the parents' attention was focused on the daughter. The boys naturally felt excluded and eventually both got into trouble and dropped out of school. The family never had a holiday and the whole week's timetable was organized around the activities of the daughter. They refused respite care and other offers of assistance to the obvious detriment of the other members of the family.

(Burger *et al.*, 1993; Luesley *et al.*, 1994). This would therefore suggest that women with learning difficulties have at least as high a risk of developing cervical cancer as women in the general population. Unfortunately, women with learning disabilities do not attend for regular cervical screening and attendance has been estimated to be as low as 8% (Mencap, 1998).

One of the national priorities outlined in *Saving Lives: Our Healthier Nation* (DoH, 1999) was the reduction in deaths from cancer, with the cervical screening programme in the forefront. Health care teams and those professionals involved with women with learning disabilities are in a prime position to ensure this group are not neglected and included in screening programmes, thereby promoting equity in service provision. However, staff must also bear in mind that some of these females may not have been sexually active and therefore screening is unnecessary. Consent to such treatments should always be sought where possible.

Clients with learning disabilities need care and time to help them live as normal a life as possible. Nurses are frequently in a unique position to assess patients' sexual needs and problems due to their close relationship with patients and their families. In addition there must be awareness when working in this area of sexuality that cultural backgrounds and practices will vary and these need to be taken into consideration (Cooper and Guillebaud, 1999). Many have been rehabilitated very successfully into the community and manage to cope well with day-to-day life events and have been able to develop close relationships, both sexual and platonic. Marriages between people with a learning disability are increasingly common and these are often stable and successful. Genetic counselling may be appropriate in some instances.

Violence against women

Child abuse

Child abuse can be verbal, emotional, physical or sexual. Verbal and emotional abuse can occur when a parent or parents continually fail to show their child love or affection. They may shout at the child, call it names or even threaten or taunt the child about sending it away or leaving it on its own. This causes the child to lose self-confidence and self-esteem and become nervous and withdrawn. Verbal and emotional abuse, although leaving no physical scars, cause psychological damage and can have far-reaching effects.

These long-term effects of child sexual abuse are extremely damaging and it may manifest in adulthood in many ways. An inability to enjoy sex, the inviting of pleasureless sexual encounters, the seeking of affection or comfort through sex, alcohol, drugs and food, severe depression, self-harm, an inability to trust people and a total loss of confidence.

Sexual misuse or exploitation of children includes three distinct activities: sexual abuse, child prostitution and child pornography. Child sexual abuse, including incest, has ceased to be a taboo subject and is increasingly discussed by the media. Naturally, though, it still continues to arouse a sense of moral and legal outrage. The actual incidence of child sexual abuse is very difficult to measure as the vast majority of cases go unreported, making it one of the most under-reported forms of crime. Fear, embarrassment and concern about the response of medical, social and legal agencies lead to this lack of reporting, although the number has increased dramatically during the past decade, possibly due to increased surveillance by the social services and better community awareness programmes.

Child sexual abuse occurs mainly within the family by a relative, but can also occur outside the family by someone known to the child (or family) or by a complete stranger. Both boys and girls are abused, and frequently it is the eldest children who are more often affected. Within a family it is more common for just one of the children to be abused and the others left alone. Young children are most at risk, partly due to the fact that they are more vulnerable and cannot seek help. Coitus is rare with younger children, but exhibitionism, fondling and masturbation are common.

Much of the abuse is by the child's parents and is more common where a cohabitant is involved

who is not related to the child but is living in the home. Younger parents are more likely to abuse their children than older parents. Sexual abuse is more commonly perpetrated by men, whilst suffocation and Munchausen's syndrome by proxy abuse are usually perpetrated by women. It is common for both parents to be involved in cases of physical abuse or neglect.

The abusing parents do not generally have an identified mental illness though many have personality traits predisposing to violent behaviour or inappropriate sexual behaviour. Men who have poor self-esteem may have considerable anxieties about their own identity and capacity. Sexual activities with children may seem easier, with less resistance to overcome, and less chance of rejection and repetition of earlier humiliation (Bentovim, 1992). Daughters who are victims of incest often suspect that although their mothers know what is going on they are too embarrassed or horrified to broach the topic with them (Cohen *et al.*, 1987).

Abuse and incest occurs in all ranks of society (Renvoize, 1982) but is more likely to be reported in those families who are socially deprived. Abuse is thought to be 20 times more likely if one of the parents has been abused themselves as a child.

Health professionals should be aware of the variety of ways in which children are abused, whether emotionally, physically or sexually, and be aware of the 'risk factors' that make a particular family more vulnerable to abuse than another (Box 6.3).

Box 6.3   Vulnerable families

◆ Disturbed family background
◆ Chaotic relationships
◆ A succession of stepfathers
◆ Previous incest or sexual deviance in the family
◆ A new male member of the household with a record of sexual abuse
◆ When the perpetrator is under the influence of alcohol
◆ Where there is, or has been, sexual rejection
◆ Paedophile sexual orientation in relation to sex rings and pornography.

Children who have been abused may have a variety of symptoms (Box 6.4). Health professionals are often the first professionals, along with teachers, who have the ability and opportunity to make accurate observations of a child they think may be abused. These observations and the action taken will determine whether the child will ultimately receive the treatment and protection required or whether the cycle of abuse will continue.

The guidance of the Joint Working Party on Child Protection (1993) advises that where a child is at risk the child's interests must always be regarded as paramount and will usually require disclosure to the relevant authority.

Child sexual abuse is neither a rarity nor a fantasy. Children who are abused may not realize that they are being abused and may think the experience is a normal part of family life. It is only when they are older and find themselves in different circumstances that they realize they have been abused. This can cause severe emotional, interpersonal and sexual problems in later life (see Chapter 5).

SCENARIO

Ann, a 49-year-old single woman, came to the menopause clinic to discuss her symptoms. The nurse learned that she had not had a cervical smear for some years and discussed with Ann the need for this investigation. While she was being examined Ann began to cry and on gentle questioning told the nurse about her early life.

Ann had been born abroad where she had lived with her parents and three elder brothers on a farm in a remote part of the country. From the age of 10 she had been regularly sexually abused by her father, her brothers and her uncles. Her mother was also abused regularly by the males in the family. It was only when she left home to obtain work that she realized what she had undergone was not a normal part of growing up.

Ann eventually came to this country and over the years she had a succession of male friends but she always terminated the relationships when they became intimate. She said that although she had a successful career, her life was lonely and unhappy. She had always wanted to marry and have children and she had neither.

She went on to explain how angry and bitter she felt about her family and how she had not seen or kept in contact with them since she left home. She said it was the first time in her life that she was able to unburden herself of the secret. Ann was given support and counselling for some considerable time in order to help her come to terms with her childhood abuse.

Abuse of women

Based on worldwide statistics, researchers estimate that as many as one in three women have been beaten, coerced into sex, or otherwise abused in their lifetime. Women are most at risk from people they know, their family members, their spouses and their friends (Heise *et al.*, 1999).

As with children there is no typically abused adult. Violence and sexual abuse happens to all types of people whether they are children, young people or adults. They can be male or female, although women are consistently more likely than men to be the targets of physical, sexual and emotional abuse. They can come from any family background, any social class or any culture. They can be highly intelligent or with a learning disability, be able bodied or disabled.

Box 6.4 Symptoms and signs of child abuse

Physical symptoms

◆ Trauma
◆ Infection
◆ Perineal soreness
◆ Vaginal discharge
◆ Anal pain or bleeding.

Emotional effects

◆ Loss of concentration
◆ Enuresis
◆ Encopresis (loss of bowel control)
◆ Anorexia
◆ Truancy
◆ Disturbed behaviour from early childhood
◆ Changes in behaviour, e.g. withdrawn or aggressive; or developing obsessive behavioural patterns, e.g. worry about cleanliness
◆ Severely self-destructive behaviour.

Sexual abuse entails all types of sexual activity, often with escalating intrusiveness. Women may be exposed to indecent acts, pornography, photography or external contact in the form of fondling, touching or masturbation. Penetrative sex can be vaginal, anal or oral.

A recent UK study of GPs, practice nurses and health visitors reported that over 80% of each professional group considered domestic violence to be a health care issue, and most health professionals believed that there was something they could do to help victims of domestic violence. However, less than 5% of each professional group reported that they routinely enquired about domestic violence. In addition GPs were least likely to request training on the issue (Richardson *et al.*, 2001). It would appear that, although domestic violence is recognized as an important health issue, many health professionals do not routinely ask about abuse experiences and do not want to conduct routine screening (Mezey, 2001).

The reluctance of health professionals to enquire directly about domestic violence has been attributed to a number of factors: lack of knowledge and training, fear of offending women, time constraints, concern about opening a 'Pandora's box' and the belief that domestic violence is not a valid health issue (Sugg and Inui 1992; Brown *et al.*, 1993). In direct contrast to this, a number of studies have shown that the majority of women are in favour of routine screening (by direct questioning) for domestic violence (Friedman *et al.*, 1992; Bacchus *et al.*, 2002; Bradley *et al.*, 2002; Richardson *et al.*, 2002).

In a survey of women attending accident and emergency departments who reported past or current abuse, 36% said that they would only divulge domestic violence if asked directly, 25% said that they would volunteer this information without being asked and 11% said that they would not report domestic violence even if asked (Hayden *et al.*, 1997). Women are more likely to disclose domestic violence to health professionals who are supportive, non-judgemental and who ask questions in a sensitive manner (Rodrigues *et al.*, 1996; Bacchus *et al.*, 2002).

It is very difficult, if not impossible, to assess how often sexual abuse occurs as studies both in the UK and other countries have shown that the vast majority of cases go unreported and of those that are reported only a small percentage ever get to court. Koss (1985) found in the USA that only 5–8% of women who had been sexually assaulted actually reported the crime. The reasons for this reluctance to report are numerous and include self-blame, fear of reprisal and lack of confidence that justice will be done. Due to an increased awareness of abuse and more open discussion there are now greater numbers of people seeking help.

The effects of violence and sexual abuse of an individual are far reaching both in the short term and with the longer-term sequelae. Violence can have a debilitating effect on a woman's health and all her future relationships whether sexual or not. Violence against women will frequently leave a 'legacy of pain' to future generations.

Many men's conception of self-worth centres on possessiveness with regard to women as partners and wives (Horder, 1997). Dobash and Dobash (1984) questioned battered women about sources of the conflicts leading to violent episodes with their partners. In 45% of cases the women cited possessiveness or sexual jealousy and a further 16% of cases centred on expectations about domestic work.

Research has shown that many separated or divorced women gave abuse by their spouse as one of the main reasons for leaving them (McLeod and Cadieux, 1980; Ellis and Ryan, 1987). For some, separation was seen as the solution to marital problems, including psychological, emotional and physical abuse. However, such a solution to the problem of spouse/partner abuse appears to have variable effects. Some women who are beaten before separation from their partners found that if they returned, the beating ceased, whilst others who had not experienced violence before separation reported that they were beaten on their return.

Female economic dependence is associated with a higher rate of severe violence within the relationship (Kalmuss and Strauss, 1982) and women are more likely to sever the relationship if they are working outside the home.

Abuse and violence against women in their own homes is a social problem and is remarkably similar across international samples. The attitude of the police and their response to domestic and sexual abuse is vital, and a number of police forces throughout the UK now have special sections that deal with such problems where the staff involved are given additional training.

Abuse in pregnancy

This is also covered in Chapter 8. Pregnancy, far from offering protection, in some cases appears to increase the risk of violence against women by their partners. During pregnancy women are vulnerable and least able to defend themselves or take evasive action. Pregnant women also appear to suffer from a disproportionate amount of abuse, with as many as one in six women suffering from physical or sexual assault during pregnancy (Flitcraft, 1995). Repeated violent assault has a detrimental effect on maternal and fetal health and physical development and in extreme cases leads to prematurity, miscarriage or fetal death (Mezey and Bewley, 1997).

Domestic violence is, in part, an attack on the woman's sexuality: injuries are often located around the breasts and, in pregnancy, around the abdomen and genitalia. The fetus is as much the target of the man's anger, hatred and envy as the woman. Pregnancy symbolizes the woman's independence from her partner and is about the only thing in the relationship that belongs to the woman alone and that she can control. Campbell (1993) has proposed four different categories of domestic violence in pregnancy:

◆ Jealousy towards the unborn child
◆ Anger towards the unborn child
◆ Pregnancy-specific violence
◆ 'Business as usual'.

It is interesting to note how often the male attempts to control the woman's reproductive powers through rationing her contraception, insisting on terminations, often in the context of jealous delusions and over-solicitous and intrusive

attendance during each obstetric or gynaecological consultation (Mezey and Bewley, 1997).

Victims of domestic violence tend not to disclose their injuries to health professionals and if injuries are detected they will often fabricate explanations. Women may not be able to get away with this during pregnancy as they have more frequent physical examinations which make bruising and injuries more difficult to hide.

Violence during pregnancy is also associated with late booking, sporadic attendance at antenatal appointments and the pregnancy being described as 'unwanted'. It is crucial that health professionals involved in the care of women during pregnancy are alert to the existence of domestic violence and its presentation and that they manage such cases with particular care.

Rape

Rape is committed when a man has sexual intercourse with a woman either knowing that she does not consent or being reckless as to whether she consents or not. Consent must be genuine and not obtained through violence, threats, fraud and coercion. It can also be termed rape if intercourse occurs with a woman who is unconscious or asleep; when the rapist impersonates the woman's partner; or where the woman is not in a position to consent on the grounds of being mentally deficient, too young or drunk.

The slightest penetration of the penis into the outer labia or vagina is sufficient to be termed rape and there is no requirement for the hymen to be broken (in the case of a virgin), nor for there to be any ejaculation of semen. An indecent assault is an assault or battery accompanied by circumstances of indecency. What 'circumstances of indecency' means has never been clearly defined but seems to refer to any overtly sexual conduct which could include kissing.

Perception in society as to what constitutes rape has varied over the years and is constantly changing even in the present day. There have been recent changes in the law and it is now possible for a man to rape his wife. Sexual assault and rape can affect any woman, irrespective of age, class and background. A high percentage of rape cases show that the rape is committed by a person who is known to the victim, and the most common place for this to happen is the victim's home. She may be attacked by more than one assailant and the sexual assault will frequently involve other acts, forcing the victim to take part in sexual activity and degrading practices against her will. One-third of all rapists have a sexual dysfunction. When a woman is attempting to end a relationship batterers are particularly likely to be violent (Websdale *et al.*, 1999) or to attempt rape (Bergen, 1996).

When rape victims first divulge what has happened to them they need gentle handling and considerable support to help them through their immediate problems. Your own reaction is vital and you should encourage the woman to talk and validate the trauma she is experiencing. Victims of rape and assault need to feel in control and they must not be pushed for details that are not immediately relevant.

Women who have been victims of rape and sexual assault may attend the accident and emergency department, their GP's surgery or family planning clinic with a variety of complaints. This can be either immediately after the assault or it may be some considerable time later (see page 184). They may request emergency contraception, a cervical smear, or a referral to the GUM clinic (Box 6.5). It is useful to observe patients carefully when they attend under such circumstances and watch the way they sit, undress and get on the couch. You should listen carefully to any remarks they make during the examination and note if they become tense or anxious. Some may refer to sexual intercourse as being a dirty activity and others may be obsessive about cleanliness and personal hygiene.

The woman may require considerable support from you not only in the short term but also in the future. Rape can have long-term effects not only for the woman involved, but also with her partner and their relationship. The victims of rape may suffer any or all of the problems listed in Box 6.6.

The services of a victim support team may be required and counselling and psychotherapy may help. With time and good care victims can slowly begin to reorganize their lives.

Most victims of rape feel dirty and their first instinct is to wash themselves and their clothing after the assault. This is something that should be strongly discouraged as important forensic evidence will be destroyed. Victims often need time to consider the implications of reporting rape or sexual assault to the police. If they report the attack, they need not necessarily have to go to court, but the information that they give to the police could be helpful when there have been instances of unsolved rape cases. Many police forces now have a 'rape suite' where the victim may be taken for forensic examination.

Police response to rape and domestic violence is crucial. The victim needs to feel believed and trusted and does not want to be made to feel any more uncomfortable than she already is. The police response will also encourage other victims to come forward and perhaps help in reducing the incidence of such abuse.

Box 6.5 Acute problems encountered with rape victims

◆ Fear of internal damage
◆ Pregnancy
◆ Sexually transmitted infection.

Box 6.6 Long-term problems suffered by rape victims

◆ Rape trauma syndrome
◆ Guilt and self-blame ('why me?' and 'was it my fault?')
◆ Sleep disorders
◆ Phobias
◆ Panic attacks
◆ Inability to concentrate and work
◆ Sexual problems
◆ Change in lifestyle
◆ Depression
◆ Drug abuse
◆ Alcoholism.

Nursing issues in dealing with
abused women

In your nursing practice you should learn to recognize the factors that increase the risk of violence towards women and know the cues that could signal abuse. You could incorporate, and enlarge upon, the following questions during your consultation with a woman who you suspect is being abused:

◆ Do you feel safe in your current relationship?

◆ Do you feel your partner controls your behaviour too much?

◆ Have you ever been sexually or physically abused, recently or as a child?

◆ Can you tell me what happened?

You should then be prepared and able to intervene in a sensitive and empowering way. Careful documentation is essential and the woman should be made aware of the various options for assistance that are available to her, including social service support, women's shelters, rape crisis helplines and support groups (see Resources). She should also be encouraged to seek the help and support of friends, relatives and neighbours where appropriate, although women are often reluctant to involve others initially.

Your initial reaction is vitally important when a client of any age first tells you that she has been sexually abused. A non-threatening, accepting and understanding attitude will reduce her sense of abnormality and encourage her to talk. Too often nurses do not know what to say in such a situation and might be tempted to 'gloss over' or ignore what they are being told. Referral to a psychologist or counsellor may be necessary as these women can take considerable time to come to terms with their abuse. It is important that your client does not feel that you are deserting her if you do decide to refer her for counselling. It will have taken her a considerable amount of courage to disclose the information to you and she must not feel that she is being 'passed around'.

Continuing nursing education on violence is essential if you are to become better equipped to provide the intervention and effective help that

women need in order to survive. Additionally you could establish contacts and links with local community agencies who support abused women and their families and exchange thoughts and ideas in order to provide greater continuity of care for your patients. These support agencies can help those who have been abused to develop safety plans, and consider ways women can protect themselves and their children from future violence.

Health workers alone cannot transform the cultural, social and legal environment that gives rise to and condones widespread violence against women. Ending physical and sexual violence requires long-term commitment and strategies involving all parts of society.

Nurses need to know how to empower women to avoid denial, reduce guilt feelings and acknowledge and recognize their past experiences, and then encourage them to move forward and take control of their own lives in the future.

Cultural and religious aspects of sexuality

What do we mean by culture? Culture can be summarized by saying that it describes patterns of learned human behaviour by which ideas and images can be transferred from one generation to another. This transfer is not through biological means. The same newborn child will grow up with a different set of cultural characteristics if it is reared in different cultural groups.

Today, in the UK, you will meet in your everyday work an increasing number of clients from different ethnic and cultural backgrounds. Each of these different cultures looks upon sex and female sexuality in different ways and a variety of cross-cultural views coexist at any one time. Religious beliefs will also affect these attitudes, especially in the case of Asians where religion is an integral part of their lives. It is more than a doctrine or a set of beliefs, and governs their way of life, attitudes and culture.

The aim of this section is to point out some of the many pitfalls that may arise by not concerning yourself with the religious and cultural aspects of the client's ethnic group and imposing, however unintentionally, your own religious and cultural beliefs. It would not be correct to assume that all members of the cultural groups mentioned will believe the same things. Many clients will have been born in this country and because of the interaction between them and other cultural groups their attitudes towards sexual matters, contraception and marriage will have changed.

Women from other cultures, particularly from the Indian subcontinent and the West Indies, tend to have larger families than those who are born in Britain (Cartwright, 1976). This does not necessarily mean that they are opposed to contraception but the advice they require needs to be culturally sensitive to their beliefs. Immigrant families are generally found in cities and they frequently live in poor, overcrowded conditions. However, because of the support system of their extended family, less use is made of social services.

English will not be the first language for many immigrant women, so communication with them may present a problem. You might think that your client has understood what you have been talking about because she has nodded and said 'Yes', but frequently she may be too embarrassed to admit her difficulty. Pamphlets in different languages should always be available, but if not, then you should give her the English language version and encourage her, as best as you can, to get someone to translate this accurately for her.

Interpreters are a considerable help in such situations and can range from a colleague in your clinical practice, a friend or relative of your client to a complete stranger to you both from an outside interpreting agency (either in person or on a telephone language line). Many interpreters are excellent and translate very accurately what you say, but it can be difficult working through a third party as some interpreters may unintentionally distort the questions you ask, and the information they give back to you from your client, and give you their own personal views.

In some areas where there is a significant number of women from another culture it has been considered worthwhile, in an attempt to overcome the language problems, to make an audio or video tape in different languages containing information about health care and contraception that women can listen to and watch whilst waiting to be seen.

It is not possible to discuss fully the special needs of all cultures and religions, but if you come across significant numbers of women from different groups in your clinical practice you should try to acquire some additional understanding of their needs. Often your patients are your best educators!

Hinduism

Hinduism is one of the oldest religions and is widely practised in India, East Africa and the West Indies. Hindu society is patriarchal and the role of the woman is subservient. Sex education is almost totally lacking and girls are expected to be virgins when they marry. Most marriages are arranged and the dowry and caste systems still exist. Men and women do not meet alone socially and are generally separated from puberty.

In Hindu culture there is a strict code of sexual morality to protect families and the community. Premarital and extramarital sex are strictly forbidden. Great shame follows the discovery of illicit liaisons and this may affect the whole family. Parents remain responsible for their children all their lives and the children are expected to obey and care for their parents when they are old.

Marriage is considered to be not just between two people but also between two families. It has to be decided whether a family is suitable and whether the son or daughter will be well treated. For the people arranging the marriage love and romance are the last things on their mind (Kapadia, 1966) and the individual's need for personal happiness is not recognized. It is quite common for families to marry off their sons first and use the dowry obtained to pay for the marriage of their daughters.

It is still frowned upon if a Hindu person does not want to marry, although some will delay marriage if they are, for example, in the middle of their education. The eldest son will usually remain with his parents after marriage and has specific religious duties within the family, especially concerning the ritual cremation of his parents after their death. A wife's first allegiance is to her husband and her in-laws and her own family takes second place. A Hindu father without a son is considered to be unlucky, and giving birth to a son will enhance a woman's status within the community.

The situation described in the scenario here is not an isolated incident and over the years all health professionals have met couples with similar problems. In our multiracial society such problems are becoming increasingly common.

Contraception for Hindus

The traditionally recommended methods of birth control for Hindus are coitus interruptus and that women should breastfeed for two years.

 SCENARIO

Two students, aged 19 years, one Hindu and the other a Sikh came to a family planning clinic. The girl requested a pregnancy test. During the initial counselling they were asked what they intended to do if the outcome of the test was positive. They said that termination of the pregnancy was their only choice. Although they said they were very much in love there was no way that they could marry each other as they were from differing religions. Were they to marry both would be cut off entirely from their respective families for life.

The pregnancy test proved positive. Both were upset and needed time to come to terms with the result. A further counselling session was arranged and they went away to consider all their options. When they returned to the clinic for their appointment they requested a termination of pregnancy. This was arranged and they were seen for counselling on three further occasions in an effort for them to accept their situation.

During these sessions they talked about their future. Their parents lived in London and the Midlands and they both lived in rented accommodation away from their parental homes. The situation they found themselves in caused them deep distress. They decided that they would not tell their parents what had happened but would use a reliable method of contraception. The methods available were explained to them and they chose to use the combined oral contraceptive pill.

In the UK there is a wide range of attitudes among Hindu women about contraception. These vary from the traditionalists who would never consider any form of birth control to the more liberal women who have been born and educated in this country and realize that the social and economic differences in Western life force them to reconsider their traditional customs.

The choice of contraception may exclude all methods that require insertion, as this is taboo in some Asian cultures. Hindu women believe that only the left hand should be used to touch their genital area and this practice would make the diaphragm difficult to use. Another reason why such means of contraception are not chosen by women of Asian cultures is that they find internal examinations shocking and humiliating and may not wish to use a method that requires one. Hindu women will only have been touched by their husbands and will be reluctant to be examined by a male doctor.

When menstruating, Hindu women cannot attend prayers and cannot carry out certain household duties, particularly preparing food and cooking. As the IUD may cause longer periods this method of contraception may not be chosen; however, the Mirena IUS is becoming an acceptable option as in most women it stops menstruation, although amenorrhoea needs careful explanation. The most popular method of contraception in Hindu communities is still the condom but the pill is becoming acceptable to the younger woman. Many Hindus are vegetarian and it is worth remembering this when teaching clients how to take the pill, as absorption may be affected due to a high-fibre diet.

General knowledge of contraception is minimal in immigrant Hindu women as there is little sex education in schools. The subject is very private and many women do not even discuss the matter with their husbands. When discussing contraception and sexual issues with Hindu women you should remember these points and approach the subject with sensitivity.

Hinduism is the most complex religious group to describe because the customs and beliefs vary widely, both regionally and from class to class.

Hindus form the smallest group of Asian migrants to Britain and those that settle are mostly from agricultural and trading groups of quite high social status. Many Tamils who have come to the UK in recent years from Sri Lanka are practising Hindus.

Islam

Islam is the religion of Muslims: a world religion that is widespread and not just confined to the Indian subcontinent. Nearly all the Muslims in Britain are from Pakistan or from Bangladesh.

Islam means 'complete submission to God' and Muslims have five codes of behaviour; these are sometimes called the five 'pillars' of Islam:

◆ There is only one God

◆ Prayers five times a day

◆ Giving money to charity

◆ Fasting from dawn to dusk during the month of Ramadan

◆ Performance of pilgrimage, especially to Mecca.

In Muslim society the roles of men and women are made clear by Islamic law and the Holy Koran. Men are responsible for all matters outside the home and for supporting the families. Women are responsible for rearing and educating children, looking after the family and running the home. Muslim boys must be circumcised before puberty. This procedure is sometimes done in Britain by a Jewish rabbi. Elsewhere it may be done by the family doctor. Circumcision for boys is legal in the UK but the circumcision of girls is illegal (see page 134).

Beliefs about women's roles and responsibilities influence Muslim parents' decisions about the education and upbringing of their daughters in Britain. It is almost impossible for a Muslim girl to participate fully in the life of her British peers and yet remain a good Muslim.

In Muslim society marriage is compulsory for both men and women and it is now illegal for a man to have more than one wife. Muslims often marry first cousins so genetic counselling may be necessary. Neither men nor women expose their bodies, and a woman should also cover two-thirds of her head.

A Muslim woman is always under the guardianship of a man; this may be her father, her husband, or her sons if she is a widow. This is considered very important in matters concerning the outside world. Within the family, both men and women share decision-making. There is a rigid formal code of behaviour between the sexes.

Contraception for Muslim women

Although there are no statements on contraception in the Holy Koran, many conservative Muslims feel that contraception interferes with God's design. The women are considered responsible for producing children and infertility can have serious implications for a couple, leading to eventual rejection and divorce. Conservative Muslim men may be most reluctant to attend fertility clinics with their wives and will feel humiliated and angry at any suggestion that they might be responsible in some way.

Opponents of family planning claim that children have been depicted in the Koran as 'great assets' and claim that the larger the number of Muslims the greater their power. Mothers and mothers-in-law still exert considerable influence on the decision-making within the household.

Confidentiality is very important for Muslims and sex is very private and rarely discussed. The woman's attitude towards sex is very reserved as the beauty of a woman is considered to be her sexual naivety. Muslim women are forbidden to fast during Ramadan and are not allowed to visit the mosque when menstruating. Therefore any method of contraception that prolongs menstruation or may cause breakthrough bleeding is unacceptable. The diaphragm may also be unacceptable as Muslim women dislike touching their genitals and may only use their left hand for this. Muslim women often refuse to have a vaginal examination within 10 days of their period and prefer intrauterine devices to be fitted when they are not menstruating. Conservative Muslim women do not have intercourse for 40 days after a baby is born.

SCENARIO

Jameela, a Muslim aged 24 years, had been married for 3 years. She regularly came to see the nurse at her GP practice in tears as her husband suffered from an erectile dysfunction. It was an arranged marriage; her husband had been born in Britain and she was born in India. Her command of the English language was limited.

Her extended family constantly wanted to know why she was not pregnant and this naturally placed her in a very difficult situation. She had not used any form of contraception as a baby was expected by both the bride and groom's family within the first year. She had undergone basic fertility investigations and her hormone levels and ovarian function appeared to be within normal limits.

After a number of counselling sessions the nurse remained unable to convince Jameela that her husband should also attend, despite the advice and information on the subject she gave Jameela to give to her husband. He refused to attend and on one occasion asked his wife to collect pills for his problem which of course the nurse was unable to supply.

Jameela told the nurse that he would not admit to any family member that the fertility problem could be his. She felt unable to talk to his family about the problem so they all blamed her for not producing a child. She was desperate and said that if she did not become pregnant soon her husband would divorce her and she would be sent back to India to her parents. This would cause her own family considerable shame and embarrassment as there would be no place for her in Muslim society without a husband and children.

Eventually Jameela managed to persuade her husband to attend the doctor to have his problem investigated. Follow-up psychosexual counselling sessions were arranged for both of them to attend.

Sikhs

Most of the Sikhs in Britain come from the Punjab, although there are a few that come to this country from East Africa. Sikhism is a relatively new religion, having developed as a reformist movement of Hinduism in the sixteenth century.

Sikhs believe in one God and, unlike Hindus, do not worship different manifestations of God. There are very few practical regulations concerning the everyday or religious activities of Sikhs. Every Sikh makes his own relationship with God and worships in his own way. Sikhism emphasizes the practical rather than the theoretical.

Sikh women are highly respected and have a great influence in important domestic and community matters. Both men and women take part in all-important religious ceremonies. Women are educated equally with men and have considerable freedom and authority although, as among Hindus and Muslims, there is a system of etiquette which influences the behaviour of the sexes in public.

It is important for a Sikh couple to have a son. In rural societies a large family with several sons ensures family prosperity and survival and is regarded as a blessing. Many Sikhs will therefore decide to continue having children until they have at least one son.

Western culture seems to have influenced Sikhs more than the previous two religious groups discussed, Hindus and Muslims. Women are allowed to work outside the home and the cultural environment. This inevitably leads to many Sikh women exercising greater influence over family affairs such as the decision to regulate family size.

Infertility is again a very important factor and, as with Hindus and Muslims, men will look upon this as the fault of the woman and they will regard any suggestion that they could be the cause as a personal affront. In some families failure to produce sons may be regarded as a reason for rejecting a wife.

Chinese

In recent years, in common with many Western countries, Britain has seen a significant increase in the number of Chinese and Vietnamese people who choose to live away from their own native country. Many of them are refugees and will have left behind members of their family and consequently feel isolated and alone. They tend to gather together in this country in small areas in an urban environment.

Almost all Chinese are Buddhists. Buddhists believe in reincarnation, and so accept responsibility for the ways in which they exercise their freedom in life, since the consequences of their actions may be seen in subsequent lives. It is therefore important that the individual behaves properly. Because there is no 'God' there is no actual worship, but the act of 'Puja' (to respect) is the Buddhist way of acknowledgement of an ideal.

Infanticide and abortion have been practised in China for thousands of years. The dowry system is still practised and up until the recent interventions in birth control unwanted female children were disposed of. At present in China no marriage is allowed before the age of 24. The laws relating to childbirth and the number of children allowed to a married couple are changing regularly. Currently a couple are only permitted one child and are given State payments and grants if they manage this. A second pregnancy frequently ends in an abortion and grants being withdrawn. Because of this restriction on family size the Chinese are usually quite aware of methods of contraception.

In Chinese culture oral contraceptives may be avoided because of the perception that 'hormones are not good for you'. The most common method of contraception used is the IUD. In China the devices are fitted without threads so they are not easily removed. However, women will occasionally have the device removed and will then pretend that it fell out unnoticed. If they have been seen to be using contraception and become pregnant due to a 'method failure' they are sometimes allowed to keep the second child. Male sterilization is widely practised and China has the highest number of vasectomies in the world.

Astrology is an important part of Chinese traditional belief and some families may want to know the precise time of birth so that the child's horoscope can be drawn up. The child is regarded as a human being from the moment of conception and, based on the lunar calendar, a Chinese baby may be considered to be 1 year old at the time of birth.

Vietnamese

Vietnamese women are completely submissive to their fathers until their marriage, at which time their loyalty and obedience is transferred to their husband and his family. If a woman becomes widowed her eldest son becomes the head of the family and she must obey him (Yick and Agbayani-Siewert, 1998). Because of these hierarchical values many women simply accept abuse as a sign of their obedience to him and his family.

In Vietnamese culture large families are traditionally a great source of pride. The size of the family is not in any way related to social status. Vietnamese women reject any argument that it is better to have small families. The appeal of family planning for them is that it enables them to space their children rather than limit their numbers.

Family planning is available in Vietnam on a limited scale and family planning campaigns are carried out by the State. Trained health workers visit towns and villages to give information and advice about contraception. Where available, the most commonly used methods are the pill, the IUD and the condom. Contraception is not freely discussed between the sexes in Vietnam.

SCENARIO

Suzy, a Chinese woman aged 31 years, was living in Britain whilst studying for a PhD and came to a family planning clinic for advice. Her husband and daughter were still living in China and she had recently visited them. The method of contraception they used was the condom. She now found that she was pregnant and visited the clinic to arrange for a termination.

During the counselling session she went on to explain that only one child was allowed to each couple in China. There was a possibility that she would have continued with the pregnancy if she could settle in this country but as her husband had a senior position in the Chinese government, his career and hers would suffer as a consequence.

The termination was arranged and at a further counselling session she wanted to know the sex of the fetus. The counsellor was unable to give her this information. Suzy told the counsellor that the sex would not have influenced her decision regarding a termination but that both she and her husband would have liked a son to carry on the family name.

She was advised on the methods of contraception available to her in this country and she chose the IUD. She was very much against using any hormonal method as she thought it was 'not natural'.

When family planning talks are arranged the audience will be either all male or all female. In your clinical practice, to avoid embarrassment it may be easier to discuss matters concerning contraception separately with the husband and wife.

If it is necessary to use an interpreter they should be of the same sex as the person to whom you wish to speak. Vietnamese are often vague about their reproductive anatomy and embarrassed to discuss it. The IUD and the pill are acceptable to some women, although the latter needs careful and adequate explanation as to how it should be used. The diaphragm is not generally available in Vietnam and some Vietnamese women in Britain are initially embarrassed at the idea of inserting and removing it. Their reluctance, coupled with the language barrier, sometimes discourages the doctor or nurse suggesting it as a possible alternative.

In recent years all forms of religious practice have been discouraged by the Vietnamese State. Because of this, some Vietnamese people feel threatened by questions about their religious beliefs and give the response they feel the most diplomatic in the circumstances. Although Vietnam has no official religion, Buddhism, Taoism and Confucianism are the three philosophical traditions that have played a significant part in the development of Vietnamese culture. Roman Catholicism was introduced to Vietnam by the French, and although the Catholic population of Vietnam is small, a significant number of Vietnamese in Britain are practising Catholics.

Asian family life and differing attitudes among Asian women

Asian society has a community-centred organization. The extended family is still the norm and may consist of unmarried sisters, brothers with their wives and families all living under the same roof. All social events are centred around the family and relatives and any problem encountered will affect the whole family. Although this close network has become more dispersed with families who have settled in Britain, the psychological factors that bind families together remain very strong.

Parenting is not, as was believed some years ago, a natural instinct; it is an acquired skill. One of the virtues of the extended family system, as seen in Asian families, lies in the parenting skills that the elder members impart to young parents (Laungani, 1989).

The Asian child has several close attachments apart from its mother and father. Whilst growing up the child acquires several role models amongst whom are its grandparents and other elders, uncles and aunts who all play an important part in the child's upbringing. Research has shown that this, combined with the close family network, produces a low incidence of child abuse.

Asian mothers rely on the experience of their elders, who have had children of their own, to learn parenting skills. All elders within Asian families are accorded special status and are very much concerned with the moral and spiritual development of the child. Children are seen as a gift from God. Asian parents foster in their children values that emphasize obedience to parental wishes and respect of their elders and teachers.

Research undertaken in Leicester and London on the Asian community has reported that Sikh and Hindu women are much more authoritative and outgoing than their Muslim counterparts (Leicester Council, 1986). Muslim women, particularly those in the Bangladeshi community, consider making decisions on contraception impossible without the approval of their partners. Muslim women prefer the pill whilst their men have a tendency to use condoms.

Sikh women, however, take more responsibility in choosing methods of contraception without encountering opposition from their husbands. Some Hindu women prefer IUDs while the Sikhs are equally happy with pills, IUDs and condoms. Sterilization is accepted on a small scale by all three religious groups.

Afro-Caribbean

The term Afro-Caribbean mainly relates to people of African descent who came to the UK from the West Indies and the Caribbean. Some of these people refer to themselves as West Indian and others as black. They have a wide diversity of family patterns depending on factors such as class, family heritage and religion.

Most Afro-Caribbeans are Christians and belong to different denominations; many in the UK are members of the Pentecostal Church. Historically in the Caribbean, families were large but nevertheless there is evidence that attitudes to family size in the UK are changing (Daud, 1992).

Under slavery, Afro-Caribbean women were encouraged to produce children but were forbidden to marry. The women, their children and the fathers of the children were the property and responsibility of the slave owner. Thus the father's place was never secure as he was not the source of provision and protection for the mother and her children. Marriage among Afro-Caribbeans nowadays is considered to be a very serious matter. A man must be able to support his wife, thus marriage in this community tends to occur later in a couple's life.

In some Afro-Caribbean cultures premarital sex is accepted. It is important for the woman to prove her fertility to her partner and illegitimacy does not carry the same stigma as it does in Western society (Hiro, 1971).

Recent studies have shown that the Afro-Caribbeans are in the category of those ethnic groups who have a genetic predisposition to hypertension. This is possibly due to increased salt intake or to hypersensitivity to salt. Therefore African and Afro-Caribbean women may be more susceptible to pill hypertension than other ethnic groups.

Acetylator status is the rate at which the body inactivates a drug. The Afro-Caribbean community have 87% slow acetylator status. A client who is of low acetylator status is likely to retain a drug longer, giving increased beneficial effects but also more prolonged side effects. If an Afro-Caribbean client complains that she cannot tolerate the pill, the above should be taken into account, and a lower-dose pill suggested. Acetylator status applies to all drugs.

The IUD is usually preferred by Afro-Caribbean clients. Most like to have normal periods and do not like menstruation to be suppressed. For those clients who suffer from sickle cell anaemia it has been shown that the injectable 'Depo-Provera' lessens the number of sickle crises. Depo-Provera has a stabilizing effect on the cell membrane in sickle cell disease which is a positive health feature. Although the combined oral contraceptive pill is not contraindicated in women with sickle cell disease it may increase the number of sickle crises (Howard, 1994).

Rastafarians

Rastafarians can be found in many parts of the world and are easily recognized by both their colourful dress and their hairstyle. They consider that they are the true Jews who will be redeemed by their return to Africa, their true home and Heaven on earth. They believe in Ras Tafari, the former emperor of Ethiopia, crowned Haile Selassie I, as a god who is also regarded as a Black Messiah.

Rastafarians follow the Old Testament teaching in that they should 'be fruitful and multiply'. Children are regarded as a blessing and are seen as a continuation of life. Contraception is unacceptable to many Rastafarians and is seen as an attempt of white-dominated society to control black fertility. They may use natural family planning (self-taught) as an attempt at birth control.

Traditionally, women are mainly responsible for childcare although many fathers are also involved. Both men and women are encouraged to develop their own potential and in many relationships there is equality, with decisions being taken jointly after discussion. Many Rastafarians are vegetarian, or avoid eating pork and drinking alcohol. They wear their hair in matted locks (dreadlocks), and often cover these with knitted caps (tams) of red, gold, green and black, the colours of the Ethiopian flag, which holds particular symbolic significance for them.

Jews

Jewish religion and culture are inextricably entwined. Judaism is based on the belief in one universal God, and the religious precepts followed are simply to worship one God, to carry out the ten commandments and to practise charity and tolerance towards one's fellow human beings.

The family is of great importance in Jewish life. In Britain today there is a wide spectrum of observance among Jews from 'reform' and 'liberal' to the ultra orthodox communities whose daily lives are guided by the code of laws contained in the five books of Moses, the 'Torah'. There are strict Sabbath laws which must be observed from 4 pm on Friday to 4 pm on Saturday. There are also a number of feast days.

Judaism is a male-centred religion. Orthodox Jewish women will dress with modesty but are unlikely to make a special request to see a female doctor. Any form of fertility control is opposed by orthodox Jewish religion because it negates the command to 'be fruitful and multiply'. Jewish belief is that the life-giving potential of semen is sacred and any form of contraception which prevents sperm and ova from meeting, or which destroys or wastes sperm is not allowed. Thus the use of barrier methods, spermicides and coitus interruptus are forbidden by the 'Halacha' (the body of the Jewish law). On the same principle, female sterilization is more acceptable than male, since it does not damage the sperm. According to other Jewish authorities, the use of the diaphragm is more acceptable because the sperm is deposited in the vagina and not wasted.

If pregnancy is considered harmful to the health of the woman then contraception may be used. In this case, the use of barrier methods and the use of oral contraception in the form of the pill are acceptable. Although the latter prevents the sperm from meeting the ova, it does not interfere with the natural act of intercourse and does not directly destroy the male sperm. The use of the IUD is permitted, with reservations based on the mechanism of action of the IUD. If it prevents fertilization it may be acceptable, but if fertilization can occur and the IUD acts by preventing implantation then it may be considered an abortifacient and thus is unacceptable.

Ambivalence about birth control among Jews stems from a tension between the prescription of the marital duty to procreate and the desire to provide adequate sexual companionship. Responsible parenthood is often seen as a more important issue for Jewish families rather than which method of contraception to use.

Marriages are usually 'arranged' and marrying anyone outside the Jewish religion is forbidden, as is extramarital sex (Thompson, 1993).

During menstruation women are considered 'unclean' and are forbidden inside the synagogue. Sexual intercourse is also forbidden at this time. This unclean state continues until seven days after menstruation when the 'Mikvah' (the ritual bath) takes place. In consequence, the IUD, which might cause longer menstruation, is not desirable.

Circumcision is performed on baby boys on the first opportunity eight days after birth. This is a Bible-based practice and is seen as a covenant with the Torah and God. Circumcision is very widely practised and causes much soul searching for out-married couples, i.e. Jew and non-Jew, as it is seen as a continuity of covenant with being Jewish.

In very orthodox circles the sexes are segregated from an early age, around 7 or 8 years, especially in educational establishments. In the home this is not so pronounced but at any social event outside the home, segregation would take place. For orthodox Jews the dietary laws are strict, and only 'kosher' food is acceptable. Milk and meat are not eaten at the same meal. Meat must be killed according to kosher ritual and is acceptable only from animals that chew the cud and have a cloven hoof, or from poultry. Pig and rabbit meat are forbidden.

Abortion is generally forbidden, but would be allowed in circumstances where the mother's health is at risk or where congenital diseases are detected in the early stage of pregnancy. Ashkenazi Jews are the main ethnic group at risk from Tay–Sachs disease. One in 25 people in this group is a Tay–Sachs disease carrier as opposed to 1 in 250 of the non-Jewish population. Tay–Sachs disease is an incurable neurodegenerative disorder caused by the deficiency of an enzyme called hexosaminidase A (Hex A), which results in the accumulation of a harmful substance in the brain. It causes early death due to progressive mental retardation and motor weakness. As there is no cure for Tay–Sachs disease, treatment focuses on the management of the various complications and on ensuring that the child is as comfortable as possible. Death usually occurs by the age of 4 years.

Catholics

The Catholic Church sees itself as the one, true, universal and apostolic Church of Christ. It teaches that there are two specific ways of fulfilling the vocation of love:

◆ Through marriage characterized by permanence, fidelity and openness to life

◆ Through virginity or celibacy.

Any alternative is viewed as an abuse of human sexuality whether intentional or through immaturity or ignorance.

Many Catholics feel caught between the tensions of the conservative position of the central Church and the current Pope on population issues and the more liberal moves to reform and modernize Catholic doctrine.

Controversy and discontent with the Church's teaching is now a reality and debate surrounding the above issues will not go away. With today's more liberal outlook, attitudes towards premarital sex and divorce are being challenged on all sides and restrictions regarding contraception are widely disregarded. All the Catholic Church's teaching on contraception refers to contraception *within* marriage so the question of contraception outside marriage does not arise.

Catholicism, however, is not opposed to family planning in its literal sense but demands self-control or abstinence to achieve this. Natural family planning is the only method of contraception that is acceptable. Catholic couples can be referred to a suitable agency to learn more about this method (see page 287).

Catholic couples tend to have larger families than other couples, as they are opposed to abortion and sterilization. According to both American and British fertility studies (Woolf, 1972; Cartwright, 1976), in reality all methods of birth control are used and abortion itself is resorted to when a woman feels she cannot face another pregnancy. Although abortion remains illegal or is heavily restricted in many countries, it is practised in most countries throughout the world. Views and values regarding elective abortion differ from one culture or religion to another, and women of all cultural groups and religious affiliations seek and obtain abortions. Some Catholic women, when they feel they have had the number of children with which they can cope, will request sterilization.

Catholics in the Republic of Ireland, who wish to practise a method of contraception not accepted by the Church, will travel miles outside their local area to seek family planning advice. Many of their family doctors are now beginning to prescribe the pill for 'menstrual irregularities' rather than as a method of contraception. Despite the prohibitions on premarital sex, pregnancy before marriage frequently occurs. About 4000 Irish women travel to Britain each year to have abortions, and others to have their baby so that their families will not discover the pregnancy.

Some priests are now leaving the decision on the use of birth control methods other than those advocated by the Catholic Church to the conscience of the woman or couple concerned.

Hispanic, Mexican, Puerto Rican and Cuban peoples are predominately Roman Catholic; they use most forms of contraception, including permanent sterilization (Amaro, 1998).

Nursing issues affecting culture and religion

The above is not a definitive list of cultures and religions. It does, however, include the main cultures and religious groups to which a significant number of your clients will belong. Not all the individuals coming from these cultures will still conform and many, particularly if they have been born and brought up in Britain, will be far more westernized than others. Practices relating to sex, marriage and the family frequently cause conflict between generations with those (usually the old) who wish to preserve traditions and those who wish to adapt and change. The more diverse the population becomes the more attitudes and practices will change.

In your clinical practice you should be aware that culture and religion can have a powerful influence on the way a woman feels about her sexuality and you should try to assess these during your initial consultations. It is also important for you to be aware of your own religious and cultural beliefs about sexuality and not let these influence you in your care of your client, particularly if they are in opposition. You should be able to demonstrate an accepting, non-judgemental attitude towards all your clients regardless of their ethnic background in order to provide the holistic nursing care they need.

Culture needs to be more clearly understood as a separate concept from religion. Culture encompasses the values, ideas, knowledge and ideologies of human beings, which develop and change. Part of change needs to include a process of reflection on beliefs, principles and behaviour to assess whether any aspect of social and customary values, knowledge and practice is standing in the way of people's better development and well-being. In the area of women's health and gender, this reflection is essential as most cultural practices are frequently referred to in sweeping statements as barriers to better health.

In reality there are traditional health practices that contribute greatly to protecting and maintaining women's health. Yet there are also practices that need to change now that there is new knowledge to show that they are not beneficial, or that other health interventions are more effective.

Female genital mutilation

Female genital mutilation (FGM) is widely practised and an acceptable norm in many African ethnic groups and in some parts of the Middle East and South-East Asia. The countries where this practice is most predominant are Somalia, Nigeria, Eritrea and Sierra Leone. Some practise it with a belief that it is a religious requirement for Muslims. However, the Holy Koran does not include a single mention of female circumcision although it refers to many issues pertaining to women such as pregnancy, childbirth, breastfeeding, divorce and menstruation. FGM is practised by Christians, Muslims and non-believers alike.

The World Health Organization (WHO, 2000) classified FGM into four types:

◆ Type 1. Excision of the prepuce, with or without excision of part or all of the clitoris

◆ Type 2. Excision of the clitoris, with partial or total excision of the labia minora which accounts for 80% of FGM (WHO, 2000)

◆ Type 3. Excision of part or all of the external genitalia and stitching/narrowing of the vaginal opening (infibulation)

◆ Type 4. Unclassified: this includes pricking, piercing or incising of the clitoris and/or labia, stretching of the clitoris and/or labia, cauterisation by burning of the clitoris and surrounding tissue. (Momoh, 1999)

The 'operation' is usually carried out under poor aseptic conditions that are likely to be unhygienic, and the infection rate is high. Ninety-five per cent of FGM is performed on girls between 1 day old and 16 years, i.e. before they become too vocal and able to understand the long-term implications. The more wealthy parents tend to use trained surgeons.

The incidence of FGM or 'female circumcision' was fairly rare in Britain until the 1970s when an increasing number of immigrants and refugees began to arrive from parts of the world where it is practised. There can be no doubt that FGM is an extreme form of physical assault on a defenceless child, which has a lifelong effect on the victim. Such mutilation of a child's genitalia, for no good medical reason, is a violation of the child's human rights and is, in effect, 'child abuse'.

In Britain it is estimated that 10,000 female children are at risk (Hedley and Dorkenoo, 1992). In 1985 the British government passed legislation that made 'female circumcision' illegal in Britain. Consequently some immigrant families take their daughters out of the UK to their home country for a 'holiday' to have this procedure carried out. A girl who is not circumcised can have difficulty finding a husband.

A woman who has undergone FGM as a child may not present until she is pregnant (childbirth and FGM is discussed on page 185). Following childbirth it is illegal to do a complete repair of the vulva so that it is restored to its previous infibulated state (Jordan, 1994). Others may present earlier with problems of non-consummation, infertility, dysmenorrhoea, recurrent urinary tract and vaginal infections and psychosexual problems. The initial consultation provides an ideal opportunity for giving information and for sensitive counselling. Sometimes a de-infibulation procedure may be decided upon after such counselling and support.

All health visitors, family planning nurses, midwives and school nurses need to be aware of this practice as they will occasionally come across women and children from other cultures who have undergone FGM. Those who come into contact with families who have cultural or racial links with countries where this practice is endemic should use their skills to advise parents of the health risks involved. Such clients require an approach that is culturally sensitive and non-judgemental.

Conclusion

This chapter has highlighted some of the situations where health professionals might find they need extra resources to enable them to help women in different circumstances. The domiciliary family planning service, where it is available, can successfully cope with many of these requirements. People with learning disabilities are encouraged to become more independent and are being cared for in the community – they need the skills of caring professionals to help them cope with their sexuality.

Women within violent relationships need sensitivity in helping them come to terms with what has happened to them and recover. Over the past few decades the UK has become a more homogeneous mix, with people from many ethnic backgrounds, cultures and religions living together in relatively small communities. Health professionals who make an effort to understand religious and cultural needs will have the bonus of being able to give holistic advice that is relevant to an individual woman's ethnic background.

Women with special needs are more vulnerable; not only do they need special care for their own individual situations but they may also have problems with many of the issues that are discussed elsewhere in this book, e.g. unplanned pregnancy, subfertility, psychosexual problems and premenstrual syndrome to name but a few. Many changes are taking place within the health service and it is important that women with special needs should receive the more individual care that they require.

Ideas for personal and professional development

- Utilize, where available, the outreach service. It is especially useful to follow up young people in care, some of whom move from place to place inside and outside your area

- Gain a deeper understanding of female genital mutilation to enable you to feel confident when confronted with a client who has undergone such a traumatic experience. Find out where to refer a woman who requests a reversal operation

- Compile a list of services and resources available for those who have been abused. Learn how to ask the right questions where abuse is suspected, and find out more about the assessment tools available

- Liaise with your local trust to find what courses are available on demographic diversity and cultural awareness. Find out how to access local interpreting services for those who need them

- Explore factors that contribute to the incidence of learning difficulties in minority ethnic populations.

Patient education points

- The outreach service is available for those who find it difficult, for a variety of reasons, to access health care

- Interpreting and translating services are available either in person or via a telephone. Utilize volunteers and staff from the community who are culturally compatible with local people: which in itself increases participation. They might be able to translate health education leaflets into other languages

- Advice, support and help are available in a confidential setting for women and children. Put posters up and have handouts available at clinics and surgeries with contact numbers and addresses

- Those with learning difficulties, and their carers, can receive non-judgemental guidance and support to enable them to express their sexual needs.

Resources

ACIA (African Community Involvement Association)
Eagle Court, 224 London Road, Mitcham, Surrey CR4 3HD
Tel: 020 8687 2400
www.acia-uk.org

Asian Women's Resource Centre
108 Craven Park, London NW10 8QE
Tel: 020 8961 5701

Buddhist Hospice Trust
1 Laurel House, Trafalgar Road, Newport, Isle of Wight PO30 1QN

Catholic Marriage Advisory Council
Natural Family Planning Service, Clitherow House, 1 Blythe House, Blythe Road, London W14 0NW
Tel: 020 7371 1341

Childline
Freepost 1111, London N1 0BR
Tel: 0800 1111 (freephone)
www.childline.org.uk
Telephone counselling service for young people who have been sexually abused.

Chinese National Healthy Living Centre
29–30 Soho Square, London W1D 3QS
Tel: 020 7837 7297

Equal Opportunities Commission
Arndale House, Arndale Centre, Manchester M4 3EQ
Helpline: 0845 601 5901
www.eoc.org.uk

Fertility UK
Bury Knowle Health Centre, 207 London Road, Headington, Oxford OX3 9JA
www.fertilityuk.org
Provides training for health professionals.

Hindu Centre (London)
39 Grafton Terrace, London NW5
Tel: 020 7485 8200

Islamic Cultural Centre
London Central Mosque, 146 Park Road, London NW8 7RG
Tel: 020 7724 3363
www.islamicculturalcentre.co.uk

London Chinese Health Resource Centre
43 Dean Street, London W1V 5AP
www.surgerydoor.co.uk

National Children's Bureau
8 Wakley Street, London EC1V 7QE
Tel: 020 7843 6000
www.ncb.org.uk
Promotes the interests and well-being of all children and young people across every aspect of their lives. Publications available.

National Spiritual Assembly of the Baha'is of the United Kingdom
www.bahai.org.uk

NSPCC (National Society for the Prevention of Cruelty to Children)
Weston House, 42 Curtain Road, London EC2A 3NH
Helpline: 0800 800500
www.nspcc.org.uk

Parents Anonymous (for parents who feel they may abuse their children)
36 Park Drive, London NW11 7SP
Tel: 020 7263 8918

Rape and Sexual Abuse Support Centre
PO Box 383, Croydon CR9 2AW
Tel: 020 8239 1122
Helpline: 020 8683 3300
www.rasasc.org.uk

Rape Crisis Federation Wales and England
Unit 7, Provident Works, Newdigate Street, Nottingham NG7 4FD
Tel: 0115 900 3560
www.rapecrisis.co.uk
Can provide details of local rape crisis centres in England and Wales.

Relate
Herbert Gray College, Little Church Street,
  Rugby CV21 3AP
Tel: 01788 573241
www.relate.org.uk
Look in the phone book for the nearest branch
  under Relate or marriage guidance.

**Rights of Women (ROW) (advice and
  referral)**
52–54 Featherstone Street, London EC1Y 8RT
Tel: 020 7251 6575
Advice: 020 7251 6577
www.rightsof women.org.uk

Samaritans
The Upper Mill, Kingston Road, Ewell,
  Surrey KT17 2AF
Tel: 020 8394 8300
www.samaritans.org.uk
Check in the telephone directory for local
  branches.

Shelter
National Helpline: 0808 800 4444
London Helpline: 020 7404 6929
www.shelter.org.uk

Sikh Missionary Society
10 Featherstone Road, Southall,
  Middlesex UB2 5AA
Tel: 020 8574 1902

**SPOD (Association to Aid the Sexual and
  Personal Relationships of the Disabled)**
This society has now closed but enquiries
  can be directed to the Outsiders helpline: 0707
  499 3527 or www.outsiders.org.uk

Survivors
PO Box 2470, London SW9 6WQ
Helpline: 0845 1221201
www.survivors.org
For male clients only who have been raped or
  assaulted.

Tamil Refugee Centre
65-66 North Square, London N9 0HY
Tel: 020 8345 6301

The Haven
Kings College Hospital, Denmark Hill, London

Tel: 020 7346 1599 from 8.30 am to 5 pm
  Monday to Friday, other times 020 7737 4000.
www.met.police.uk/the havens/haven

Victim Support
Cranmer House, 39 Brixton Road,
  London SW9 6DZ
Enquiries: 020 7735 9166
Support line: 0845 30 30 900
www.victimsupport.com

Vietnamese Refugee Group
West Library, Bridgman Road, London N1 1BD
Tel: 020 7607 6271

Visitation Committee
c/o Office of the United Synagogue, Woburn
  House, Upper Woburn Place, London WC1
Tel: 020 7387 4300

Women & Girls Network
PO Box 13095, London W14 0FE
Tel: 020 7610 4345
For women/girls who have experienced
  violence, sexual/physical/emotional.

Women's Aid
PO Box 391, Bristol BS99 7WS
Tel: 0118 944 4411
www.womensaid.org.uk
Provides support and temporary refuge for
  women in violent relationships – mental,
  physical or sexual abuse.

Women's Health
52 Featherstone Street, London EC1Y 8RT
Tel: 020 7251 6333
Helpline: 0845 125 5254
www.womenhealthlondon.org.uk
Can provide leaflets about women's health,
  disabilities and black women's health issues.

Useful websites

www.disabilitynet.co.uk
Details of many UK organizations and charities.

Domestic Violence, Crime and Victims Bill
www.parliament.the-stationery-office.co.uk

Sexual Offences Act 2003
www.hmso.gov.uk/acts2003/20030042

Further reading

Family planning

ALLEN, I. (1991) *Family Planning and Pregnancy Counselling Projects for Young People*. London: PSI Publications.

CHRISTOPHER, E. (1987) *Sexuality and Birth Control in Community Work*. London: Tavistock, pp. 234–54.

RCN (1993) *Domiciliary Family Planning Special Needs*. London: RCN.

Learning disabilities

COOPER, E. and GUILLEBAUD, J. (1999) *Sexuality and Disability: A Guide for Everyday Practice*. Oxford: Radcliffe Medical Press.

CRAFT, A. and CRAFT, M. (1985) *Sex and the Mentally Handicapped: A Guide for Parents and Carers*. London: Routledge & Kegan Paul.

FRAZER, J. (1991) *Contraception: Birth Control, Family Planning, 'Learning to Love'*. A set of simple booklets on sexuality for young people with learning difficulties who have minimal reading skills. London: Brook Advisory Service.

GUNN, M.J. (1991) *Sex and the Law: A Brief Guide for Staff Working with People with Learning Difficulties*, 3rd edn. London: Family Planning Association.

SIMS, A. and OWENS, D. (1993) *Psychiatry*, 6th edn. London: Baillière Tindall.

THOMPSON, T. and MATTHIAS, P. (1992) *Standards and Mental Handicap: Keys to Competence*. London: Baillière Tindall.

Sexual abuse

BANCROFT, L. and SILVERMAN, J.G. (2002) *The Batterer as Parent, Addressing the Impact of Domestic Violence on Family Dynamics*. London: SAGE Publications.

BASS, E. and DAVIS, L. (1990) *The Courage to Heal: A Guide for Women Survivors of Child Sex Abuse*. London: Mandarin.

BRYANT-JEFFERIES, R. (2003) *Counselling a Survivor of Child Sex Abuse*. Oxford: Radcliffe Medical Press.

CORBY, B. (2000) *Child Abuse Towards a Knowledge Base*. Buckingham, Philadelphia: Open University Press.

DORKENOO, E. (1992) *Female Genital Mutilation: Proposals for Change*. London: Minority Rights Group.

FINKELHOR, D. (1984) *Child Sex Abuse*. New York: Macmillan.

FROST, M. (1999) *Clinical Issues in Domestic Violence*. London: Nursing Times Monographs.

HOSKEN, F.P. (1994) *Genital Sexual Mutilation of Females*, 4th edn. Lexington, MA: Women's International Network.

LIGHTFOOT-KLEIN, H. (1991) *Prisoners of Ritual: An Odyssey into Female Genital Circumcision in Africa*. London: Howarth Press.

LIVITNOFF, S. (1992) *The RELATE Guide to Sex and Loving Relationships*. London: Vermillion.

VIANO, E.C. (1992) *Intimate Violence: Interdisciplinary Perspectives*. Washington, DC: Hemisphere.

WYRE, R. and SWIFT, A. (1990) *Women, Men and Rape*. London: Hodder & Stoughton.

Cultural aspects

AHMED, L. (1992) *Women and Gender in Islam*. New Haven: Yale University Press.

BERKOVITS, D. (1992) *A Guide to Jewish Practice for Nurses and Medical Staff*. London: Federation of Synagogues.

CASHMORE, E. (1984) *The Rastafarians*. London: Minority Rights Group.

COOMBE, V. and LITTLE, A. (1986) *Race and Social Work: A Guide to Training*. London: Tavistock.

EISLER, R.M. and HERSEN, M. (2000) *Gender, Culture, and Health*. Mahwah, NJ: Laurence Erlbaum.

FONG, L.C. and WATT, I. (1994) Chinese health behaviour: breaking barriers to better understanding. *Health Trends* **26**(1):14–15.

HENLEY, A. (1979) *Asian Patients in Hospital and at Home*. Bath: Pitman Press.

HENLEY, A. and SCHOTT, J. (1999) *Culture, Religion and Patient Care in a Multi-ethnic Society*. London: Age Concern Books.

HORNSBY-SMITH, M.P. (1991) *Roman Catholic Beliefs in England: Customary Catholicism and Transformations of Religious Authority*. Cambridge: Cambridge University Press.

OWEN COLE, W. (1991) *Moral Issues in Six Religions*. London: Heinemann.

RAWAF, S. and BAHL, V. (1998) *Assessing Health Needs of People From Minority Ethnic Groups*. London: Royal College of Physicians.

RCN (Royal College of Nursing) (1994) *Female Genital Mutilation: The Unspoken Issue*. London: RCN.

SHEIKH, A. and GATRAD, R. (2000) *Caring for Muslim Patients*. Oxford: Radcliffe Medical Press.

SPITZER, J. (2003) *Caring for Jewish Patients*. Oxford: Radcliffe Medical Press.

THOMPSON, R. (1993) *Religion, Ethnicity and Sex Education: Exploring the Issues*. London: National Children's Bureau.

References

AMARO, H. (1998) Women in the Mexican-American community; religion, culture and reproductive attitudes and experiences. *Journal of Community Psychology* **16**:6–20.

BACCHUS, L., MEZEY, G. and BEWLEY, S. (2002) Women's perceptions and experiences of routine enquiry for domestic violence in a maternity service. *British Journal of Obstetrics and Gynaecology* **109**:9–16.

BENTOVIM, A. (1992) *Trauma. Organised Systems – Sexual and Physical Abuse within Families*. London: Karmac.

BERGEN, R.K. (1996) *Wife Rape; Understanding the Response of Survivors and Service Providers*. Thousand Oaks, CA: Sage.

BRADLEY F., SMITH, M., LONG J. and O'DOWD, T. (2002) Reported frequency of domestic violence: cross sectional survey of women attending general practice. *British Medical Journal* **324**:271–4.

BROWN, J.B., LENT, B. and SAS, G. (1993) Identifying and treating wife abuse. *Journal of Family Practice* **36**:185–91.

BURGER, M.P. *et al.* (1993) Cigarette smoking and human papillomavirus in patients with reported cervical cytological abnormality. *British Medical Journal* **306**(6880):749–52.

CAMPBELL, J.C. (1993) Why battering during pregnancy? *Clinical Issues in Woman's Health Nursing* **4**:343–9.

CARTWRIGHT, A. (1976) *How Many Children?* London: Routledge & Kegan Paul.

CHRISTOPHER, E. (1980) Domiciliary family planning – a service described and assessed. *British Journal of Family Planning* **6**.

COHEN, T.B., GALENSON, E., VAN LEEUWEN, K. *et al.* (1987) Sexual abuse in vulnerable and high risk children. *Child Abuse and Neglect* **11**:461–74.

COOPER, E. and GUILLEBAUD, J. (1999) *Sexuality and Disability: A Guide for Everyday Practice.* Oxford: Radcliffe Medical Press.

CRAFT, A. (1990) *Sex Education for Individuals with a Mental Handicap.* London: Novum.

CRAFT, A. and CRAFT, M. (1985) *Sex and the Mentally Handicapped: A Guide for Parents and Carers.* London: Routledge & Kegan Paul.

DAUD, S. (1992) Abortion, contraception and ethnic minorities in the UK. *Planned Parenthood in Europe* **21**(3):9–12.

DOBASH, R.E. and DOBASH, R.P. (1984) The nature and antecedents of violent events. *British Journal of Criminology* **24**:269.

DoH (Department of Health) (1992) *The Health of the Nation.* London: The Stationery Office.

DoH (1999) *Saving Lives: Our Healthier Nation*, White Paper. London: HMSO.

ELLIS, D. and RYAN, J. (1987) *Lawyers and Post Separation Women Abuse: The Relevance of Social Support.* A report submitted to the Department of Justice, Ottawa, Canada, and the Laidlaw Foundation.

FLITCRAFT, A. (1995) From public health to personal health. Violence against women across the lifespan. *Annals of Internal Medicine* **123**(10), 800–2.

FRIEDMAN, L.S., SARNET, J.H., ROBERTS, M.S., HUDIN, M. and HERIS. P. (1992) Inquiry about victimization experiences. *Archives of International Medicine* **152**:1186–90.

HAYDON, S.R., BARTON, S.D. and HAYDON, M. (1997) Domestic violence in the emergency department: how do women prefer to disclose their issues? *Journal of Emergency Medicine* **15**:447–51.

HEDLEY, R. and DORKENOO, E. (1992) *Child Protection and Female Genital Mutilation: Advice for Health, Education and Social Work Professionals.* London: Forward, 38 King Street, WC2 8JT.

HEISE, L., ELLSBERG, M. and GOTTEMOELLER, M. (1999) Ending violence against women. *Population Report* Series L, No. 11.

HIRO, D. (1971) *Black British, White British.* Harmondsworth: Penguin.

HORDER, J. (1997) *Provocation and Responsibility.* Oxford: Clarendon Press.

HOWARD, R. (1994) Contraception and sickle cell disease. *IPPF Medical Bulletin* **28**(4):3–4.

JOINT WORKING PARTY OF THE DEPARTMENT OF HEALTH, BRITISH MEDICAL ASSOCIATION AND CONFERENCE OF MEDICAL COLLEGES (1993) *Child Protection: Medical Responsibilities.* London: BMA.

JONES, M. (1998) The grand protocol shake-up. *Practice Nursing* **9**(10).

JORDAN, J. (1994) Female genital mutilation (female circumcision). *British Journal of Obstetrics and Gynaecology* **101**:94–5.

KALMUSS, D. and STRAUSS, M.A. (1982). Wife's marital dependency and wife abuse. *Journal of Marriage and the Family.* **44**:277–86.

KAPADIA, K.M. (1966) *Marriage and Family Life in India.* Bombay: Oxford University Press.

KOSS, M.P. (1985) The hidden rape victim: personality, attitudinal and situational characteristics. *Psychology of Women Quarterly* **9**:193–212.

LAUNGANI, P. (1989) *Asian Perspectives in Child Abuse: A Proposed Paradigm Shift.* London: New Quest, p. 76.

LEATHARD, A. (1985) *District Health Authorities Family Planning Services in England and Wales.* London: FPA.

LEICESTER COUNCIL (1986) *Religious Background of Asians in Leicester*, city survey.

LUESLEY, D., BLONFIELD, P., DUNN, J., SHAFI, M., CHENOY, R. and BUXTON, J. (1994) Cigarette smoking and histological outcome in women with mildly dyskarotic smears. *British Journal of Obstetrics and Gynaecology* **101**(1):49–52.

McCARTHY, M. (1993) Sexual experiences of women with learning difficulties in longstay hospitals. *Sexuality and Disability* **11**(4):277–86.

McGUIRE, A. and HUGHES, D. (1995) *The Economics of Family Planning Services.* London: FPA.

McLEOD, L. and CADIEUX, A. (1980) *Wife Battering in Canada: The Vicious Circle.* Ottawa.

MENCAP (1998) *The NHS – Health for All?* London: Mencap.

MEZEY, G. (2001) Domestic violence in health settings. *Current Opinion in Psychiatry* **14**:543–7.

MEZEY, G.C. and BEWLEY, S. (1997) Domestic violence and pregnancy. *British Medical Journal* **314**:1295.

MOMOH, C. (1999) Female genital mutilation: the struggle continues. *Practice Nursing* **10**(2).

NHSE (National Health Service Executive) (1998) *Report on the Supply and Administration of Medicines under Group Protocols.* Health Service Circular HSC 1998/051. Leeds: NHSE.

RENVOIZE, J. (1982) *Incest: A Family Pattern.* London: Routledge & Kegan Paul.

RICHARDSON, J., FEDER, G., ELDRIGE, S., CHUNG, W.S., COID, J. and MOOREY, S. (2001) Women who experience domestic violence and women survivors of childhood sexual abuse; a survey of health professionals' attitudes and clinical practice. *British Journal of General Practice* **51**:468–70.

RODRIGUES, M.A., SZKUPINSKI, S. and BAUER, H.M. (1996) Breaking the silence. *Archives of Family Medicine* **5**:153–8.

ROYAL COLLEGE OF NURSING (1991a) *Standards of Care in Family Planning Nursing.* Harrow: Scutari.

ROYAL COLLEGE OF NURSING (1991b) *Family Planning Manual for Nurses.* Harrow: Scutari.

SIMS, A. and OWENS, D. (1993) *Psychiatry*, 6th edn. London: Baillière Tindall.

SUGG, N.K. and INUI, T. (1992) Primary care physicians' responses to domestic violence. Opening Pandora's Box. *Journal of the American Medical Association* **276**:3157–60.

THOMPSON, R. (1993) *Religion, Ethnicity and Sex Education: Exploring the Issues*. London: National Children's Bureau.

WEBSDALE, N., TOWN, M. and JOHNSON, B. (1999) Domestic violence fatality reviews: from a culture of blame to a culture of safety. *Juvenile and Family Court Journal* **50**(2):61–74.

WOOLF, M. (1972) *Families Five Years On*. London: HMSO.

WORLD HEALTH ORGANIZATION (WHO) (2000) Fact sheet No. 241. www.who.int/mediacentre/factsheets.

YICK, A.G. and AGABAYANI-SIEWERT, P. (1998) Perceptions of domestic violence in a Chinese American community. *Journal of Interpersonal Violence* **12**:832–46.

7: Young People and Sex

Catriona Sutherland

OBJECTIVES

This chapter should help you understand:

◆ How the law affects young people with regard to contraception, abortion and other related issues ◆

◆ The current situation concerning sex education in schools ◆

◆ That young people have many needs when seeking advice but that their greatest anxiety is that confidentiality will be broken ◆

◆ The extra problems that peer group pressure can exert, with particular regard to eating disorders. ◆

Introduction

Young people have their own special needs both as a generic group and as individuals. These needs – particularly in the areas of sex education, contraception, advice and counselling – can only be met with special services that are accessible and relevant to them.

This chapter is intended to help you to extend your knowledge and skills in relation to the needs of young women. The particular skills needed include sensitivity, the ability to listen, respect for others, being non-judgemental and well informed.

The term 'young woman' is generally used throughout, in preference to girl, teenager, child or adolescent.

Legal issues affecting under-16s

Age of majority

The Family Law Reform Act 1969 in England and Wales reduced the age of majority from 21 to 18. This means that young people of 18 and above can vote and marry without the consent of their parents.

Section 8 of this Act puts the age of medical majority at 16. Therefore young people, once 16, can consent to their own surgical, medical or dental treatment without reference to their parents. This means that a young woman of 16 can consent to use any method of contraception or to have an abortion.

Contraception advice and treatment to under-16s

Contraceptive advice and treatment to under-16s is lawful. In 1974 the Department of Health and Social Security issued a Memorandum of Guidance (DHSS, 1974) which stated that a doctor was: 'not acting unlawfully provided he acts in good faith in protecting the girl from the harmful effects of intercourse'.

In 1980 the DHSS issued a revised memorandum which stressed the hope that the doctor: 'will always seek to persuade the child to involve the parent or guardian'. The wording of this memorandum made it quite clear that it would be the normal procedure to obtain parental consent, and to do anything else would be exceptional. There was considerable concern about the interpretation of this advice and the understanding of what was to be thought 'exceptional'. A resolution to this confusion took many years.

141

Then in 1980 Mrs Victoria Gillick sought an assurance from her local Area Health Authority (AHA) that her daughters under 16 years would not be given contraceptive advice or treatment without her consent. This assurance could not be given. In 1982 Mrs Gillick looked for a High Court ruling against her AHA and the DHSS. This ruling went against her, and in 1984 she went to the Appeal Court.

As a result of the Gillick case, there was a ruling from the House of Lords in 1985. This ruling was felt, once and for all, to have clarified that the giving of contraceptive advice to under-16s was not unlawful. In 1986 the DHSS issued a Health Circular specifying that when giving contraceptive advice and/or treatment to under-16s certain guidelines should be used. The guidelines, commonly known as the Fraser Guidelines, stated that contraceptive advice could be given, without the knowledge of parents, provided the doctor was satisfied:

(i) that the girl, regardless of age, will understand the doctor's advice;

(ii) that they cannot persuade her to inform or to allow him/her to inform the parents that she is seeking contraceptive advice;

(iii) that she is very likely to begin or to continue having sexual intercourse with or without contraceptive treatment;

(iv) that unless she receives contraceptive advice or treatment her physical or mental health or both are likely to suffer;

(v) that her best interests require him/her to give contraceptive advice, treatment or both without parental consent.

What this means is that young people under 16 are legally able to consent, on their own behalf, to any surgical, medical or dental procedure provided, in the doctor's opinion, they are capable of understanding the nature and possible consequences of the procedure.

It is important for persons under 16 seeking contraceptive advice to be aware that the doctor is legally obliged to discuss the value of parental support. However, it does not have to go any further than a discussion and the doctor must respect the young person's confidentiality. The professional codes of nurses and other health professionals also place a duty on them not to disclose information about individual patients. A whole practice policy will include reception and administration staff. In other settings the right to confidentiality will also include youth workers and health promotion workers. It may be useful to explain to those under 16 that confidential information may be shared within the team.

Obviously it would be best for a young woman to have the support of her parents at this significant stage in her life. However, her own wishes are more important. Establishing a trusting relationship with the doctor or nurse will do more to promote health than the refusal to see the young woman without involving her parents. Not all young women have caring families and many have very difficult family relationships. Some are abused; some want to protect their parents; some are desperate for their own independence; some just want to make some very mature decisions with privacy.

◆ 'If I have to tell, my dad would chuck me out. That's what he did with my older sister.'

◆ 'If you tell my mum she will try to stop me from seeing my boyfriend. But it won't make any difference and I may have to leave home.'

◆ 'I can't tell my parents. They are having terrible fights at the moment and my dad is threatening to leave. If I told them it would only make things worse and my dad would blame my mum.'

The publicity and discussion generated during the Gillick case greatly affected the accessibility and availability of contraceptive advice to under-16s. Many young women still mistakenly believe that if they ask for advice the doctor will insist that their parents are informed. It is vital that health care workers continue to stress this point to all those seeking advice who are under 16 years old.

Consent to treatment

Consent to treatment can be implied, spoken or written.

(DoH, 1990)

Implied consent is mainly a non-verbal communication that the patient consents to undergo an examination or treatment. She may roll up her sleeve to have her blood pressure taken; she may remove the relevant clothing, voluntarily, and lie on the couch to have a cervical smear taken. This is a valid form of consent, but there can still be problems. There may be a misunderstanding between the patient and the nurse about what the nurse is proposing to do. She may not be aware of the intention of the nurse.

A young woman may put out her arm to have a blood sample taken, but has she consented for each test that may be carried out on that sample? She may not know that she is going to be tested for HIV.

Spoken, or *verbal, consent* is what most nurses rely on in their day-to-day work. For example, you may simply ask 'Have you come for your smear test?' and receive the reply 'Yes'.

Care needs to be taken that assumptions are not being made that the procedure is understood. This may be particularly true of young people. The nurse needs to ensure that the young woman understands the purpose of the procedure, what has and has not been done. The limits of the procedure need to be explained and understood. For example, a routine blood test for anaemia will not tell the patient her blood group or if she has HIV; a cervical smear test is not taken to detect a vaginal infection and does not routinely include a pelvic examination.

When asking for consent for a procedure an open question, rather than a closed one, will usually elicit a more useful response. For example, even though the nurse suspects that the woman has booked for a cervical smear, the open question 'What can I do for you today?' may get the response 'You know that I have come for my smear'. However, it may get 'I don't know, I received a letter telling me to come' or 'I was told I couldn't have any more pills until I had been to see you', and neither of these replies could be construed as giving consent to any procedure.

Written consent is rarely used in non-hospital settings. Although a signed consent form may provide evidence that the patient has given consent, the fact that the form has been signed does not itself make the consent legally valid (McHale, 1998).

If a person under the age of 18 refuses to consent to treatment, it is sometimes possible for their parents or the courts to overrule that decision. This can only happen on the basis that the welfare, both physical and psychological, of the young person is paramount. The psychological effect of having the decision overruled would have to be taken into consideration.

The age of consent

Sexual Offences Act 2003

The Sexual Offences Act 2003 became law in May 2004 and applies to England and Wales only, with some sections extending to Northern Ireland and Scotland.

The Act contains:

◆ Stronger protection for children, for vulnerable people and for the public

◆ Stronger penalties for sexual violence

◆ Stronger penalties to deal with sexual exploitation

◆ Equality in the law for men and women

◆ Clarification in the position of advising children on sexual matters.

The key changes make all forms of sexual activity for under-16s illegal. The same laws will cover both heterosexual and homosexual relationships. The intention is to protect young people from new offences such as 'grooming'.

Research shows that almost 35% of girls and more than 50% of boys will have had some form of sexual experience short of intercourse before the age of 16 (Brook, 2003). Therefore, the result could be that by making all forms of consensual sexual activity unlawful for under-16s a large proportion of the population will effectively be criminalized. There have been concerns that health professionals and others would be unable to provide confidential sexual health advice and treatment to young people.

The Teenage Pregnancy Unit at the Department of Health has issued advice and clarification (TPU, 2003):

◆ The Act will not prevent the provision of confidential advice and treatment to young people under 16, including those under 13

◆ A person is not committing an offence when acting for the purpose of:

(i) protecting the child from sexually transmitted infection, or

(ii) protecting the physical safety of the child, or

(iii) preventing the child from becoming pregnant, or

(iv) promoting the child's emotional wellbeing by the giving of advice

◆ There is no offence as long as the purpose is not to cause or encourage an offence or the child's participation in it

◆ For the first time the exception covers not only health professionals, but also others who act to protect the child, e.g. teachers, Connexions Personal Advisers, teenage advice columnists, parents, other relatives and friends.

Abortion

A young woman under 16 can consent to a termination of pregnancy even if her parents have refused consent. The circumstances surrounding this would generally be considered most exceptional. Equally, a termination of pregnancy cannot be carried out against an under-16's wishes, even if her parents have consented. Young women in such circumstances inevitably need considerable support and counselling in helping them reach a decision (see also page 214).

Homosexuality

The Sexual Offences (Amendment) Act 2000 finally lowered the age of consent for homosexual acts between males to 16 years, provided both consent and the act takes place in private, in England, Wales and Scotland. The age of consent remains at 17 years in Northern Ireland.

The only law relating to female homosexuality is that of indecent assault. Lesbian acts are therefore legal, provided both women consent and are aged 16 or over.

The Children Act 1989

The Children Act 1989 brings together for the first time the public and private law relating to children. The most important principle of the Children Act is that the welfare of the child is the paramount consideration. Parents have new rights and responsibilities under the Act. However, children under 16, whether or not they are 'in care', can give or refuse their own consent to medical treatment depending on their capacity to understand the nature of the treatment.

Sex education

Sex education is not just about sex. It is about knowledge, information and understanding. It is about feelings and relationships. It is about empowering young people to make safe decisions regarding their sexual health. It is about having a high self-esteem. It is about being assertive. It is about being enabled to make important personal choices. It is about life.

What is sex education for?

Sex education is a lifelong process of acquiring information and skills, forming attitudes, beliefs and values about sexual relationships, identity and intimacy. This process starts informally with parents and carers, long before any formal sex education takes place in school (Sex Education Forum, 1997a).

There is evidence that those people who are better informed and have a higher self-regard will make better choices about their sexual health. Conversely, poor information about sexual matters helps to confirm feelings of guilt, which may be damaging to relationships. Massey (1990) suggests that ignorance is likely to perpetuate prejudice in such matters as sexism, homosexuality and unplanned pregnancy.

Where do young people get their sex education?

Most young people acquire their knowledge of sex from their parents and families, from their friends, from the media and from their schools.

Young people's experiences of sex education is that it is 'too little, too late and too biological'. The people they most want to talk to them about sex are their parents. However, their parents are very unlikely to talk to them about sex and relationships, particularly if they are boys (Sex Education Forum, 1997b).

Parents

Ideally sex education should be part of the whole learning process. It should not be a formal topic to be tackled when a child reaches a particular age, but accepted as a part of everyday life. Questions should be answered and information given by parents within the family context. The depth of the questions and the complexity of the information to be given grows as the child matures and develops.

Allen (1987) found that most parents believe that their children should have adequate sex education, as do the young people themselves. Although parents feel that, ideally, this information should come from them – a survey by the Schools Health Education Unit (1994) supports this – they often feel ill-equipped to provide the information and education, and consider that school is the best place for this to be given in a carefully planned setting.

Parents may feel that they are not the right people to provide sex education for a number of reasons. It could be that they feel embarrassed and consider that they are ill-equipped and ill-informed for answering questions about sex and sexuality. The majority of parents also felt their own sex education was poor or non-existent.

What most parents would like is a partnership with the schools. Parents have clear views on the topics they wish the schools to cover, which include basic bodily changes, pregnancy, contraception and AIDS. A significant number of parents believe that the schools should have the sole responsibility for covering sex education.

◆ 'I can't talk to my daughter about that, it's much too embarrassing.'

◆ 'Where can I find out what I should tell them? My mother never told me anything and I don't know how much to tell at what age.'

◆ 'They find out what they need to know when the time comes.'

Friends

Every young person receives some sex education from their friends and many young people will ask their friends for advice even though they are aware that these friends themselves may be, for the most part, ill-informed. At its best the advice is informative, helpful, supportive and safe, but at its worst it can be a mish-mash of rumour and hearsay. Such bad advice can help to perpetuate the myths and misconceptions that surround sex and is not always helpful, and may indeed be harmful.

◆ 'My friend says that you always start your pills seven days after your period.'

◆ 'My boyfriend says that I can't get pregnant if he does not come inside me.'

◆ 'I didn't know about the morning after pill, but my friend knew what to do and where to go.'

◆ 'My boyfriend says I can't ask him to wear a condom, it would mean that I didn't trust him.'

◆ 'My friend knew where to go for a pregnancy test.'

The media

Parents are often worried about the influence of pornographic videos and magazines. In books, newspapers and magazines there are constant references, both in words and pictures, to sex and sexuality. These references reinforce and perpetuate stereotypical behaviour and prejudices. Some magazines run useful 'agony aunt' pages, which often give straightforward and factual advice about situations that young women often feel too embarrassed to ask their friends and parents about. The anxieties may be about periods, masturbation, physical changes, sexual feelings or how to handle difficult sexual situations and how to say 'no'. As long as the information is correct then these columns have a useful function.

Schools

All schools must now have an up-to-date sex and relationship education policy. It is generally accepted that this should be firmly rooted as part of a programme of 'the personal, social health education and citizenship framework'.

What actually happens in individual schools varies enormously. At one end of the scale, a school may not have a policy, and may only be compelled to formulate one and consider formal sex education in response to a crisis, for example when a pupil becomes pregnant. At the other end of the scale, a school may have an excellent policy, and a well-planned and executed programme that is being regularly evaluated and altered in response to local or current needs (Box 7.1).

In the majority of schools it is the teachers who carry out sex education – usually an interested biology teacher. This may be why there is often a purely biological emphasis to sex education, paying little attention to aspects that concern sexuality and relationships. Sex education and related topics are not part of the teacher training programme and consequently many teachers feel ill-equipped to tackle the subject.

Some schools ask a professional from outside to come in and 'do' sex education. However, they may be given totally unrealistic targets of what to cover in the time available. It has been known for a professional to be asked to go in and speak to 35 14-year-olds for a total of 40 minutes and to cover menstruation, contraception, pregnancy, drug abuse, HIV and AIDS in this time.

Some teachers are very proprietorial about the teaching of sex education and are unwilling to share this subject with health professionals. However, other schools have an excellent relationship with professionals such as school nurses, family planning nurses or sex education outreach workers.

Some local authorities employ sex education outreach workers, who can help with the development of a sex education policy, programme development and teacher training. The outreach

worker is there to support the teachers, not to take the work away from them. In one area, a youth worker reported, 75% of the pupils said they would prefer to have an outside speaker, rather than a teacher from the school. Over recent years there has been an increase in the number of outreach workers as local authorities, hospital trusts and other agencies realize that they need to go out to where the young people are to give advice, rather than wait for them to go to their doctor or a clinic when it is often too late.

Outreach workers, who also work with young men, aim to reach young people out of school, through youth clubs, young mothers' groups, tuition centres, the probation services and young people with special needs, which may include the young homeless. It was hoped that these initiatives

---

Box 7.1   Sex education

Some comments from young people on their experience of sex education:

◆ 'I can talk to my mum about anything. I can't remember being sat down and told the facts of life, or anything like that. We would just discuss new topics when they came up. I never felt that any big deal was being made of it.'

◆ 'When we had our sex education the teacher seemed really embarrassed. I think we all knew more than him.'

◆ 'It was really stupid when we did our sex education. The boys all sat in a group and said ignorant, macho things. They made it impossible for us girls to join in and ask questions. All it did was show themselves up.'

◆ 'It was brilliant the way they did sex education in our school. They had someone in from outside. She came several times. We would break up into small groups, where we would work on all sorts of topics. You feel more comfortable in a little group, you can say all sorts of things and not feel stupid.'

◆ 'They do your sex education much too late. It should have to start while you are in junior school.'

◆ 'Sex education classes never tell you what you really want to know.'

◆ 'One thing we did in sex education was how to recognize difficult situations. Then we worked on how to be assertive. We did work on how to say "no" to things we didn't like. It was really helpful and I think it taught the boys something.'

would help reduce the pregnancy rate in the under-16s as outlined in *The Health of the Nation* (DoH, 1992).

Whatever the policy and however much schools feel that they have 'dealt with' sex education, young people continue to start sexual activity at an early age (Box 7.2).

Wellings *et al.* (1995) found that, in the UK, 16- to 19-year-olds who had received school sex education were no more likely to have intercourse before the age of 16 than those who had not. More importantly, they were more likely to have used a method of contraception. The Dutch have a very effective sex education programme which has led to a well-informed young population with a low teenage pregnancy rate. There is no national curriculum in schools, but sex education is compulsory, and starts at a much earlier age than in the UK.

Francis (1994) found that there appear to be three main differences between the UK and the Netherlands concerning the provision of sex education:

◆ The Dutch have a much more accepting attitude to teenage sexuality and the need for contraception

◆ Young people are given more consistent messages from the government, the media and the schools about contraception: 'pill scare' stories are rare

◆ Young people know they can trust their doctor and are given the same degree of confidentiality as adults.

None of this leads to sexual activity starting at an earlier age. In fact, the emphasis is one of individual choice and personal responsibility for safer sexual behaviour. One outcome of this has been the 'double Dutch' method of contraception, i.e. the use of the pill and condoms as protection against pregnancy and also infection.

Additionally young men are specifically targeted for sex education in the Netherlands as it was considered that in the past their needs had been overlooked and sex education was mainly for young women. This is in contrast to the experience of many young men in the UK: e.g. 'All I got on sex education in school was a 30-minute film on having a baby. And I'm gay.'

Another good European initiative was the French decision to make emergency contraception available in all schools directly from the school nurse. Unfortunately in 2000 the French courts declared that this enterprise was illegal and young people could only receive emergency contraception on prescription or in a family planning clinic. In the UK, arrangements have been made to make emergency contraception more easily available in non-traditional settings, and at selected pharmacies without a prescription. This should make it easier for many people, particularly the young.

Emergency contraception is available free from:

◆ GPs

◆ Family planning clinics

◆ Brook centres

◆ NHS walk-in centres

◆ Most sexual health/GUM clinics

◆ Some accident and emergency departments

◆ Some pharmacies.

Young women over 16 can buy emergency contraception from many pharmacies, but the cost is around £25.

Box 7.2 Some statistics about young people and sex

◆ Among those aged 16–19 the average age of first sexual intercourse is 17 years

◆ Nearly 20% of 16- to 19-year-old women had first sexual intercourse before the age of 16

◆ The average age for first sexual experience (not intercourse) is 14 for young women

◆ Those who have their first sexual intercourse before the age of 16 are less likely to use contraception that first time and are more likely to have more partners in the future, than those who first have sex after the age of 16

◆ Half of those who have sex before the age of 16 do not use contraception, compared to one third of those aged over 16 (CES, 1998)

◆ 10% of clients seen at London Brook Advisory Centres in 1998/9 were aged under 16.

Teenage pregnancy

Teenage pregnancy and motherhood are important issues because young women are at higher risk of experiencing adverse health, educational, social and economic outcomes (Fullerton *et al.*, 1997). Truancy, low academic achievement and poor sex education are all factors implicated in this high rate (Westall, 1997).

Analysis of a wide range of statistics has identified that while the rate of teenage sexual activity has increased steadily and consistently over the last four decades, the corresponding underlying trend in teenage fertility has been downward, though not consistently so (Wellings and Kane, 1999).

The UK has the highest rate of teenage pregnancies in Western Europe. In an attempt to reduce this, the *Health of the Nation* document (DoH, 1992) set a target 'to reduce the number of conceptions among the under-16s by at least 50%' by the year 2000. Unfortunately this target was not achieved, although teenage conceptions have started falling in recent years (ONS, 2004) (see Figure 7.1).

The Social Exclusion Unit was set up to investigate ways to reduce teenage pregnancy. Their report (Social Exclusion Unit, 1999) allocated £60 million to halve the teenage pregnancy rate (especially in the under-16s) in England by 2009. They advocated improved coordination of local and national initiatives, improvements in sex education and contraceptive services, encouragement and support of vulnerable pregnant teenagers and teenage parents into education, training and employment, and employing other solutions to combat the risk of social exclusion for them and their children. Teenage boys have also been targeted. The Teenage Pregnancy Unit was formed to implement the Social Exclusion Unit's report on teenage pregnancy.

The Independent Advisory Group on Teenage Pregnancy was set up in 2000 to provide advice to the Government and to monitor the overall success in reducing teenage pregnancy and increasing the participation of teenage parents in education, training and work. Sure Start Plus projects have been created to coordinate support packages for teenage parents including tailoring midwifery, health visiting support and help with returning to education, training or employment.

Legislation and official guidance concerning sex education

In 1986 the report of Her Majesty's Inspectorate supported the teaching of sex education. The HMI report states:

> the importance of sexual relationships in all our lives is such that sex education is a crucial part of preparing children for their lives now and in the future as adults and parents.

In England and Wales sex education, including information about under-16s, homosexuality and abortion, is compulsory in all state maintained secondary schools. The DfE recommends that all primary schools should have a sex and relationship education programme tailored to the age and physical and emotional maturity of the children.

The sex and relationship policy should be drawn up by the governing body and be available to parents and for inspection. The policy should be developed in consultation with parents and the wider community, and must include how they will teach the relevant National Curriculum science topics and how they will provide sex and relationship education as part of PHSE (personal, health and social education).

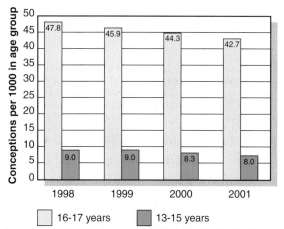

Figure 7.1 Conception rates 1998–2001 (ONS, 2004).

The local authority then has the obligation to see that the school curriculum is one which:

(i) promotes the spiritual, moral, cultural, mental and physical development of pupils at the school and of society; and

(ii) prepares such pupils for the opportunities, responsibilities and experiences of adult life.

Section 28 of the Local Government Act 1988 amended Section 2 of the Local Government Act 1986, and prohibited local authorities from promoting homosexuality by teaching or publishing material. However, the Department of the Environment advised that Section 28 only applied to the local authorities and not to schools. This is because school governors have been given the responsibility for decisions on sex education in their own schools. The Section was finally repealed in 2003. 'This notorious piece of legislation gave legitimacy to discrimination and homophobic bullying, confused teachers, deprived young people of their rights and was extremely bad for the sexual health of the nation' (fpa, 2004).

By 1993 legislation ensured that all maintained schools should provide sex education (including education about HIV and AIDS and other sexually transmitted infections) to all registered pupils. These schools should all have an up-to-date written policy available to all parents. Any sex education should be given: 'in such a manner as to encourage young people to have regard to moral considerations and the value of family life'.

Parents of a pupil can withdraw their child from all or part of the sex education programme except where this forms part of the National Curriculum.

The National Curriculum

Health education, of which sex education may be a part, is named as one of five cross-curricular themes in the National Curriculum. None of these themes is compulsory, unlike the 10 core subjects that are. Sex education is only compulsory when it forms part of the science core subject.

The health education theme in the National Curriculum is broken down into nine components:

◆ Substance abuse and misuse
◆ Sex education
◆ Family life education
◆ Safety
◆ Health-related exercise
◆ Nutrition
◆ Personal hygiene
◆ Environmental aspects of health education
◆ Psychological aspects of health education.

Guidance is given over appropriate topics and areas of study at key stages (which are only compulsory at key stage 4). The key stages relate to age groups (Box 7.3).

Over the years stories and rumours about the provision of sex education have abounded. Sensational stories appear in the popular press about inappropriate information being given to children who were too young to understand.

Box 7.3 Examples of guidance on sex education for pupils at key stages 2, 3 and 4

Key stage 2 (age 7–11)
Pupils should 'begin to know about and have some understanding of the physical, emotional and social changes which take place at puberty.'

Key stage 3 (age 11–14)
Pupils should 'understand that organisms (including HIV) can be transmitted in many ways, in some cases sexually; be aware of the range of sexual attitudes and behaviours in society.'

Key stage 4 (age 14–16)
Pupils should 'consider the advantages and disadvantages of various methods of family planning in terms of personal preference and social implications; recognize and be able to discuss sensitive and controversial issues such as conception, birth, HIV/AIDS, child rearing, abortion and technological developments which involve consideration of attitudes, values, beliefs and morality; be aware of the need for preventive health care and what this involves; be aware of partnership, marriage and divorce and the impact of loss, separation and bereavement; be able to discuss issues such as sexual harassment in terms of their effect on individuals.'
See Box 7.4 for curriculum details.

This information is frequently reported as being of a near pornographic nature. The truth is usually that a responsible teacher or health professional was answering direct and explicit questions by pupils as accurately as possible.

Effective sex and relationship education is essential if young people are to make responsible and well-informed decisions about their lives, and so the teaching of it should be firmly rooted in the framework for PHSE (DfEE, 2000). The guidance document was produced because there was much uncertainty about what sex and relationship education was and how it should be taught.

The three main elements of sex and relationship education include:

◆ Attitudes and values
  ◆ learning the values and individual conscience and moral considerations
  ◆ learning the value of respect, love and care
  ◆ exploring, considering and understanding moral dilemmas.

◆ Personal and social skills
  ◆ learning to manage emotions and relationships confidently and sensitively
  ◆ learning to make choices based on an understanding of difference and with an absence of prejudice
  ◆ developing an appreciation of the consequences of choices made
  ◆ learning how to recognize and avoid exploitation and abuse.

◆ Knowledge and understanding
  ◆ understanding human sexuality, reproduction, sexual health, emotions and relationships
  ◆ learning about contraception and the range of local and national sexual health advice, contraception and support services
  ◆ learning the reasons for delaying sexual activity, and the benefits to be gained from such delay
  ◆ the avoidance of unplanned pregnancy.

Box 7.4 Extracts from the National Curriculum for schools in England since September 2000

Age 5–7

Recognize that bullying is wrong.

Age 7–11

Teaching should include:

◆ Information about the consequences of anti-social behaviour including bullying and racism
◆ Information about the changes that puberty brings.

Sex education is discretionary in primary schools. Should governing bodies decide to provide sex education:

◆ The policy must be available to parents
◆ Teaching should be appropriate to the age and maturity of the pupils
◆ Parents should be able to view the materials used.

Age 11–14

Teaching should include:

◆ The basic facts and laws on illegal substances and the risks associated with misused prescribed drugs
◆ Information about human reproduction, contraception, HIV and sexually transmitted infections and high risk behaviours
◆ The means to practise ways of resisting pressure which threatens their own safety and well-being
◆ Information about the effects of prejudice, discrimination and stereotyping
◆ Some basic interpersonal relationship skills
◆ Information about the roles and responsibilities of parents.

Age 14–16

Teaching should include:

◆ Information about the health risks associated with alcohol and drug misuse, early sexual activity and pregnancy
◆ Where and how to seek advice and help in making safer future choices about good parenting and its value to family life.

Some relevant extracts from the National Curriculum that came into force in 2000 are listed in Box 7.4.

Organizations such as the Sex Education Forum provide advice, information and resources to support the provision of effective sex education.

Confidentiality

Many young people (particularly those under 16) are reluctant to seek medical help or contraceptive advice as they fear that a consultation will not be confidential and will be mentioned to others.

The Shorter Oxford English Dictionary defines confidential as: 'Spoken or written confidence; enjoying another's confidence; entrusted with secrets.'

The Nursing & Midwifery Council (NMC) gives guidance to nurses through the Code of Professional Conduct (NMC, 2002). Clause 5 of the code states 'as a registered nurse or midwife, you must protect confidential information' and summarizes that the following principles concerning confidentiality apply:

◆ A patient or client has the right to expect that information given in confidence will be used only for the purpose for which it was given and will not be released to others without their permission

◆ You should recognize each patient's or client's right to have information about them kept safe and private

◆ If it is appropriate to share information gained in the course of your work with other health or social work practitioners, you must make sure that as far as it is reasonable, the information will be kept in strict professional confidence and be used only for the purpose for which the information was given

◆ You are responsible for any decision that you make to release confidential information because you think that this is in the public's best interest

◆ If you choose to break confidentiality because you believe that this is in the public's best interest, you must have considered the situation carefully enough to justify that decision

◆ You should not deliberately break confidentiality other than in exceptional circumstances.

The nurse's duty to protect patient confidentiality does not have the same authority as the law (Medical Defence Union, 1992). This means that for a nurse the duty of confidentiality is an ethical one, rather than a legal one.

A patient should be able to speak with total freedom to their doctor, nurse or to any other health care professional. This freedom can only come from the trust that the patient has in that particular professional to respect their confidentiality. A person under 16 should expect the same duty of confidentiality as any other person.

A patient may be afraid that personal and private information will be revealed to other people. This anxiety is particularly prevalent in young people. If they fear that their trust will not be respected then they may not ask for medical help or else may not pass on information that is relevant to their medical care. Consequently this may mean that a young woman may not be truthful about her age, she may not reveal that she is taking a specific medication or she may not seek advice for a vaginal discharge.

 SCENARIO

Rebecca, aged 18, came to see the nurse at the clinic several times. The first time she came she said that she had had two epileptic fits, which had been extensively investigated and no cause found. She was put on drug therapy that she did not take. At the clinic she was prescribed a higher dose contraceptive pill to counter the effects of the antiepileptic. After she had had several repeat visits to the clinic she told the nurse that the drug Ecstasy had caused the fits. She did not want her GP to know, so she pretended to continue taking the medication.

A doctor may refuse to give advice or treatment to a person under 16 years if he or she believes that the young person cannot understand what the advice or treatment may involve. Even if a young person is considered too immature to give valid consent, the consultation should still remain confidential. Most doctors will respect the confidentiality of those asking for contraceptive advice. However, the suspicion remains that a few doctors, because of their personal beliefs, would breach confidentiality with someone under 16 years. The difficulty for the young person lies in the ability to distinguish between those they feel they can and cannot trust. The consequences of a breach of confidentiality may be devastating to a young person.

◆ 'When I was 16 I went to my doctor for a pregnancy test. The doctor told my mum I was pregnant. Before I could say or do anything I had had an abortion. I had a bad time for a couple of years after that; I went a bit wild. I behaved very badly and took a lot of serious risks. It may have been the right decision, but it wasn't my decision. I can't talk to my mum now.'

The British Medical Association, General Medical Services Committee, Health Education Authority, Brook Advisory Centres, Family Planning Association and Royal College of General Practitioners issued a joint guidance note for doctors in 1993 (BMA *et al.*, 1993). The note spells out clearly that disregarding confidentiality, except in the most exceptional circumstances, is a serious breach of professional ethics. The fear of such a breach is a serious anxiety to many young women, although there is, in fact, very little evidence that these breaches are made. It has usually happened to 'a friend of a friend'!

◆ 'I can't go and see my doctor about going on the pill. He is a very good friend of my parents and would be bound to tell my mum.'

◆ 'My friend went to the doctor for the pill. He said she had to tell her mum first.'

◆ 'I went to make an appointment at my doctor's for family planning. The receptionist said that I was too young.'

The only way to counter such anxieties is for health professionals to repeat, again and again, that all consultations are confidential, whatever is said in them. The only exception to this could be if during the course of a consultation there is a suspicion of sexual abuse or other danger, either to the young woman or to someone else. She must be warned at that stage that it may be necessary to break her confidence.

All general practices are expected to have a confidentiality policy, which should be publicized in the practice information leaflet and through a confidentiality statement displayed in the waiting room. In addition, all practice staff are expected to participate in training around confidentiality.

Needs and attitudes of young people

Young people have a good idea of the kind of help and advice that they want. The majority know that there is birth control and have a reasonable knowledge of the different methods of contraception. However, many, especially young men, do not know where clinics are or where to go for help. Young people are clear about what they need and would like from a contraception clinic or youth session, which should be confidential, accessible, relevant, professional, non-judgemental and sensitive. These criteria, although relevant to medical consultations at any age, are particularly pertinent for young people. A campaign in 2002 jointly supported by the Royal College of General Practitioners and the Royal College of Nursing, 'Getting it right for teenagers in your practice', was aimed at improving young people's access to health services.

Confidential

A review of the relevant literature (Gleeson *et al.*, 2002) demonstrates that this is still considered to be one of the most important issues for young people. Though confident in many ways, some still doubt the total confidentiality of the clinics or consultations with their GP. Young people fear that the doctor will write or speak to their parents or that they will be forced to speak to their parents themselves.

Accessible

The timing of the session is important. A lunchtime session may be helpful, but not if pupils are unable to leave school premises. After-school sessions are popular, but not so useful in rural areas, where a young person may miss the only bus to take them home if they stay behind.

In urban areas after-school, early evening and Saturday morning sessions are convenient, as these are often held at times when their absence from home can easily be explained:

◆ 'My mum thinks that I'm out shopping with my friend.'

◆ 'They think that I've gone to visit my Nan; I'll go on to see her when I leave here.'

◆ 'My mum thinks that I have stayed on at an after-school club.'

For some young people the precise location of a clinic may be important. Some may have the confidence to walk in, off the street, into a clearly signposted youth advice session or contraception clinic, and are not worried about anyone seeing them, whilst others would prefer the relative anonymity of a health centre, where they may be going to see other health care professionals such as the dentist or chiropodist. Some prefer to see their doctor in a group practice, where they may also be going for advice about their acne or ingrowing toenail.

There has been much collaborative work done to improve young people's access to services; for example:

◆ An inner city general practice with a dedicated young people's clinic offering contraceptive and sexual health advice to young people not registered at the practice

◆ Nurse-led services in youth clubs

◆ Mobile contraceptive and sexual health clinics (Clinic in a Box) making services available in non-traditional settings (youth clubs and sports and leisure facilities)

◆ Sessions in secondary schools and sixth form colleges, run by individual school nurses, or working with family planning nurses and youth workers

◆ One-stop-shops for young people in sexual health clinics.

Obviously, young people can only access services that they know about and can reach. Some services can be accessed through the use of mobile phones, text messaging and the Internet. It is also necessary to consider the needs of those in different situations; for example, those who are:

◆ With physical and mental disabilities

◆ Looked after

◆ Homeless.

Relevant

Young people want any service that is offered, whether by their own doctor or a clinic, to be relevant to their needs. They do not want to be just given condoms and told 'not to do it'. Young people want to discuss and have advice on a wide range of topics including:

◆ Contraception

◆ Pregnancy

◆ Abortion

◆ HIV/AIDS

◆ Sexuality

◆ Incest

◆ Sexual abuse

◆ Genetic disorders

◆ Menstruation

◆ STIs

◆ Weight and eating problems

◆ General health issues

◆ Psychological issues

They also want and need the freedom to discuss relationships. These relationships may be with girlfriends, boyfriends, or parents and family. Their parents may be having their own relationship difficulties which they may want to talk about or there may be anxieties about drugs or alcohol, with their schooling or where they are living.

Professional

Young people want help from people who are professional, up-to-date, well informed and who understand the needs of the local community, e.g. having the clinic open at a time and in a place that is accessible to all (some young women may be closely chaperoned by parents or relatives), or knowing that all staff are trained and informed of the cultural impact on sexual behaviour and contraceptive choice that comes from different ethnic groups.

They want help from those who have total integrity as far as confidentiality and legal issues are concerned. In short, they want help from someone they can trust to have their best interests as a priority. They also want help from someone who is friendly and sympathetic.

Non-judgemental

At the heart of training in youth advice and family planning is the strong belief that any involvement with young people should be non-directive and non-judgemental. You should not make assumptions and moral judgements. Obviously, we all have opinions and prejudices, and have some areas of practice with which we feel uncomfortable. But what is important is that we are aware of these feelings and recognize the primacy of the young person's own situation. No one knows why a young person has come to a clinic until that person says the words. Even then, why they say they have come may not be the reason why they have really come. You need to remember that you are there to help young people to make their own decisions and to learn to take responsibility for their own actions. Young people want to feel good about having come to ask for help. They do not want to feel put down or intimidated; to be made to feel guilty or bad. It needs to be acknowledged that the young person has made a big step in coming to ask for help, often a very difficult decision to take. For many it will be the first mature decision that they have made and they want to be listened to and they do not want to be talked down to or patronized.

Sensitive

Young people can find it very difficult to ask for what they want, or indeed what they think they want. This difficulty may be caused by embarrassment or come from ignorance. For example, a young woman may ask you for a pregnancy test, when what she really needs is emergency contraception, and vice versa. It is essential that you use appropriate language, language that is clearly understood by both parties, and, as far as possible, reflects the young woman's level of knowledge. The language used must not increase her possible anxiety, particularly during the first visit.

All this has to be achieved while not appearing to be patronizing, but friendly and approachable.

Young people will not come to clinics and ask for help if their needs are not met; or if they come once, they will not return and will certainly not encourage their friends to attend if they did not feel welcome. They are also less likely to persist with their chosen method of contraception or to use it correctly if they felt uncomfortable during the consultation (Hutchinson, 1993; Williams, 1994).

◆ 'I didn't like the clinic I went to. I felt stupid when I didn't understand what they were on about.'

◆ 'I thought I was going to be lectured to and made to feel small. But it wasn't like that at all.'

◆ 'They explained everything to me, then let me decide.'

◆ 'It was really embarrassing having to explain what had happened. But I understand that it was necessary. I went away feeling much better.'

◆ 'They treated me like an adult, not like a silly kid.'

◆ 'I really trust the clinic. There's a counsellor to talk to if you have other problems. I would tell any of my friends to go there.'

◆ 'My mum took me to the doctor's. They did talk to her, but they made it clear that any decisions were mine. That was brilliant.'

Service provision

In an effort to reduce teenage pregnancies many GP surgeries and family planning clinics are setting up specially designated young people's clinics. If you are involved in setting up a session or clinic for young women in your locality it is important to research fully the needs of young people in your area. You will need to arrange:

- Staff who understand and are sympathetic to young people's needs
- An informal atmosphere and convenient location
- An appropriate time of day, possibly after school
- Provision for 'drop-in' (no appointment) sessions
- Publicity emphasizing that the service is totally confidential
- Provision of a professional, comprehensive service
- Availability of on-the-day appointments (e.g. for emergency contraception or contraceptive injection).

While this is what should be available to women of any age group, it is particularly important that it is provided for young women because they tend to be more vulnerable and may lack the verbal skills or initiative to seek advice further afield. If they are too frightened to go to a clinic, or if they go and their expectations are not met, or if they are treated insensitively and do not return, then they may be 'lost' for years at a time of need.

A study in the Trent region showed that general practices with female doctors, young doctors, or more nurse time had lower teenage pregnancy rates (Hippisley-Cox *et al.*, 2000). Such findings may have implications for the mix of health professionals within primary care when planning for the future.

Sex and sexual needs and anxieties

Sexuality is thinking about it. Sex is doing it. Sexuality is the interest in sexual activity. This interest develops during the adolescent years, and sexual feelings usually develop earlier in girls than in boys. Along with this interest a range of needs and anxieties emerge.

The sexual needs and anxieties that young women have can be many and varied and stem from a variety of sources:

- Some come from the way in which a young woman has been brought up, from her family life and in particular from the way her mother has influenced her view of herself as a female (see Chapter 1)
- Some come from the pressures and influences of friends and peers
- Some come from the pressures and influences of society, much of it through the media, which frequently gives conflicting, confusing and complex messages about the role, status and value of young women in society.

The anxieties may be to do with physical changes, with relationships, with sexual relationships, and with sex itself.

The change of body shape at puberty may cause many fears and anxieties and young women need to find a way of accepting their alteration in body image. The transformation from child's body to womanly body appears effortless for some, but for others it turns into a long, hard and awkward process. Breasts and hips may seem to be too big or too small and there may be too much or too little body hair. Greasy skin, spots and acne can be a considerable problem, giving rise to a loss of confidence.

Periods usually start at 12–13 years, but they may start as early 9 or as late as 16 or 17 and you need to be able to reassure young women that this is normal. Everyone feels that their own experience of puberty is unique. How a young woman views her periods is very much influenced by how her mother has prepared her for them. So ideas about pain, bad blood, the 'curse' and smell are negative. There can be difficulties and anxieties regarding different types of sanitary protection. There may be practical problems with privacy at school, particularly if she starts her periods while still at junior school. For some young women (and their mothers) there may be fears about attempting to use tampons. You may find that you are in a position to offer sensible and constructive advice, e.g. practising with the smallest or different types of tampon, with and without an applicator, perhaps using a lubricant and giving reassurance that the tampon cannot get lost. Some young women have problems with period pains and premenstrual syndrome and need to be given help with both these problems.

Some young women are very shy, and lack the maturity and social skills to make relationships. Some are fearful of rejection with friends of either sex. Often, a young woman may be ambivalent about her sexuality – unsure whether or not she is a lesbian. It may be difficult to determine the difference between a 'crush' and real sexual feelings.

The majority of sexual anxieties and needs are to do with sex itself. How a young woman feels about sex is influenced by her family, her friends and by society. How she feels may also be determined by what sexual experiences she has already had. These experiences may include rape, sexual abuse, incest and sexual harassment. Any of these experiences may be in the background of a young woman coming for help for the first time.

There may be particular reasons why a young woman wants a sexual relationship at this time. It may be a mature, planned decision about a deepening and loving relationship. It may be an act of defiance, intended to shock. It may reflect a need for someone to love her. It may be the only way for her to leave her family or home.

Some young women have a lack of knowledge about what sex really is. There are anxieties about vaginal penetration; this can be to do with the size they think their vagina is and the size they think their boyfriend's penis is. They may have been influenced by having had problems using tampons.

◆ 'My mother said that she was very small inside. She said everything was always very difficult. When I was born she had to have a 'Caesar'. She says that I am just like her. I'm really worried that my boyfriend won't be able to get inside me.'

◆ 'The third time I went out with my boyfriend he told me that his penis was 8 inches long. We hadn't talked about having sex at that time. I want to have sex with him, but I'm frightened it'll hurt. Why did he have to tell me about his size?'

There is ignorance about what an orgasm is and how to achieve one. This is hardly surprising, considering that most young women's early sexual experiences are at the hands of equally inexperienced young men and usually only last for a few minutes – if that long! It can take trust, experience and a reasonably relaxed location to make sex fulfilling: requirements that may not be met whilst fearing that parents might return home at any minute or which takes place on the back seat of a car.

If penetration is difficult for any reason there is the fear of being labelled 'frigid'. This is a term that is usually used by men to describe women, totally disregarding any ineptness or lack of sensitivity that they might have.

Most of the anxieties young women have about sex are to do with communication and with being able to negotiate with a boyfriend about what feels right for her. This may be saying 'no' to a sexual relationship at this particular stage or with this particular person. It may be to do with saying 'yes', but needing to be able to discuss issues of contraception and safer sex first. Mutual respect can be shown by not using these topics as an issue or a weapon, but demonstrating the need to discuss them as a partnership.

Some of the problems surrounding sex are compounded by not having a common language and by using words that are not clearly understood by all concerned. 'Making love' may only mean kissing to one person, whilst to another it means mutual masturbation, and to a third, penetrative vaginal sex. 'Oral sex' may be just kissing, or merely talking about sex. If a clearly understood vocabulary is used then issues of contraception, safer sex and sexual relationships can be negotiated.

No assumptions should ever be made about anyone's level of knowledge. Terms like 'contraception', 'birth control' and 'family planning' may not be understood.

◆ 'I don't want to go to a family planning clinic yet. I'm not thinking of planning a pregnancy and family for a number of years.'

A young woman may come asking for help because she thinks she may need contraception or perhaps emergency birth control. But she may be quite unsure as to whether or not she has had penetrative sex. Sensitive questioning is needed to assess the present risks and help her make decisions for the future.

Perhaps the main area of anxiety for young women is pregnancy. You should remember that young people are individuals and studies show that there is no simple model of sexual behaviour that will enable health professionals to target those at risk of unplanned pregnancy (Woodward, 1995). Teenage pregnancy is a complex problem and you should try to acknowledge and recognize young people's individuality in your dealings with them.

Sometimes a young woman will choose to become pregnant, or at least make no effort to stop becoming pregnant. This may be for a variety of reasons, she:

◆ May see it as a way of demonstrating her independence

◆ May feel that she is showing devotion to her boyfriend

◆ May be desperate for someone of her own to love

◆ May have nothing better to do: no status, no expectations

◆ May be worried about infertility, not because she wants a baby now, but because she wants to be sure that she can when she wants to.

Sometimes a young woman will deliberately become pregnant and then have an abortion, just to demonstrate her fertility. You may find that this is more likely to occur in some cultures than others.

For most, though, the main anxiety is to prevent pregnancy at this time in their life, although for a few it is because they never, ever want a pregnancy.

◆ 'I'm really worried about becoming pregnant. I take my pills very carefully. I never forget them. And I don't let my boyfriend come inside me. What else can I do?'

◆ 'It would be an absolute disaster if I got pregnant for the next two years. I must use the best, safest birth control. But there mustn't be any side-effects.'

There may be anxieties about being examined, and about having a smear test. Some young women believe that if they go to a clinic or to their GP and ask about contraception, then a vaginal examination is a prerequisite for using any contraception. Yet many of these young women are virgins. A few think the examination is some kind of punishment for their sexuality and a procedure that has to be endured. If you can pick up this anxiety and explain the situation the relief expressed can be enormous. Someone showing extreme anxiety about being examined, or always coming up with an excuse for postponement, needs to be considered carefully. It is an opportunity to reveal underlying psychosexual problems or difficulties (see also page 88).

The same anxieties apply to the smear test, which many young women mistakenly believe they should have as soon as they become sexually active. You can use telling them that they do not need to have smear test until they are 20 (or 25 under the new guidelines) as an opportunity to talk about a wide range of health-related issues, including menstruation, sexually transmitted infections, AIDS, smoking, diet, as well as any relevant family history. For many young women this will be the first time that they have had an opportunity to take responsibility for their own health, and make their own decisions.

Your own attitudes at this initial consultation may have an enormous impact on how the young woman views her future sexuality and it is vitally important that you appear relaxed and comfortable whilst discussing sex so that she can pick up these positive feelings from you. Hopefully, if she feels confident and comfortable then she will encourage her friends to visit for similar advice. Her first examination and/or smear should be carried out in a calm, private situation and the procedure fully explained. Many women dread vaginal examination later in life as their first experience of this was uncomfortable, intrusive, insensitive and rushed.

Some young women are prescribed the oral contraceptive pill for dysmenorrhoea or menorrhagia, or to 'regulate' their periods, and they have anxieties about being examined.

An examination and smear on a virgin is not necessary, as long as there is no concern about any underlying pathology.

Peer group pressure

Peer group pressure can vary enormously and cover a range from subtle, almost subliminal messages through to heavyweight pressure that might almost be called bullying.

Most young people want to fit into a group. They value the opinions and style of their friends and want to be accepted and valued by the group. This may lead them to be pressurized into behaving in certain ways, to conform to group standards. On one level this pressure may be no more than to wear certain clothes or to have a particular hairstyle, but on another level there may be pressure to become involved in dangerous and/or illegal activities.

Young women can also be incredibly supportive of each other. They may see that one of their friends is in trouble and will bring her in for help and advice.

Smoking

Peer group pressure to smoke is common amongst teenagers. It is not unusual to find that a group of friends will be either all smokers or all non-smokers; boys being more influenced by their peers than girls and girls being more influenced by parental smoking. Some young women see smoking as a way of controlling or reducing their weight (Camp *et al.*, 1993). In fact, some research has shown that smokers have a significantly higher body mass (Townsend *et al.*, 1991). This may be explained by smokers drinking more alcohol, taking less exercise and having a less organized diet.

The most recent statistics (DH, 2003a) found that:

◆ In 2001, 27% of adults in England aged 16 and over smoked cigarettes; 25% of women and 28% of men

◆ In 2002, 10% of children aged 11–15 smoked cigarettes regularly; 11% of girls and 9% of boys.

Dieting

Many young women feel that they have to conform to an ideal body shape. They may try to achieve this through 'dieting', disorganized eating, smoking or by increasing the exercise that they take (see later in this chapter).

Alcohol

The peak age for experimenting with alcohol is 13–15 years. By 13 years 90% of young people have had some alcohol. Most recent data (DH, 2003b) find:

◆ In 2001, 15% of women aged 16 and over drank on average more than 14 units a week

◆ In 2002, 24% of pupils in England aged 11–15 had drunk alcohol in the previous week.

Family influences are strong here with young people who see family views as strict and repressive being likely to drink more (see also page 54).

One of the dangers of excessive drinking is the greater likelihood of unprotected and/or unplanned sex. In these circumstances not only is there a high risk of pregnancy but also of infection. There may have been no rational, careful consideration before intercourse.

Drugs

The same is also true for drugs. The vast majority of 15- and 16-year-olds will have been offered drugs. Solvent abuse is also dangerous, but cheap, and appears to be more common with boys than girls. Young people think they are knowledgeable about drugs: the types, availability, effect and cost. Drugs are very much part of current youth culture and they may be used much more than alcohol.

◆ 'The bars at the clubs don't make any money these days. That's because almost everyone is taking drugs.'

The most recent data (DH, 2003c) find:

◆ In 2002 among 11- to 15-year-olds in England and Wales:

  ◆ 11% had taken drugs that year; 6% of 11 year olds compared to 36% of 15 year olds

- Cannabis was the most commonly reported drug
- 1% had tried heroin, 1% had used cocaine
- In total 4% had used class A drugs in the last year.
- In 2002 among 16- to 24-year-olds in England and Wales:
  - 30% had used drugs in the last year and 19% in the last month
  - 27% had used cannabis, 7% ecstasy, 5% amphetamines, 5% cocaine, 4% poppers and 1% crack
  - In total 9% had used class A drugs
  - The use of cocaine and ecstasy had increased significantly since 1994 (from 1% to 5%, and from 4% to 7%, respectively).

There are new programmes, both in primary and secondary schools, aimed at educating young people about the dangers of drugs. In some areas there are exciting initiatives to try and combat the problem such as a 'drug' bus that tours with information. In the Netherlands a drugs prevention programme is running very successfully in Amsterdam's primary schools, with plans for it to be set up in other Dutch cities. It is hoped that the scheme will have the same level of success as the Dutch sex education programme.

With drugs, as with alcohol, there are known health risks. As a result of the loss of inhibition, there are the risks of unplanned, unprotected or even unwanted sex. As a health professional you could offer advice about drug safety (Box 7.5).

Sexual health

Young people are a significant risk group, and are more likely to have higher numbers of sexual partners, use barrier methods inconsistently and are more likely to become reinfected after being diagnosed with and treated for an initial STI.

Gonorrhoea
According to data (HPA, 2003):

- During 2002 in England, Wales and Northern Ireland the highest rates were in 16- to

---

Box 7.5 Advice to give young people about drug safety

This should better be described as 'how to minimize the risk'. These are some suggestions:

- If taking ecstasy don't drink any alcohol, but do drink plenty of water otherwise heat exhaustion can follow
- Make use of needle exchange programmes and do not share 'works'
- Do not take hallucinogenic drugs when you are alone, and if in a group have one person not tripping
- Do not do cocktails of drugs, in the same way you do not mix drinks
- Remember, if on drugs your judgement will be affected and you may put yourself in an unsafe situation personally, sexually (with unplanned, unprotected or even unwanted sex) or both.

19-year-old females and 20- to 24-year-old males
- 40% of all diagnoses in females were in those under 20 years.

Chlamydia
According to data (National Statistics, 2003):

- *Chlamydia* is the most common sexual infection
- Cases are rising steadily
- Highest rates are seen in young people, especially women under 25 years
- In 2002, 16- to 19-year-old females had the highest rate (almost 1% in this age group)
- It is an important reproductive health problem, because 10–30% of infected women develop pelvic inflammatory disease (PID).

Sex

There is pressure to be sexually active, or to appear to be sexually active. A young person can be made to feel immature, unattractive and boring if they do not become sexually active. Unfortunately there is often little planning in their early sexual encounters. The younger a person is when they have their first sexual experience, the less likely they are to use any contraception.

Peer pressure can also influence the kind of contraception that they can or cannot use.

◆ 'You mustn't use the pill, it makes you fat.'

◆ 'You can never have a coil if you have never had a baby.'

◆ 'My friend says I must change my pill. She says that her pill is much better because it costs more than mine.'

◆ 'We didn't use a condom because I was told that you only get pregnant if you have an orgasm. I've never had an orgasm.'

◆ 'He says he can't use a condom because they are all too small for real men.'

A practice nurse relates:

We have a young woman in the practice that was pregnant, with twins, when she was still 17. She has great influence with a group of other young women, and a number of them became pregnant too. Now that she has had the babies and has chosen to use reliable contraception, we are hoping that her friends can be encouraged to make similar choices.

Bullying

Woolfson (1989) suggests that with girls bullying is likely to be verbal, while with boys it tends to be physical. There is no accurate information on the nature and extent of bullying, but estimates suggest that 10–25% of pupils are directly affected, either as victims or as bullies themselves (Friend, 1992). This is probably a considerable underestimation particularly since bullying can now be carried out by e-mail and by text messaging.

Head teachers now have a specific duty to draw up measures to prevent all forms of bullying among pupils (DfEE, 1998), and to encourage pupils and parents to come forward if there is a problem. Effective anti-bullying strategies should form part of a school's discipline and behaviour policy. The DfEE has produced an anti-bullying pack for schools – *Bullying: Don't Suffer in Silence* (1994). There are guidelines issued by teaching organisations. There are some excellent examples of different policies and methods for dealing with bullying, including peer counselling. Despite this, many schools still maintain that they do not have any bullying and so have no need for a policy.

Self-harm

Some young people self-harm in different ways as a response to the stress they are experiencing (Young Minds, 2004); for example, problems to do with

◆ Race, culture or religion

◆ Money

◆ Bullying

◆ Growing up

◆ Sexuality

◆ Friends

◆ Bereavement

◆ Housing

◆ Pressures at school or work

◆ Pressure to fit in.

Society's expectations

Apart from the peer group pressure to be at the best school, in the best class and to achieve the best results, pupils also feel the pressure of society's expectations, even in the most supportive and unpressurized family or school. Some pupils will become physically ill in the build-up to exams. There is often an enormous pressure on them to achieve; some parents have very unrealistic or inflexible expectations of their children's potential. They want their children to do well academically, perform well at sport, have additional skills and interests, and to have a good group of friends.

There is pressure from both parents and schools for young people not to smoke or drink, not to become involved in drug taking or solvent abuse, and yet young people often feel that they have far greater knowledge in these areas than their parents. Parents want there to be no question about their child's sexual orientation and many would ideally want their child's relationships to be non-sexual. All these pressures may come from parents who smoke and drink themselves, who may take 'recreational' drugs, who are not always honest, and who may have adulterous relationships. It is no wonder that their children are experiencing very conflicting and confusing messages. As so often with young people, it is a case of 'do what I say, not what I do'.

◆ 'I really wanted to talk to my parents about my boyfriend, but I can't. My dad's having an affair with another woman, and my mum's in a terrible state.'

Your role as a health care professional is to listen. The young person needs to trust that you are there for her, to support her, to be non-judgemental and to value her concerns. If this is forthcoming then you can help her.

Young lesbians

Young women are not generally seen as sexual beings in their own right. They are often perceived to need a man to be sexual, and that if they are lesbians they are only infatuated with another girl and they can be 'cured' by a real man. As with gay young men, young lesbians have problems with coming out. Many lack any support from family and friends, and have experienced great personal difficulty. Many young lesbians find it difficult to come out until they leave home. Most find information about advice groups, social groups, etc., from any of the various 'listings' publications.

Eating disorders

Anorexia nervosa and bulimia nervosa are the eating disorders most likely to be encountered in young people. There are also binge eating disorders.

Eating disorders develop as outward signs of inner emotional or psychological distress or problems (Eating Disorders Association, 2004). They become the way that some people cope with difficulties in their life. Eating or not eating is used to help block out painful feelings.

Anorexia nervosa

Anorexia is a serious illness affecting perhaps as many as 1% of secondary schoolchildren (Crisp

et al., 1976). As many as 10% of these pupils may die as a result of the illness. This means there could be as many as 10,000 schoolgirl anorexics in the UK. The Eating Disorders Association suggests that approximately 1 in 500 women between the ages of 15 and 25, or around 6000 people a year in Britain require treatment. In addition, some research suggests that 1 in 50 of university students is affected with an eating disorder. This number rises to 1 in 14 of students at dancing and modelling schools, where the 'ideal' body shape is seen as being ultra slim (Slade, 1984).

The typical anorexic is a female in her mid- to late teens, although the disease can manifest itself at an earlier as well as at a much later age. Males form only 10% of anorexics. The majority of anorexics appear to start 'slimming' because they believe, rightly or wrongly, that they are overweight. However, unlike the average 'dieter' who gives up after a time, the anorexic persists until there is an abnormal weight loss. The longer they persist the more abnormal their thinking and reactions become (Bruch, 1978). Bruch describes anorexia as 'the relentless pursuit of excessive thinness'.

Many anorexics in order to achieve their 'ideal' body weight resort to the use of laxatives so that they lose another pound or two. Once weight has been lost, young women will frequently also have amenorrhoea as the body attempts to conserve energy for the basic activities of life.

There appears to be a genetic predisposition that gives anorexics a specific personality; they are likely to be perfectionists with obsessive compulsions, who are very determined. This type of personality means that when they encounter difficulties they respond by starving themselves. The difficulties may be anything from a chance remark about their weight, exam pressure, and family problems, to sexual abuse. The response is to take control in the only way they know. Anorexia is not just about food; it is about doing something perfectly.

Anorexics make an abnormal response to what others might consider a normal but upsetting situation. For example, a young woman turned down by ballet school might decide that if she loses weight then the school will offer her a place after all. A young woman may be anxious about how she will do in her exams; losing weight may be something that she can do very well. A young woman's father may die; so she loses weight to stay a little girl and not grow up. For some it may be a way of avoiding some of the problems of adolescence, particularly those to do with developing sexuality, adolescence being a time of uncertainty and self-consciousness (Palmer, 1989).

Anorexia may be the response of some young women to the profound changes in their lives. It may be a demonstration that they are self-sufficient, independent and have no needs.

Common signs and symptoms of anorexia nervosa are listed in Box 7.6.

Bulimia

Bulimia is characterized by overeating followed by self-induced vomiting. The amount of food consumed in a bingeing session can be enormous. In addition, excessive exercise and the taking of laxatives and diuretics are used to keep weight down.

The condition usually starts between the ages of 15 and 24 years. It is thought that about 3% of women will be affected at some stage in their lives, but because of the secretive nature of the condition this has to be a conservative estimate. As with anorexia, bulimia may be the response to stressful life events. However, where anorexics

---

> **Box 7.6**   Signs and symptoms of anorexia
>
> ◆ Abnormal desire to be thin
> ◆ Abnormal weight loss – and covering up this weight loss with baggy clothes
> ◆ Distorted body image (thinking of herself as fat), even when obviously underweight
> ◆ Obsession with food, calories and cooking, but denial of dieting
> ◆ Obsession with exercising, sometimes for hours at a time
> ◆ Low self-esteem and lack of confidence
> ◆ Isolation from friends
> ◆ Use of laxatives/vomiting
> ◆ Amenorrhoea
> ◆ Lanugo (an excess of fine body hair)
> ◆ Feeling cold.

> **Box 7.7**   Signs and symptoms of bulimia
>
> ◆ Irregular periods
> ◆ Fear of fatness
> ◆ Binge eating, often huge amounts of food, most commonly in secret
> ◆ Normal weight
> ◆ Regular self-induced vomiting
> ◆ Possible use of large doses of laxatives and/or diuretics
> ◆ Tooth decay.

'choose' to starve themselves, bulimics need to show that they are coping and capable, and so keep their chaotic eating a secret (Lawrence and Dana, 1990).

Signs and symptoms of bulimia are listed in Box 7.7.

Causes

There are various theories as to the origins of the two conditions anorexia and bulimia. These origins include:

◆ Pressures of society

◆ Family pressures, in which the meal becomes the arena for family problems

◆ Child sexual abuse

◆ Depression

◆ Stress, particularly a reaction to some distressing event

◆ Biological changes, as a way of controlling and avoiding physical, bodily changes

◆ Genetic predisposition

◆ Needs, which may be in conflict to upbringing.

Whatever the causes, it is now recognized that more is needed than force-feeding the young woman until her weight is 'normal'. Treatment may consist of behavioural, psychodynamic or family therapy, living in a therapeutic community, self-help groups, diet and nutritional advice or any combination of these. Therapy is seen as the only way of trying to resolve the underlying problems that manifest themselves as an eating disorder. Whatever the methods used, two elements are necessary to achieve a satisfactory outcome. The first is the woman having a desire to change, although some may have mixed feeling about 'giving up' their illness (EDA, 2004). The second is the woman having an understanding of the trigger for her disordered eating habit, e.g. a disturbed family relationship (Abraham and Llewellyn-Jones, 1992).

Treatment and prognosis

Unfortunately, there are few specialist eating disorders units in this country; they are mainly located in psychiatric units or hospitals. The prognosis appears to be related to the length of time the disorder has been present; the earlier the condition is recognized and treatment started, the better the outcome.

The majority will recover, but it may take many years. How good the recovery is may be variable: a good outcome being measured by the maintenance of a normal weight and regular menstruation. The young woman with anorexia may be easier to identify because of her extreme weight loss, but the young woman with bulimia may more readily come and ask for help.

A school nurse reports:

◆ 'If a pupil has anorexia then it is her friends who will come and tell you and ask you to do something. If the pupil has bulimia, then she is very likely to come and ask for help herself'.

The consequences of untreated or inadequately treated anorexia or bulimia can be very serious, the effects being broadly grouped depending on whether there is starvation, vomiting or laxative abuse (Box 7.8). One mother says of her daughter: 'She eats too little to live, but too much to die.'

Your role when encountering young women with eating disorders is to be sensitive to the clues that might indicate that there is an eating problem. These clues may be:

◆ Wearing an inappropriate amount of baggy clothing
◆ Anxiety about menstruation
◆ Delayed onset of menstruation
◆ Excessive thinness
◆ Unexplained weight loss
◆ Fainting or dizziness.

> **Box 7.8** Potential damage to health from eating disorders
>
> **Anorexia**
> ◆ Severe constipation
> ◆ Osteoporosis
> ◆ Muscle wasting
> ◆ Severe electrolyte imbalance
> ◆ Death.
>
> **Bulimia**
> ◆ Mouth ulcers
> ◆ Tooth decay and gum disease
> ◆ Stomach and bowel disorders
> ◆ Hair loss
> ◆ Hypokalaemia causing cardiac arrhythmias
> ◆ Muscle weakness
> ◆ Kidney damage.

When you have identified someone at risk of an eating disorder good health promotion may be all that is necessary. Having calculated the young woman's body mass index (BMI) (see page 41), which should be between 19 and 24.9, you can then advise her of a healthy eating programme. You should be able to discuss the risks to her health of chaotic eating and be able to discover some of her anxieties and her level of understanding of her situation. With this information you should be able to determine if the young woman needs to be referred on for expert professional treatment.

Conclusion

Government strategies have meant that the health situation regarding young people is constantly changing. New targets for reducing the teenage pregnancy rate, although appearing unrealistic at first, are achievable if the experiences of our European counterparts are used alongside local initiatives to improve sex education, and greater publicity about the availability of sexual health information. Young people need to know where they can seek sexual health advice preferably before embarking on a sexual relationship, but sex for young people is often unplanned and impulsive so adequate information about emergency contraception also needs to be available.

Having read this chapter you will appreciate many of the difficulties young people experience whilst growing up. Young women will seek your professional help and advice which should be confidential and given in a professional, supportive and non-judgemental manner. If you appear relaxed and comfortable when dealing with young people then they will pick up positive messages from you and encourage their friends to attend. Not only do young people learn from you but you can also learn from them about their needs so that the service you offer can be improved for others. After all, sex and sexuality are human pleasures and you should be able to enjoy your sexual health work with young people.

Patient education points

● Explain your confidentiality policy at the start of consultations. Why not put a poster in the waiting area?

● Many clients are confused about swabs and smears. Always remember to explain the differences

● Discuss some techniques for remembering to take pills regularly, e.g. keep with a toothbrush

● Identify barriers to effective condom use and explore ways to overcome them

● Discuss ways in which they can negotiate with a partner not to have sex.

Resources

Brook Advisory Centres
Tel: 0800 0185 023
www.brook.org.uk

Childline
Tel: 0800 1111
www.childline.org.uk
Department of Health
www.doh.gov.uk

Drugs in Schools Helpline
0345 366666

Eating Disorders Association
103 Prince of Wales Road,
   Norwich NR1 1DW
Adult helpline (over 18 years): 0845 634 1414
Youthline (up to and including 18 years):
   0845 634 7650
www.edauk.com

fpa
2–12 Pentonville Road, London N1 9FP
Tel: 020 7837 5432 (switchboard)
Helpline: 0845 310 1334 (England and Wales);
   0141 576 5088 (Scotland)
www.fpa.org.uk

Kidscape (preventing bullying and child abuse)
2 Grosvenor Gardens, London SW1W 0DH
Tel: 020 7730 3300

Ideas for personal and professional development

● Is your practice/place of work young people friendly? Do you offer services for them? Is it easy for them to access these services?

● What guidelines are available within your clinical practice regarding the medical treatment for under-16s? Do you operate within Gillick/Fraser guidelines? If not, you need to address this issue with your manager

● Compile a list of local services specifically for young people, e.g. sexual health, contraception and teenage pregnancy; drugs, alcohol and smoking; careers advice and education; housing; crime and legal services; general health and well-being

● Find out what your local priorities are and what strategies have been developed to implement any policies. Do you need additional training to carry out new work?

● Do you have a child protection policy? Find out who your local officer is and what training is available

● Does your experience with patients show evidence of good practice in providing sex education at local schools? You could meet with your local school nurses to discuss local issues.

Helpline: 08451 205 204
www.kidscape.org.uk
National Drugs Helpline
Tel: 0800 77 66 00
www.talktofrank.com

Office for National Statistics
www.statistics.gov.uk

Playing safely (the NHS guide to sexually transmitted infections)
Tel: 0800 567 123
www.playingsafely.co.uk

Sex Education Forum
Based at National Children's Bureau,
    8 Wakley Street, London EC1V 7QE
Tel: 020 7843 6000
www.ncb.org.uk/sef

Sexwise
Tel: 0800 28 29 30
www.ruthinking.co.uk
Teenage Health Freak
www.teenagehealthfreak.org

Teenage Pregnancy Unit
www.doh.gov.uk/teenagepregnancyunit

Young Minds Trust
102–108 Clerkenwell Road, London EC1M 5SA
Tel: 020 7366 8445
www.youngminds.org.uk

Further reading

BRYANT-JEFFERIES, R. (2003) *Counselling Young People.* Oxford: Radcliffe Medical Press.
BULL, D. (2000) *What Every Girl Should Know.* Salisbury: Element Books.
BURNINGHAM, S. (1994) *Young People Under Stress: A Parent's Guide.* London: Virago.
CHAMBERS, R., BOATH, E. and WAKLEY, G. (2000). *Tackling Teenage Pregnancy: Sex, Culture And Needs.* Oxford: Radcliffe Medical Press.
DONOVAN, C., SUCKLING, H. and WALKER, Z. (2004). *Difficult Consultations With Adolescents.* Oxford: Radcliffe Medical Press.
fpa 4 girls. London: fpa.
McPHERSON. A. and MACFARLANE, A. (1989) *I'm a Health Freak Too!* Oxford: Oxford University Press.
McPHERSON, A., DONOVAN, C. and McFARLANE, A. (2002) *Healthcare of Young People.* Oxford: Radcliffe Medical Press.

NOONAN, E. (1993) *Counselling Young People.* London: Routledge.

References

ABRAHAM, S. and LLEWELLYN-JONES, D. (1992) *Eating Disorders: The Facts*, 3rd edn. Oxford: Oxford University Press.
ALLEN, I. (1987) *Education in Sex and Personal Relationships.* London: Policy Studies Institute.
BMA *et al.* (British Medical Association, General Medical Services Committee, Health Education Authority, Brook Advisory Centres, Family Planning Association and Royal College of General Practitioners) (1993) *Confidentiality and People Under 16: A Joint Guidance Note.* London.
BROOK (2003) MPs Reject Amendments to Sexual Offences Bill: press release. London: Brook (wwwbrook.org.uk).
BRUCH, H. (1978) *The Golden Cage: The Enigma of Anorexia Nervosa.* London: Open Books.
CAMP, D.E., KLESGES, R.C. and REYLEN, G. (1993) The relationship between body concerns and adolescent smoking. *Health Psychology* **12**:29.
CES (Contraceptive Education Service) (1998) *Young People: Sexual Attitudes and Behaviour.* Factsheet No. 7. London: CES.
CHILDREN ACT (1989) London: HMSO.
CRISP, A.H., PALMER, R.L. and KALUCY, R.S. (1976) How common is anorexia nervosa? A prevalence study. *British Journal of Psychiatry* **128**:549–54.
DfEE (Department for Education and Employment) (1994) *Bullying: Don't Suffer in Silence.* London: HMSO.
DfEE (1998) *Schools Standards Framework Act.* London: HMSO.
DfEE (2000) Sex and Relationship Education Guidance.
DH (Department of Health) (2003a) Statistical Bulletin 2003/21: Statistics on smoking: England, 2003. London: DH (www.doh.gov.uk).
DH (2003b) Statistical Bulletin 2003/20: Statistics on alcohol: England, 2003. London: DH (www.doh.gov.uk).
DH (2003c) Statistical Bulletin: Statistics on young people and drug misuse: England, 2002. London: DH (www.doh.gov.uk).
DHSS (Department of Health and Social Security) (1974) *Family Planning Service Memorandum of Guidance.* Issued with circular HSC(IS)32, May.
DoH (Department of Health) (1990) *A Guide to Consent for Treatment*, HC (90). London: DoH.
DoH (1992) *The Health of the Nation: A Strategy for Health.* London: HMSO.
EATING DISORDERS ASSOCIATION (2004) What is an eating disorder? www.edauk.com.
FAMILY LAW REFORM ACT (1969) London: HMSO.
fpa (2004) Goodbye to Section 28: Campaigns Winter Bulletin 2004 www.fpa.org.uk/news.
FRANCIS, C. (1994) Sex education for teenagers in Holland. *Nursing Standard* **15**:27.
FRIEND, B. (1992) Blighted childhood. *Nursing Times* **88**:18.
FULLERTON, D., DICKSON, R., EASTWOOD, A. and SHELDON, T. (1997) Preventing unintended teenage pregnancies and reducing their adverse effects. *Effective Health Care* **3**:1–12.

GLEESON, C., ROBINSOM, M. and NEALE, R. (2002) A review of teenagers' perceived needs and access to primary health care: Implications for health services. *Primary Health Care Research and Development* 3:184–93.

HIPPISLEY-COX, J., ALLEN J., PRINGLE, M. *et al.* (2000) Association between teenage pregnancy rates and the age and sex of general practitioners: cross sectional survey in Trent 1994–7. *British Medical Journal* **320**:842–5.

HMI (Her Majesty's Inspectorate) (1986) *Health Education from 5 to 16 (Curriculum Matters)*. London: HMSO.

HPA (Health Protection Agency) (2003) Epidemiological Data – Gonorrhoea (www.hpa.org.uk/infections).

HUTCHINSON, F. (1993) Contraceptive needs of young people. *British Journal of Sexual Medicine* **10**.

LAWRENCE, M. and DANA, M. (1990) *Fighting Food: Coping with Eating Disorders*. London: Penguin.

LOCAL GOVERNMENT ACT (1988) London: HMSO.

MASSEY, D. (1990) School sex education: knitting without a pattern? *Health Education Journal* **49**:134.

McHALE, J. (1998) Consent to treatment: general principles. In McHale, J., Tingle, J. and Peysner, J. (eds) *Law and Nursing*, Chapter 5. Oxford: Butterworth-Heinemann.

MEDICAL DEFENCE UNION (1992) *Confidentiality*. London: MDU.

National Statistics (2003) Sexual health: chlamydia rates continue to rise (www.statistics.gov.uk/CCI).

NMC (2002) *Code of Professional Conduct*. London: NMC.

ONS (Office for National Statistics) (2004) *Health Statistics Quarterly* **21**:51 (www.statistics.gov.uk).

PALMER, R.L. (1989) *Anorexia Nervosa: A Guide for Sufferers and their Families*, 2nd edn. Harmondsworth: Penguin.

ROYAL COLLEGE OF GENERAL PRACTITIONERS, ROYAL COLLEGE OF NURSING (2002). *Getting It Right For Teenagers In Your Practice*. RCGP: London.

SCHOOLS HEALTH EDUCATION UNIT, UNIVERSITY OF EXETER (1994) *Young People in 1993*. Exeter: HEU.

SEX EDUCATION FORUM (1997a) *Ensuring Entitlement: A Sex Education Charter*. Forum factsheet No. 14. London: National Children's Bureau.

SEX EDUCATION FORUM (1997b) *We're Talking About Sex Education*. Leaflet. London: National Children's Bureau.

SEX EDUCATION FORUM (1997c) *Teaching About Contraception*. Forum factsheet No. 13. London: National Children's Bureau.

SEXUAL OFFENCES (AMENDMENT) ACT (2000): Age of Consent; Home Office Circular 46/2000. London (www.homeoffice.gov.uk).

SEXUAL OFFENCES ACT (2003) Key messages. London: Teenage Pregnancy Unit (www.info.doh.gov.uk/tpu/tpu/nsf).

SLADE, R. (1984) *The Anorexia Nervosa Handbook*. London: Harper & Row.

SOCIAL EXCLUSION UNIT (1999) *Teenage Pregnancy*. London: The Stationery Office (www.cabinet-office.gov.uk/seu/1999/Teenpar/index.htm).

TEENAGE PREGNANCY UNIT (2003) www.info.doh.gov.uk/tpu.

TOWNSEND, J., WILKES, H., WILKES, A. and JANIS, M. (1991) Adolescent smokers seen in general practice: health, lifestyle, physical measurements, and response to anti-smoking advice. *British Medical Journal* **303**:949.

WELLINGS, K. and KANE, R. (1999) Trends in teenage pregnancy in England and Wales: how can we explain them? *Journal of the Royal Society of Medicine* **92**(6):277–82.

WELLINGS, K., WADSWORTH, J., JOHNSON, A.M., FIELD, J., WHITAKER, L. and FIELD, B. (1995) Provision of sex education and early sexual experience: the relation examined. *British Medical Journal* **311**:417–20.

WESTALL, J. (1997) Poor education linked with teen pregnancies. *British Medical Journal* **314**:535.

WILLIAMS, E. (1994) Contraceptive compliance among young people. *British Journal of Sexual Medicine* May/June:12.

WOODWARD, V. (1995) Why do teenagers fall into the pregnancy trap? *Modern Midwife* August:15–18.

WOOLFSON, R. (1989) Bullying at school: part 1 – the nature and extent of the problem. *Health at School* **4**:152.

YOUNG MINDS (2004) What makes people so stressed? www.youngminds.org.uk.

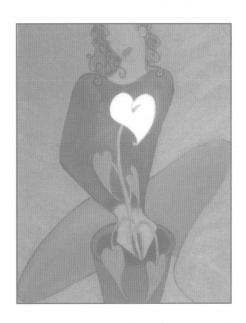

Fertility

8: Sexuality During and After Pregnancy

Gillian Aston

OBJECTIVES

This chapter should help you understand:

◆ How sexuality, sexual relations and sexual activity during the childbearing continuum are influenced by biological, psychological and social variables ◆

◆ How changes in body image, especially during pregnancy, may affect sexuality ◆

◆ That health professionals need to be aware of and address their own attitudes towards sexuality during the childbearing continuum ◆

◆ The importance of exploring with women and their partners that there is no normal pattern of sexual behaviour during pregnancy and following childbirth ◆

◆ That care planning should focus on the needs of the individual woman and couple. ◆

Introduction

Childbearing is intricately bound up with a woman's sexuality and sexual health. However, the activities of sex and reproduction are surrounded by a whole series of complicated emotions and meanings. Throughout life, the way individuals respond to and feel about their sexuality changes as their lives undergo transition. The changes associated with pregnancy, childbirth and the transition to motherhood have a special significance, representing one of the most fundamental periods of change that a woman will experience. As McNeill (1994) says, 'a woman's sexual expression and sexual health is intimately linked to her self-image, her well-being, her personal circumstances and the social context in which she develops and lives'.

The relative contributions of the feelings and experiences noted above 'have not been adequately studied and thus cannot be quantified'. Nevertheless, it can be seen that central to sexual health and the childbearing continuum are individual experiences, personal histories and all the bits and pieces of our unique existences (Carter, 1979).

Biological and psychological factors influence sexuality throughout all stages of life. During pregnancy and following childbirth these factors are completely interwoven. The physical changes that occur during pregnancy and childbirth and the experiences involved while caring for a baby can, according to Alder (1994),

> have a considerable effect on both sexual behaviour and sexual feelings. Psychological changes in role, identity and self image also affect sexuality. These interact so that the

experience of being pregnant, giving birth and breast-feeding may also depend on feelings about sexuality.

Literature for health professionals on sexuality following childbirth and during early motherhood is still relatively scarce. Sex during early parenthood has been described as 'one of our last taboos' (Dye, 2002; Dixon *et al.*, 2000). Fortunately more literature is available on sexuality during pregnancy but the majority, including articles from the popular media, tend to focus on and portray bleak and depressing pictures of sexual relationships. Oakley (1979) makes a similar point: 'I have tried to show the positive side, but of course it is to some extent true that the best news is bad news: happiness doesn't hit the headlines because it is boring'.

Some may feel that this chapter also perpetuates a negative image of sexuality during the childbearing continuum. However, it is important for the reader to gain an understanding of the complexities involved, the need for integrated approaches as well as the need for more work on sexual health during pregnancy, labour and following childbirth.

Pregnancy: A time of transition

Pregnancy is a normal life event which involves considerable adjustment by the parents. Oakley (1979) has criticized much of the research that has focused on adjustment or 'adaptation' to pregnancy and argues that it reduces pregnancy to a symbol of conforming to cultural definitions of femininity. She suggests that it is not natural that all women should like and enjoy being mothers with all the constraints that motherhood puts on 'normal' life. Nevertheless, the transition to parenthood can be seen as a developmental crisis or a critical event in adult life (Clulow, 1982) with different degrees of stress involved. Apart from affecting the pregnant woman, the stress also affects her partner and their relationship.

A first pregnancy produces the greatest change. As Taylor (1992) pointed out, pregnancy represents the end of freedom and a dramatic change in lifestyle. It also has a dramatic effect on a couple's sense of identity, communication patterns and role behaviour. During pregnancy, concerns about finance are naturally a common problem. If the woman has been in employment she has to make decisions about whether to continue after the baby is born. There may be legitimate concern about whether the couple can afford to lose one income. Feelings of guilt can be evoked in the pregnant woman as she attempts to resolve the competing demands of career and family and listens to the conflicting advice from friends and relatives. Although a neglected area of research, evidence indicates that relationships with female friends may change during pregnancy or significantly influence the experience for the pregnant woman (Leifer, 1980).

The relationship between the pregnant woman and her partner encompasses a complex web of tangled emotions. The results of a study conducted by Taylor (1992) suggest that fears about the relationship are probably quite common experiences. Taylor reports that: 'In some cases, men feel that their relationship with their partner assumes a secondary position compared with their partner's relationship with their unborn child'.

This finding has been corroborated by other studies. Shapiro (cited in Taylor, 1992) also suggests that fear of losing this relationship plays a significant role in the tendency for some men to have an affair during their partner's late pregnancy. Feelings of rejection were cited as the main motivational factor for affairs at this stage. The ability of men to confront such fears is clearly important for both partners and for their relationship during pregnancy.

The transition and adjustments that are made during the first pregnancy are affected by the ability of both parties to come to terms with changes in their social roles and status. As Clulow (1982) puts it: 'the transition from wife to mother, or husband to father, is an integral part of the transition from two to three'.

Stress in pregnancy

A degree of personal stress is a common feature of most pregnancies. Anxiety, often accompanied by a revival of past conflict, depression, worries, mood lability, impaired concentration, a reawakening of early childhood relationships and experiences of mothering, as well increased dependency and altered spatial orientation have all been identified in studies of normal antenatal clinic populations (Raphael-Leff, 1991). There are a number of other factors, often unrelated to the pregnancy itself, which can affect the woman's ability to adjust and come to terms with her pregnancy. They impose added burdens and add to the stress and anxieties of pregnancy, which in turn may affect sexuality and sexual health.

Women who have to cope with moving house, changing or losing their jobs when they are expecting a baby may find it difficult to cope with the demands of pregnancy. Whilst these events would cause some anxiety and confusion in the lives of everybody, as Raphael-Leff (1991) says, 'When these life events occur alongside the emotional upheaval of pregnancy, they increase the sense of disorientation and interrupt the psychological work of pregnancy by presenting intrusive or, at times, conflicting demands for readjustment'.

Unexpected and painful distressing events can also impinge on a woman's coping ability. Bereavement in the family, eviction or dismissal as well as events associated with the pregnancy such as threatened miscarriage, negative results of a fetal diagnostic test or death of a twin *in utero*, are associated with an intrusion into the natural emotional adjustments and processes of pregnancy. Raphael-Leff (1991) suggests that these events can invoke feelings of anxiety, grief, rejection, emptiness and loss just at a time when the woman is physically and psychologically geared to receptivity, hopefulness and fulfilment. Women who find themselves alone following death, divorce, separation or abandonment by their partners are especially vulnerable. In addition to the pregnancy they are coping with an extremely distressing emotionally charged and often unforeseen life event. Women who have not chosen to become single mothers are likely to have their distress compounded by feelings of lack of control over their future destiny and dissolution of their partnership at the very time when it was about to expand into a family (Raphael-Leff, 1991).

An increasing number of women turn to complementary therapies to help them cope with stress during pregnancy and childbirth. Such therapies include massage, aromatherapy, reflexology, acupuncture, hydrotherapy and osteopathy (see Chapter 4). Counselling and advice on the many ways to reduce stress will be appreciated by both the woman and her partner and are comprehensively covered by Tiran and Mack (2000) in their book *Complementary Therapies for Pregnancy and Childbirth,* 2nd edition.

Support during pregnancy

Studies have emphasized the need for pregnant women to feel supported at home, at work and in their relationships. It has been suggested that if a woman perceives she has emotional support this then buffers the effects of life changes (Jones and Jones, 1991). Pines (1993) suggests that during pregnancy interpersonal conflicts can be exacerbated by the emotional changes that occur as a result of pregnancy. These include mood swings, introversion, extreme sensitivity and tiredness as well as changes in sexual patterns.

The father of the child is also likely to undergo emotional changes which can also affect the mother. Taylor (1992) is critical of the dearth of literature concerning men's feelings and experiences in areas related to pregnancy and states that: 'Many men are completely unprepared, both emotionally and intellectually, for the birth of their child(ren). Men have feelings and experiences in relation to issues which are often dismissed as women's matters'.

The question here then is what kind of support is he able to offer? 'The fact that a woman does have a partner, need not imply that she is supported. A husband may be present in the flesh but emotionally absent' (Raphael-Leff, 1991). Oakley (1979) demonstrated the profound emotional shock posed by the transition into first-time motherhood. The women in this study said it was good to take part in the research as they thought the process of interviewing was a socially supportive experience. Women welcomed the opportunity to talk about the things that concerned or delighted them. They also found it was a positive relief to unburden themselves of critical feelings and experiences.

It is important for health care professionals to attempt to identify women with inadequate emotional support as well as to help all pregnant women make the most of the resources available. The demands of single parenthood without adequate emotional, practical and financial support will increasingly need to be borne in mind. As Oakley (1992) points out:

> The norm that behind every pregnant woman there is a supportive husband working and ready to supply emotional companionship, domestic help and financial resources, will increasingly be a piece of cultural mythology. The old label 'marital status' is becoming a poor guide to women's living circumstances. Whether a woman is legally married or not does not inform her health care providers, either about her household arrangements, or as to the social, financial and emotional support available to her.

As we discuss later, it is also important for health care professionals not to assume that a woman is heterosexual and to expect that her main source of support during and after pregnancy will be a man. Increasing numbers of lesbian couples are choosing to become parents (Garcia, 2003).

Domestic violence and pregnancy

Domestic violence has been defined as physical, sexual or emotional violence from an adult perpetrator directed towards an adult victim in the context of a close relationship. In the majority of incidences this will mean domestic violence from a man to his wife, ex-wife, female partner or ex-partner (Home Office, 2003). Violence and abuse, which may be sexual, can begin within a relationship at any time. However, studies indicate that it may begin or worsen during pregnancy and that attacks on the breasts, abdomen and genitals are common during pregnancy (Bewley and Gibbs, 2000). On average a woman will have been attacked 35 times before she reports domestic violence and that may frequently amount to many years of torture (Byrne, 1994).

As well as the physical injuries inflicted upon women by violent men, the psychological effects of domestic violence have been shown to be profound. Anxiety, depression, shame, guilt and a low self-esteem are just some of these effects. Not surprisingly, women who are the victims of violent men 'May be quite frightened during sexual intercourse and will not be in a position to refuse unwanted activities nor will they be able to express their own needs' (Walton, 1994). Campbell and Alford (1989) examined the timing of sexual attacks in their sample of 115 battered women. Approximately half reported being raped by their partners while they were physically ill, and 46% were forced immediately following a hospital discharge, and most importantly this was usually after childbirth. Another study of 159 battered women found that almost half (45.9%) had been forced into sex by their intimate partner or ex-partner (Campbell and Soeken, 1999). Women who had been sexually assaulted had higher scores on negative health symptoms, gynaecological symptoms, and risk factors for homicide. The number of sexual assaults was significantly correlated with depression and a negative body image. The study suggests that body image is the aspect of self-esteem damage that is affected particularly from forced relationship sex.

Awareness of domestic violence and pregnancy has now been raised and midwives and health professionals must be alert to the problem, take heed and address the issues involved. If domestic violence is suspected then women need to be advised on the organizations and services available for practical and emotional support.

Other children

Children can bring women much happiness and joy but childrearing can also be very stressful and tiring. This can add to the complex emotional and physical adjustments a woman makes during and after pregnancy. Little or no support, shortage of money and a lack of childcare facilities to give the mother a break can result in an emotional crisis. The mother of the twenty-first century is more likely than her own mother to have other relatives to care for, as well as her own children. She is also much more likely to have paid employment of her own. Negotiating and resourcing childcare arrangements can be another stress and burden experienced by women during pregnancy (Aston and Pacanowski, 1999). A mother nowadays is frequently trying to juggle the multiple roles of being a carer for elderly relatives, a loving wife or partner, a multiple orgasmic lover, a successful career woman, as well as being a devoted mother. Tiredness and looking after other children, as well as the home, may lessen sexual libido and make sexual intercourse, understandably, a low priority.

Pregnancy and sexuality

Myths and misconceptions

The relationship between sexuality and pregnancy, childbirth and the puerperium (the first 6 weeks after the birth) is historically replete with cultural stereotypes, false universals, myths and various 'taboos'. What is intriguing is the deep imprint these powerful and pervasive beliefs have on attitudes about sexuality during pregnancy. Kitzinger (1985) points out that pregnant women frequently fear that sexual intercourse may provoke miscarriage or premature labour or in some way damage the fetus, and as a result feel that they should abstain from sexual intercourse. She goes on to report that some men have expressed fear of breaking the 'bag of water' during sexual intercourse, whilst others believe that they could damage the baby or precipitate labour:

> It is almost as if they feel that to keep themselves under restraint will help make the pregnancy go well; as if their self control will somehow 'guard' the pregnancy. These beliefs are remarkably similar to those held in Third World societies, where taboos are enjoined on a father in order to ensure the well-being of a baby whilst it is still in the uterus.
>
> (Kitzinger, 1985)

Recent research conducted in Nigeria on aspects of male sexual behaviour during pregnancy supports the comments noted above. Onah *et al.* (2002) found that personal beliefs significantly affected sexual relationships between Nigerian husbands and their pregnant wives. As a result one-third of husbands engaged in extramarital

relationships as a way to satisfy their unmet needs during pregnancy.

Is pregnancy sexy? The question is an important one because within its answer lies the whole range of society's attitudes towards pregnancy, sexuality and towards women. Reamy and White (1987) stated that pregnant women are not seen as sexually attractive and societal norms stress that sexual desires, responses and activities should not occur during pregnancy. This observation is interesting as it suggests that it is not nature that makes sex and pregnancy a taboo combination, but cultural and society's attitudes towards pregnancy. Such an observation does, however, need to be counterbalanced as Wallace (1989) remarks that:

> There seems to be a vast difference between what pregnant women might actually feel and what society thinks they should feel. There is an over-riding ethos in our culture that pregnancy may make women feel fat, unattractive, sick, tired, fragile, neurotic or 'blooming', but the one thing that seems scarcely imaginable is that it might make us feel sexy.

Other explanations to account for the contradictory and confusing aspects of pregnancy and sexuality have been offered. Contratto (1980) argues that one of the most pervasive beliefs that still exists in Western culture (although little information exists on who holds the belief) is that 'good mothers are generally asexual'. She suggests that many women have successfully internalized the identity of asexual motherhood. This quote from a mother of two small infants is used by Contratto to make the point: 'You're writing a paper on maternal sexuality? What in God's name is that?' Contratto proposes that many women who are pregnant or are new mothers are 'intensely uncomfortable with their own sexuality, consciously or unconsciously and as a result experience considerable psychological pain'. This could have far reaching effects on their relationships. A second explanation has been offered by Ussher (1989) to account for the confusion and contradictions regarding sexuality which women have to face when they become pregnant. She argues that it is the inevitable result of the way women are categorized:

Individual women are inevitably positioned at either end of the dichotomy: good/bad, madonna/whore, feminine/career-orientated, and their position is often determined by their reproductive status. Thus, the woman who is pregnant or a mother cannot be a good mother and a sexual person at the same time, both madonna and whore; women's sexuality is dangerous and threatening and is therefore at odds with the stereotype of the good mother.

The preceding discussion suggests that the deep internalizing of societal attitudes and the categorization of women may affect sexuality and sexual relations during pregnancy. However, if pregnant women are not too embarrassed by cultural mores to admit it, 'their libido, sexual activity and sexual responsiveness can reach heights previously uncharted' (Black, 1994).

Sexuality issues for the pregnant woman

Pregnancy is a unique time in a woman's life. She experiences dramatic alterations in her physiology, her appearance and her body, as well as changes in her social status which all occur simultaneously. Psychic and social changes also exist for both partners in the relationship. Pregnancy can either disrupt the relationship between a couple or can deepen and strengthen it (Kitzinger, 1982). According to Kitzinger, sexual interaction is one facet of the relationship which is often affected. Research has shown that relationship satisfaction and emotional closeness are strong predictors of sexual desire and sexual satisfaction during and after pregnancy (De Judicibus and McCabe, 2002). Further illuminating insights into the meaning of sexual satisfaction in pregnant women has been provided by a study conducted in Taiwan, Republic of China (Lee, 2002). The results revealed four essential themes as women said:

◆ That sexual satisfaction improved their sense of self-identity
◆ They felt empowered through sexual relations
◆ A strengthening of the marital bond
◆ Positive reinforcement of the value of sexuality.

Several empirical studies have described a decrease in sexual desire, frequency and satisfaction in women during pregnancy (De Judicibus and McCabe, 2002; Orji *et al.*, 2002; von Sydow *et al.*, 2001; Oruç *et al.*, 1999; Bogren, 1991; Barclay *et al.*, 1994). This decrease is usually most marked in the third trimester of pregnancy and least in the second. Masters and Johnson (1966) reported increased sexual desire and sexual satisfaction during the second trimester compared to before pregnancy. They also found that decreased desire during the first trimester was only true for women expecting their first baby.

The study conducted by Jones (1990) found that a large number of pregnant women reported a loss of libido. The findings suggest that affection and reassurance between partners rather than physical contact is important. In this study pregnant women reported that they felt restricted because of their size and that positions for sexual activity and intercourse were limited. This observation is particularly interesting as it could indicate a lack of education from health care professionals; this problem can be overcome by discussing different positions for sex or other ways of experiencing sexual satisfaction. Researchers appear to agree that coital frequency declines during pregnancy and they link this to a woman's declining sexual interest and the discomfort caused by advancing pregnancy (De Judicibus and McCabe, 2002; Barclay, 1990). The pattern and intensity of this decline is not clear. Studies have also reported a linear decline in sexual interest and activity over successive trimesters (Alder, 1994).

Unfortunately, many studies of sexuality during pregnancy have methodological flaws (Sayle *et al.*, 2003). However, what is important is that there is no 'norm' of sexual behaviour, particularly with regard to pregnancy (Coppens, 2002). Sexual behaviour varies between individuals. During pregnancy the desire and needs of couples for sexual intimacy and activity constantly go through a process of redefinition and change.

The physical and emotional adjustments of pregnancy can cause changes in body image, fatigue, mood swings and sexual activity. The woman's changing shape, emotional status, fetal activity, changes in breast size, pressure on the bladder and other discomforts of pregnancy result in increased physical and emotional demands. These can produce stress on the sexual relationship of the pregnant woman and her partner. As the woman's appearance and emotional status change during pregnancy, her partner may react with confusion, fear or anxiety, wondering how his relationship with her will be affected.

Being pregnant is not all sexually negative. Walton (1994) acknowledges that, freed from the fear of pregnancy, many couples find that 'it is the greatest turn-on ever. The woman feels fulfilled and magnificent and the man feels proud and protective'. A satisfying sexual relationship during pregnancy contributes to satisfaction and happiness by strengthening ties of caring, mutual respect, pleasure and intimacy.

Physiological changes

Many physiological changes occur during pregnancy. The hormones oestrogen and progesterone act together to evoke marked pelvic vasocongestion. Vaginal congestion occurs because of increased vascularity and venous stasis. The venous congestion of pregnancy can result in a heightened manifestation of all aspects of sexual intercourse. The orgasm may be heightened and the vaginal lumen becomes smaller, thus gripping the penis tighter (Walton, 1994). However, vasocongestion can also predispose pregnant women to discomfort during sexual intercourse. Reamy and White (1985) state that:

> The progressive deep pelvic congestion of pregnancy and its associated pressure can be aggravated by sexual intercourse; tumescence becomes increasingly exaggerated, prolonged and progressively less responsive to orgasm.

Vulval varicosities and haemorrhoids may be precipitated and aggravated by pregnancy. Labial vasocongestion and distension is also exacerbated by varicosities and by the pregnant state, making some routine activities such as walking very uncomfortable and the idea of sex seem impossible.

Body changes and body image

During pregnancy major body changes occur with startling rapidity. Such changes inevitably mean that adjustment has to be made to what constitutes a 'normal body image'. There is very little research focusing directly on women's views of their body changes or of their size during pregnancy. Nevertheless, the few studies that do exist indicate that the focus on women's physical appearance changes during pregnancy, and that they are generally viewed differently by men. For example, Price (1988) notes that there is a shift away from women being viewed as 'seducers' to being viewed as 'producers' during pregnancy. For some women body image during pregnancy is viewed in a very positive light: 'your body metamorphoses into this magnificent spectacle – loose and open and warm' (Miller, 1995).

The way a pregnant woman feels and experiences her body during pregnancy can affect her sexuality. It has been suggested that some women have very positive feelings about their bodies, whilst others are more negative, especially during the last three months of pregnancy (Raphael-Leff, 1993). Tiredness, the changes that occur in the breasts, backache, as well as frequency of micturition are just some of the physical changes that can affect sexual activity. According to Kitzinger (1985) some women have distorted views of their bodies during pregnancy: 'They feel bigger than they really are or believe that their partners must find them ugly, when in fact, men often delight in pregnant women and find their physical changes exciting and beautiful'.

However, there is evidence of considerable dissatisfaction with pregnancy due to the connotations that fatness has with being unattractive (Wiles, 1994). Such findings provide evidence of the importance of physical attractiveness in women's self-esteem. According to Jones (1999) the 1990s was the decade of the 'designer' protuberance as articles, pictures and 'sexy shots' of the bodies of pregnant pop stars, celebrities and supermodels were published in the media. However, there are studies which suggest that pregnant women in general do not identify with contemporary media imagery of the pregnant body (Grogan, 1999; Kent, 1998) as stretch marks and 'drooping breasts' have been identified as important concerns in study samples.

As already mentioned, a woman's sexual health is intimately linked to her own self-image and this needs to be acknowledged and discussed with women by midwives during pregnancy. Sexual positions to increase comfort as the pregnancy progresses as well as alternative non-coital modes of sexual expression, such as manual partner stimulation and masturbation, should be explored with the pregnant woman and her partner. Women who are expecting a multiple birth may have particular concerns and anxieties about physical restrictions because of their size.

Negative feelings regarding body image during pregnancy have been identified (Jones, 1990). Yet, as Jones points out 'By paying attention to a woman's thoughts, feelings and perceptions about her body, we can help her adapt to her changing situation'.

Sexual intercourse during pregnancy

The Bible advises against it and Hippocrates maintained that it could lead to abortion (Main *et al.*, 1993). The British tradition in antenatal care in relation to intercourse in pregnancy has historically been one of 'avoidance' (Nicolson, 1990). However, in the recent guidelines for the antenatal care of healthy pregnant women maternity care professionals are advised to inform pregnant women that sexual intercourse in pregnancy is not known to be associated with any adverse outcomes (National Institute for Clinical Excellence, 2003). Several studies have examined the relationships between sexual intercourse, uterine contractility and pre-term labour with conflicting results (Sayle *et al.*, 2001). You are recommended to read the review of the studies by Andersen and Fuchs (1993) and their analysis of the difficulties of carrying out well-designed studies on sexual activity in pregnancy and pre-term birth. Orgasm, with or without sexual intercourse, has been reported to be associated with premature rupture of membranes, especially during late pregnancy and with a slow fetal heart rate (Ekwo *et al.*, 1993). Pregnant women frequently fear that sexual intercourse may provoke miscarriage or premature labour or damage the fetus, and so feel they should abstain (Savage and Reader, 1984).

Evidence from the study of 158 pregnant women by Oruç *et al.* (1999) suggests that these fears are pervasive. They found that 24.5% of their sample reported avoiding intercourse throughout pregnancy, 49.1% avoided it sometimes and 26.4% stated that they had never had avoidance behaviour. The reasons for avoidance behaviour were 'it can harm the baby' (49.1%), 'it can cause abortion' (25.2%), 'my sexual desire decreased' (22.6%) and 'I have physical difficulties' (22.0%). Clearly these findings have implications for maternity and health care professionals, as validation of experiences, acknowledgement of concerns and fears can do much for their avoidance or amelioration.

The findings of a study conducted by Mills *et al.* (1981) of the sexual activity of 10,477 women during pregnancy led them to conclude that sexual intercourse with orgasm up to term has no ill-effects on the outcome of pregnancy. Savage and Reader (1984) confirmed this, finding no significant increase of fetal distress in women who continued to be sexually active throughout pregnancy. Another finding of the study was that 27% of the women respondents noted uterine contractions following orgasm. The majority reported these as always or sometimes painful. Once painful contractions had been noted after orgasm, women reported having sexual intercourse less frequently or ceasing altogether. The avoidance of sexual intercourse or the avoidance of orgasm should be differentiated and explored. The warning signs indicative of abstaining from sexual intercourse and seeking professional advice also need to be discussed (Box 8.1).

Box 8.1 Indications to abstain from sexual intercourse during pregnancy (Guana-Trujillo and Higgins, 1987)

- Vaginal bleeding
- Placenta praevia
- Premature dilatation of the cervix
- Rupture of membranes
- History of premature delivery
- Multiple pregnancy
- Engaged fetal head.

The physical effects of sexual intercourse in pregnancy should be discussed by health professionals with the woman or the couple. Any advice on sexual intercourse or abstinence during pregnancy needs to explore non-penetrative sex, sexual intercourse and orgasm. Alder (1994) has argued that there is a wide variation of sexual behaviour and that couples should be aware that there is no normal pattern, as frequency, quality and satisfaction vary throughout the lifespan. Any notion that 'normal' sexual activity requires penetrative sex should be dispelled and alternatives ranging from kissing and cuddling to masturbation can be discussed.

It could be argued that more information is needed regarding the relative importance of female orgasm and sexual intercourse on uterine contractility (Main *et al.*, 1993). Nevertheless, it would seem appropriate for health professionals to suggest back massage or back rubbing as a way of attempting to relieve discomfort caused by prolonged contractions of orgasm, especially during the third trimester.

Sexual intercourse is often stated to be a natural method of induction of labour (Tomlinson *et al.*, 1999). Although it is not known if sexual intercourse at term influences the onset of labour, there are several theoretical reasons why it may (Tomlinson *et al.*, 1999; Andersen and Fuchs, 1993). Any study on whether sexual intercourse at term is implicated in the onset of labour would pose practical and ethical difficulties. However, a recent survey to assess the interest of women and men regarding the role of sexual activity and the onset of labour, found that the majority of the sample indicated that if sexual intercourse did influence the onset of labour, then it would have an effect on sexual activity at term (Tomlinson *et al.*, 1999).

Dyspareunia in pregnancy

How frequent and problematic is dyspareunia among pregnant women? In a study conducted by Reamy and White (1985) of 52 married women throughout pregnancy, dyspareunia appears to be far from incidental and becomes increasingly prevalent as pregnancy progresses. By the third trimester of pregnancy 12% of the women were experiencing painful sexual intercourse more than half the time. Correlations were found between happiness about being pregnant, anxiety about the pregnancy or the impending delivery, and the women's perceived attractiveness to their husbands. Additionally, the authors reported that just over one-third of the women respondents reported having stopped intercourse altogether; the specific reasons for this were not identified.

Another study of the effects of pregnancy on the sexuality of 158 pregnant women also found that dyspareunia was common in the study group (Oruç *et al.*, 1999). Women in the first trimester had a significantly lower rate of dyspareunia compared to the other two trimesters. Twenty-six per cent of respondents claimed to have had dyspareunia throughout pregnancy, 36% sometimes and 38% reported no dyspareunia at all. Pregnancy was also found to have a negative effect on orgasmic quality. Dyspareunia and a decrease in orgasmic quality both influenced the frequency of sexual intercourse. Coital frequency was found to decline as the month of the pregnancy increased.

Multiple physical and psychosocial factors have been identified that influence the occurrence of dyspareunia during pregnancy (Box 8.2). You are recommended to read the article by Morris and Mukhophadyay (2003) as it reviews the causes of dyspareunia and outlines assessment and management of the problem.

Dyspareunia and avoidance of sexual intercourse demands a systematic evaluation by health care professionals. Sexual health and sexual responses are dependent upon the interaction between physiological and psychosocial systems. Reamy and White (1985) point out that pregnant women need to be given permission to feel sexual and to be sexual. They also need to know that emotional and sexual fluctuations during pregnancy are to be anticipated and are normal. Disclosure of sexual symptoms including dyspareunia, and its systematic evaluation and treatment, are important considerations during pregnancy and at any stage of a woman's life. The physical causes for the problem should not be overlooked, neither should the psychological causes be neglected.

> **Box 8.2** Causes of dyspareunia during pregnancy (Reamy and White, 1985)
>
> **Physical factors**
>
> ◆ Pelvic vasocongestion
> ◆ Vaginal congestion and reduced lubrication
> ◆ Subluxation of the symphysis pubis and sacroiliac joints
> ◆ Retroverted uterus – particularly during the first weeks of pregnancy
> ◆ In late pregnancy, weight of partner on the gravid uterus
> ◆ Deep engagement of the fetal head
> ◆ Chorioamnionitis
> ◆ Candidal infection
> ◆ Sexually transmitted *Trichomonas vaginalis*
> ◆ Genital herpes and genital warts.
>
> **Psychosocial factors**
> *Intrapersonal*
>
> ◆ Anxiety and fear
> ◆ Vaginismus
> ◆ General emotional state
> ◆ Tiredness
> ◆ Self-esteem
> ◆ Body image
> ◆ Sexual guilt.
>
> *Interpersonal*
>
> ◆ Hurt and anger between the expectant parents
> ◆ Deficient communication and trust between the expectant parents.

Effects on relationships

Research into sexuality and pregnancy has predominantly focused on the female partner and ignored the male partner and the relationship. Barclay *et al.* (1994) claim that when research into sexuality ignores social context and relationships its usefulness is limited. The findings of their study of couples experiencing a first pregnancy provide an example of the effects on sexuality during the changes of pregnancy.

A substantial decline in sexual interest amongst the women, which was not matched by their male partners, was identified. This was reflected in a marked reduction in the frequency of sexual intercourse and in the range of sexual activities. Concern and guilt about the loss of sexual interest and responses to the approach of partners was expressed by some women. The need for holding, cuddling, kissing and physical affection was seen as important for a number of women. This was especially important during the later part of pregnancy. Breast tenderness, a perceived loss of physical attractiveness and their ability to maintain the interest of partners in them as women were some of the reasons articulated by the women in the study. The authors found that 76% regularly practised fellatio and cunnilingus (oral sex) and 12% of males regularly practised anal intercourse during pregnancy. Another key observation was that 28% of the men interviewed did not always achieve orgasm during sexual intercourse (Barclay *et al.*, 1994). It should be stressed to couples that the forceful blowing of air into the vagina during foreplay and oral sex should be avoided particularly during pregnancy as it may cause air embolism (Robinson, 1998).

These findings suggest that the mismatch of female sexual interest levels in pregnancy could present a challenge to stable partnerships (Barclay *et al.*, 1994; Taylor, 1992). During assessment and planning maternity care, professionals need to gather information about sexual activity before and during pregnancy. The comfort level around sexual activity and the interest and concerns of partners should be discussed. Guidance on the individual differences and variations in sexual response during pregnancy should be given whether asked for or not. Alder (1994) suggests that most couples will find that they have different levels of interests and patterns of sexual activity at different stages of their lives. She notes that:

> Accepting variations in sexuality would relieve the pressure to behave in what may be perceived as the normal pattern of sexual behaviour, and allow each individual couple to find their own level of sexual activity.

By giving permission to talk about and then normalize sexual experiences, professionals can then aim to enhance the sexual experience of pregnancy and the relationship for those most intimately involved. For some women sex during pregnancy can be a more enriching and fulfilling experience: 'The necessity of finding new positions (there are plenty if you apply as much concentration as you would to finding a parking space) adds spice. And orgasms seem more intense and happen more easily' (Miller, 1995).

The findings of Barclay *et al.* (1994) highlighted that a woman's loss of self-esteem and perceptions of loss of physical attractiveness are very real to her. Black (1994) points out that:

> Knowing this, one can recommend rear-entry (a tergo) positions to the couple. As the woman's back remains slim when on view to her partner, the knee-chest position and its variants provide good support and relaxation for the pregnant body.

Research has identified that sexual functioning during pregnancy continues, albeit in varying degrees. However, it has also identified that maternity care professionals are often either inadequate in their efforts or do not provide enough information about sexual activity and sexual intercourse during pregnancy (Guana-Trujillo and Higgins, 1987; Savage and Reader, 1984). Moreover, it has been shown that women welcome information about sexual activity and sexual intercourse during pregnancy.

When planning care for pregnant women you should be able to address this need but must be aware of your own sexual feelings and attitudes towards sex during pregnancy and give accurate and informed advice. If avenues of communication are open regarding sexual intercourse and sexual activity during pregnancy, any fears and myths the pregnant woman and her partner may have can be dispelled. You can then identify areas in which more information is required and give factual, non-judgemental advice. The findings of Oruç *et al.* (1999) highlight the importance of this as 35.5% of pregnant women sampled stated that they knew nothing about sexuality during pregnancy, and 41.3% stated that they only had a limited knowledge. However, knowledge about sexuality during pregnancy did not affect sexual desire or the frequency and avoidance patterns of sexual intercourse.

Assessment for care planning needs to include the biological and psychosocial variables that can affect sexuality. This includes knowledge about pregnancy and effects of pregnancy on sexuality and sexual behaviour; attitudes towards and the feelings about pregnancy; as well as attention to the concerns of the partner. Questions that could highlight some of these issues have been identified and include the following:

◆ 'What have you heard about sex during pregnancy?'

◆ 'What do you feel about sex during pregnancy?'

◆ 'How do your feelings and ideas about sex differ from your partner?'

◆ 'Most women experience changes in sexuality and their sexual relationship during pregnancy – what changes, if any, have taken place in your sexual relationship?'

Such enquiries will encourage information exchange regarding sexuality and may enable women to share their attitudes, experiences and concerns (Reamy and White, 1987).

Sexuality issues for the health professional

Pregnancy and the transition to motherhood for most heterosexual women is both the consequence of having had a sexual relationship with a man, and an enactment of ascribed gender roles. It is a manifestation of their sexuality (Nicolson, 1990). However, it is important for health care professionals to remember that not all their clients will be heterosexual. According to a study of the health care experiences of self-identified lesbians, health care professionals usually assume that their female clients are heterosexual (Robertson, 1993). Other research has indicated that this is a major hindrance in effective therapeutic communication with health care providers (Garcia, 2003; Burns, 1992). In a meta-analysis of the research about lesbian health care Stevens (1993) states that: 'Lesbians believed that health care providers were generally condemnatory toward and ignorant about them … upon disclosure of their lesbian identity they experienced many kinds of mistreatment.'

Such findings and negative ramifications are serious issues that all health care providers must address (Cronin, 2004; Wilton, 1999). An increasing number of lesbian women are choosing to bear children (Kenney and Tash, 1993). There are different routes to pregnancy for lesbians but 'like any other path to parenthood, they are all emotionally intense' (Martin, 1993). Pregnancy can be a very isolating experience for lesbian women. It is often assumed that the pregnant lesbian woman is a single mother, which is a painful negation of her identity (Burns, 1992). This assumption marginalizes and negates the position of the lesbian who is supporting her partner and is going to co-parent. According to Burns (1992) 'she might well be placed in the position of the caring friend'. As with heterosexual couples, adjustment to the physical and psychological changes during pregnancy may require lesbian couples to adapt or modify their roles and relationship. Yet the lack of acknowledgement of the parental role of the non-biological parent is a poignant difference (Kenney and Tash, 1993). Maternity care professionals need to include the female partner during care provision and acknowledge the change in the life of the co-parent.

In order to provide appropriate assistance and support to lesbian childbearing couples it is important to affirm their values and relationship. Saffron (1999) makes some very sensitive and helpful suggestions about the kinds of things lesbians have said they either found helpful or would have been appreciated in the context of midwifery and maternity care. Such suggestions include the use of open questions with gender-neutral terms, such as 'Is there someone you would like to include in your antenatal care?' It is crucial to not only learn more about their maternity and health care concerns but also to avoid acting on the assumption that all women are heterosexual. Kenney and Tash (1993) comment that:

> Lesbians would like to be understood and accepted if they reveal their identity and not feel that they might be rejected and possibly mistreated. Health care providers who adopt an open, sensitive and non-judgemental attitude and are willing to listen to and respect lesbians as intelligent women with feelings will be sought out by this group.

The research that exists on sexuality and pregnancy and the relationship between maternity and sexuality is often confusing and contradictory. A lot of the work is anecdotal but one thing the studies all have in common is that they usually raise more questions than answers (Contratto, 1980). Many studies have documented the inadequacy of health care professionals in taking account of the sexuality of those in their care. There is also evidence of their reluctance to take an adequate sexual history (Belfield, 2004; Gribbin, 2003). These are important findings because childbearing is intimately bound up with a woman's sexuality and all midwives and other health care professionals must learn to address this issue if they aspire towards holistic care for their patients (Aston, 1994).

Midwives are the health professionals who are principally involved with women during the process of childbearing. Although Contratto (1980) argues that discussion of maternal sexuality makes virtually everyone anxious, Sedgwick's (1994) study of midwives challenges this view and reports that midwives felt sexual discussions with clients should be part of their normal role. The midwives also identified that it was important for them to have knowledge about the sexual aspects of the childbearing continuum. However, the majority of midwives found their training on sexual issues either inadequate or non-existent and that it had not prepared them for professional practice. Formal teaching on sexual matters to help their practice was seen as valuable by 91% of the midwives surveyed. Nevertheless, in spite of this most of the midwives did discuss sexual issues with their clients and attempted to meet the needs of women in this respect.

Sexual health problems and pregnancy

Various conditions are commonly associated with pregnancy. Although they may be perceived as 'minor ailments' they can be a source of considerable distress and adversely affect sexual health. To promote sexual health during pregnancy, sensitive approaches and questioning are essential in order to minimize any embarrassment.

In this discussion the more common conditions affecting pregnant women are included. The issues surrounding HIV infection in relation to pregnancy are manifold and are not explored in this chapter, but the scenario in Chapter 2, page 23 highlights some interesting questions. For more information see the book *HIV in Pregnancy and Childbirth* by Jane Kennedy (2003).

Physiological vaginal discharge

Physiological vaginal discharge is the result of secretions from Bartholin's and Skene's glands and from the endocervix. Epithelium shed from the vagina and lactobacilli, the latter maintaining an acidic vaginal environment to protect against infection, are also present. The vaginal micro-environment changes with age, mostly in response to alternations in oestrogen and progesterone. An increase in vaginal secretions has been reported in pregnancy and is known as leucorrhoea. The normal leucorrhoea of pregnancy is whitish to clear in colour and should not cause soreness, irritation or an offensive odour (Walton, 1994). During pregnancy, any woman with a discharge different from leucorrhoea needs to be referred to a doctor. In pregnancy the vaginal pH is 3.8–4.4. Symptoms relating to candidiasis (thrush) occur more frequently in pregnancy due to increased vaginal glucose and glycogen and also due to the changing hormonal balance.

Candidiasis (thrush)

Candida albicans is the usual cause of 'thrush'. It is the most common fungal species found in the vagina, where it often exists commensally. Candidiasis most frequently presents as a thick, white, curd-like discharge or sometimes as a watery vaginal discharge associated with vulval irritation and vaginal soreness. Dyspareunia is a common complaint (Roth, 1999). Hormonal influences appear to have an important role in its occurrence and pregnant women have been reported as having a higher incidence of asymptomatic colonization and symptomatic candidiasis (Woolley, 1994). Other predisposing factors have been identified and include diabetes, broad-spectrum antibiotic therapy which can reduce

commensal bacteria, especially lactobacilli, and immunosuppressive therapy (Woolley, 1994; Uthayakumar *et al.*, 1994). Women complaining of recurrent vulvovaginal candidiasis should have a thorough examination and be investigated for glucose intolerance and anaemia. Individuals with chronic mucotaneous candidiasis have been shown to have abnormal iron metabolism and low iron stores (Woolley, 1994). The woman's sexual partner should also be investigated as some men can get balanitis (Uthayakumar *et al.*, 1994).

Candida infection is characterized by severe vulval itching, which is often worse during the night. The infection can make a woman lose sleep and become exhausted and run down. On examination, the vulva and vagina appear inflamed. Although 'thrush' can be diagnosed on the basis of history alone, provided that the woman has a single stable partner, diagnosis is made on microscopy of wet preparations or Gram-staining of vaginal secretions (Uthayakumar *et al.*, 1994; Woolley, 1994). Treatment and self-help measures that the woman can use are discussed in Chapter 14.

The urinary system

In pregnancy there are changes in the physiological and functional anatomy of the urinary system. Pelvic organs are displaced and the relationship between the bladder and the uterus and vagina are subtly altered. The changes are caused by hormonal and endocrine factors, compression of the ureters by the gravid uterus and fetus, as well as circulatory changes. These changes can predispose pregnant women to urinary tract infections (Roth, 1999). As a result it is also common for pregnant women to have symptoms of urinary frequency and stress incontinence. Frequent nocturia can disrupt sleep patterns and affect fatigue levels and sense of well-being. Genuine stress incontinence is associated with pregnancy. The reported prevalence during pregnancy ranges from 23% to 67% and after childbirth from 6% to 31% (Mason *et al.*, 1999). Estimations of prevalence vary as a result of methodological differences among studies. Pelvic floor exercises have been shown to be effective if commenced within the third trimester of pregnancy and continued after childbirth. Ideally pelvic floor exercises should continue throughout life (see also page 495).

Urinary incontinence has significant social and psychological consequences and can have a profound effect on sexuality and sexual health (see Chapter 17). Genuine stress incontinence is associated with the leaking of urine during sexual intercourse, commonly on penetration (Kelleher *et al.*, 1993). During care planning and assessment, you will need to ask your client if she leaks urine during sexual intercourse so that you can offer appropriate treatment, support and interventions, such as pelvic floor exercises. Other important factors associated with urinary incontinence and sexual health are the reaction of the pregnant women and her partner, the embarrassment, and the effect on her libido and self-esteem. Results of an interview study of 42 women who experienced urinary stress incontinence up to one year after delivery (Mason *et al.*, 1999) identified that few women had sought advice or professional care for their symptoms. Restrictions placed on the women, the worry or continual awareness stemming from the condition, and feelings of embarrassment were the major concerns of the respondents. Some women indicated that they did not want their sexual partners to find out that they were incontinent and they were worried about leaking urine during sex. Dyspareunia secondary to urine dermatitis can also add to the distress of women suffering with urinary incontinence (Kelleher *et al.*, 1993).

Haemorrhoids

Haemorrhoids are varicose veins in and around the anus and are particularly common during pregnancy. They are often a joke subject to those who do not suffer from them and are not usually talked about in 'polite' company. Women with haemorrhoids may suffer in painful and embarrassed silence (Thompson, 1994) before seeking medical help. Haemorrhoids can develop during pregnancy because of venous dilatation and reduced peripheral resistance due to the hormonal influence of progesterone. Previous haemorrhoids, constipation and the woman's

weight may also be contributory factors. Haemorrhoids can worsen during the second stage of labour and can also be troublesome during the puerperium.

Rectal bleeding, itching and soreness around the anus, discomfort during defecation and a mucous discharge are signs and symptoms associated with haemorrhoids. Any woman with rectal bleeding should be referred to the doctor as it may be due to other conditions. During pregnancy, women need to be advised to take appropriate action to avoid constipation. A high-fibre diet and plenty of fluids is the best preventative action. Iron pills could be a cause of constipation. Relief may be obtained from ice cubes or ice packs or from special creams available over the counter. The discomfort and irritation of haemorrhoids may be eased by wearing loose, cotton underwear or applying a pad soaked in witch hazel.

Sexuality and pregnancy loss

Infertility

Infertility and infertility investigations can affect a sexual relationship. The need to take basal temperatures, time intercourse for the fertile period and undergo post-coital tests can be particularly disruptive (see Chapter 10). Levels of happiness and satisfaction within a sexual relationship may also vary during the various stages of infertility investigations. It has been suggested that couples with 'normal' sexual functioning prior to a diagnosis of subfertility may develop decreased coital frequency, orgasmic dysfunction or mid-cycle male impotence (Pepperell and McBain, 1985). However, there is also evidence that marital and sexual difficulties in couples undergoing infertility investigations may be relatively uncommon (Edelmann and Connolly, 1994). This finding needs to be interpreted with caution as it may be due to an element of self-selection among the client group. It may be that only couples with stable relationships get as far as seeking medical help in their efforts to conceive, and that those whose relationships are not so secure do not go so far as to seek infertility advice. Infertility may serve to improve a marital and sexual relationship by bringing a couple closer together, providing the problem is acknowledged by both partners as one that they share and which should be faced together (Edelmann and Connolly, 1994).

Miscarriage

Miscarriage is the commonest complication of pregnancy and affects 25% of all women who conceive a pregnancy. Recurrent miscarriage, defined as three or more consecutive losses of pregnancy, affects approximately 1% of all women (Clifford and Regan, 1994). The risk of a further miscarriage has been shown to increase after each successive pregnancy loss. This distressing problem can have a marked effect on sexual feelings and sexual relations. Barclay *et al.* (1994) identified that a previous miscarriage or episodes of bleeding intensified the fear of miscarriage during pregnancy. As a result, frequency of sexual intercourse and the variety of sexual activities that couples found acceptable was markedly reduced.

Fear of miscarriage can result in the pregnant woman perceiving sex as a direct threat to the baby. The partner may also feel that he poses a threat to the pregnancy (Orji *et al.*, 2002). Kitzinger (1985) points out that: 'any couple who feel like this interact negatively each triggering off further anxiety in the other'. However, there is little evidence to suggest that sexual intercourse and miscarriage are related in the absence of other problems (Kitzinger, 1985). Kitzinger states that 'no studies have been done to show whether not having sexual intercourse in early pregnancy helps to avoid miscarriage, though many people think this must be so'. Pregnant women are often advised by doctors to abstain from sexual intercourse if they have previously miscarried or threaten to do so in their current pregnancy. Bleeding in pregnancy is alarming and women therefore feel safer avoiding sexual intercourse (Sen and Esen, 2003; Savage and Reader, 1984). It is important to inform pregnant women when any suspected risk period is over, so that sexual intercourse can resume. Lack of communication of this fact can result in the woman feeling guilty if she does have sexual intercourse without 'medical permission'.

Fear of miscarriage may result in the couple abstaining from sexual activity throughout pregnancy, 'assuming that a ban on intercourse means a ban on all sexual activity' (Kitzinger, 1985). Again, it will be helpful to advise women of other ways of enjoying sex without having penetrative sex.

It is important for health care professionals to be acutely sensitive to the feelings evoked by miscarriage in a subsequent pregnancy. Barclay *et al.* (1994) highlighted the deep-rooted fear that couples felt in the context of their sexual relationship. In an editorial comment on the study, Black (1994) makes the point:

> Despite having assured some couples that sexual activity would be all right in this pregnancy, no amount of convincing may alter the contrary opinion of either or both partners, where there has been a previous pregnancy loss or episode of bleeding. One can only reassure such couples that if they experienced a genuinely satisfying sexual relationship beforehand, that it will return once this baby arrives safely.

Bereavement

Research on sexuality and sexual intercourse following perinatal death has largely been neglected. The difficulties of re-establishing a loving, sexual relationship following the death of a baby comes mainly from primary sources, namely mothers' personal anecdotes and experiences (Mander, 1994). Mander draws attention to the fact that enjoyment of human contact, even that quite independent of lovemaking, may be too much to ask of a grieving patient. There is evidence to suggest that following the death of a baby sexual intercourse may not be resumed until the couple are planning another pregnancy. Mander (1994) suggests that: 'Differing patterns and rates of grieving may compound this difficulty because one partner is unable to respond to the other's tentative advances.'

Other factors also have a bearing on sexual intercourse during the process of grieving. Sexual intercourse may seem as a reminder of the birth and also of the death. Borg and Lasker (1982) suggested that the pleasure of making love may be regarded as inappropriate. This may be due to 'previous memories of lovemaking which began their baby's brief existence being a carefree and joyful time' (Mander, 1994). Couples may regret their inability to give each other intimate and loving support at this difficult time. However, the removal of anxieties about performance and conception may be a relief for some couples (Borg and Lasker, 1982). Another important aspect to be considered which could impact on sexuality is depression. A study of women whose previous pregnancy ended in stillbirth reported higher levels of depression and state anxiety than matched controls during the next pregnancy and at one year postnatal (Hughes *et al.*, 1999). Women who had conceived within 12 months after loss were more vulnerable than women with longer time since loss.

Childbirth and sexuality

Women approach labour and childbirth with a mixture of emotions ranging from happiness and excitement about their new baby to apprehension and fear. These anxieties can cover many aspects of childbirth.

◆ Will I be alright in hospital amongst strangers?

◆ Will I be able to cope with the pain?

◆ Will I be able to remain within my birth plan?

◆ Will my new baby be normal?

◆ How will my other children left at home cope?

If there is a positive outcome to all these anxieties then a woman will often feel the whole experience of childbirth has been an enriching fulfilment of her hopes. Her relationship with her partner will be enhanced and this can facilitate attachment to her new baby.

Although labour and birth are often associated with pain and anxiety, the experiences and feelings evoked are also closely linked to sexuality and sexual health. Kitzinger (1985) described the experience of birth for some women as:

the most intensely sexual feeling a woman ever experiences, as strong as orgasm, even more compelling than orgasm. Some women find it

disturbing because it is sexual and they feel out of control as the energy floods through them and they can do nothing to prevent it.

Drawing on her personal experiences, Southern (1994) also addresses the links between the process of childbearing and sexuality:

Even if labour does not directly evoke sexual feeling in the woman, the process of childbearing must surely indirectly evoke sex. How are babies conceived? And how are they born? The reproductive organs are sexual organs and I do not believe that women can expose themselves and open up to give birth without making this connection.

Given that childbirth and sexuality are related, as well as the many personal experiences and dimensions encompassed under the term sexual health, this discussion will only focus on just some of the issues associated with women and sexual health during labour and childbirth.

Childbirth following sexual abuse

Sexual abuse is covered more fully in Chapters 5 and 6 but some issues that are relevant to childbirth are discussed in this section.

One of the most consistent findings to emerge from recent work has been clear evidence of the significance of childbirth in evoking personal sexual experiences (Barlow and Birch, 2004). As Southern (1994) points out: 'Some women's experiences of sex will have been invasive and traumatic as a result of rape, incest or some other sexual abuse'. In assessing this important and often neglected area of women's lives, Kitzinger's (1992) study of 39 women survivors of childhood sexual abuse draws attention to the kinds of feelings and vulnerability stirred up during childbirth. Kitzinger reported that over half of the respondents were reminded of their experiences of sexual assault by internal examinations, cervical smears, dental examinations, but of particular significance was the process of childbirth. Women explained that they had felt 'lack of control over their own bodies', 'helpless in the hands of another person', 'depersonalized' and other similar feelings during childbirth. Such feelings had reminded them of the feelings and indignities associated with the abuse all over again.

Kitzinger's analysis also acknowledged that childbirth may be a significant experience because of extra-medical factors:

> Pregnancy and giving birth involve feelings about one's body – how it looks and feels and whether it is 'good' enough. Women often feel that their body has been deformed or ruined by abuse, or that it betrayed them by attracting the abuser or sexually responding to his touch. Childbirth may either confirm or challenge these perceptions.

It is not only women who have been sexually abused who may find childbirth experiences traumatic and distressing. Other such women are those who have previously undergone invasive obstetric or gynaecological procedures (RCOG, 1997; Clement, 1994). Vaginal examinations have also been identified as difficult for women with a history of miscarriages, terminations and stillbirths.

So it is important that midwives and other health professionals create an environment during pregnancy and labour that facilitates optimal conditions and the potential for a more satisfying experience for all women (Hall, 2002). Care givers will often not know of a previous experience of sexual abuse, and without individualized care and continuity of carer 'women are unlikely to disclose experiences of abuse. Even in optimal conditions, some women will choose not to share this information' (Clement, 1994).

A common thread that runs through the literature is that midwives, doctors and health professionals should ensure that the care they offer 'counteracts rather than reenacts the violation of women's bodies' (Kitzinger, 1992):

> Childbirth can be an opportunity for women to relate to their bodies in new ways, to experience them as powerful, competent and creative. Some women whom I interviewed spoke positively of the care with which midwives, doctors, and nurses responded to their needs. A gentle examination, a listening ear, and a respectful approach can all help women to overcome alienation from their bodies. Sensitivity on the part of the staff who understood and validated their distress, provided information, and offered practical support was vital in helping women through such experiences.

Female genital mutilation and pregnancy

Female genital mutilation damages the health of women, and because it interferes with their sexuality it is a sexual health issue (see also pages 134 and 368). During labour and childbirth great sensitivity as well as cultural awareness is important, in order to give appropriate care and psychological support for women who have undergone any form of female genital mutilation, especially infibulation. Omer-Hashi (1994) suggests that all infibulated women should be expected to have fears about labour and birth complications. Specialist antenatal clinic services have found that assessment prior to labour of whether problems are likely to occur during childbirth have made a significant contribution to the health and emotional well-being of women during labour and delivery. The provision of information and counselling on de-infibulation for women and their partners during pregnancy has been a crucial part of this maternity care provision (McCaffrey, 1995).

There is a dearth of research literature available on the sexual and psychological effects of severe forms of genital mutilation when compared to studies and case reports on the physical complications during childbirth. Dyspareunia and lack of satisfaction from sexual intercourse are frequently reported in the available literature (for an excellent analysis of sexuality, studies on marital sex, and discourse on the clitoris, see Boddy, 1998). A syndrome of chronic anxiety and depression 'arising from worry over the state of their genitals' and other sexual health issues has been observed in many infibulated women (Toubia, 1994). When performing an examination during labour on any woman who has been mutilated, it is important that health care professionals 'should control their facial expression and shock at her distorted genitalia so as not to hurt her self esteem' (Omer-Hashi, 1994).

Vaginal examinations and other interventional procedures (such as applying fetal scalp electrodes, performing fetal blood sampling) can be difficult, painful or impossible in some cases. A normal birth may also not be possible. However, there is evidence to suggest that 'where physicians are not trained to deal with infibulated women unnecessary caesarean section which can be avoided with a simple de-infibulation performed with the woman under a local anaesthesia' is causing increasing concern (Toubia, 1994).

It is important that midwives and other health professionals are knowledgeable and comfortable about female genital mutilation, its variations and potential complications (Royal College of Midwives, 1998; London Black Women's Health Action Project, 1999). During labour and childbirth may not be the optimal time to establish whether or not a woman has been infibulated.

The *Policy on Female Genital Mutilation* (1999) by the London Black Women's Health Action Project suggests that the provision of NHS services for reversal of female circumcision is only on an *ad hoc* basis. It also reports that women are hampered from seeking medical help because of their language problems, feelings of shame, fear of being ridiculed and ignorance about the availability of services.

Although de-infibulation can be performed during pregnancy or labour, early deinfibulation is associated with decreased pain during labour and a shorter period of postpartum recovery (Omer-Hashi, 1994).

Men and birth

The effects of the presence of men during childbirth and the implications for sexual relationships in the short and long term are contentious issues. Michel Odent proposes that the father's presence at the birth has long-term implications for sexual attraction 'which needs mystery' (Boseley, 2000). Shannon (1993) argues that although 90% of births are now attended by fathers 'in the midst of all the superlatives, some local difficulties are beginning to emerge'. These include pressure, guilt, trauma, fears and 'damage to the relationship between the mother and father'. Although a survey of 441 men who were present at birth identified that women were the biggest influence on the decision to be present during childbirth (86%), the majority (93%) of men said they wanted to be there. The experience was described as 'wonderful' by 64%;

29% described feeling of being 'scared', whilst only 9% admitted to being 'upset' by events that occurred in the delivery room (Royal College of Midwives, 1994).

There is little documented information and research in professional literature about the short- and long-term effects for both partners and their sexual relationship after a shared birth experience. However, O'Driscoll (1994) draws attention to psychosexual problems that could be traced back to men witnessing birth. Hall (1993) also points out that:

> No one should deny that childbirth is painful, and to watch someone you love in excruciating pain and be unable to do anything about it may have a devastating effect on a man. If the birth becomes complicated, as with forceps delivery, men have been known to become totally switched off sexually and need counselling for many months through fear of putting his partner (and himself) through the experience again.

Lewis (1999) described a father who was refusing to have sex with his partner 12 months after delivery because he could not bear the possibility of her going through another birth experience.

 SCENARIO

Tanya had a normal vaginal delivery of her first baby three weeks previously. When the midwife visited her at home she seemed worried, and told the midwife that because her husband had been at the birth and had witnessed her pain and distress during labour she was anxious about whether his feelings towards her would change. She talked about whether he would still find her attractive and she feared that his witnessing the birth could have an effect on their sex life. The midwife validated Tanya's concerns and gave her the opportunity to discuss the potential impact of having a new baby on their relationship. During the discussion that followed, the midwife gave Tanya information on sexual intercourse following delivery and advised her that it would probably be helpful if Tanya and her husband could talk openly about any fears, anxieties and concerns that they both had about sex. The midwife reflected upon the interaction with Tanya and recognized that her concerns are fairly common and should have been anticipated.

The issues are complex and there are no clear answers. Yet the implications and significance for sexual relationships and sexual health must be taken into account by midwives and health professionals. Individual couples should be encouraged to discuss their fears and feelings about what is right for them as individuals, as well as what is right for them as a couple and their relationship, during labour and childbirth. O'Driscoll (1994) suggests that as: 'being present at the birth may cause long-lasting harm to the relationship men should not be coerced into staying'. She also highlights the importance of the recognition of the needs of individual men and women. She suggests that 'sexual matters with both partners should be discussed openly at preparation classes and during postnatal care' with both partners. About this last point O'Driscoll comments that: 'midwives should educate both partners about the anatomy of the vagina and its marvellous ability to stretch and return to normal size'.

In a positive vein, there is evidence to suggest that the father's presence during delivery can be beneficial and that his presence adds to the enjoyment of birth for both parents, as well as strengthening the relationship between them (Lewis, 1999; Clulow, 1982). Labour and childbirth are events of pivotal significance for both partners and their psychosexual life, and should be openly discussed.

Postnatal sexuality

Studies of the sexual behaviour and sexual health of women after childbirth have indicated that they are influenced by profound psychological, interpersonal, social and biological variables (Morof et al., 2003; Stewart-Moore, 2000; Corkhill, 1996; Demyttenaere et al., 1995). Research suggests that there are four main factors that appear to have a detrimental impact on sexuality during the first 12 weeks following delivery:

◆ Postnatal depression
◆ Maternal fatigue
◆ Dyspareunia
◆ Breastfeeding.

Aspects of these will be raised in this discussion. Once again there is evidence that midwives and other health professionals often fail to address adequately sexuality and sexual relations following childbirth. Studies have shown that only 25% of men received information about resuming sexual relations following childbirth (Royal College of Midwives, 1994). Another study found that although most women had been given advice about contraception after the birth (75%), only a few (24%) had the opportunity to talk about sex after childbirth during the pregnancy. Women also reported that following childbirth they had been left to deal with changes and potential problems in their sexual relations on their own without support (National Childbirth Trust, 1994).

Studies of when women resume sexual intercourse following childbirth show that this varies a great deal (Alder, 1994). The majority of women appear to resume sexual intercourse by 8 weeks postpartum. In a longitudinal study of the sexual behaviour of postnatal women the median time to restarting sexual intercourse and contraception was 6 weeks (Glazener, 1997). Women who reported perineal pain, depression or tiredness experienced problems related to sexual intercourse more often than those who did not. During the first couple of months after delivery, breastfeeding was associated with less interest in intercourse. Although many women reported problems with intercourse, the number who expressed the need for help or advice was small (7–13%). Glazener suggests that health professionals should be aware of the high prevalence of postnatal sexual problems, prepare women before birth, have a high index of suspicion postnatally and be responsive to any problems that might occur (Glazener, 1997).

The study by Robson et al. (1981) also found that about a third had resumed intercourse by 6 weeks after delivery and nearly all had done so by 12 weeks after delivery. However, many women were having intercourse less frequently at 12 weeks (77%) and 1 year after delivery (57%) compared to before they became pregnant. This study concludes that, overall, childbearing diminishes sexual activity and enjoyment for at least a year after delivery. Another study, which provides new data on the postnatal sexual health of 484 primiparous women, will give little comfort to women. Reports on male perspectives of postnatal sexual health are still awaited. The study by Barrett *et al.* (2000) showed that over 80% of women experienced at least one postnatal sexual problem in the first 3 months after birth, and two-thirds were still experiencing problems at 6 months. Dyspareunia, vaginal dryness and loss of libido were very common. Only a minority of the respondents reported receiving information about sexual health from maternity and health care professionals. Rates of consultation for problems with sexual intercourse were low.

However, positive aspects of sexual activity after childbirth have been reported as many women have described feeling that whatever time they chose to resume sex was the right time for them. Others have reported improvement in their sex lives and relationships following delivery: 'My sexuality has blossomed with motherhood, my erotic responses have been enhanced not damaged' (Miller, 1995). Some of the reasons that have been offered are:

◆ Feeling less inhibited
◆ Being more relaxed
◆ Having a better body image.

In addition, women have also commented that sex may be less frequent but of better quality. This was summed up by one respondent as 'Quantity down – quality up' (National Childbirth Trust, 1994).

Several authors have reported that women are anxious about their bodies in the early weeks and months following childbirth. Studies have consistently reported that body image is closely linked with sexual attractiveness, and after childbirth women have said that they felt pressure from their sexual partners to regain their figures and to be slender, in order to maintain their sexual relationship (Grogan, 1999). Having a 'flabby belly' and 'droopy breasts' have been identified as specific causes of dissatisfaction (Grogan, 1999). Other causes of anxiety often attributed by respondents are perineal pain and soreness,

as well as a decreased sense of attractiveness (Reamy and White, 1987).

The physical demands made by a new baby and the stress of new parental roles, responsibilities and fatigue place particular demands on the emotional reserves of women (*Prima Baby Magazine*, 2002; Felstein, 1998; Tobert, 1990) creating anxiety and frustration in a couple. Nicolson (1990) in her study of the experiences of women in the transition to motherhood reported that a reduction in intimacy and quality of adult couple relationships was exacerbated by men's perceived secondary role in childcare and their lack of understanding of their partner's daily routine combined with her increased investment in the mothering role. Tiredness can compromise the coping ability of a new mother and affect her libido. The impact of tiredness on the sexual responses of women during pregnancy and postpartum should not be underestimated. It is clear from the findings of a recent study that fatigue had a profound impact on libido and measures of sexuality during pregnancy and at 12 weeks and 6 months postpartum (De Judicibus and McCabe, 2002).

For our purposes, these findings are important because the birth of a baby may herald a time of discord, relationship problems and sexual dissatisfaction (von Sydow, 2002; Reamy and White, 1987). Moreover, it has been found that sexual and marital therapists often report that their clients say that their sexual problems first became apparent at the time of the birth of their first child (Alder, 1994). A recent study of couples completing their first or second pregnancy reported a reduction in the number of episodes of sexual activity 8 months after the birth of their baby (Dixon *et al.*, 2000). Around 50% of first-time parents described their sex life as 'poor' or 'not very good', and 17% said they wanted help with their sexual problems. Primiparae most commonly complained of lack of libido and tiredness. For multiparae, tiredness appeared to be a more significant factor than lack of libido, and 7.5% of second-time parents said they would like help with sexual problems. It could be argued that if there was greater understanding and more realistic expectations of the demands and what is involved in becoming a parent, some of these problems could be avoided. Although Alder (1994) states that:

> When there is important change in role and accompanying physical demands it is not surprising that there may be communication problems. If the male partner feels unable to express his feelings about the baby and partner's changing role and the woman is too tired and anxious about the baby to give him attention, there is ample opportunity for failure of communication.

Whilst these factors may have some relation to, and impact on sexual health and the relationship between the woman and her partner following childbirth, they are not the whole story. There is also a gender issue and Van Wert (1991) reminds us that all too often the way the 'problem' of changed sexual relations after childbirth between partners is constructed, is that it is the woman's 'problem and fault':

> To hear couples tell the tale, the halt in sexual relations is usually the woman's fault. Men say they are ready, they have always been ready, but the women have changed, feel too tired or ugly, won't tolerate the barest of touches, or reject them outright. Women blame themselves as well, having succumbed to culturally instilled guilt for failing to fit the role models shown in books, movies and mass advertising.

It is clear that social and contextual factors influence the dynamics of interpersonal relationships and the sex life of a woman after having a baby (Walton, 1994). However, there are also physical causes that may affect libido and sexual health following childbirth.

Following childbirth the resumption of intercourse and sexual activities needs to be discussed with the woman and couple. In 1998 the deaths from air embolism during sexual intercourse of two women, both in their twenties and both within 8 days following a spontaneous vaginal delivery of their third and fourth child respectively, were reported in the medical press and the media (Batman *et al.*, 1998; Boseley, 1998). One couple had used the missionary position for sex and the other pair had used rear entry

(knee-chest) position. In the case of the latter, the postmortem showed the woman had taken amphetamines (Batman *et al.*, 1998). The authors of the medical report concluded that, 'whilst cases of fatal air embolism during the puerperium are rare, we feel it would be wise to warn mothers, without causing undue alarm, that intercourse could be dangerous in the early days of the puerperium' (Batman *et al.*, 1998). Not surprisingly, these remarks left maternity care professionals rather anxious and concerned about potential risks and what advice they should give to parents, as they underscored previous views that couples are best advised to resume intercourse as and when they feel is appropriate for them.

Following an analysis of the literature on air embolism caused by intercourse and sexual activities in the puerperium (and pregnancy), Robinson (1998) notes that what maternity and health care professionals could say to couples is that, although death is rare, 'they should wait until bleeding stops, and in any case should avoid deliberately blowing air into the vagina and avoid using a knee-chest position for any activity (including sex) in the early days. It could also be that what a couple did safely after the birth of their first may be less safe after the third or fourth'.

It is important to determine what knowledge and concerns the woman and her partner have about their sexual relationship. Evans (1992) suggests that:

> By establishing what knowledge the couple already have the midwife will then be able to use this as a basis for further education, to prepare parents for the physical and emotional reactions they may encounter when resuming sexual intercourse and to enable them to respond appropriately to problems.

However, midwives and other health professionals need to initiate the giving of such information as women may be reluctant to ask. Robson *et al.* (1981) found that many women did not mention sexual difficulties to their general practitioners or obstetricians during pregnancy and at three months after delivery 30% of the women respondents said that they would have liked sexual counselling and would have found it beneficial.

A discussion of the normality of fluctuations of sexual interest and enjoyment following childbirth is a crucial part of professional care planning.

> Alternative coital positions and non-coital options for the intimate expression of affection and mutual pleasure can do much to enrich the quality of the pregnancy, the birth experience, and the marital and family bond.
>
> (Reamy and White, 1987)

Several factors contribute to sexual health following childbirth. McConville (1994) argues that following childbirth: 'Women are certainly under pressure to get back to "normal" (i.e. "sexual") as soon as possible after birth'. However, sexual relations and sexual activity after childbirth cannot be isolated from the psychological and sociological adjustments that are required by the woman and her partner. The effect of fatigue, as a result of coping with the demands of a new baby, on libido and sexual activity should not be underestimated. Riley (1989) reports that reduced sexual desire, resulting in lowered frequency of sexual intercourse, is not uncommon following childbirth. This can result in disharmony in the relationship, which may further inhibit the resumption of satisfactory and mutually satisfying sexual activity. The common causes of concern that have been reported over the resumption of sexual intercourse include the risk of damage to a healing episiotomy scar, damage to internal organs and the abdominal wound following caesarean section, as well as the risk of infection. Riley (1989) suggests that: 'Perhaps some of the sexual and emotional problems encountered in the postnatal woman can be prevented by adequate preparation'.

Postnatal women and their partners need to know what to expect when resuming sexual intercourse and how any discomfort can be prevented. They also need advice on contraception during the puerperium and safer sex. Health professionals also need to inform women and their partners what *not* to expect, e.g. excessive pain, persistent lack of desire, so that they will know what is abnormal and when to seek help.

Box 8.3 Common causes of postnatal dyspareunia (Lee, 1994)

◆ Decreased vaginal lubrication which may be associated with breastfeeding or with decreased sexual arousal

◆ Inflammation and infection, e.g. granuloma, Bartholin's abscess

◆ Sensitive hymenal tags/skin tags following malalignment of perineal repair

◆ Contracture/scarring of the perineum

◆ Vaginismus due to expectation of pain with intercourse.

Postnatal dyspareunia

Health professionals need to ask women about painful intercourse as it appears that postnatal superficial dyspareunia is not uncommon. Postnatal superficial dyspareunia has been defined as painful sexual intercourse following childbirth, excluding those women who have experienced persistent dyspareunia in their nulliparous state and/or have dyspareunia of a known psychosexual origin (Lee, 1994). The common causes are listed in Box 8.3.

Potential sources of discomfort should be identified, e.g. an episiotomy incision or caesarean section wound. Signorello *et al.* (2001) found that women whose babies were delivered over an intact perineum reported better outcomes in terms of the frequency and severity of postpartum dyspareunia compared to women who had been delivered by obstetric instrumentation. Although little research has been published on caesarean section and postnatal sexual health, a recent review of what evidence there is, revealed that contrary to popular opinion women who undergo caesarean section can experience postnatal sexual problems (Barrett and McCandlish, 2002). These authors concluded that whilst women with caesarean section may experience fewer sexual problems than those women with vaginal births in the short term, there appears to be very little difference by six months post delivery.

Advice on coital positions such as side-to-side and female superior positions which minimize episiotomy soreness may be helpful. Gentle insertion of a clean finger into the vagina and massage may help promote relaxation as well as enable women to check the healing process and any residual soreness. Gels for vaginal lubrication, especially for women who are breastfeeding, may be helpful, if there is vaginal dryness. Information regarding pelvic floor exercises may be beneficial, as such exercises increase cognitive awareness of vaginal sensation and tension, promote healing, strengthen the muscles and improve vaginal tone (Reamy and White, 1987). Increasing age and parity are associated with progressive denervation of the pelvic floor muscle and consequently stress incontinence and prolapse. To some degree 80% of mothers are affected and one study showed that perineal squeeze pressure had not returned to normal at 8 weeks post-delivery (Smith cited in Lee, 1994). A need for the correct teaching and subsequent review of pelvic floor exercises has been identified (Lee, 1994).

Although this distressing condition progressively resolves for most women, a significant group are left with a persistent problem. Health professionals need to include the topic in parenthood and health education programmes. Myths surrounding birth may need to be dispelled to make accurate information available. It is important to listen, advise and support women and to know when to refer them for further counselling or advice.

Postnatal depression

Psychiatrists argue that postnatal depression is affected by environmental and social factors, but endocrinologists postulate that ovarian hormones may be responsible for the occurrence of depressive illness in women at times of profound hormonal change, e.g. after pregnancy, premenstrually and during the climacteric. Studd (1992) suggests that these three depressive disorders constitute a triad of oestrogen-responsive psychiatric pathology.

Postnatal depression affects 1 in 10 women in the first year following childbirth. The condition usually begins in the first few weeks following delivery and can last for weeks, months or for more than a year (Biggerstaff, 1999). Postnatal depression is often a silent and hidden disorder and the condition is frequently overlooked by health professionals. According to Pitt (1991) the symptoms include: 'anxiety, irritability, fatigue, and a demoralizing sense of failure to cope with consequent feelings of guilt and reduced confidence and self esteem'.

Another key feature of postnatal depression is loss of libido which may put further strain on a relationship. Pitt (1991) states that: 'There is usually little interest in sex which may further strain a marriage already overcast by the new mother's troubled preoccupation and apparent lack of responsiveness'. Demyttenaere *et al.* (1995) also suggest that loss of sexual interest may be a sign of postnatal depression. Recent research has shown that sexual health problems are common after childbirth in both depressed and non-depressed women (Morof *et al.*, 2003). However, these researchers reported that depressed women are less likely to have resumed sexual intercourse at 6 months. This finding is in line with other studies: for example, De Judicibus and Mccabe (2002) found that depression was an important predictor of reduced sexual desire during pregnancy, and of reduced frequency of intercourse at 12 weeks postpartum.

One study has reported that fathers are more likely to have postnatal depression at both 6 weeks and 6 months postpartum if their partners also suffer from postnatal depression (Ballard *et al.*, 1994). Other studies have shown a link between the maternity 'blues' and postnatal depression. The blues have been described as transient episodes of low mood which typically occur around the fourth or fifth day after childbirth. They occur in at least 50% of mothers and normally lift within 1 or 2 days. The blues, however, can be severe and may merge into postnatal depression.

In order to support the woman and her partner health professionals must recognize and be able to deal with postnatal depression. This is an important part of our role as the onset of postnatal depression can be insidious and many women are not aware of what is wrong with them. It may be difficult for women to admit how miserable they are feeling due to embarrassment or feelings of guilt. Jebali (1993) suggests that: 'Guilt is very common among new mothers

Box 8.4 Postnatal depression and puerperal psychosis

The Scottish Intercollegiate Guidelines Network (2002) have published an evidence-based guideline on diagnosis, screening and prevention of postnatal depression and puerperal psychosis. Website address: www.sign.ac.uk/guidelines/fulltext/60/section2.html.

◆ All women should be routinely assessed during the antenatal period for a history of depression
◆ Postnatal depression should be treated
◆ Psychosocial interventions should be considered when deciding on treatment options
◆ Puerperal psychosis should be managed in the same way as other psychotic disorders, but with consideration given to drug therapy regarding breastfeeding and in pregnancy
◆ Medication should be at the lowest possible dose for the shortest period necessary.

and is usually internalized; the woman may eventually convince herself that she is a bad mother and therefore a bad person'. According to Jebali, it is also not culturally acceptable to admit to feeling unhappy as a new mother.

As a health professional you need to ask women how they really feel, and also ask them whether they have felt depressed during the first few weeks following childbirth. The Edinburgh Postnatal Depression Scale (EPDS) has been found to be a valuable screening test. Further information on the utilization of the EPDS and postnatal depression is given in Box 8.4. Treatment with antidepressants may be helpful, but more important is ensuring that the woman has sustained regular support and counselling. Pitt (1991) asserts that: 'The most important step in the provision of support is ensuring involvement of the husband, family, and if the patient agrees, friends'.

Women with severe postnatal depression have been helped with high-dose oestrogen replacement therapy and it has been shown that such therapy significantly reduces depression scores and accelerates recovery (Gregoire *et al.*, 1996).

Midwives, health visitors and general practitioners as well as other health professionals are ideally placed to recognize the onset of depression in new mothers. They are also in the unique position to initiate whatever help, support and therapy is considered appropriate.

Breastfeeding and sexuality

It has been suggested that in 'contrast to the close association between "breasts and sex", "breastfeeding and sex" are not supposed to go together ... they are cultural chalk and cheese' (McConville, 1994). Breastfeeding women and their sexual partners may lose the desire for sex whilst others may find that breastfeeding has the effect of enhancing sex. Breastfeeding women may feel particularly fatigued and exhausted, 'which is never good for sex' (McConville, 1994; Stewart-Moore, 2000). McConville comments that this can be distressing, usually for the male partner, and engender resentment, especially if the couple have had no prior warning that this may occur. Given this background, it is surprising to find that 'men are rarely considered when breastfeeding issues are discussed' (Jackson, 2000). This indicates the need for more discussion on sexuality and men's attitudes to breastfeeding. As Alder (1994) stated:

> Some sexual partners may find breastfeeding by their partners arousing, others will be indifferent, and a few will find it offensive. Most women enjoy the pleasurable sensation of a baby suckling but some women may feel guilty. Their partners may resent it, either because they regard the women's breasts as their property, or because breastfeeding is an activity which they cannot share.

The physiological mechanisms and the psychological experiences associated with breastfeeding can reduce sexual interest and arousal. Breast tenderness and fear of milk leakage is associated with sexual inhibitions in lactating women and may reduce sexual desire in their partners (Hames cited in Alder, 1994). Painful intercourse, which may be related to low oestrogen levels, is more common in women who exclusively breastfeed when compared to women who bottle-feed their babies (Alder, 1994). Lactational atrophic vaginitis (a condition typically associated with the hypoestrogenic state of menopause) has recently been identified as an under-reported and under-researched phenomenon in breastfeeding women (Palmer and Likis, 2003). Symptoms include discomfort with urination, vaginal itching and dryness, and dyspareunia. Sexual arousal which can accompany breastfeeding may engender feelings of guilt and anxiety in the woman. McConville (1994) argues that 'a deep and meaningful silence about the sensual or sexual pleasure which can accompany breastfeeding' pervades.

Explanations about factors that may influence sexuality and breastfeeding need to be offered. There are myths such as, 'you cannot get pregnant whilst breastfeeding and if you have not started your periods' which may need to be dispelled. Maternity and health care professionals need to discuss the efficacy of lactational amenorrhoea and other methods of contraception with breastfeeding women (see page 294). Sexual activity and sexual intercourse may be a low priority during breastfeeding. However, for some couples, breastfeeding is 'a time to enjoy breasts and a woman's sexuality in a deeper way than ever before' (McConville, 1994).

Conclusion

Sexuality and sexual health during pregnancy, childbirth and the postnatal period is affected by many different variables and contexts. For example, love, gentleness, kissing, passion, body freedom, freedom from fear, lack of coercion, communication, emotional involvement, manual skills and cooperative contraception have all been identified as important aspects of women's sexuality (von Sydow, 2002; Tiefer, 1995). Health professionals must take into account when planning care the needs and personal experiences of the individual woman and her partner.

In this chapter there is a clear demonstration of the need for health professionals to address their own attitudes, knowledge and skills about and towards sexuality and the childbearing continuum, in order to provide holistic care (Glazener, 1997; O'Driscoll, 1998; Curtis and Dunn, 1996). The relationship between women's sexual health and body image, especially during pregnancy and after childbirth, is an important aspect of assessment and care planning.

An increasing number of studies are highlighting the impact that fatigue and depression can have on relationships and the sexual health of women. Health care professionals should explore the influences of changes that occur during and after pregnancy. Their role is to prepare couples for change and to help them survive the changes that having a baby brings. Women and their partners need information about the normality of the fluctuations of sexual interest and enjoyment

Ideas for personal and professional development

- Explore the leaflets and written information about sexuality during and after pregnancy that are in your practice area: are there any gaps? Are they up to date? In what languages are they available?

- Research which sources of information about sex during pregnancy, women have said they have used

- Find out if women have a six-week 'postnatal check' after the birth of their babies, and identify information that is needed regarding contraception, sexuality and sexual relations

- Reflect upon whether you are able to talk about and involve men/fathers/partners in discussions about pregnancy and sexuality.

Patient education points

- Pregnancy and having a baby can have a positive impact on sexual health and well-being for both partners in the relationship

- There is no normal pattern of sexual behaviour during and after pregnancy but adaptation and change in sexual relations is common and should probably be expected

- The meaning of body image and the possible effect on sexual activity should be explored from a woman-centred perspective

- Women need to know what to expect and what not to expect regarding fatigue and postnatal depression. Most importantly they need to know where to get support and help.

during pregnancy and following childbirth. It is possible to build up a gloomy picture of sexuality in relation to the childbearing continuum; however, for many women childbirth enhances and intensifies their sexual pleasure. Health care professionals are in the unique position to care for the sexual health of women during pregnancy, childbirth and family beginnings, which should be a positive experience for all those most intimately involved.

Resources

Action on Puerperal Psychosis
Queen Elizabeth Psychiatric Hospital,
    Birmingham B15 2QZ
Tel: 0121 678 2361
www.bham.ac.uk/app

Association for Post-Natal Illness (APNI)
145 Dawes Road, Fulham,
    London SW6 7EB
Tel: 020 7386 0868
www.apni.org

La Leche League of Great Britain
PO Box 29, West Bridgford, Nottingham
    NG2 7NP
Tel: 0845 120 2918
www.laleche.org.uk

National Childbirth Trust
Alexandra House, Oldham Terrace, Acton,
    London W3 6NH
Tel: 0870 770 3236
www.nctpregnancyandbabycare.com

Women's Aid Federation of England
PO Box 391, Bristol BS99 7WS
Tel: 0177 944 4411(administration)
www.womensaid.org.uk
Women's Aid National Helpline: Tel: Freephone
    – 24 Hour National Domestic Violence
    Helpline: 0808 2000 247

Further reading

ALTENEDER, R.R. and HARTZELL, D. (1997) Addressing couples' sexuality concerns during the childbearing period: use of the PLISSIT model. *Journal of Obstetric, Gynecologic, and Neonatal Nursing* 26(6):651–8.

BARTELLAS, E., CRANE, J.M., DALEY, M., BENNETT, K.A and HUTCHENS, D. (2000) Sexuality and sexual activity in pregnancy. *BJOG: An International Journal of Obstetrics and Gynaecology* 107(8):964–8.
CARROLL, N.M. (2000) Providing gynecological and obstetric care for lesbians. *Contemporary Reviews in Obstetrics and Gynecology* 12(1):75–9.
DAVIS, E. (2002) Sex after the baby comes. *Midwifery Today–International Midwife* 62:11–14.
KENNEDY J. (2003) *HIV in Pregnancy and Childbirth* London: Elsevier Science.
LEROY, M. (1994) *Pleasure: The Truth About Female Sexuality*. London: Harper Collins.
MILLER, J. (1983) *Happy As A Dead Cat*. London: Women's Press.
NICOLSON, P. and USSHER, J. (eds) (1992) *The Psychology of Women's Health and Health Care*. London: Macmillan.
TIEFER, L. (1995) *Sex Is Not a Natural Act and Other Essays*. Oxford: Westview Press.
TIRAN, D. (2000) *Clinical Aromatherapy for Pregnancy and Childbirth*. Edinburgh: Churchill Livingstone.
TIRAN, D. and MACK, S. (eds) (2000) *Complementary Therapies for Pregnancy and Childbirth*, 2nd edn. London: Baillière Tindall.

References

ALDER, B. (1994) Postnatal sexuality. In Choi, P.Y.L. and Nicolson, P. (eds) *Female Sexuality, Psychology, Biology and Social Context*. Hemel Hempstead: Harvester Wheatsheaf.
ANDERSEN, L.F. and FUCHS, F. (1993) Sexual activity and preterm birth. In Fuchs, A.R., Fuchs, F. and Stubblefield, P.G. (eds) *Preterm Birth: Causes, Prevention and Management*, 2nd edn. New York: McGraw-Hill, pp. 161–72.
ASTON, G. (1994) The construction of pregnant women and HIV. Paper presented at *AIDS' Impact*, 2nd International Conference on Biopsychosocial Aspects of HIV Infection, Brighton.
ASTON, G. and PACANOWSKI, L. (1999) The changing social context of parenting. In *Transition to Parenting: An Open Learning Resource for Midwives*. London: Royal College of Midwives Trust.
BALLARD, C.G., DAVIS, R., CULLEN, P.C., MOHAN, R.N. and DEAN, C. (1994) Prevalence of postnatal psychiatric morbidity in mothers and fathers. *British Journal of Psychiatry* 164(6):782.
BARCLAY, L. (1990) Sexuality and pregnancy. Paper presented at the International Confederation of Midwives 22nd International Congress, Kobe, Japan.
BARCLAY, L., McDONALD, P. and O'LOUGHLIN, J.A. (1994) Sexuality and pregnancy: an interview study. *Australian and New Zealand Journal of Obstetrics and Gynaecology* 34(1):2.
BARLOW, J. and BIRCH, L. (2004) Midwifery practice and sexual abuse. *British Journal of Midwifery* 12(2):72–5.
BARRETT. G. and McCANDLISH R. (2002) Caesarean section: better for your sex life? A review of the evidence. *MIDIRS: Midwifery Digest* 12(3):377–9.
BARRETT, G., PENDRY, E., PEACOCK, J. et al. (2000) Women's sexual health after childbirth. *BJOG: An International Journal of Obstetrics and Gynaecology* 107(2):186–95.

BATMAN, P.A., THOMLINSON, J., MOORE, V.C. and SYKES, R. (1998) Death due to air embolism during sexual intercourse in the puerperium. *Postgraduate Medical Journal* **74**(876):612–13.

BELFIELD, T. (2004) What we say *and* how we say it … *Journal of Family Planning and Reproductive Health Care* **30**(1):11.

BEWLEY, C. and GIBBS, A. (2000) Domestic violence and pregnancy: a midwifery issue. In Alexander, J., Roth, C. and Levy, V. (eds) *Midwifery Practice: Core Topics 3*. London: Macmillan Press, pp. 100–12.

BIGGERSTAFF, D. (1999) Postnatal depression. *Practice Nursing* **10**(8):22–4.

BLACK, J.S. (1994) Sexuality and pregnancy: an interview study. Editorial comment. *Australian and New Zealand Journal of Obstetrics and Gynaecology* **34**(1):1.

BODDY, J. (1998) Violence embodied? Circumcision, gender politics, and cultural aesthetics. In Dobash, R.E. and Dobash, R.P. (eds) *Rethinking Violence Against Women*. London: Sage Publications, pp. 77–110.

BOGREN, L.Y. (1991) Changes in sexuality in women and men during pregnancy. *Archives of Sexual Behaviour* **20**(1):35.

BORG, S. and LASKER, J. (1982) *When Pregnancy Fails*. London: Routledge and Kegan Paul.

BOSELEY, S. (1998) Sex soon after childbirth can kill. *The Guardian*, 1 October (No. 47297), p. 12.

BOSELEY, S. (2000) Being there. *The Guardian*, 18 January (No. 47710) pp. 4–5.

BRITISH MEDICAL ASSOCIATION (1998) *Domestic Violence: A Health Care Issue?* London: BMA.

BURNS, J. (1992) The psychology of lesbian health care. In Nicolson, P. and Ussher, J. (eds) *The Psychology of Women's Health and Health Care*. London: Macmillan.

BYRNE, J. (1994) *When Home is Where the Hurt Is*. London: BBC Radio Two Social Action Team and the Women's Aid Federations.

CAMPBELL, J.C. and ALFORD, P. (1989) The dark consequences of marital rape. *American Journal of Nursing* **89**(7): 946-949.

CAMPBELL, J.C. and SOEKEN, K.L. (1999) Forced sex and intimate partner violence: effects on women's risk and women's health. *Violence Against Women* **5**(9):1017–35.

CARTER, A. (1979) *The Sadeian Woman – An Exercise In Cultural History*. London: Virago.

CLEMENT, S. (1994) Unwanted vaginal examinations. *British Journal of Midwifery* **2**(8):368.

CLIFFORD, K.A. and REGAN, L. (1994) Recurrent pregnancy loss. In Studd, J. (ed.) *Progress in Obstetrics and Gynaecology*, Vol. 11. Edinburgh: Churchill Livingstone.

CLULOW, C.F. (1982) *To Have and To Hold Marriage. The First Baby and Preparing Couples for Parenthood*. Aberdeen: Aberdeen University Press.

CONTRATTO, S.W. (1980) Maternal sexuality and asexual motherhood. *Signs: Journal of Women in Culture and Society* **5**(4):766.

COPPENS, M. (2002) Sexual intimacy during pregnancy. *Midwifery Today–International Midwife* **62**:21–4.

CORKHILL, A. (1996) Effects of the birth of a first baby on a couple's sexual relationship. *British Journal of Midwifery* **4**(2):70.

CRONIN, A. (2004) Gender and sexuality. In Stewart, M. (ed.) *Pregnancy Birth and Maternity Care: Feminist Perspectives*. London: Elsevier Science.

CURTIS, P. and DUNN, K. (1996) Sex and sexuality. *Modern Midwife* **6**(5):26.

DE JUDICIBUS, M.A. and McCABE, M.P. (2002) Psychological factors and the sexuality of pregnant and postpartum women. *Journal of Sex Research* **39**(2):94–103.

DEMYTTENAERE, K., GHELDOF, M. and VAN ASSCHE, F.A. (1995) Sexuality in the postpartum period: a review. *Current Obstetrics and Gynaecology* **5**(2):81.

DIXON, M., BOOTH, N. and POWELL, R. (2000) Sex and relationships following childbirth: a first report from general practice of 131 couples. *British Journal of General Practice* **50**(452):223–4.

DYE, M. (2002) Sex and the motherhood myth. *Midwifery Today–International Midwife* **62**:20.

EDELMANN, R.J. and CONNOLLY, K.J. (1994) Reproductive failure and the reproductive technologies: a psychological perspective. In Penny, G.N., Bennett, P. and Herbert, M. (eds) *Health Psychology A Lifespan Perspective*. Chur, Switzerland: Harwood Academic.

EKWO, E.E., GOSSELINK, C.A., WOOLSON, R., MOAWAD, A. and LONG, C.R. (1993) Coitus late in pregnancy: risk of preterm rupture of amniotic sac membranes. *American Journal of Obstetrics and Gynecology* **1**(1):22–31.

EVANS, K. (1992) Getting back to nature. *Modern Midwife* **2**(1):14.

FELSTEIN, I. (1998) Sexual management after the second baby. *British Journal of Sexual Medicine* **25**(2):12–13.

GARCIA, T.C. (2003) Primary care of the lesbian/gay/bisexual/transgendered woman patient. *International Journal of Fertility and Women's Medicine* **48**(6):246–51.

GLAZENER, C.M. (1997) Sexual function after childbirth: women's experiences, persistent morbidity and lack of professional recognition. *British Journal of Obstetrics and Gynaecology* **104**(3):330–5.

GREGOIRE, A.J.P., KUMAR, R., EVERITT, B., HENDERSON, A.F. and STUDD, J.W.W. (1996) Transdermal oestrogen for treatment of severe postnatal depression. *Lancet* **347**(9006):930–3.

GRIBBIN, C. (2003) Managing psychosexual problems: essential skills for gynaecological consultations. *Current Obstetrics & Gynaecology* **13**(4):244–9.

GROGAN, S. (1999) *Body Image: Understanding Body Dissatisfaction in Men, Women and Children*. London: Routledge.

GUANA-TRUJILLO, B. and HIGGINS, P. (1987) Sexual intercourse and pregnancy. *Health Care for Woman International* **8**(5):339.

HALL, J. (1993) Attendance not compulsory. *Nursing Times* **89**(46):69.

HALL, J. (2002) Understanding sexuality in midwifery practise. *Midwifery Today–International Midwife* **62**:47.

HOME OFFICE. (2003) *Safety and Justice: The Government's Proposals on Domestic Violence*. London: Her Majesty's Stationery Office.

HUGHES, P.M., TURTON, P. and EVANS, D.H. (1999) Stillbirth as risk factor for depression and anxiety in the subsequent pregnancy: cohort study. *British Medical Journal* **318**(7200):1721–4.

JACKSON, K.B. (2000) Women, men, breastfeeding and sexuality. *British Journal of Midwifery* **8**(2):83–6.

JEBALI, C.A. (1993) A feminist perspective on postnatal depression. *Health Visitor* **66**(2):59.

JONES, A. and JONES, K. (1991) Accepting motherhood. *Nursing Times* **87**(20):58.

JONES, D. (1999) Pop belly. *The Sunday Times Magazine*, 28 February, pp. 32–40.

JONES, K. (1990) Expectant fears. *Nursing Times* **86**(15):36.

KELLEHER, C.J., CARDOZO, L.D., KHULLAR, V., WISE, B. and CUTNER, A. (1993) The impact of urinary incontinence on sexual function. *Journal of Sexual Health* **3**(7):186.

KENNEDY, J. (2003) *HIV in Pregnancy and Childbirth*. London: Elsevier Science.

KENNEY, J.W. and TASH, D.T. (1993) Lesbian child-bearing couples' dilemmas and decisions. In Stern Noerager, P. (ed.) *Lesbian Health: What Are the Issues?* London: Taylor & Francis.

KENT, E. (1998) *A Study to Explore Women's View of their Body Image During the Third Trimester of Pregnancy.* Unpublished BSc(Hons) midwifery dissertation. King's College, University of London.

KITZINGER, J.V. (1992) Counteracting, not reenacting, the violation of women's bodies: the challenge for perinatal caregivers. *Birth* **19**(4):219.

KITZINGER, S. (1982) Sexuality in pregnancy. *British Journal of Sexual Medicine* **9**:44.

KITZINGER, S. (1985) *Woman's Experience of Sex*. London: Penguin Books.

LEE, B. (1994) It all started after I had my baby. *Journal of the Royal Society of Medicine* **87**(10):639.

LEE, J.T. (2002) The meaning of sexual satisfaction in pregnant Taiwanese women. *Journal of Midwifery & Women's Health* **47**(4):278–86.

LEIFER, M. (1980) Pregnancy. *Signs: Journal of Women in Culture and Society* **5**(4):754.

LEWIS, C. (1999) Transition to fatherhood. In *Transition to Parenting: An Open Learning Resource for Midwives*. London: Royal College of Midwives Trust.

LONDON BLACK WOMEN'S HEALTH ACTION PROJECT (1999) *Strategy Policy on Female Genital Mutilation: FGM is a World-Wide Issue*. London: London Black Women's Health Action Project.

MAIN, D.M., GRISSO, J.A., SNYDER, E.S., CHIU, G.Y. and HOLMES, J.H. (1993) The effects of sexual activity on uterine contractions in pregnancy. *Journal of Women's Health* **2**(2):141.

MANDER, R. (1994) *Loss and Bereavement in Childbearing*. Oxford: Blackwell Scientific.

MARTIN, A. (1993) *The Guide to Lesbian and Gay Parenting*. London: Pandora.

MASON, L., GLENN, S., WALTON, I. and APPLETON, C. (1999) The experience of stress incontinence after childbirth. *Birth* **26**(3):164–71.

MASTERS, W.H. and JOHNSON, V.E. (1966) *Human Sexual Response*. Boston: Little, Brown.

McCAFFREY, M. (1995) Female genital mutilation: consequences for reproductive and sexual health. *Sexual and Marital Therapy* **10**(2):189–200.

McCONVILLE, B. (1994) *Mixed Messages Our Breasts in Our Lives*. Harmondsworth: Penguin Books.

McNEILL, E. (1994) Blood, sex and hormones: a theoretical review of women's sexuality over the menstrual cycle. In Choi, P.Y.L. and Nicolson, P. (eds) *Female Sexuality: Psychology, Biology and Social Context*. Hemel Hempstead: Harvester Wheatsheaf.

MILLER, L. (1995) We did it. And it was good. *The Guardian*, 7 March.

MILLS, J.L., HARLAP, S. and HARLEY, E.E. (1981) Should coitus late in pregnancy be discouraged? *The Lancet* **11**(8238):136.

MOROF, D. BARRETT, G. PEACOCK, J. VICTOR, C. MANYONDA, I. (2003) Postnatal depression and sexual health after childbirth. *Obstetrics & Gynecology* **102**(6): 1318–25.

MORRIS, E. and MUKHOPHADYAY, S. (2003) Dyspareunia in gynaecological practice. *Current Obstetrics & Gynaecology* **13**(4): 232–8.

NATIONAL CHILDBIRTH TRUST. VICTOR, C. and BARRETT, G. (1994) Is there sex after childbirth? *New Generation* **13**(2):24.

NATIONAL INSTITUTE FOR CLINICAL EXCELLENCE (2003) Antenatal care: routine care for the healthy pregnant woman. Clinical Guideline 6. London: National Institute for Clinical Excellence.

NICOLSON, P. (1990) Sexuality and the transition to motherhood: an impossible dilemma? Paper presented at the 10th Annual Merseyside Conference on Clinical Psychology, Chester College.

OAKLEY, A. (1979) *Becoming a Mother*. Oxford: Martin Robertson.

OAKLEY, A. (1992) The changing social context of pregnancy care. In Chamberlain, G. and Zander, L. (eds) *Pregnancy Care in the 1990s*. Carnforth: Parthenon Publishing.

O'DRISCOLL, M. (1994) Midwives, childbirth and sexuality 2: men and sex. *British Journal of Midwifery* **2**(2):74.

O'DRISCOLL, M. (1998) Midwives discover sex. *The Practising Midwife* **1**(4):27–9.

OMER-HASHI, K.H. (1994) Commentary – female genital mutilation: perspectives from a Somalian midwife. *Birth* **21**(4):224.

ONAH, H.E., ILOABACHIE, G.C., OBI, S.N., EZUGWU, F.O. and EZE, J.N. (2002) Nigerian male sexual activity during pregnancy. *International Journal of Gynecology & Obstetrics* **76**(2):219–23.

ORJI, E.O., OGUNLOLA, I.O. and FASUBBA, O.B. (2002) Sexuality among pregnant women in South West Nigeria. *Journal of Obstetrics and Gynaecology* **22**(2):166–8.

ORUÇ, S., AYSEN, E., LAÇIN, S., ADIGÜZEL, H., UYAR, Y. and KOYUNCU, F. (1999) Sexual behaviour during pregnancy. *Australian and New Zealand Journal of Obstetrics and Gynaecology* **39**(1):48–50.

PALMER, A. and LIKIS, F.E. (2003) Lactational atrophic vaginitis. *Journal of Midwifery & Women's Health* **48**(4):282–4.

PEPPERELL, R.J. and McBAIN, J.C. (1985) Unexplained infertility: a review. *British Journal of Obstetrics and Gynaecology* **92**(6):569.

PINES, D. (1993) *A Woman's Unconscious Use of Her Body. A Psychoanalytical Perspective*. London: Virago.

PITT, B. (1991) Depression following childbirth. *Hospital Update* **17**(2):133.

PRICE, J. (1988) *Motherhood: What It Does To Your Mind*. London: Pandora.

Prima Baby Magazine (2002) Having a baby cuts your love life in half. *Prima Baby*, December, pp. 17–18.

RAPHAEL-LEFF, J. (1991) *Psychological Processes of Childbearing*. London: Chapman and Hall.

RAPHAEL-LEFF, J. (1993) *Pregnancy: The Inside Story*. London: Sheldon Press.

REAMY, K.J. and WHITE, S.E. (1985) Dyspareunia in pregnancy. *Journal of Psychosomatic Obstetrics and Gynaecology* **4**(4):263.

REAMY, K.J. and WHITE, S.E. (1987) Sexuality in the puerperium: a review. *Archives of Sexual Behaviour* **16**(2):165.

RILEY, A.J. (1989) Sex after childbirth. *British Journal of Sexual Medicine* **16**(5):185.

ROBERTSON, M.M. (1993) Lesbians as an invisible minority in the health services arena. In Stern Noerager, P. (ed.) *Lesbian Health: What Are the Issues?* London: Taylor & Francis.

ROBINSON, J. (1998) Dying for sex? Intercourse in the puerperium. *British Journal of Midwifery* **6**(11):732–3.

ROBSON, K.M., BRANT, H.A. and KUMAR, R. (1981) Maternal sexuality during first pregnancy and after childbirth. *British Journal of Obstetrics and Gynaecology* **88**(9):882.

ROTH, C. (1999) Sexually transmissible and reproductive tract infections in pregnancy. In Bennett, V.R. and Brown, L.K. (eds) *Myles Textbook for Midwives*, 13th edn. London: Churchill Livingstone, pp. 329–50.

ROYAL COLLEGE OF MIDWIVES (1994) Men at birth. News Release NR279/11/94. London: Royal College of Midwives.

ROYAL COLLEGE OF MIDWIVES (1998) *Female Genital Mutilation (Female Circumcision), Position Paper Number 21.* London: Royal College of Midwives.

ROYAL COLLEGE OF OBSTETRICIANS AND GYNAE-COLOGISTS (1997) *Intimate Examinations: Report of a Working Party.* London: RCOG Press.

ROYAL COLLEGE OF PAEDIATRICS AND CHILD HEALTH (1998) *Intercollegiate Working Party for Enhancing Voluntary Confidential HIV Testing in Pregnancy: Reducing Mother to Child Transmission of HIV Infection in the UK.* London: Royal College of Paediatrics and Child Health.

SAFFRON, L. (1999) Meeting the needs of lesbian clients. *The Practising Midwife* **2**(11):18–19.

SAVAGE, W. and READER, F. (1984) Sexual activity during pregnancy. *Midwife, Health Visitor and Community Nurse* **20**(11):398.

SAYLE, A.E. SAVITZ, D.A. and WILLIAMS, J.F. (2003) Accuracy of reporting of sexual activity during late pregnancy. *Paediatric and Perinatal Epidemiology***17**(2):143–7.

SAYLE, A.E. SAVITZ, D.A., THORP, J.M., HERTZ-PICCIOTTO, I. and WILCOX, A.J. (2001) Sexual activity during late pregnancy and risk of preterm delivery. *Obstetrics & Gynecology* **97**(2):283–9.

SCOTTISH INTERCOLLEGIATE GUIDELINES NETWORK (SIGN) (2002) Postnatal depression and puerperal psychosis. *Guideline 60 Section 2: Diagnosis, screening and prevention.* Edinburgh.

SEDGWICK, L.R. (1994) Midwives' view on discussing sexual issues with clients. Unpublished BSc(Hons) midwifery dissertation. King's College, University of London.

SEN, S. and ESEN, U.I. (2003) Maternal collapse and coagulopathy following sexual intercourse in pregnancy. *Journal of Obstetrics and Gynaecology* **23**(2):205.

SHANNON, D. (1993) Fathers in hard labour. *Independent on Sunday*, 24 October.

SIGNORELLO, L.B., HARLOW, B.L., CHEKOS, A.K. and REPKE, J.T. (2001) Postpartum sexual functioning and its relationship to perineal trauma: a retrospective cohort study of primiparous women. *American Journal of Obstetrics and Gynecology* **184**(5): 881–90.

SOUTHERN, M. (1994). Labour and sexuality. *Midwifery Matters:* **61**:5.

STEVENS, P.E. (1993) Lesbian health care research: a review of the literature from 1970 to 1990. In Stern Noerager, P. (ed.) *Lesbian Health: What Are the Issues?* London: Taylor & Francis.

STEWART-MOORE, J. (2000) Sexual health in the postnatal period. In Alexander, J., Roth, C. and Levy, V. (eds) *Midwifery Practice: Core Topics 3.* London: Macmillan Press, pp. 83–99.

STUDD, J.W.W. (1992) Oestrogens and depression in women. *British Journal of Hospital Medicine* **48**:211–13.

TAYLOR, V.J. (1992) Pregnancy: a shared experience? Men's experiences and feelings about their partner's pregnancy. *Journal of Advances in Health and Nursing Care* **2**(2):59.

THOMPSON, J. (1994) *Haemorrhoids The Facts.* Brentford: SmithKline Beecham, Consumer Healthcare.

TIEFER, L. (1995) *Sex Is Not a Natural Act and Other Essays.* Oxford: Westview Press.

TIRAN, D. and MACK, S. (eds) (2000) *Complementary Therapies for Pregnancy and Childbirth*, 2nd edn. London: Baillière Tindall.

TOBERT, A. (1990) Sexual problems in pregnancy and the postnatal period. *Midwife Health Visitor and Community Nurse* **26**(5):177.

TOMLINSON, A.J., COLLIVER, D., NELSON, J. and JACKSON, F. (1999) Does sexual intercourse at term influence the onset of labour? A survey of attitudes of patients and their partners. *Journal of Obstetrics and Gynaecology* **19**(5):466–8.

TOUBIA, N. (1994) Female circumcision as a public health issue. *New England Journal of Medicine* **331**(11):712.

USSHER, J.M. (1989) *The Psychology of the Female Body.* London: Routledge.

UTHAYAKUMAR, S., SHAH, P.N. and SMITH, J.R. (1994) Vaginal discharge. *Update* **49**(3):155.

VAN WERT, W.F. (1991) Sex after childbirth. *Mothering* **60**(summer):115.

VON SYDOW, K. (2002) Sexual enjoyment and orgasm postpartum: sex differences and perceptual accuracy concerning partners' sexual experience. *Journal of Psychosomatic Obstetrics & Gynecology* **23**(3):147–55.

VON SYDOW, K. ULLMEYER, M. and HAPP, N. (2001) Sexual activity during pregnancy and after childbirth: results from the Sexual Preferences Questionnaire. *Journal of Psychosomatic Obstetrics & Gynecology* **22**(1):29–40.

WALLACE, R. (1989) A pregnant pause. *The Guardian*, 5 December.

WALTON, I. (1994) *Sexuality and Motherhood.* Hale: Books for Midwives Press.

WILES, R. (1994) 'I'm not fat, I'm pregnant': the impact of pregnancy on fat women's body image. In Wilkinson, S. and Kitzinger, C. (eds) *Women and Health Feminist Perspectives.* London: Taylor & Francis.

WILTON, T. (1999) Towards an understanding of the cultural roots of homophobia in order to provide a better midwifery service for lesbian clients. *Midwifery* **15**(3):154–64.

WOOLLEY, P. (1994) Diagnosis and management of vaginal infections. Part 2. *British Journal of Sexual Medicine* **21**(3):16.

9: Unplanned Pregnancy

Kati Gray

Kati Gray

OBJECTIVES

This chapter should help you understand:

◆ The practical and emotional aspects of an unplanned pregnancy ◆

◆ The difficulties surrounding decision-making ◆

◆ The legal and moral considerations surrounding abortion ◆

◆ Different abortion procedures ◆

◆ Professional dilemmas ◆

◆ The role of the health professional. ◆

Introduction

When a woman has an unplanned pregnancy it can be a shocking and deeply disturbing experience. An unplanned pregnancy is not a single entity in itself, but is usually preceded and followed by many incidents (of greater or lesser complexity) which together form the whole experience. This multiplicity of events and the process of addressing and understanding them are what will be discussed in this chapter.

Practical issues, such as giving the results of a pregnancy test, the law relating to abortion and abortion procedures, will be considered along with more emotional concerns. What an unplanned pregnancy means, how to make a decision about it and what the impact of that decision will be upon a woman's life are not questions to which there are practical or general answers. Every woman's experience of pregnancy is a personal one. For whilst many women have unplanned pregnancies, the circumstances each of them faces, what pregnancy means to her, and what she decides to do about it involve emotions and experiences that belong uniquely to her. Many women go through this experience in confusion and isolation, feeling desperately in

need of help but not knowing where to go. The aim of this chapter is to enable you, as a health professional, to think about the practical and emotional aspects of unplanned pregnancy. Reflecting upon some of the issues discussed may facilitate and support you in your work with a woman who has, or had in the past, an unplanned pregnancy. The care of a woman in this situation can be greatly enhanced by your skilled nursing intervention, and using your expertise in this area of women's health care can also be a richly rewarding (albeit challenging) experience for you.

Defining unplanned pregnancy

When a woman has an unplanned pregnancy it is important to be clear about what this means for her as an individual. Health professionals may assume that the woman has been foolish, unlucky or careless; that her pregnancy is unwanted or that she secretly desired to be pregnant; that she ought/ought not to continue the pregnancy because of her personal circumstances; and that a decision about the pregnancy must be made quickly. On the other hand, the pregnant woman may experience a mixture of emotions such as shock, despair, anger, excitement and relief simultaneously, and consequently any hope of making a decision based on her own needs and desires may seem slim indeed.

In the midst of the potential ambivalence and confusion surrounding unplanned pregnancy it is important that you recognize that some unplanned pregnancies may have occurred 'accidentally on purpose', and that many are most definitely not unwanted. The meaning of unplanned pregnancy can only be revealed and understood in relation to an individual pregnant woman. For whilst women with unplanned pregnancies share a common reality, their experiences of that reality and their thoughts and feelings in relation to it are always deeply personal. There is no 'right' way to feel about an unplanned pregnancy. What is important is that any woman in this situation is able to discover what her feelings are.

Confirming pregnancy

A woman may suspect, feel, hope for or fear pregnancy before she comes to the clinic or surgery. Often she will have used a home pregnancy testing kit, or paid a chemist to do a test for her. Therefore, when she first comes to the clinic it is helpful to establish whether a test has been done previously, and what the result was.

Obtaining this information gives the woman the opportunity to begin speaking about her reactions to being pregnant, and offers you an initial insight into her emotional response to her possible pregnancy.

In some clinics it is the policy to carry out a pregnancy test for every woman, regardless of the result of any previous test. If this is the case, it is important to explain this to her (along with the possibility of a false positive or false negative result) so that she understands the reason for the procedure. When such explanations are not given, a woman may feel that she is being disbelieved or mistrusted, or that her physical experience of pregnancy is being dismissed.

Whether a previous test has been done or not, it is necessary to inform the woman of the arrangements regarding testing (and the policy relating to giving test results) at the particular clinic she is attending. For example, whilst many clinics now offer a 'walk-in' pregnancy testing service with results available in minutes, at others it may take several days before the results can be given as the tests are sent outside the clinic to be processed.

Some clinics require the woman to make an appointment with a medical practitioner in order to be given results, whilst at others it is the nurse who fulfils this role.

Explaining the process at the outset not only avoids misunderstanding and confusion, but allows the woman to consider whether what is available at the clinic meets her individual needs.

For a number of reasons a woman may not want the result of her pregnancy test at the time she submits it. She may have come to the clinic alone but want her partner, friend or a relative to be with her when she is given the result. Or she may be on her way to work, place of study or another appointment, and not feel it is appropriate to know the result at that particular time. She may have a baby or young child in her immediate care and therefore not feel able to deal with the impact of having her pregnancy confirmed.

Alternatively, she may feel that she needs to know whether or not she is pregnant immediately and is not prepared to wait several days before the result is available.

Once the service offered at the particular clinic she is attending has been explained, the woman is in a position to choose how she wishes to proceed. You can then discuss with her the appropriate course of action. The clinic's service may be what the woman expects and wants, but if not then alternatives need to be discussed and found. Testing at another clinic, where results are available more quickly, or another appointment when her partner or friend can be present, or when she feels it would be a more appropriate time to know the result, are all possibilities that you could consider.

Unplanned pregnancy can result in a woman feeling powerless and out of control. Enabling her to exercise choice about how and when she has her pregnancy confirmed can be the first stage in the process of her regaining a sense of control within this situation, and also in her life.

Giving a pregnancy test result

When required to tell a woman what the result of her pregnancy test is, you should first give some thought to the setting. Whether a 'walk-in' service or one where she is returning for the result, the woman should be offered a quiet private space in which to sit with you. It is a courtesy to have a box of tissues available within her reach and a bin in which she can easily deposit any used tissues. (If she does begin to cry, tissues should not be pushed towards her as she may take it as a signal to stop crying and 'pull herself together'.)

If you know in advance that the woman is coming for a pregnancy test result, extra time should be allowed if possible. This way neither the woman nor you will be under pressure to 'get on with it' or hurry the interaction. Asking her what she thinks the result is or what she wants it to be is preferable to saying 'It's positive', 'I'm sorry to tell you …', 'I'm afraid that …', 'You're going to be a mum'. The difficulty with such statements is that they do not take account of the woman's feelings and reveal a lot about your own. For the pregnant woman, the agenda and tone of the interaction will have been set for her, rather than by her.

Alternatively, if you have already ascertained the woman's feelings about a result this will then allow her to set the agenda. She may say 'I'm terrified that …', 'I just know that …', 'I just don't know …', 'If I am, I'll …' – any of which may give you an indication of how best to continue.

The value of this approach is that you are *responding* to the thoughts and feelings of the woman rather than *leading* the interaction between you.

Once the pregnancy has been confirmed the woman should be allowed time to reflect upon this result. If she is distressed and crying she should be allowed to cry; if stunned into silence, the silence should be respected; if shouting about the unfairness or awfulness of it all, she must be allowed to express these feelings. Even for a woman who has long suspected that she is pregnant, having the pregnancy confirmed can be a shocking and extremely distressing experience. Whilst for the woman who had no idea that she was pregnant, being told that she is may make no sense to her at all. Women in this situation can need several hours or days before they are able to respond and react in any logical way.

Having an unplanned pregnancy confirmed means that a decision about the pregnancy has to be made. However, unless the woman is especially clear in her thoughts or has already made her decision, it is always appropriate to offer her another appointment. Not only does this provide invaluable time for her to consider and reflect upon her feelings but it also provides an opportunity for her to discuss her pregnancy with her partner, family or friends. It is also a way for you to enable the woman to create space and time in which to think.

Women with unplanned pregnancies often feel very alone and that they should have already made a decision. By offering another appointment you are conveying two very important messages. First, that there is time for the woman to think about her pregnancy and to discuss her thoughts and feelings with others if she wishes. Second, that there is someone in a professional capacity willing to help her and therefore she does not have to manage alone.

Whilst it is often the case that a woman does not feel she wants or needs a second appointment, this in no way detracts from the value of the message conveyed when the offer is made. Moreover, given the degree of shock, disbelief and despair that the woman may experience when her pregnancy is confirmed, it may be unrealistic to expect a considered decision at this stage.

The meaning of unplanned pregnancy

Before a decision can be made about her pregnancy, the woman needs to understand what becoming pregnant at this stage of her life means for her. Pregnancy may mean that contraception has failed; that a woman is fertile despite previously being told otherwise; that she had sexual intercourse when she was not expecting to and therefore was not using contraception; that she wanted to know whether she could conceive and was 'testing' her fertility; that she wants a baby; that life is chaotic and difficult and preventing pregnancy the least of her concerns.

The possible meanings of pregnancy are numerous but are always unique for the individual pregnant woman. Understanding what pregnancy means for her involves the woman being able to explore her thoughts and feelings about it, as well as the circumstances in which she became pregnant. This can be a difficult process, not least because the woman may have feelings she considers to be contradictory or mutually exclusive. It is only by acknowledging or addressing these feelings that the meaning of this specific pregnancy for this particular woman can be revealed.

The difficulty for you can be in acknowledging and tolerating the confusion and distress of the woman, whilst avoiding telling her what her pregnancy means and what she should do about it. This can be particularly difficult when the woman asks such questions as 'What do you think I should do?' or 'What's going to be best for me, please tell me?' or 'I can't decide – what would you do in my position?'

In situations such as these it is vital to remind yourself that your role is not to tell her what to do. It is to enable her to understand what her pregnancy means and then to make her own decision about it. Whilst you can help her to explore the meaning of her pregnancy, you cannot tell her this meaning and you should not tell her what to do about it. Clearly, some women with an unplanned pregnancy will find this process much more difficult than others. Furthermore, individual life situations vary and some are far more complex than others.

A woman for whom contraception has failed within a stable, supportive relationship may feel clear about making a decision to continue her pregnancy or to have an abortion. Even so she may value the opportunity to discuss the meaning of her pregnancy, and her feelings about it, with you. She may also need practical information about antenatal care or abortion. It is important for both of you that she has, and continues to receive, the help and support she needs and is comfortable with whatever decision she has made.

Another woman may be pregnant as a result of not using contraception. This could mean that her pregnancy is the result of rape or coercive intercourse, or that she refuses or does not feel able to take control of her own fertility. She may not have any stable or supportive relationships in her life and may feel completely unable to understand or make a decision about her pregnancy.

Abortion is an issue that most people have an opinion about, but in fact nobody can be certain about their own reaction until they themselves are pregnant, and have to make a decision about whether to continue the pregnancy. Thus, a woman who has always supported a woman's right to choose an abortion and who has used contraception believing that should it fail she would choose to have an abortion, finds she cannot make that decision for herself. Similarly, a woman who has always been fiercely opposed to abortion and said that it would never be a choice she would make, can have an unplanned pregnancy and realize that abortion is the only suitable option. Another woman may say she is having an abortion because it is what her partner/mother/family or medical practitioner thinks is right for her, whilst another may simply say 'I have no choice, I have to do it'.

In these, and numerous other similar situations, it is of paramount importance that a woman recognizes she always has a choice, and that she makes that choice herself, based on her own needs and desires. For some women this is an extraordinarily difficult task and you may both recognize that the complexities involved need to be addressed before any decision about her pregnancy can be made.

If you feel it is appropriate and possible for you to address these issues with her, then it may be feasible to offer a series of appointments to explore her feelings. However, your work environment (clinic lay-out, lack of private rooms, heavy caseload, 10-minute appointments, etc.), your expertise being in other areas (e.g. practice nursing, family planning, women's health, rather

SCENARIO

Anna, a 19-year-old university student, presented at her local clinic requesting an abortion. She said that her partner had said that he would support her, but she knew that this was 'just words' and he had offered no care or support since she became pregnant. She went on to say that her mother would 'go mad' and her stepfather would 'throw me out of the house' if they knew she was pregnant.

Recognizing that Anna was talking about others but not herself, the counsellor asked how she felt about her pregnancy. Anna began to cry and said that she wouldn't be able to live with herself if she had an abortion, but that she could see no way of being able to continue her pregnancy as a single, unsupported student.

The counsellor suggested that, given her feelings, she should not proceed with making arrangements to having an abortion at this time, and instead offered two more counselling appointments. During these, Anna was able to explore her own feelings about her pregnancy, and the reasons why she felt so influenced by the (fantasized) reactions of her family. As a result she chose not to have an abortion, and felt very positively that continuing her pregnancy was right for her – if not for others.

than in-depth psychological and emotional counselling) and your own personal feelings may make such extended work impossible. Should this be the case, the woman should be told that although you recognize her need to discuss and try to resolve some of the complex issues, you are unable to do this with her. (This should be said using words with which you feel comfortable and are natural for you.) You can then offer to refer her to someone who has the necessary training, experience and time to do this work with her. It is helpful to have a regularly updated list of counsellors and support agencies that you can give her if, after discussion with you, a referral seems appropriate. Any cost and restrictions of the service should also be discussed prior to referral.

Referring on can be a vital aspect of the woman's care and can relieve you of a potential burden that would be impossible to cope with in your current professional role and practice.

Personal needs – professional responsibility

Unplanned pregnancy and abortion are not just professional clinical issues but also involve personal private feelings. For both male and female health professionals pregnancy, childbirth, subfertility, miscarriage, parenthood or the decision to be childless are personal issues as well as professional ones. Therefore it is of paramount importance that when working with women or couples with unplanned pregnancies you are clear about your own feelings and attitudes.

Working professionally does not mean that you are not entitled to your own views and feelings. However, it does mean that you have a responsibility to reflect upon them, and to ensure that your personal feelings neither influence nor inhibit the treatment of patients.

Clearly there are times when it may be impossible to work with women contemplating abortion; for example, if you have just had a baby, an abortion or a miscarriage, are recently bereaved, or if you are trying to conceive or are having fertility treatment. Any of these life events are likely to mean that you are very involved in your own emotional responses and possible confusion. To expect to deal with the emotions of a woman with an unwanted pregnancy who is considering an abortion is at best unrealistic, and at worst harmful for you and your patient.

The interests of the patient and yourself will best be served by referring her to someone else who is not emotionally vulnerable in the way you are at present. Not only does this ensure that the patient gets the care she needs (from someone who is able to focus on her emotional state whilst temporarily putting their own emotions to one side) but it relieves you of a potentially painful and distressing burden. When we are emotionally distraught, the emotions of others are much more difficult to tolerate and it may be impossible not to become critical and judgemental in our work.

Referring on in situations such as those mentioned above ensures you are acting professionally in the interests of the patient and in the interest of your own well-being – which is of no less importance. It is, of course, equally important to refer on when for religious, ethical or moral reasons you choose not to become involved in the treatment of a woman seeking an abortion.

Decision-making

Counselling is an important part of the decision-making process for a woman with an unplanned pregnancy. Whilst counselling is not about giving advice, or telling the woman what to do, it does provide a space for her to explore her thoughts and feelings about her pregnancy (no matter how confused or conflicting they may seem). Thus counselling facilitates an understanding of the meaning of pregnancy for each individual woman and can provide the emotional support necessary for her to be able to make a decision.

Counselling should be offered with someone who has appropriate training and experience and who has no emotional investment in the woman's decision. Therefore, family, friends, GP, the medical practitioner agreeing to perform an abortion, reproductive health or practice nurse that the woman may know well, or any other individual with whom she has similar contact cannot adequately fulfil the counselling role. Family and friends are likely to be emotionally involved themselves; GPs and other medical practitioners may have conflicting interests. The counsellor should be someone the woman does not know personally, and to whom she feels able to speak freely, honestly and confidentially without being concerned about needing to apologize, to protect or to convince them. The skill of the counsellor lies in being able to deal with the confusion and distress of the pregnant woman, to hear the ambiguities and covert desires in what she says, and to be able to keep personal feelings and opinions out of the interaction between them.

The degree of distress and confusion felt by women with unplanned pregnancies varies greatly but there are few who do not welcome the opportunity of discussing the pregnancy and their feelings about it. Being someone whom the

SCENARIO

Kathy, a 28-year-old, came to the clinic with her partner, Pete, saying that she did not want an abortion but needed to know the gestation of her pregnancy. Pete appeared agitated, and the nurses in the clinic were alarmed and upset by his apparently aggressive behaviour.

When they were seen by the counsellor, Kathy began to talk about the difficulties within their relationship as she experienced it. They live together with their four-year-old son. Pete doesn't work and does little or no childcare or work in the home to help Kathy. He spends a lot of time (particularly during the evenings) away from home. Kathy works, and maintains the home whilst caring for their son. She wants their relationship to change and would like to marry Pete. Pete refuses to get married, saying he doesn't see the point, and although he accepts Kathy's accounts of his behaviour within the relationship, he does not see it as a problem.

The counsellor asked each of them what they saw the future of their partnership as being. Kathy began to cry and said she could not continue in this way. When asked what implications she thought this had for her pregnancy, she replied she could not continue it. At this point Pete became very angry and began shouting about how all she wanted to do was to get rid of his baby. The counsellor asked him to sit down and stop shouting. She said that she could see that he was angry and very upset and invited him to say what he wanted. He related his own disturbed and deprived history, and said it had left him determined to survive and to put himself first. The counsellor observed that this is what Kathy found difficult within the relationship, and wondered whether he believed they could reach some compromises, where neither had to be first all of the time. Pete responded by saying that he was not going to change, and that all of this was beside the point. The counsellor suggested that couple or individual psychotherapy would be a way of addressing these difficulties. Both were rejected as unnecessary and irrelevant by him.

At this point the counsellor asked Kathy what she wanted to do, and she replied that unless Pete was willing to acknowledge and address their difficulties, and to make a commitment to her, she saw no future for the relationship. She also said she did not feel able to continue her pregnancy and a week later had an abortion.

Kathy and Pete were in a very difficult and painful situation: they both had needs which were not being met. However, Pete's refusal to consider change, or to seek help, left Kathy feeling that there was no future for the relationship. Perhaps having an abortion was (albeit unconsciously) her way of ensuring the end of the relationship.

woman does not know and who will have no involvement with either her continuing pregnancy or abortion enables the counsellor to fulfil an important role that other health care professionals cannot reasonably be expected to. Counselling is offered by all the major charitable agencies and clinics (see Resources), by an increasing number of NHS services, and also by some reproductive health clinics and GP practices. It is essential that women know these services are available and that they have clear information about how to access them. A woman should be able to request, and receive, counselling as soon as she feels she needs to, and for some women several counselling sessions may be necessary before they feel able to make a decision.

No woman should proceed with an abortion unless she feels able to acknowledge that this is the choice *she*, personally, has made and feels comfortable with. Once she has had an abortion she cannot alter that decision and decide to continue her pregnancy. Therefore, if there is any doubt about whether an abortion is what she wants, or feels she must choose, a woman should be offered further counselling and more time to think about her choices.

In working with women with unplanned pregnancies, you may feel under great pressure to encourage or facilitate them in making a decision about whether or not to have an abortion which is an option only up to a certain stage of pregnancy for most women (see below). However, it is important to remember that a woman who ultimately cannot decide to have an abortion is making a decision to continue her pregnancy – albeit vicariously. In short, there is no necessity for a woman to be pushed or rushed into deciding to have an abortion, as *not* making that decision could be the most important decision of all.

Abortion and the law

On 27 October 1967 royal assent was given to the Abortion Act and it became law on 27 April 1968. This Act of Parliament made abortion legal only under certain circumstances (Box 9.1).

Box 9.1 Circumstances under which abortion is allowed under the Abortion Act 1967

1. The continuance of the pregnancy would involve risk to the life of the pregnant woman greater than if the pregnancy were terminated.
2. The continuance of the pregnancy would involve risk of injury to the physical or mental health of the pregnant woman greater than if the pregnancy were terminated.
3. The continuance of the pregnancy would involve risk of injury to the physical or mental health of the existing child(ren) of the family of the pregnant woman greater than if the pregnancy were terminated.
4. There is substantial risk that if the child were born it would suffer from such physical or mental abnormalities as to be seriously handicapped.

The Abortion Act of 1967 did not incorporate a time limit within which legal abortion must be carried out, but the Infant Life Preservation Act of 1929 states that it is a criminal offence to terminate a viable pregnancy. Viability was taken to be from the 28th week of pregnancy, and therefore to comply with the terms of the 1967 Act, an abortion had to be carried out before the 28th week of pregnancy.

Before an abortion could take place, the Act stated that two medical practitioners were to be in agreement that the pregnant woman's request for abortion met with one, or more, of the criteria listed in Box 9.1. Over 98% of induced abortions in Britain are undertaken because the pregnancy threatens the mental or physical health of the woman or her children (RCOG, 2000).

On 1 April 1991 the Human Fertilization and Embryology Act (1990) amended the 1967 Abortion Act in the following two ways:

◆ A time limit for abortion was incorporated in the Act and this was set at 24 weeks of pregnancy
◆ The time limit stated in the Infant Life Preservation Act (which previously applied in all circumstances) was removed where there was considered to be risk to the life of the pregnant woman; risk of permanent

damage to the mental or physical health of the pregnant woman; or risk that the child would be seriously handicapped.

Opponents of the legalization of abortion believe it is ethically or morally wrong, and that legalizing abortion leads to women aborting pregnancies they would otherwise carry to term. However, these beliefs are not borne out by research. The question of whether or not abortion is morally acceptable can only properly be decided by the pregnant woman; making abortion illegal does not prevent women having abortions. A report published in 1947 estimated that there were 100,000 illegal abortions annually in England and Wales (Chance *et al.*, 1947), and other researchers have drawn similar conclusions (Francome, 1977). Moreover, enquiries into maternal deaths revealed that mortality in England and Wales due to illegal abortion fell from 77 during 1961–63 to 1 in 1979–81, and to zero since 1981 (DoH, 1998).

It is evident that whilst making abortion legal does not interfere in any way with a woman's right to choose to continue her pregnancy, the criminalization of abortion does little to prevent a woman who does not wish to be pregnant from having an abortion, even though exercising this choice may cost her life. It is a sobering thought that worldwide, between 70,000 and 100,000 women a year die as a result of illegal or unsafe abortion (Ferriman, 1999).

The fact that abortion in the UK has been legal for nearly 40 years does not mean that all women have equal access to NHS abortion services. The interpretation of the clauses of the Act is liberal by some medical practitioners and extremely strict by others. District medical officers are under no obligation to provide abortion services and this means that while in some areas women requesting abortions are seen and treated swiftly within their local NHS service, for others NHS services are at best restricted and at worst non-existent.

In Scotland in 2002, 99.8% of abortions were performed in NHS premises (Information and Statistics Division of the NHS in Scotland, 2004). In contrast, the proportion of abortions paid for by the NHS health authorities in England and Wales in 2001 varied with an overall average of 76.3% (Office for National Statistics, 2002). Women who have no access to NHS services are left with little choice but to consult one of the charitable or private agencies. This is not only costly in financial terms (the lowest current fee for early medical or surgical abortion being £380) but often involves the women travelling many miles to the nearest charitable or private clinic.

The overall abortion rate for women resident in England and Wales remains relatively stable, although there appears to have been a very small increase over recent years. In spite of the often expressed contrary view, there is no such thing as 'abortion on demand' in the UK. To have a legal abortion means the criteria of the Abortion Act have to be fulfilled and that two medical practitioners have to consent to a woman's request for an abortion. For women in areas where there is no NHS provision of abortion services, it also requires a considerable financial outlay and a great deal of determination to find the appropriate agencies.

Abortion procedures

When a woman has had her pregnancy confirmed, received counselling, had medical consultations and had time to consider the choices available to her, she may decide to abort her pregnancy. Where NHS services are available, this can be done at a local hospital. Where there is not adequate NHS provision or when a women has the financial resources to allow her to choose where to be treated, she may be seen by one of the independent providers. Whether in the NHS or private sector, the method by which the abortion is carried out is usually defined by the gestation of her pregnancy (Box 9.2).

Induced abortion is one of the most commonly performed gynaecological procedures in Great Britain, with around 186,000 terminations performed annually in England and Wales and around 11,500 in Scotland. The highest numbers are performed on those in their late teens and 20s,

> **Box 9.2** Methods of abortion for different gestations (RCOG, 2004)
>
> **Early abortion**
> ◆ Early aspiration (with strict protocols), < 7 weeks
> ◆ Suction termination of pregnancy (STOP), 7–15 weeks
> ◆ Medical termination of pregnancy (MTOP), 4–9 weeks.
>
> **Mid-trimester and late abortion**
> ◆ Dilatation and evacuation (D and E), 15–24 weeks
> ◆ Late medical abortion using Mifepristone and multiple doses of prostaglandin (this regimen is unlicensed), 13–24 weeks.

although many under 16s and perimenopausal women also request a termination (Figure 9.1). At least a third of British women will have had an abortion by the time they reach the age of 45 (RCOG, 2004).

The Royal College of Obstetricians and Gynaecologists (RCOG) issued evidence-based guidelines in 2000 on the care of women requesting abortion, which were revised in 2004. These state that all women seeking an abortion are entitled to a fast and efficient service that includes a choice of procedures, screening for sexually transmitted infections (or antibiotics to prevent problems after the abortion) and contraceptive advice.

Early abortion

Early aspiration abortion

Within the independent sectors it is now possible for women to have an abortion within a very short timeframe (sometimes referred to as 'lunchtime abortions'). This can be performed at gestations below 7 weeks using electric or manual suction. To increase confidence that the gestation sac has been removed, protocols include safeguards such as the magnification of aspirate and follow-up serum βhCG estimation. Whilst for some women this quick procedure has many advantages and will be a positive choice, it is not so for all women. For example, the women who has only recently discovered her pregnancy may still be in a state of panic and shock. Unable to think clearly about her feelings and choices, swift treatment within an environment which, by its very structure, may offer little reflective time and minimal support carries with it the risk of too prompt and, ultimately for the woman, wrong treatment.

Similarly, a woman who has very little by way of emotional resources and support may find the rapid and very short progression through a hospital or clinic environment a lonely and isolating experience, which potentially could complicate her process of recovery. Therefore, whilst being a welcome addition to services available to women requesting abortion, these 'lunchtime' services are not appropriate for all women.

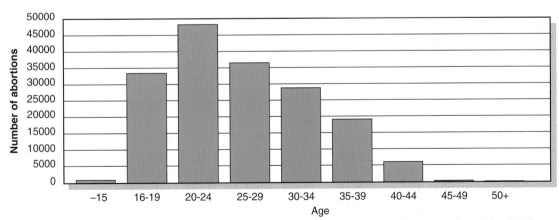

Figure 9.1 Number of abortions by age in England and Wales, 2001 (Office for National Statistics, 2002).

Suction termination of pregnancy (STOP)

A STOP can be carried out under local or general anaesthesia and is usually a day-case procedure up to around 13 weeks of pregnancy. In Scotland in 2002, 65.5% of abortions were performed before 10 weeks gestation and a further 27.5% between 10 and 13 weeks (Information and Statistics Division of the NHS in Scotland, 2004).

The woman is admitted to the hospital or clinic having had nothing to eat or drink for at least 6 hours. The Royal College of Obstetricians and Gynaecologists recommend that cervical preparation with a single vaginal preparation containing prostaglandin, e.g. misoprostol, or other cervical dilation agent is 'beneficial prior to suction termination and should be routine if the woman is aged under 18 years or at a gestation of over ten weeks' (RCOG, 2004). In reality, procedures vary, e.g. some consultants do not do this for a multiparous woman. She is taken to the operating theatre where either local anaesthesia is administered to the cervix (this is not usually offered after 9 weeks of pregnancy) or she has a general anaesthetic. The surgeon then dilates the cervical canal sufficiently to allow insertion of an aspiration cannula into the womb. Vacuum aspiration using negative pressure then removes the pregnancy. The procedure takes approximately 10 minutes and is followed by a 2 hour recovery period prior to being discharged. There is rarely any necessity for the woman to remain at the hospital or clinic overnight, but she will be advised to rest for 24–48 hours afterwards.

There should be no major pain or discomfort following the procedure, but mild analgesia is usually prescribed for uterine cramp or pain, should it occur. On the day of the operation, or the following day, 95% of women will bleed, but this should not be heavier or last longer than a normal menstrual period. If the bleeding becomes heavy or prolonged, the vaginal discharge begins to smell offensive, there is a sudden rise in body temperature or the symptoms of pregnancy persist, the woman should consult a medical practitioner at the hospital or clinic where the abortion took place, her GP practice, or her local accident and emergency department. Routine medical follow-up after the procedure is advisable to establish that a successful recovery has been made and to give the woman the opportunity to ask any questions that are important for her now that the physical process is complete.

Most women feel physically able to resume their usual daily activities 48 hours after the operation. However, emotional recovery can take longer and some individuals might need more time before resuming work, study, childcare etc.

Medical termination of early pregnancy (MTOP)

Since 1991 it has been possible for women in the UK to have medical abortions. Although at present this option is not widely available in the NHS, it is offered by the majority of independent clinics.

In Scotland in 2002, 49.8% of abortions were performed medically, compared with 16.4% in 1992 (Information and Statistics Division of the NHS in Scotland, 2004). The rate in England and Wales however is lower, with only 12.3% of abortions performed medically in 2001 (Office for National Statistics, 2002).

Medical abortion is commonly known as taking 'the abortion pill' or RU 486. This is not a very accurate description as it involves more than simply taking a pill.

For MTOP to be an option a woman must be:

◆ Under 35 years old if she smokes (if over 35 years she must be a non-smoker)

◆ Generally fit and healthy

◆ Her last menstrual period must be less than 63 days prior to treatment.

Having had counselling and medical consultations, the woman is given one tablet of mifepristone 200 mg (Mifegyne) to take whilst at the hospital or clinic. She is then able to go home. Two days later she returns to the hospital or clinic and is given a vaginal preparation containing prostaglandin, e.g. misoprostol, or other cervical dilation agent. Mifepristone acts by blocking the effects of progesterone (a hormone necessary for the continuation of pregnancy), whilst the prostaglandin tablets or other agent causes the cervix to soften and dilate, the uterus to contract and the pregnancy to be expelled.

Having taken the original mifepristone tablet, the woman can spend that day and the following one in her usual way – working in or outside the home. During this time some women may have some bleeding and period-like pains, but it is unlikely that the abortion itself will occur.

When she returns to the hospital or clinic 48 hours later for the vaginal tablet insertion, she will have to remain there until the medical abortion is complete. It will usually take 6-8 hours before vaginal bleeding starts and the process is complete. She is then able to go home.

For many women, being able to continue their usual daily activities having taken the tablets, and the process being complete without the need for anaesthesia or surgical intervention, makes MTOP particularly acceptable. It is a relief for them not to have to wait for, and then undergo, a minor operation, and they usually feel much more in control of what is happening during the abortion than women who have a surgical termination.

Although it seems unlikely to become the treatment of choice for the majority of women seeking abortions, MTOP is a valuable addition to the options available. As with any treatment option, women need to be informed about not only the potential advantages but also of the potential problems with MTOP (Box 9.3).

However, once a woman has been told about these factors, and possible outcomes, she is then free to make an informed choice about whether this particular method of abortion is acceptable to and appropriate for her.

MTOP enables a woman to obtain an abortion in the very early stages of pregnancy and is ideal for a woman who is clear about not wanting to continue her pergnancy. This factor can greatly reduce both the impact of an unwanted pregnancy on day-to-day living and the emotional burden of unwanted pregnancy. It is regarded as a valuable development in women's health care by both the providers and the users of abortion services.

Guidelines from RCOG in 1997 recommended MTOP as the method of choice for women less than 7 weeks pregnant, and that MTOP should be a choice for those between 7 and 9 weeks pregnant. Some centres are now offering MTOPs at gestations from 9 to 12 weeks and Stewart et al. (2003) conclude that this appears to be an acceptable method of termination in the late first trimester.

In 1999 the Family Planning Association and the Population Council held a seminar on induced abortion. In England and Wales, women present later for abortion than in Scotland. As MTOP is only available up to 63 days gestation, this has an obvious impact on providing services and choice for women. The seminar concluded that in order to make MTOP a genuine choice for woman there needs to be:

◆ An increase in women's awareness of MTOP

◆ New training for abortion service providers

◆ A reduction in waiting times for appointments

◆ More flexible procedures, e.g. reducing the number of visits to the clinic

◆ Enthusiastic staff to implement MTOP.

It is hoped that in the future MTOPs may take place at home for carefully selected women. They would be given the mifepristone in hospital and then insert the misoprostol 2 days later at home. The pregnancy would then be expelled at home. In such cases it would be imperative that the woman should be given a contact number in case of problems.

Mid-trimester and late abortion

Mid-trimester abortions are those carried out between 13 and 18 weeks and late abortions are those which take place from 19 weeks onwards. In 2001, 21,495 women in England and Wales had

---

Box 9.3   Potential problems with MTOP

◆ There is a 5% chance that the procedure will be unsuccessful and therefore that a surgical abortion will be necessary

◆ A third of women experience extreme discomfort, having had the vaginal pessary and may require strong analgesia

◆ Sometimes women find seeing the expelled contents of the womb distressing.

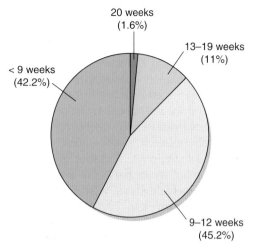

Figure 9.2 Percentage of abortions by gestation weeks, residents of England and Wales, 2002 (Office for National Statistics, 2004).

a mid-trimester or late abortion, accounting for 12.6% of all abortions performed (ONS, 2002) (see Figure 9.2).

For most of these women, for some reason there has been a delay in recognizing their pregnancy (Box 9.4).

However, there are other factors that can contribute to women seeking abortions after 12 weeks of pregnancy:

◆ Lack of access to reproductive health services

◆ Poor access to general health care services

Box 9.4 Reasons for delay in recognizing or acknowledging pregnancy

◆ Young women may be unaware of where to go for help when they first realize they are pregnant, or else may be too frightened or embarrassed to seek help

◆ Older women can assume that missed periods mean the beginning of the menopause rather than the beginning of pregnancy

◆ Sometimes women fail to acknowledge pregnancy because of their precarious or unstable life situations

◆ Women may bleed slightly during early pregnancy and wrongly assume that this is a normal period and not realize they are pregnant. (See Scenario in Chapter 2.)

◆ Unsympathetic GPs (who may refuse to refer a woman for an abortion)

◆ Poor local resources for addressing the needs of a woman with an unplanned pregnancy

◆ Insufficient information about services and options available

◆ Where antenatal screening has detected a fetal abnormality

◆ Where the woman has recently been given medical information about her own health, e.g. positive HIV result or cancer.

The decision to end a pregnancy is one that few women reach easily. Whilst early abortion can be difficult to decide upon and come to terms with, the more advanced a woman's pregnancy, the greater the potential difficulties she is likely to experience – both emotional and physical.

A woman having an abortion because of fetal abnormality is likely to have planned her pregnancy and wanted the baby. The knowledge of a fetal abnormality means that she is faced with difficult and painful decisions: to continue her pregnancy, knowing her baby will be severely mentally and/or physically handicapped and may even die shortly after birth, or to abort this planned and wanted pregnancy and with it all the desires, plans and love that she has attached to it. Whether there is fetal abnormality or not, a woman having a mid-trimester or late abortion has been pregnant for several months and may even have felt the fetus moving inside her uterus. These factors add to the emotional difficulty of deciding to have an abortion as she may feel by this stage she is aborting a baby and not just a pregnancy.

Physical complications arising from abortion increase after 15 weeks of pregnancy (Clayton *et al.*, 1986) and it may not be possible for the abortion to be done as a day-case procedure, so a longer stay may be required in the hospital or clinic.

Having had counselling and medical consultations and decided that she wishes to proceed with an abortion, the woman will be admitted to the hospital or clinic. All of the standard preoperative tests will have been carried out prior to admission, together with a pelvic ultrasound scan to establish the precise gestation of her pregnancy. There are two procedures for performing mid-trimester and late abortions: dilatation and evacuation (D and E) and medical abortion with mifepristone and prostaglandins.

Dilatation and evacuation (D and E)

Prior to going to the operating theatre the woman is given a cervical preparation to soften her cervix, thereby making dilation easier. Once she has been given a general anaesthetic the surgeon gently dilates the cervix and then the contents of the womb are evacuated. When this procedure is carried out, the surgeon is careful to ensure that all fetal and placental material is removed as retained products can cause haemorrhage and infection. This procedure may be followed by an overnight recovery period at the hospital or clinic. As long as postoperative complications do not develop, follow-up can be with the woman's GP or local reproductive health clinic.

Complications can occur at the time of surgery from tearing of the cervix (although this is less of a problem with the use of cervical preparations) or perforation of the uterus; and postoperatively, due to retained products of conception or infection. In the longer term, damage to the cervix during the operation can lead to cervical incompetence during future pregnancies, thus increasing the risk of miscarriage.

The procedure for mid-trimester and late abortion varies from district to district and hospital to hospital. There are some gynaecologists who are willing (and, more importantly, skilled enough) to perform mid-trimester and late abortions vaginally, whilst the woman is under general anaesthesia. For the majority of women this is understandably the treatment of choice. However, this procedure requires considerable skill on the part of the surgeon and particular dedication on the part of all staff working in the operating theatre. Whilst it may make the process easier for the pregnant woman, these late surgical abortions can undoubtedly be far more demanding and distressing for healthcare staff to witness.

To avoid this stress for health professionals there has been a growing trend for some units to perform medical terminations up to 20 weeks of pregnancy, although mifepristone is not licensed for use this late is pregnancy.

Late medical abortion

A late medical abortion may be performed on a young woman in the second trimester of pregnancy (whose cervix is soft and therefore more susceptible to tearing and damage), or an older woman whose pregnancy is advanced by more than 18 weeks.

The following regimen, although unlicensed, is optimal for mid-trimester medical abortion: mifeprisone 200 mg orally followed 36–48 hours later by multiple doses (vaginal or oral) of prostaglandin (RCOG 2004).

Observations of pulse, blood pressure, uterine contractions and cervical dilation are maintained. Analgesia is offered if the woman finds the process painful or too uncomfortable, and she will usually be offered fluids orally.

It is not possible to predict for an individual woman how long it will take before the prostaglandin causes uterine contractions strong enough to expel the pregnancy. However, most women are expected to abort within 12–20 hours. If there is any concern that there may be retained products of conception she may be taken to the operating theatre for an evacuation of the uterus under general anaesthesia.

Some centres aim to start early morning so that the woman aborts by late afternoon or evening. Following this she will have a recovery period at the hospital or clinic before being discharged. As with surgical abortion, routine follow-up can be with her GP or reproductive health clinic.

Post-abortion follow-up

Many women choose follow-up care with their GP practice or reproductive health clinic rather than returning to the hospital or clinic where they had their abortion. This may be because a woman prefers to be seen by someone she knows in familiar surroundings. Alternatively there may be reasons for her not wanting to return to the place where her abortion was carried out:

◆ If she felt she was treated unsympathetically or disrespectfully it is unlikely she would wish to return

◆ If the process was painful, complicated or distressing she may be reluctant to seek further care from that source

◆ If the hospital or clinic was a great distance or difficult to reach from her home it may be impractical for her to return.

Conversely, a woman who has had a positive experience with staff and an uncomplicated treatment from a local service may also be unwilling to return for follow-up care. She may find it just too painful to return to the building where her abortion was performed and she may fear either the memories it could evoke, or being overwhelmed by sadness or grief. She may also dread a re-emergence of the physical symptoms of pregnancy, or even a temporary desire to still be pregnant; whilst for a woman for whom the decision to have an abortion was particularly difficult, going back to the hospital or clinic could be like 'returning to the scene of the crime'.

So for all these reasons, and more, you may find yourself in your clinical setting being responsible for the follow-up care of a woman who has recently had an abortion. Of course her physical recovery or lack of it is a medical matter, but by asking about her health, whether the post-abortion bleeding has stopped, and if the symptoms of pregnancy have abated, you could help to establish whether or not further medical intervention is necessary. If it seems clear that her pregnancy has ended and that there are no physical complications following the abortion, you could then ask the woman how she is feeling generally. For some women, this invitation to speak about how they are feeling is a vital aspect of follow-up care. It may also be the first time anyone has asked her how she is feeling.

A woman who has postoperative complications may feel physically unwell, confused and angry. She may not understand what is happening and could believe that her physical complications are due to something she has done, or failed to do. The opportunity to talk about her feelings and to have the necessary explanations about the problems she is experiencing, and their treatment, is extremely valuable.

No matter how clear a woman feels about her decision to have an abortion, post-operative complications often give rise to feelings of guilt and self-doubt. 'Did I do the right thing?' 'Is this my punishment for having an abortion?' 'Am I still pregnant?' are all questions that a woman may repeatedly ask herself, and ask you. They are not questions you should attempt to answer (except perhaps the one about remaining pregnant) but you should allow the woman the opportunity to talk about her own responses to her questions. For example, how does she judge whether or not she did the right thing, and what does that judgement mean for her? Or, if she does feel she is being punished for having an abortion, why does she think she should be punished, and by whom? It is through exploring the meaning of her questions with her (as opposed to giving your own answers to them) that the woman will be able to find an emotional context in which to place her experience of abortion.

Whether she has complications or not, a woman may find it extremely helpful to discuss her feelings after having an abortion (even though she may not request, or require, formal post-abortion counselling). An appointment for a post-abortion medical check, for contraceptive supplies or a cervical smear can all provide an opportunity for you to discuss with her whatever feelings about her abortion she may have.

In the days immediately afterwards many women feel extremely sad and tearful and often talk about feelings of emptiness, or of feeling nothing. In talking with these women, you may discover that in their own individual ways they are engaged in the process of mourning. Freud in 1915 wrote that when we suffer a loss we mourn, and mourning involves feelings of loss, grief and sadness, losing interest in the world around us, being preoccupied with whatever (or whoever) is lost and constantly seeking its (or their) return. The statement that 'Those who mourn may mimic madness to the observer's eye', aptly expresses not only the feelings of the woman who is mourning, but also those of people who come into contact with her at this time. Yet this is no madness. The fact that abortion is a loss which the woman has chosen in no way mitigates her feelings of loss and sadness. The emotional well-being of each one of us is dependent upon being able to mourn during times of loss (see also page 106). It is a slow, painful process, but for most it reaches an end, and the woman is able to resume day-to-day living, having ceased to mourn.

Sadly, for some grief does go wrong, and mourning can become depression. If a woman is still struggling with feelings of loss and grief many weeks or even months after her abortion, she should be offered referral to a formal counselling service. This will give her the opportunity to discuss her feelings with someone who is trained for this work, and able to offer the time and support she requires.

Of course, it may not always be immediately obvious that a woman is having emotional difficulties following an abortion, but these difficulties may be expressed in other ways. For example, a woman may be reluctant to have a pelvic examination or a cervical smear taken. She may not come for, or may cease requesting, contraceptive supplies, and she may become overanxious about vaginal infections or pelvic pain and discomfort. Sensitive questioning may reveal that she is having problems maintaining a sexual relationship (or has even stopped any kind of sexual activity altogether) since her abortion. At the time of requesting an abortion, or immediately afterwards, it is very common for a woman to say she does not want contraceptive supplies because she does not ever intend having sexual intercourse again. Happily, for most women this is not an intention that endures! For those who have not felt able to resume sexual relationships, referral to a counselling service may be the most appropriate and helpful form of treatment.

In the longer term, unresolved grief and sadness about an abortion may re-emerge during a later pregnancy; at the time of her first child's birth; pre- or post-hysterectomy; during the menopause; and following a daughter's pregnancy, abortion or first child being born. A woman receiving treatment for gynaecological cancer may have her recovery impeded by unresolved feelings about a previous abortion or abortions. She might have unconscious thoughts that she is being punished, or that she was damaged in some way by the abortion procedure. Such thoughts can be deeply troubling to her, especially if she has not had children at the time of her diagnosis and treatment. The anniversary of her abortion, or the expected birthday of her potential baby, are dates a woman may remember many years later and, in some cases, for the rest of her life.

This may mean that a woman attending a reproductive health clinic, an antenatal clinic, a well-woman clinic or GP surgery may need the issue of past abortion to be addressed, regardless of how long ago it was, and of her age and her current reason for attending the clinic. The fact that unresolved grief does not go away (thus a woman may continue to suffer many years later) means that the grief is accessible, can be worked with and the woman helped. Your awareness of this, together with sensitive picking up on clues about sexual difficulties, depression, etc., can be the first step toward a woman being able to overcome her difficulties following an abortion – no matter how long after this may be.

Professional dilemmas

If for personal, religious or ethical reasons you feel unable to actively participate in the care of a woman undergoing an abortion you still have a professional responsibility to ensure that the woman receives the nursing care and help she requires (Royal College of Nursing, 1997).

Abortion is always a regrettable and sober matter, for pregnant women and health care professionals alike. It is undertaken for reasons that are considered and deeply personal for the woman concerned, and believed to be authentic and proper by those providing abortion services. However, there are some circumstances where you may feel the understandable dilemmas about abortion to be greater than usual (Box 9.5).

Chapter 2 discusses an ethical dilemma regarding a woman who presented for a late abortion.

Repeat abortions

Women who have repeated abortions present perhaps the greatest challenge of all. You may feel angry at what you believe to be their irresponsibility, frustrated because they fail to use adequate contraception and distressed because there appears to be little that you (or anyone else) can do to help them avoid unwanted pregnancy.

One unwanted pregnancy may be considered a mistake, two seen as unfortunate but, after that, compassion and empathy often begin to run out. It is even believed that women who have several abortions may simply be using abortion as a form of contraception. Sadly for the minority of women (and in the UK they are a minority) who present for repeat abortions, little in their lives tends to be simple.

Some women have repeat abortions because they have repeated failures with contraception. The pill does not suit them, the IUD caused pelvic problems, they conceived whilst using the diaphragm, their partner is allergic to latex, etc. It is a regrettable fact that in the twenty-first century we still do not have safe, effective contraception that is suitable for every woman who wants it.

Other women have repeat abortions because each time they become pregnant their relationship founders and they do not feel able to continue a pregnancy unsupported. Some women conceive as a result of forced intercourse within an abusive relationship. They did not want or plan to have sexual intercourse and therefore were not using (or were prevented from using)

contraception. There are also women who repeatedly become pregnant because they never use contraception, and who then go on to have abortions because they have no wish to have a baby or to be a mother. The desire to be pregnant (whether conscious or unconscious) is not necessarily the same as the desire to have a baby and to be a mother. Whilst acknowledging and understanding this difference is a complex and difficult process, it is worth while remembering that for some women this difference does exist.

Another reason why some women repeatedly become pregnant whilst not using contraception is that for them life is chaotic and a constant struggle. Taking control in any area of their lives may feel impossible and that often includes control of their fertility. There is no single reason why women are willing to risk pregnancy but have no wish to have a baby, or why chaos and struggle are the ruling forces of women's lives. What individuals in these situations need is skilled help to enable them to begin to understand what their repeat pregnancies and abortions may mean. Through understanding what is being expressed by her actions, a woman will hopefully be enabled to discover that she can make other choices, including the choice to control her fertility or to allow herself to become a mother.

Whilst it may not be possible for you to address these complex issues, an awareness of them (together with an effort to see the woman you are working with as an individual whose personal and unique life experiences have brought her into your care) may enhance your capacity to engage professionally with a woman requesting repeat abortions.

Under-16s

When a young woman who is not yet 16 becomes pregnant there are legal considerations as well as medical ones that have to be taken into account. Legally, a young woman under 16 cannot become pregnant. In reality sexual activity may begin long before they are 16 and, unfortunately, this may result in an unplanned pregnancy. Before any decisions are made about her pregnancy a young woman should be offered counselling with a trained counsellor. The paradox of a 'child' making a decision about an 'adult' predicament has to be accepted by the counsellor, and the wishes of the young woman must be seen as paramount. It may take several counselling sessions before the fear, confusion and distress felt by the young woman can be worked through. At all times her right to confidentiality must be respected (unless a child protection issue is suspected) and she should be assured that contact will not be made with parents/guardian, GP or anyone else, without her consent.

The circumstances in which she became pregnant, whether she has a regular partner and what support (if any) she currently has, must all be addressed, together with what it is she wants to do now that she is pregnant. Every pregnant woman has the right to choose whether to continue her pregnancy or to have an abortion, and this right applies equally to those under 16. If the wishes of her parents/guardian conflict with her own, then the counselling process must address this. If she does not want her parents/guardian to know about her pregnancy and decides to have an abortion, this can be legally carried out as long as the medical practitioner is satisfied that she/he has done all that is possible to encourage parental involvement, and that the young woman is mature enough to understand the consequences of her choice and the abortion procedure.

Young women often present later in pregnancy (see page 209), and therefore clear information about what abortion entails and what to expect afterwards is an important aspect of care. This may be part of the role you are called upon to fulfil, so ensure you have all the necessary information to hand when seeing her. Ask if there are any questions she wishes to ask and do not be afraid to check whether she feels she has had enough time to discuss things with a counsellor, doctor or anyone else involved in her care. It may be worth while suggesting that she asks a parent/guardian, partner or friend to go with her to the hospital or clinic, and encourage them to ask questions on her behalf, if necessary.

The experience of pregnancy and abortion may leave a young woman feeling different to and separate from her peer group and thus unable to utilize her usual support network. Therefore, a follow-up appointment is an important opportunity for her to be able to discuss her feelings. If you are offering the follow-up care, be aware that young women do not mourn or grieve any less than older women, and that because they have returned to school or college after an abortion it does not mean that life is 'back to normal'.

A young woman may feel she has to protect her family, friends and others from her grief, or else she may feel so guilty and embarrassed herself that she does not want others to see her emotions. A follow-up appointment allows you to establish whether she is physically and emotionally well after her abortion, as well as to address the important issue of future contraception. If you do not feel that the service in which you work is able to meet the needs of a young woman pre- and post-abortion, she can always be referred to a dedicated young person's reproductive health service (see Resources).

Finally, it can be very difficult to work with a pregnant under-16-year-old, particularly if you have teenage children yourself. Parental emotions may take over and you find yourself asking 'What would I do in this situation?' or feeling that 'I'd want to know', 'I'd want to help'. However, it is not as a parent that this young woman is seeking your help but as a professional upon whose skills and objectivity she is depending. If you find the conflict between your experience as a parent and your professional role too great, you should not attempt to work with this young woman. Referring her to someone else at the initial stages will be the best thing for both of you.

Women who are HIV positive

It is not within the scope of this chapter to address all the health issues relating to a woman being HIV positive; however, a brief consideration of some issues concerning pregnancy is appropriate.

When a woman who is HIV positive has an unplanned pregnancy, she faces all the dilemmas that any other woman in this situation may experience, but, in addition, her pregnancy raises issues concerning her own health and the health of her baby (if she decides to continue her pregnancy).

Every woman who has an unplanned pregnancy has a right to receive the help and support relevant to her, to enable her to make a decision about her pregnancy. A woman who is HIV positive may assume (and may find that others assume) that she has to have an abortion, and therefore that there is no decision-making process to be gone through. This assumption is not justified on medical grounds, and it is likely to inhibit the pregnant woman's exploration of her thoughts and feelings about her pregnancy. A woman who is HIV positive may need your time and support, in the same way any other woman with an unplanned pregnancy does. However, if she has specific concerns about the effects of pregnancy upon herself, and her potential baby, she should be referred to specialist services.

A woman who is HIV positive may already be in contact with health professionals, and may wish to seek information and support from them, as part of the decision-making process in relation to pregnancy. In addition there are self-help groups and organizations that she could contact.

Whilst an important factor in the decision-making process, a positive HIV status should not be seen by you as *the* issue in your work with this woman. Like any other woman with an unplanned pregnancy, she may be shocked, distressed, need time to think and need to speak with a partner, family or friends (as well as needing sound impartial medical information) before a decision can be made. Moreover, like every other pregnant woman, the decision whether (or not) to continue the pregnancy must be hers.

Abortion following subfertility treatment

Occasionally, a woman who has been receiving treatment for subfertility problems will become pregnant, only to request an abortion. Whatever her personal reasons for this request, it is clearly an indication that something, somewhere is wrong.

It may be that in the months or years since treatment began her desire in relation to having a baby has lessened or ceased. The idea of pregnancy and motherhood may have been attractive but the reality much less so. A woman may become pregnant with someone other than her regular partner and, in spite of her desire for a child, feel unable to continue this particular pregnancy. The pregnancy may have occurred at a time when she was relinquishing all hope of pregnancy or when she (or her partner) were about to change jobs, home, country of residence, or face some similar major life upheaval.

Whatever the reason for her abortion request the woman must also reassess her desire for future pregnancy. If the probability of future conception is low, is abortion the right thing for her? Once the forthcoming life-events have taken place, is not being pregnant going to be what she wants? Do she and her partner need to reassess their desire for a child? Should she continue with fertility treatment? Addressing these issues while she is still pregnant will enable the woman to make a clear informed choice about this particular pregnancy and about future treatment and conception.

Liaison with the hospital or clinic that she attends for fertility treatment may be valuable for her, as could joint appointments for her and her partner. It may take more than one appointment before she (or they) can begin to think clearly about her current situation and the implications of her request for an abortion. Do not hesitate, therefore, to offer more than one appointment with you or, if you feel her particular situation requires more formal help, to suggest referral for counselling.

Fertility treatment is about becoming pregnant; abortion is about ceasing to be pregnant. For a woman who is in receipt of the former to be requesting the latter, indicates that somewhere between the two, things have become very confused. Your willingness to recognize this and the offer of time for discussion could enable a woman to begin to address, and perhaps resolve, some of that confusion.

Abortion for fetal abnormality

A woman who has decided to have an abortion because of fetal abnormality is likely to be in the second or third trimester of her pregnancy. She is also probably choosing to abort a pregnancy that was planned and a baby that was wanted. This can only add to the difficulties and distress involved in reaching the decision to have an abortion.

Where there is a known risk of abnormality or hereditary life-threatening disease a woman and her partner may have received genetic counselling. However, this does not mean that the emotional aspects of abortion will have been addressed. Knowing the risks involved and the chances of carrying a healthy pregnancy to term does not make the choices a woman faces any easier, or mean that an abortion has been prepared for. You should be aware that this may not be the first time this woman has become pregnant, only to be told that her pregnancy is not healthy and thus decided to have an abortion.

In addition to the guilt she may feel for wanting to 'keep on trying' to have a healthy baby, a woman also has to deal with the loss of her unhealthy ones. This loss is not only physical but is also a loss of her hopes, her plans and of her 'family' – that she may in fact never have. For all women pregnancy is a symbolic as well as a physical and emotional experience. The symbolism of a deformed, disabled or diseased baby is extremely powerful and distressing and, for a woman who may never be able to have the healthy baby or family she desires, it may feel symbolic of a whole aspect of her life, and of herself.

The fact that a woman at risk of having a pregnancy with a fetal abnormality may be seen in designated antenatal clinics or diagnostic units does not mean that she is any less in need of your skilled help than other women before or after an abortion. Indeed, she may greatly value the opportunity to speak with someone whom she may see as being less focused on the process of testing and diagnosis, and therefore more able to discuss feelings, rather than facts, about her pregnancy.

Fostering and adoption

An unplanned pregnancy may be unwanted but unwanted pregnancy does not always result in abortion. For many reasons a woman may not wish, or feel able, to care for a baby but she may also know that abortion is not an option for her. Continuing pregnancy to term and giving up the baby for fostering or adoption is a choice few women make since the Abortion Act became law. It does, however, remain an option that is open to women with an unplanned pregnancy and for some it is the choice they make.

A woman considering continuing her pregnancy and then having her baby fostered or adopted needs to ask questions and to know facts. Therefore, it is vital that she discusses these options with social workers, childcare and legal professionals. She needs to know what the process involves, what her rights are throughout (and afterwards, in relation to her child), and how to halt the process once it has begun, should she so choose.

Having an infant fostered or adopted is a serious step to take. A woman may not realize that she is ultimately relinquishing all her rights in relation to her child and she needs time to consider the impact of this choice upon her own life, as well as her child's.

In your work with women with unplanned pregnancy, fostering and adoption are options that you should bear in mind and may perhaps choose to raise with some women. Any woman who then wishes to give serious consideration to these choices should be referred to the appropriate agencies and charities in the first instance (to ensure that she gets adequate accurate information), and then to the appropriate professionals.

When working with older women across the spectrum of women's health care, it is important to remember that any one of them who had an unplanned pregnancy before the 1967 Abortion Act may have had a baby adopted, not out of choice but rather because there was no other option available at that time. For these women grief about their lost – usually first – child is often compounded by the awfulness of not knowing anything about their son or daughter – where they are or who they have become. A woman who has had this experience may be in no less need of help than a woman who has had an abortion.

Contraception

Any woman requesting an abortion does so because she feels unwilling or unable to continue her pregnancy and/or care for a baby. With the possible exception of women who have been raped and those for whom fetal abnormality was detected, this usually means that the woman neither wishes to be pregnant at the present time nor in the near future. In order that she receives complete care at this time the issue of contraception must be addressed.

It can be advantageous if a woman has been able to decide on her future contraception before she has her abortion. If she would like an intrauterine device or an intrauterine system, many clinics will fit these at the time of the abortion thus saving the woman having another gynaecological procedure. If the injection is chosen, this can be administered before she leaves the clinic or if she requests the pill then a supply can be given in advance so that she can start taking it immediately. Initiating contraception so promptly can make some women feel more in control of a situation where they had previously felt powerless.

At what stage this issue is raised, and by whom, is a moot point, and it would be inappropriate to lay down hard and fast rules, as clearly contraception is not just a practical matter. The circumstances in which a woman became pregnant, how she feels about her decision for an abortion and the existence (or not) of a current sexual relationship will all affect her thoughts and feelings about contraception. It would be negligent in the extreme for contraception not to be discussed at some point during the process of confirming an unplanned pregnancy and having an abortion. However, for the individual woman the appropriate time for this discussion varies greatly.

Before the decision about her pregnancy has been made, when she is emotionally distraught, or immediately before or after the abortion procedure, are times when a discussion about contraception is wholly inappropriate. At any other stage of the process the issue may be raised, and not infrequently it is the woman herself who raises it. Deciding on a method of contraception means that clear information must be available, together with specialist help and advice (see Chapter 11). If it is a professional who raises the issue, this should always be at a time appropriate to the individual woman and in the form of an offer of help (as opposed to a requirement of the referral to the hospital or clinic, or the abortion being carried out). For whilst it is an essential aspect of her care at this time, it is one which needs to be approached with sensitivity and skill.

Conclusion

An unplanned pregnancy can cause confusion and despair in pregnant women and health care professionals alike. Pregnant women may despair of ever getting the support and care that they need; the professionals may feel confused by their emotional response to this situation, and wonder what help they can usefully give. Yet a willingness by you, the professional, to reflect honestly upon your own feelings whilst allowing those of the pregnant woman to be central can enable this confusion and despair to be transformed. Using your skills to facilitate the woman's thinking and speaking about the dilemma she is currently facing, and ensuring that she has all the factual information she wants, can bring relief and promote well-being where previously there seemed to be only pain and anguish.

An awareness of the practical issues, together with a determination to avoid assumptions, decision-making on the woman's behalf and judgements about her and her situation, can facilitate a potentially disastrous life-experience becoming one that is negotiated without long-term suffering. It can be a demanding area of work, and you should refer on without hesitation if the impact upon you feels too great, or the situation too complex. Yet it is also a field where your skills are invaluable, and using them can be a rewarding and fulfilling experience for you; whilst for your patient, the efforts made on her behalf bring benefits both profound and enduring.

Ideas for personal and professional development

- Find out about your local TOP services. What is offered, how do women access the service and are there any restrictions within the service?

- Where are specialist services located, e.g. for young women or women who are HIV positive? Familiarize yourself with access information and, if possible, identify a named contact within the service with whom you could liaise

- Be aware that a past TOP may be a painful issue which affects women's emotional response to pelvic examination, pregnancy, menopause, fertility and other health problems

- Think about your own thoughts and emotional responses to TOP and pregnancy. Is it a difficult area of work for you? If so, can you identify why? If it is a subject you feel very passionately about can you explore that, either alone or with colleagues?

Patient education points

- There are lots of myths and misinformation about TOP. Ensure women have accurate and relevant information prior to, and after, the procedure

- Similarly, women may wrongly assume they cannot continue a pregnancy (too old/young; taking medication; not entitled to maternity benefits; etc.). Ensure individual women have appropriate and accurate information relevant to their needs

- Check that contraceptive issues have been sensitively and relevantly addressed. Some women do not have good information; others do not understand their menstrual cycle and fertility issues

- Help is available. Make sure women know whom to contact if they suspect they are pregnant or if they want to arrange a TOP, post-TOP counselling or other psychological support.

Resources

Charitable abortion services

British Pregnancy Advisory Service
Austy Manor, Wootton Wawen, Solihull, West Midlands B95 6BX
Tel: 01564 793225
Actionline (local rate): 08457 304030
www.bpas.org

Marie Stopes
153–157 Cleveland Street, London WIP 5PG
Central booking (local rate): 0845 3001212
Freephone: 0800 716 390
www.mariestopes.org.uk

Counselling and advisory services (A = advice; C = counselling)

Belfast Family Planning Association (C)
Tel: 02890 325488

Breakthrough for Women (C)
4th Floor, 30 Bell Street, Glasgow G1 1LG
Tel: 0141 552 5483
Provides pregnancy counselling and post-abortion counselling.

British Association for Counselling and Psychotherapy (A and C)
35-37 Albert Street, Coventry CV1 2SG
Tel: 0870 443 5252
www.bacp.co.uk
(Send SAE for information on local services.)

Irish Family Planning Association (C)
5–7 Cathal Brugah Street, Dublin 1
Tel: 00351 8780366

United Kingdom Council for Psychotherapy (C)
167–169 Great Portland Street, London W1N 5FB
Tel: 020 7436 3002
www.psychotherapy.org.uk
Can provide details of registered psychoanalysts and psychotherapists throughout the UK.

Women's Health (A)
52–54 Featherstone Street, London EC1Y 8RT

Tel: 020 7251 6333
Health enquiry line: 020 7251 6580
www.womenshealthlondon.org.uk
Publications, consultancy, health advice and
telephone support.

Young people's services

Brook Advisory Centres
National Office Tel: 0800 0185023
Helpline: 020 7617 8000 24-hour recorded
information helpline
www.brook.org.uk
Will provide details of local clinics nationwide
providing contraception, abortion advice,
counselling and health information.

Rape crisis centres

Rape Crisis Centre
www.rapecrisis.co.uk
Details of rape crisis centres throughout
the UK.

Rape and Sexual Abuse Group
PO Box 908, London SE25 5EL
Tel: 020 8239 1122
Helpline staffed Monday–Friday 12.00–14.30
and 19.00–21.00; Saturday, Sunday and
Bank Holidays 14.30–17.00

Fetal abnormality

Antenatal Results and Choices (ARC)
73–75 Charlotte Street, London W1P 1LB
Tel: 020 7631 0280/0285
Pre-and post-abortion advice and support.

Adoption and fostering

British Agencies for Adoption and Fostering
Skyline House, 200 Union Street,
London SE1 0LX
Tel: 020 7593 2000
Information about adoption and fostering and
details of agencies nationwide.

Post Adoption Centre
5 Torriano Mews, Torriano Avenue,
London NW5 2RZ
Tel: 020 7284 0555

Support for continuing pregnancy

Department of Social Security
Freephone: 0800 666 555
Confidential information and advice about
welfare benefits.

Gingerbread
7 Sovereign Close, Sovereign Court, London
E1W 3HW
Tel: 020 7488 9300
www.gingerbread.org.uk
Self-help groups for one-parent families
plus information about groups
nationwide.

Life
5 Goodwins Court, off St Martin's Lane,
London WC2N 4LL
Tel: 020 7240 1275
www.lifeuk.org
An anti-abortion agency that offers free
counselling and advice to women who are
willing to continue their pregnancy.
Centres nationwide.

National Childbirth Trust
Alexandra House, Oldham Terrace,
London W3 6NH
Tel: 0870 7703236
Enquiries: 0870 4448707
www.nct-online.org
Antenatal classes, postnatal support groups,
information, advice and counselling.
Nationwide groups.

**National Council for One Parent
Families**
255 Kentish Town Road, London NW5 2LX
Tel: 020 7428 8707
www.oneparentfamilies.org.uk
Information and advice on housing,
welfare benefits and all other aspects
of single parenthood.

One Parent Families, Scotland
13 Gayfield Square, Edinburgh EH1 3NX
Tel: 0131 556 3899
Helpline: 0800 018 5026
www. opfs.org.uk

Further reading

FREED, L. and SALAZAR, P.Y. (2001). *A Season To Heal: Help and Hope For Those Dealing With Post-Abortion Stress.* Nashville: Cumberland House Publishing.

MUNDIGO, A. and INDRISO, C. (1998) *Abortion In The Developing World.* London: Zed Books.

STOTLAND, N.L. (1998). *Abortion: Facts and Feelings – A Handbook For Women and the People Who Care About Them.* Arlington: American Psychiatric Publishing.

References

CHANCE, J. *et al.* (1947) *Backstreet Abortion?* London: Abortion Law Reform Association.

CLAYTON, S.G., LEWIS, T.L.T. and PINKER, G.D. (eds) (1986) *Gynaecology by Ten Teachers.* London: Edward Arnold.

DoH (Department of Health) (1998) *Confidential Enquiries into Maternal Deaths 1994–96.* London: The Stationery Office.

FERRIMAN, A. (1999) Medical abortion still not available in most countries. *British Medical Journal* **319**:1091.

FRANCOME, C. (1977) Estimating the number of illegal abortions. *Journal of Biosocial Science* **9**(4):467–79.

FREUD, S. (1915) *Mourning and Melancholia,* Standard edition Vol XIV. London: Hogarth Press.

HFEA (Human Fertilization and Embryology Authority) (1990) *Human Fertilization and Embryology Act 1990.* London: HMSO.

INFORMATION AND STATISTICS DIVISION OF THE NATIONAL HEALTH SERVICE IN SCOTLAND (2004) *Abortion Statistics* 2002. www.isdscotland.org.

OFFICE FOR NATIONAL STATISTICS (2002) *Abortion Statistics: Legal Abortions Carried Out Under the 1967 Abortion Act in England and Wales, 2001, Series AB no. 28.* London: The Stationery Office.

OFFICE FOR NATIONAL STATISTICS (2004) *Health Statistics Quarterly,* Spring 2004. London: The Stationery Office.

ROYAL COLLEGE OF NURSING (1997) *Guidelines on the Termination of Pregnancy.* London: RCN.

ROYAL COLLEGE OF OBSTETRICIANS AND GYNAECOLOGISTS (1997) *Induced Abortion, Guideline no. 11.* London: RCOG.

ROYAL COLLEGE OF OBSTETRICIANS AND GYNAECOLOGISTS (2000) *The Care of Women Requesting Induced Abortion, National Evidence-Based Clinical Guidelines no. 7.* London: RCOG.

ROYAL COLLEGE OF OBSTETRICIANS AND GYNAECOLOGISTS (2004) *The Care of Women Requesting Induced Abortion: Evidence-Based Clinical Guidelines no. 7.* London: RCOG Press.

STEWART, P., FLETCHER, J. and SHARMA, A. (2003) Medical termination of pregnancy in the late first trimester. *Journal of Family Planning and Reproductive Health Care* **29**(4): 243–4.

10: The Management of Subfertility

Mary Power

OBJECTIVES

This chapter should help you understand:

◆ The many causes of subfertility ◆

◆ The investigations required to establish a cause ◆

◆ The many complex assisted reproduction techniques that are available ◆

◆ How the stress of subfertility can affect a relationship. ◆

Introduction

Couples are classified as subfertile if pregnancy has not occurred after one year of regular, unprotected intercourse. About one in six couples seek specialist help because of difficulty in conceiving, although this figure includes some trying for a second pregnancy (Hull *et al.*, 1985; Randall and Templeton, 1991).

As women become older their fertility decreases, and as they are born with their eggs already *in situ* in their ovaries, a woman of 40 years is therefore releasing eggs that are also 40 years old. These eggs may be of poor quality, with reduced capacity for fertilization and implantation. Sperm, on the other hand, are being produced all of the time from puberty and generally take about 3 months to mature; thus men tend to remain fertile until a much later age.

In general, human fertility is relatively inefficient, largely being a matter of chance. Like trying to throw a six with a dice, you may be lucky first time but there is no guarantee that you will succeed, even after many attempts. Therefore, many couples who have been trying to conceive for only a year or two actually have normal fertility and will eventually conceive without help. Some 80–90% of fertile couples will have

achieved a pregnancy after 12 months, and 95% will have done so within two years (Cooke *et al.*, 1981; Vessey *et al.*, 1986). Others will have a real cause for their subfertility, however, and therefore all deserve to be investigated. It is thought that one-third of subfertility problems are attributed to the female, one-third to the male and one-third to both of them.

Subfertile couples are under tremendous pressure and are by nature secretive, considering their problems to be very personal. This is exacerbated by the fact that some of them suffer from unexplained subfertility, which probably constitutes between 20 and 25% of all cases of subfertility. This lack of explanation can become a nightmare for both the couple and their clinician. Thus the couple, desperate for a baby, are often beset by feelings of inadequacy and guilt and many are subjected to pressures from both family and friends. They frequently have to endure comments from relatives and colleagues such as, 'So, when are you going to start a family?' and are often unsupported in coping with the emotional trauma of such remarks. As their problem becomes more long-standing they may begin to blame one another, with consequent marital disharmony. Subfertility, therefore, is not only a physical disease but also a social one, affecting both individuals and society in general.

223

Normal physiology

Semen needs to be ejaculated close to the cervix. Sperm penetrate the cervical mucus, leaving the seminal fluid behind in the vagina. The sperm are stored in the mucus in the cervical canal for a day or two, and released in a steady stream to swim towards the Fallopian tube to meet the egg. When the egg follicle in the ovary is fully grown it ruptures to release the egg, which had previously been loosely attached to cells lining the follicle. The egg is picked up by the finger-like fimbria of the tube and is guided along the tube between the folds of its lining, which has microscopic cilia which beat towards the uterus.

Fertilization of egg and sperm occurs within the tube, and the newly fertilized egg, now called an embryo, begins to divide and subdivide into 2, 4, 8 cells, etc. It remains in the tube for several days before reaching the uterus and, once there, it begins to implant itself in the endometrium, approximately 7 days after ovulation. Following implantation, the embryo is then able to grow in size.

Soon after implantation, the hormone HCG (human chorionic gonadotrophin) from the embryo can enter the woman's bloodstream and so stimulates the ovarian follicle (now called a corpus luteum) to continue functioning and producing the hormone progesterone. This in turn continues to support the endometrium and prevents menstruation occurring, at which time a pregnancy test can detect the presence of HCG.

Causes of subfertility (Figure 10.1)

Female problems

Female problems may be due to failure to produce eggs, or irregular release of eggs from the ovary. Abnormal or blocked Fallopian tubes, endometriosis or hostile cervical mucus are other frequent causes of subfertility.

Ovulation

Overall, ovulatory problems are the commonest cause of subfertility. These usually arise as a

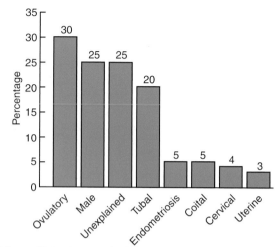

Figure 10.1 Causes of subfertility. Note that the numbers do not add up to 100% because some couples will have more than one cause. Source: The Lister Hospital.

result of hormonal imbalance either within the hypothalamus, the pituitary gland or in the ovaries. Common causes of this include stress, excessive exercise, weight loss, excessive prolactin production and polycystic ovarian disease.

Follicular development in the ovary is dependent upon the pituitary gland secreting the hormone FSH (follicle-stimulating hormone). If the pituitary gland is failing, for whatever reason, then follicular development will cease. This could be due to pituitary tumours or, very rarely, to pituitary infarction following postpartum haemorrhage.

Polycystic ovarian disease is a common condition in which there are a number of small cysts on the surface of the ovary, and also a hormonal imbalance. It is associated with absent or irregular periods, but may also occur in women with a normal menstrual cycle. It has been estimated that approximately 22% of women with regular menstrual cycles have polycystic ovaries and, in fact, about 85% of women with irregular periods will have polycystic ovaries, and 93% of those with hirsutism as well as irregular periods will suffer from polycystic ovarian disease.

The major problem with polycystic ovaries is that instead of one dominant follicle developing, multiple small follicles try to develop but none of them reach maturity. This is associated with an increased level of the hormone LH (luteinizing hormone). There could also be an elevation in the level of the male hormone testosterone. This condition is associated with infrequent ovulation, poor quality oocytes and a higher miscarriage rate.

Ovarian failure affects 1% of the female population under the age of 40 years. This condition could be primary ovarian failure, as in Turner's syndrome, or ovarian dysgenesis, in which a woman is born without any ovarian function. These women are normally diagnosed early in life as there will be no secondary sexual development. Secondary ovarian failure may be due to a premature menopause or may occur following surgery (bilateral oophorectomy), chemotherapy or radiotherapy.

Women with anovulatory subfertility may present with amenorrhoea (primary or secondary), anovulatory menses (oligomenorrhoea or irregular cycles) or luteal insufficiency, with regular menstrual cycles but low or undetectable serum progesterone in the luteal phase. The causes of ovulatory failure are summarized in Box 10.1.

Tubal blockage

Tubal blockage can occur as a result of any infection which ascends into the Fallopian tubes, or which descends to the tubes from other sites in the peritoneal cavity, such as the appendix. It will also arise as a result of sterilization procedures.

The Fallopian tubes have a delicate internal structure which, if damaged, may impede the transport of the egg, thus preventing fertilization. If the fimbrial end of the tube is affected, the pick-up of the egg may be impaired. More extensive damage to the tube may result in complete blockage.

Salpingitis may occur following sexually transmitted infections such as chlamydia or gonorrhoea and can also follow puerperal sepsis (a common cause in the Third World). Severe endometriosis is also associated with tubal damage and impairment. In the majority of cases tubal surgery for the correction of blockage or severe adhesions has been superseded by *in vitro* fertilization (IVF). There is an increasing trend to remove moderate and severely damaged Fallopian tubes prior to attempting IVF, particularly in the presence of hydrosalpinges due to an increased risk of ectopic pregnancy and low success rate after IVF in women with tubal damage.

Hostile cervical mucus

Only at the time of ovulation will the cervical mucus allow the free passage of sperm. At all other times, this passage is obstructed by hormonally induced changes in the mucus. Some women have antibodies against sperm within their mucus and in these women, even at times of ovulation, sperm are often unable to pass through the cervical canal. The most common cause of poor cervical mucus is, in fact, infrequent ovulation.

Uterine conditions

There are several uterine factors that can interfere with sperm transport and the secure implantation of the fertilized egg. These include fibroids, polyps or an abnormally shaped uterus. The uterus may be bicornuate or it may contain a septum, and all of these may inhibit implantation or cause a high rate of miscarriage. Tuberculosis and other chronic infections may affect the endometrium and thus prevent implantation.

Box 10.1 Causes of ovulatory failure

Primary ovarian failure
◆ Genetic, e.g. Turner's syndrome.

Secondary ovarian failure
◆ Premature menopause
◆ Diseases of gonadotrophin regulation
  hyperprolactinaemia
  weight loss
  excessive exercise
◆ Gonadotrophin deficiency
  pituitary tumour
  pituitary infarction
◆ Polycystic ovarian syndrome
◆ Bilateral oophorectomy
◆ Chemotherapy
◆ Radiotherapy.

Endometriosis

Endometriosis arises when tissue that normally lines the uterus (endometrium) is found in other sites in the pelvis (see also page 539). At menstruation, bleeding occurs from this tissue and can give rise to pain and dyspareunia. Endometriosis is found in approximately 25% of women undergoing infertility investigations and is usually identified at laparoscopy. In only 5%, however, is the endometriosis the prime cause of infertility. The majority of women with endometriosis will have mild disease not affecting the ovaries or the Fallopian tubes. With moderate and severe endometriosis, however, there may be a disruption of the anatomy of the Fallopian tubes and ovaries, due to the presence of scar tissue. Endometriosis is also associated with cysts on the ovaries, and these may prevent ovulation from occurring.

Male problems

Abnormalities in the semen are primarily due to a defect in sperm production by the testicles. The cause is usually unknown, but occasionally may be associated with previous infections, excessive drinking or smoking, or simply to stress. The presence of a varicocoele, a condition in which there is an increase in the blood flow around the testicles due to dilated veins, may lead to a rise in the temperature around the testicles, affecting sperm production and motility. Failure to produce sperm is occasionally hormonal and this is normally associated with the absence of secondary sexual characteristics and impotence.

Certain drugs and the administration of radiotherapy may also have a detrimental effect on the production of sperm, as can severe viral infection such as mumps.

Obstruction or absence of the vas deferens is an important cause of male subfertility. In this situation, sperm and semen production are normal but there will be no sperm in the ejaculate. Obstruction of the vas may follow infection such as tuberculosis, and may also follow trauma to the testicle. There is also an association between congenital absence of the vas and cystic fibrosis.

Antisperm antibodies may be present in the semen, and these attack the sperm and inhibit their motility. This condition commonly occurs following reversal of a vasectomy, but may also be related to previous infections or injury.

Sexual problems

The couple may not be having intercourse very frequently due to pressure of work, stress or other factors. Vaginismus or even non-consummation of the relationship may be causes, or there may even be serious psychological factors which need to be identified and treated with as much understanding and sensitivity as the physical problems that are more generally found.

Basic investigations

A couple who are concerned should be seen and counselled, regardless of the duration of their subfertility. Very often couples who present at an early stage have particular concerns, or they themselves perceive they have a problem which is worth discussing. Seeking help is often a very difficult step for them, and it may take a lot of courage to discuss something about which they feel deeply embarrassed or upset. Patients are all different in their needs, some merely require reassurance that they are doing everything correctly, whereas some want active treatment. If the woman is over 37 years, however, it is advisable to refer them to a specialist centre sooner rather than later, as time may be at a premium.

General indications for referral to a specialist clinic are listed in Box 10.2.

Box 10.2 Indications for referral to specialist clinic

- Women over 35 years with 6–12 months' subfertility
- Women with a one-year history of subfertility
- Elevated FSH indicating ovarian failure
- Failure to respond to clomiphene
- Possibility of tubal or pelvic disease
- Abnormal semen analysis
- Negative post-coital test.

History and examination

A full medical history should be taken from both partners, and this should include any previous history of pregnancy or miscarriage. Previous methods of contraception will also need to be recorded. The menstrual history is of great importance and the length of time between each menstrual period should be noted, as should the frequency of intercourse. Even questions as basic as, 'Are you making love?', 'How often?' and 'Do you know when your fertile period is?' should always be asked and can help give a better overall view of the problem.

A general examination of the woman should include weight, height, blood pressure and abdominal examination. A cervical smear and *Chlamydia* screening should be performed where appropriate, along with a pelvic examination.

At the initial appointment lifestyle factors are discussed. Attention to weight is important. If the woman's body mass index (BMI) it is found to be high (>25 kg/m) then advice regarding diet and exercise should be given. If the BMI is very high (>30 kg/m) then onward referral to a dietician is appropriate. It is important to stress the fertility benefits of reducing weight to an overweight woman, including improved pregnancy rates. Women who are significantly underweight have an increased risk of miscarriage, premature labour and intrauterine growth retardation.

Advice should also be given on reducing smoking and alcohol intake. Evidence indicates that women who smoke reduce their chance of a successful pregnancy by approximately 40% compared with non-smokers (Hughes *et al.*, 1992). In men, smoking is known to lower the sperm count, but there is no convincing evidence to show that this reduces their fertility. Women who drink more than 10 units of alcohol per week reduce their chance of conception compared with those who drink less than 5 units.

Rubella immunity should be confirmed and women should be reminded to take a daily dose of folic acid to reduce the risk of neural tube defect.

Hormonal profile

Preliminary investigations should be organized for the woman, the most important being to confirm ovulation by taking blood in the mid-luteal phase of her cycle for assay of progesterone. If the cycle is irregular, varying from 28 to 50 days, then weekly plasma progesterone estimations should be carried out starting on day 21. However, it should be emphasized that these results can only be interpreted in relation to the timing of the next menstrual cycle.

Temperature charts are of limited use, and couples should be discouraged from completing them. They may or may not provide evidence of ovulation, but many couples experience unnecessary anxiety and worry because their temperature charts do not follow the textbook pattern, despite the fact that there is a normal menstrual cycle and proven ovulation.

Another method of detecting ovulation is the use of commercially available LH urine testing kits. These are simple to use home kits similar to pregnancy test kits, and testing is normally performed around the time of expected ovulation in order to detect the early signs of mid-cycle LH rise. Long-term use of the LH predictor kits, however, should be discouraged as they place additional stress on both partners at a time when stress levels may already be very high. They also take away from the pleasure of making love and tend to turn it into a more functional, mechanical act that can rapidly take over from the normal loving relationship the couple used to enjoy.

In women with amenorrhoea, the important investigations are measurement of serum FSH, prolactin levels and an oestrogen assay. The main purpose of a serum FSH measurement is to exclude primary ovarian failure, in which FSH concentrations are invariably elevated.

A common cause of secondary amenorrhoea is hyperprolactinaemia, therefore a serum prolactin is also vital. Stress may result in transient and, in some cases persistent, hyperprolactinaemia, therefore further measurements should be undertaken. If hyperprolactinaemia is confirmed, underlying causes including primary hypothyroidism should be excluded, therefore the TSH (thyroid-stimulating hormone) should be evaluated. Finally, it may be necessary to perform a CT scan to eliminate a pituitary tumour.

Where the woman has an irregular cycle it is necessary to carry out an LH assay, which is characteristically high in women suffering from polycystic ovarian disease.

Ultrasound scan

A pelvic ultrasound scan is now an essential investigation in the treatment of subfertility. It allows for accurate assessment of the size and shape of the uterus and ovaries, and polycystic ovaries are mainly diagnosed using this procedure. Other ovarian cysts can also be demonstrated, e.g. chocolate cysts, which are associated with endometriosis. A scan can also detect the presence of uterine fibroids, polyps and other uterine abnormalities.

Semen assessment

Semen analysis forms a fundamental part of the assessment of the subfertile couple. As male subfertility constitutes at least a third of all causes of subfertility, this simple test should be performed at the very beginning of subfertility investigations, although there is still uncertainty about the minimum values associated with fertility or with the ability to fertilize human oocytes. The World Health Organization's standards for 'normal' semen samples, and the minimum parameters which should be reported are listed in Box 10.3.

Volume

Seminal fluid makes up the vast proportion of the ejaculate and is composed of secretions mainly from the prostate gland and the seminal vesicle. If the volume is exceedingly low (<0.5 ml) part of the ejaculate may be entering the bladder

(retrograde ejaculation). In this case, a post-ejaculatory urine sample should be obtained, centrifuged and examined for the presence of spermatozoa.

Concentration

The number of sperm present is a good indication of spermatogenesis. Concentrations below 10 million are associated with marked impaired fertility.

Motility

Recently ejaculated spermatozoa are actively motile and able to swim with a forward progressive motion. However, motility decreases with time after ejaculation, therefore the time at which the sample is produced is relevant to the assessment. If all of the sperm are immotile, the use of lubricants for producing the sample or exposure to excessively high temperatures should be excluded. Agglutination or clumping of the spermatozoa may be due to the presence of anti-sperm antibodies.

Morphology

Samples of semen that contain large numbers of poorly structured spermatozoa have reduced fertilizing capacity, and are associated with subfertility.

White blood cells

Samples with an increased white cell count should be screened for infection.

Sperm mucus interaction

Sperm mucus interaction can be tested by performing a PCT (post-coital test), a screening test for sperm function and mucus receptivity. The PCT is technically simple to perform, but timing and experience are needed for it to be reliable and therefore it should be performed in a specialist fertility unit. The mucus must be obtained in the pre-ovulatory phase if the test is to give valid information.

The couple are asked to come to the clinic, having had intercourse 6–8 hours earlier. A sample of mucus is removed from the cervical canal and

---

Box 10.3 WHO criteria for minimal normal semen parameters

◆ Volume 2–5 ml
◆ Concentration greater than 20 million/ml
◆ Motility greater than 40% motile
◆ Morphology greater than 40% normal forms
◆ White blood cells less than 1 million/ml.

placed on to a glass slide. Whilst this is being done, the stretchability of the mucus is noted, as is the amount of sperm present. A completely normal post-coital test will show very flowing, 'stretchable' mucus containing a significant number of moving sperm.

The most common cause for a poor post-coital test is inaccurate timing in the cycle Indeed, most clinicians feel that the PCT no longer has a place in modern fertility investigations as it is invasive and difficult to time correctly.

Hysterosalpingogram

The patency of the Fallopian tubes can easily be checked by performing a hysterosalpingogram (HSG), which is carried out on an outpatient basis. An HSG is an X-ray during which a dye is passed through the cervix, uterus and Fallopian tubes. If the dye is seen to pass easily into the abdominal cavity, then the tubes are said to be clear. It has the advantage of outlining the uterine cavity, allowing for the diagnosis of intrauterine fibroids and adhesions. The test does not, however, provide any information about the relationship between the tubes and ovaries. Nor does it identify the presence or absence of pelvic adhesions.

Laparoscopy

Once the couple have been referred to a specialist fertility centre, any remaining investigations not already performed can be arranged. When no abnormality has been detected on the initial investigations of either partner, a diagnostic laparoscopy is often carried out. This is an important part of a thorough investigation, and should not be delayed but should be regarded as a primary investigation, where indicated. The great advantage of a laparoscopy is that it allows the surgeon to obtain a direct view of the pelvic organs, thereby permitting a much more accurate assessment of their condition. The patency and integrity of both Fallopian tubes is determined under direct vision and a dye test performed (see page 553). The presence of adhesions around the tubes and ovaries can be easily detected, and their significance assessed. Other problems such as endometriosis and fibroids will also be revealed, and definitive therapeutic procedures can be performed under direct vision using the laparoscope. Such procedures include the removal of adhesions, ablation of endometriotic spots and drilling of the ovarian capsule in patients who suffer from polycystic ovarian disease.

Hysteroscopy

Examination of the uterine cavity with a hysteroscope is a valuable investigation where there is a history of repeated miscarriage or where the HSG suggests that the shape of the cavity is irregular. During this procedure, a good view of the uterine cavity is obtained. Both tubal openings can be seen, and any intrauterine abnormalities diagnosed. In some cases minor surgical procedures can also be performed under direct vision, such as the removal of intrauterine polyps or the resection of intrauterine fibroids. Intrauterine adhesions can also be removed.

Unexplained subfertility

When investigations have been completed and no satisfactory explanation has been found, the couple is said to be suffering from unexplained subfertility. A high standard of investigation is required, and the diagnosis should only be suggested when all standard investigations have been completed.

The other aspect of unexplained subfertility is that there are factors which affect the subfertile couple which are either still unknown to medicine or are untestable using all conventional methods for investigating fertility. Although there may be evidence of ovulation occurring, such as an elevated serum progesterone or a rise in basal body temperature, the egg may still be retained within the corpus luteum. In this condition, all signs of ovulation will be positive yet the oocyte will not reach the site of fertilization: as yet, it is not easy to detect this condition.

The testing of tubal patency by HSG or even laparoscopy only informs us that the woman has patent tubes, but it does not confirm that the oocyte pick-up mechanism of the Fallopian tubes is intact. Knowledge of this pick-up mechanism is very limited, and there is no suitable way yet to test for it.

Treatment

If the primary investigations are normal, couples should be encouraged by an explanation of the normal chances of conception, and they should be given advice on the correct timing of intercourse and how to detect pre-ovulatory cervical mucus. At the time of ovulation, due to increasing oestrogen levels, the mucus is a very profuse, clear, watery secretion and many women are aware of these changes. If the woman is unable to detect mid-cycle cervical mucus, ovulation may be predicted with the help of a urinary LH kit.

Apart from the problem of ovarian failure virtually all ovulation disorders are treatable with drug therapy, the most commonly used being clomiphene. Treatment starts within the first five days of the period, and continues for five days. Ovulation will usually occur 5–13 days after the last tablet of clomiphene has been taken.

If a pregnancy does not occur following 3–6 months of clomiphene therapy or where the level of oestrogen is low, the treatment of choice is FSH (follicle stimulating hormone), for example Gonal-F. This is administered by subcutaneous injection, and careful assessment of the ovarian response to therapy must be made in specialist centres. The objective of this form of treatment is the production of one or two mature follicles. In patients treated with FSH, careful monitoring by means of ultrasound scan is important to detect hyperstimulation and, therefore, prevent multiple pregnancies.

Patients with tubal blockage may be advised to have tubal microsurgery, or else be referred directly for IVF.

Endometriosis can be treated either surgically through the laparoscope, or by using medication. The objective of drug treatment in endometriosis is to induce a period of amenorrhoea, which will hopefully give the condition time to heal. The most commonly used drugs presently are LHRH (luteinizing hormone-releasing hormone) analogues, e.g. Zoladex.

Couples whose infertility is caused by a male factor may be referred to an andrologist to further investigate causes of semen abnormality. In some cases, minor surgical procedures or drug treatment may help to improve semen quality. Assisted conception in the form of intrauterine insemination (IUI), IVF, gamete intrafallopian transfer (GIFT) or micromanipulation remains the only treatment available for the majority of patients with male factor subfertility.

Human Fertilization and Embryology Authority (HFEA)

The Human Fertilization and Embryology Authority (HFEA) was set up in 1991 to license and regulate clinics which provide:

◆ IVF
◆ GIFT – where donated sperm or eggs are used in treatment
◆ Storage of gametes or embryos.

The HFEA also licenses clinics that carry out research involving human embryos. Whilst its principal task is to monitor IVF clinics, the HFEA's other statutory functions are:

◆ To publish a code of practice which provides guidelines to clinics on how they should carry out licensed activities
◆ To keep a confidential register of information about donors, all couples undergoing IVF treatment and children born from these treatments
◆ To give advice and information to licensed clinics
◆ To give advice and information to couples seeking fertility treatment, to donors and to the general public.

The HFEA inspects all licensed treatment centres annually to ensure centres achieve and adhere to the high standards set out in the code of practice.

The HFEA publishes a range of information leaflets on issues relating to infertility treatments, including a yearly report on the success rates of each IVF centre. This report also provides National Data Statistics.

The most recent publication of the Patient's Guide reported an overall live birth rate of 25.1% in women under the age of 38 and 21.8% in women of all ages. The guide also contains advice to prospective couples about the questions they should ask and the information that should be made available to them, to enable them to decide on which clinic to choose for their treatment. It is emphasized that pregnancy and take-home baby rates alone do not constitute a successful and popular clinic – friendly, compassionate and professional staff providing an excellent overall standard of care can make a huge difference to the patients who enter into this field of medicine.

NHS or private treatment

There are far more private clinics offering advanced infertility management than there are NHS programmes. Although many NHS clinics offer infertility investigations and treatment they have long waiting lists and do not necessarily offer the full range of treatment options. It is estimated that 75% of fertility treatment in the UK is carried out by the independent sector, a significant amount of it on behalf of the NHS.

Until recently a 'post code lottery' existed in the UK in which couples in certain areas were denied NHS fertility treatment that was freely available to couples elsewhere in the country. The National Institute of Clinical Excellence (NICE, 2004) published guidelines that fertility treatment should be available free on the NHS for women between the ages of 23 and 39. This would end the postcode lottery and provide fairer access to fertility treatment. As well as recommending a limited number of IVF cycles, NICE have also issued guidelines for the assessment and treatment of couples with infertility problems. As NHS funding is limited, the needs of couples may not be met and many will still require private treatment.

Women over the recommended age will also be forced into the private sector where they can be seen without a long wait for a first appointment and without lengthy delays for treatment.

Private treatment can be very expensive and is rarely covered by private health insurance and, of course, there is no guarantee that the outcome will be successful. When choosing a clinic, women should check on success rates that a clinic has with achieving a pregnancy, although all results must be looked at with caution as they might compare different age groups of women.

Assisted reproduction techniques

The advent of assisted conception techniques has dramatically changed the treatment of prolonged subfertility. Since the birth of the world's first baby following IVF and embryo transfer in 1978, IVF has been improved and simplified.

Other forms of assisted conception such as IUI, GIFT and zygote intrafallopian transfer (ZIFT) have also been developed. The general principles involved in all these techniques are as shown in Box 10.4.

The factors responsible for increased success in the course of the last decade are better ovulation induction regimens, improved ultrasound-guided oocyte recovery, optimal embryo culture conditions and, finally, the facilities of cryopreservation. Although a success rate very close to that of natural conception can be achieved, there still remains a higher risk of spontaneous abortion in pregnancies achieved by these means. Even so, assisted conception has brought new hope to childless couples who have no natural prospects of achieving a pregnancy, and for whom all other measures have failed.

Box 10.4 General principles of assisted conception techniques

◆ Induction of multiple follicular development
◆ Preparation of a sperm sample of reasonable count and mobility
◆ Bringing the gametes together in order to enhance the chance of fertilization.

There is an increased demand for assisted conception. The factors contributing to this are:

◆ A trend towards childbearing at a later age, which increases the years of exposure to toxins or infections, as well as an age-related reduction in fertility

◆ A greater public awareness of the availability and scope of such services

◆ The availability of new technology and drugs for the treatment of previously hopeless cases of subfertility.

Pre-treatment assessment

Adequate time for consultation of both partners is important to decide upon the best available options and to assess the most suitable treatment for the individual couple. They must fully understand not only their chances of success, but also the possibility of an unsatisfactory response to medication and, therefore, cancellation of the cycle. They must also appreciate that there is a possibility that the eggs may fail to fertilize, that the embryos may fail to implant and that even if a pregnancy does result, this may sadly end in miscarriage.

Intrauterine insemination

IUI involves the injection of washed sperm into the uterine cavity via the cervix, using a fine plastic catheter. It is a painless procedure which takes only a few minutes, and is performed on an outpatient basis.

IUI is useful when:

◆ The female partner has a cervical mucus problem – the mucus may be scanty or hostile to the sperm and with IUI the sperm will bypass the cervix and enter the uterine cavity directly

◆ The male partner suffers from retrograde ejaculation, in which the semen travels backwards into the bladder instead of through the penis – with IUI, a sample of urine is collected and the sperm removed and prepared for insemination

◆ The male partner suffers from impotence or anatomical abnormalities of the penis such as an uncorrected hypospadias, or if the man is paraplegic

◆ There is unexplained subfertility, since the technique of IUI increases the chances of the eggs and sperm meeting – this is also an inexpensive alternative to GIFT, especially for younger couples, and is a reasonable first choice of treatment

◆ The couple are using donor sperm.

The insemination cycle

Insemination may be carried out in a natural menstrual cycle, but by combining it with ovarian stimulation it is often possible to achieve a higher pregnancy rate per cycle. This involves taking fertility drugs to stimulate the ovaries to produce more than one egg. The growth of the egg follicle is monitored by ultrasound and when it has reached the appropriate size, ovulation is triggered by administering HCG (Profasi, 10,000 units; or Pregnyl, 10,000 units). The IUI is then performed some 36–40 hours following administration of the HCG.

The insemination procedure

It is necessary to prepare sperm prior to IUI, as 'neat' untreated semen contains prostaglandins which can be highly irritant to the uterus and can cause a 'shock-like' reaction, resulting in severe abdominal pain and collapse.

Sperm for IUI is prepared by either simple washing or by using a sperm separation technique to isolate the motile fraction. The final preparation is drawn into a sterile catheter and introduced into the uterus via the cervical os.

Success rates with IUI

Generally, the chance of conceiving in one treatment cycle is approximately 10–15%, and the cumulative conception rate is approximately 40% over five or six treatment cycles. The success rate depends upon several factors. First, the cause of the subfertility problem; for example, men with a normal sperm count who are unable to have intercourse have a much higher chance of success than couples who are undergoing IUI with poorer sperm counts. If the woman is 35 years of age or more, the chance of a successful pregnancy is significantly reduced. If IUI is going to prove successful, it usually does so within six treatment cycles. If a pregnancy has not resulted in this time, the chance of IUI working is remote, and the couple should be encouraged to explore other possibilities. IUI is a relatively simple and inexpensive form of treatment, and is often attempted before moving on to more expensive and invasive options. Repeated cycles of insemination without success can prove extremely stressful to couples, however, and close support for them is essential.

Donor sperm

The use of donor sperm is an option that should be offered when the semen characteristics of a male presenting with subfertility are such that it is unlikely a pregnancy will be achieved.

It is used to treat couples in which the male partner has either no sperm, or a very low sperm count. It is also recommended in cases where the male partner is known to be a carrier of a hereditary disease. Couples, in which the male partner has a low sperm count, are currently offered micromanipulation as a primary course of treatment with increasingly successful outcomes. Some couples, however, opt to use donor insemination for either financial or ethical reasons.

All couples considering donor insemination should be referred for counselling.

Counselling

It is most important that the medical, legal and emotional implications of donor insemination are fully understood by the couple undergoing the treatment. Counselling gives the couple an opportunity to explore their feelings in relation to the male partner's subfertility, and its implication on their relationship. The couple will also need to consider telling the child of its origins, at what age this might be done and how it might be best presented. It is important to ascertain if they have already confided in friends or relatives about their condition, and what their plans might

be to discuss it in the future with others. It is entirely up to the parents to tell the child the circumstances of its birth; however, there is always the burden of secrecy which the parents have to bear for the rest of their lives. The current trend is to encourage openness, as secrets are difficult to keep and it can also be argued that it is the child's right to know of its origins; however, many parents still choose secrecy. Patient support groups can be useful to couples in this situation, as they can share experiences and develop an understanding of each other's problems.

A group called Donor Conception Network (see Resources) has been formed to help couples undergoing donor insemination treatment and has produced a book entitled *My Story* in order to help parents tell their children of their origins.

Laws governing donor sperm

This treatment is governed by the HFEA, which requires that all sperm donors and couples receiving donor sperm are registered with the HFEA. The sperm donor has no parental rights or legal obligations towards any children resulting from treatment using his sperm. Couples undergoing donor insemination are required to sign a consent form prior to treatment, in which the male partner acknowledges that he is the legal father of any child born as a result of donor insemination.

Recruitment, selection and screening of donors

Most sperm donors are recruited from medical schools, local colleges and businesses, and must be aged between 18 and 55 years (Human Fertilization and Embryology Act, 1990). All potential donors are required to complete a questionnaire giving details about their physical characteristics as well as data about their medical and family history

Urethral cultures are performed for gonorrhoea and *Chlamydia*, and serological tests are carried out for HIV-1, HIV-2, hepatitis B surface antigen, hepatitis C, syphilis and cytomegalovirus.

Subject to the information acquired, a semen sample will then be required for analysis and if this specimen reaches the required standard, it will be cryopreserved: all semen used for donor insemination is quarantined for a minimum of 180 days prior to use. Live births from any one donor are restricted to ten under HFEA regulations, in an effort to reduce the risk of consanguinity.

A survey (Golombok and Cook, 1994) revealed that only 25% of all men wishing to become sperm donors are accepted, and that the most common reason for rejection is suboptimal semen analyses. A payment of up to £15.00 per donation as well as reasonable expenses is currently allowed under HFEA guidelines. Golombok and Cook report a widespread feeling amongst fertility centres that should these payments cease, approximately 80% of sperm donors would be lost.

Method of treatment

The method of treatment with donor sperm depends on the cause of subfertility. If there is no evidence of a fertility problem with the woman, then IUI may be a suitable form of treatment. However, there may also be indications for GIFT or IVF.

Psychological effects

Couples undergoing donor insemination often have psychological reactions which can be difficult to cope with. The sense of isolation is even more than with other forms of subfertility, since many couples do not tell anyone they are undergoing donor insemination. The male partner may feel inferior, insecure and jealous, and even wonder whether he will be able to 'father another man's child'. The female partner may in turn be resentful about having to undergo treatment for a problem which is medically not her own.

The involvement of a completely unknown third party in the form of the donor sperm can make coping with the pregnancy especially difficult. Fantasies may occur about the unknown donor, and anxieties may arise as to whether the child will be normal and what it will look like. It is therefore important that the couple do not rush into treatment with donor sperm, but also explore the alternative options.

In vitro fertilization

In vitro is the Latin term for 'in glass', which quite literally describes the technique of IVF: fertilization performed outside the body in a Petrie dish. It first reached public awareness in 1978 with the birth of the first so-called 'test tube baby', Louise Brown. It is a process in which the woman's eggs are collected from her ovaries, fertilized in the laboratory with her partner's sperm and, when normal embryo development has occurred, replaced in her uterus.

In early days, the indications for IVF treatment were absent, blocked or irreparably damaged Fallopian tubes. Subsequent developments led to IVF also being used to help couples with other problems such as male subfertility, endometriosis, unexplained subfertility and cervical factors. Essentially, IVF may be an option for any subfertile couple in whom less aggressive forms of subfertility therapy have been unsuccessful.

Finally, IVF may also be employed as a means of obtaining diagnostic information in severe forms of male subfertility as well as idiopathic subfertility, as it is the ultimate test to assess a couple's potential to achieve fertilization. No other test is currently available to determine this potential.

When IVF was first used successfully, a single egg was obtained during a natural menstrual cycle, without the use of drugs to stimulate follicular development. It was later found that the pregnancy rate was higher when several embryos, rather than just one, were transferred. Since then, it has become standard practice in most IVF centres to give the woman medication to stimulate her ovaries, in order to allow the development of more than one follicle.

The basic steps in the performance of IVF are ovarian stimulation, egg collection and embryo transfer.

Ovarian stimulation

Medication starts early in the cycle to enhance the growth and development of the ovarian follicles which have been naturally selected for that cycle. The medication is administered over a period of 10–12 days, and the ovaries are scanned at regular intervals during this time to ensure that they are responding to the medication. Hormone assays for oestradiol may also be performed to indicate oocyte maturation. When specific criteria have been met, HCG 10,000 units is given to encourage final egg maturation and induce ovulation. Egg retrieval is performed 36–40 hours later.

Ovarian stimulation is initiated with a variety of different medication protocols. Those commonly used are HMGs (such as Menogon) and FSH (Gonal F) as well as LHRH analogues (Suprefact, Suprecur). The function of the LHRH analogue is to take complete control of the woman's ovarian function, by preventing her from producing FSH and LH naturally. It also prevents a pre-ovulatory LH surge from occurring, and therefore avoids spontaneous ovulation.

There are a number of protocols for the administration of the LHRH analogue. In the 'long' protocol, the analogue is given for approximately 10 days to desensitize the pituitary gland. Once this has occurred, daily injections of FSH are commenced to stimulate the ovaries. Both the LHRH analogue and the FSH are continued until the eggs are mature enough for egg collection to be undertaken. In the 'short' protocol, both the analogue and the FSH are started together at the beginning of the menstrual cycle. This protocol is suitable for patients who have a previous history of poor response to the medication. The analogues are available either as a nasal spray or a subcutaneous injection. The most recent advance in ovarian stimulation has been development of the GnRH antagonist (Cetrotide) which achieves more immediate suppression of the pituitary gland and avoids some of the side effects related to the LHRH analogue like headaches and hot flushes.

HMG and FSH are available only in the form of intramuscular or subcutaneous injections. It may in some cases be appropriate to teach the woman how to administer the injection herself, and some partners may also be willing to learn. Couples who do their own injections tend to find the whole procedure less stressful, as this avoids the inconvenience of their visiting the clinic or attending their GP surgery on a daily basis,

therefore diminishing the intrusion of the treatment in their daily lives.

Unfortunately, not all patients respond ideally to a given medication protocol. If the ultrasound and hormone monitoring reveal a suboptimal response in terms of follicular development, the cycle may be cancelled as the chances of pregnancy will be reduced. The medication protocol may be adjusted, and a new cycle can be attempted at a later date. If the couple feel very strongly about proceeding even when it is likely that only one or two eggs will be collected they will be allowed their right to go ahead with the treatment.

Possible side effects of the drugs. Whilst taking the drugs, some women experience mild unpleasant symptoms, but these are normally short-lived and are no cause for concern. They can include hot flushes, headaches, irritability and feelings of depression.

Despite careful monitoring, a small percentage of women may develop a mild or severe form of overstimulation to the drugs, where too many follicles may develop. The ovaries will be enlarged and symptoms such as nausea, vomiting, abdominal pain and swelling may occur. Under these circumstances the cycle should be abandoned, and the woman should be carefully monitored by a fertility specialist.

Very rarely, in about 1% of cases, a more serious form of hyperstimulation may occur, where the woman notices a reduction in urine output and shortness of breath along with the previously mentioned symptoms. These complications require hospital admission to restore fluid balance and to monitor progress.

Egg collection

Egg collection is performed vaginally using ultrasound guidance. This is performed under a general anaesthetic or with the woman only mildly sedated.

With this procedure, an ultrasound probe is inserted into the vagina in order to visualize the ovaries, and a fine hollow needle is then guided directly into the ovaries and the eggs are aspirated.

A laparoscopic egg collection may be required in certain cases where it is difficult to access the ovaries from the vaginal route.

Egg identification and insemination. As the follicles are aspirated, the follicular fluid obtained is immediately taken to the laboratory where it is examined, and the eggs identified. Once evaluated for the level of maturity, the eggs are transferred to a special culture medium in preparation for insemination. In the meantime, a sample of the partner's sperm is prepared by a washing technique to remove the seminal plasma and separate out the healthy sperm.

About 100,000 motile sperm are added to each egg approximately 4–6 hours following egg collection, to allow fertilization to take place. The exact length of time the eggs are incubated before the sperm are added depends upon the maturity of the eggs. Generally, 80% of mature eggs will be fertilized in the absence of a male problem. Fertilization should occur within 18–24 hours of insemination.

Once fertilization has occurred two pronuclei can be identified. The embryos are allowed to continue developing to a two-cell or four-cell stage before transfer back into the uterus (Figures 10.2 and 10.3).

Embryo transfer (ET)

Embryos are transferred though the cervix into the uterus using a fine plastic catheter 48–72 hours after egg collection. This is a painless procedure, and no anaesthetic is required.

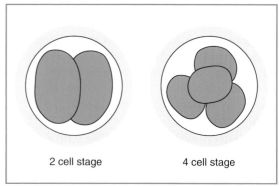

Figure 10.3   Embryos 2 days after egg collection.

Usually, two or three embryos are transferred in order to increase the chances of pregnancy. Under HFEA guidelines, clinics are not allowed to transfer more than two embryos in women under the age of 40 and no more than three in women over that age, in order to reduce the risk of multiple pregnancy.

Following ET the woman is allowed to carry on with her normal routine, as there is no evidence to suggest that resting increases the chances of becoming pregnant. ET is often regarded as the culmination of many weeks of treatment, and the emotional significance of it to the couple should not be ignored.

Blastocyst transfer

Recent developments in laboratory techniques allow us to observe the development of embryos for a longer period before transfer. Up until recently embryos were transferred to the uterine cavity two to three days after egg collection. However, in a normal physiological situation, the embryo would still be in the Fallopian tube at this developmental stage. An increasing number of studies report that embryo transfer on day five (at the blastocyst stage) give significantly higher rates of pregnancy (Marek, 1999; Gardener and Lane, 1997). Culturing embryos to the blastocyst stage allows the selection of embryos with proven developmental capacity, and their greater implantation potential means that fewer embryos need be transferred. This has the prospect of reducing the multiple pregnancy rate.

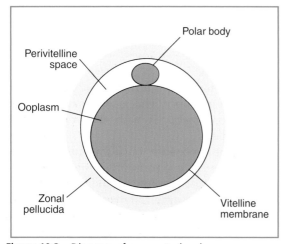

Figure 10.2   Diagram of an oocyte (egg).

The disadvantage of prolonged culture *in vitro* is that, in some cases, no embryos will develop to the blastocyst stage and there will be no embryos to transfer.

Embryo freezing

In many cases, more than three embryos are fertilized. Those embryos not transferred may be cryopreserved and stored for future treatment should the first attempt be unsuccessful, or indeed to try to achieve a second pregnancy. These embryos may be transferred at the appropriate time in a natural cycle, without the need for drugs and surgery, and are replaced 2–3 days following natural ovulation.

The chance of success using frozen embryos is less than when using fresh, as some or all of the embryos may not survive the freezing/thawing process. It is therefore important that the couple are carefully counselled on the chances of conception and the costs involved. They are also required to sign a consent form giving the clinic permission to freeze their embryos and also to determine the fate of these, should anything happen to either or both partners.

Embryos can legally be kept in storage for only 5 years, except in exceptional circumstances.

Gamete intrafallopian transfer

GIFT offers an alternative treatment to IVF for women who have patent Fallopian tubes. The first stages of the treatment are similar to those for IVF, namely ovarian stimulation with hormone treatment, monitoring of follicular growth and administration of HCG to induce final maturation of the eggs. It is from here on that the GIFT procedure differs from IVF.

The eggs are collected laparoscopically. They are examined for maturity, and the two most mature eggs are mixed with the prepared sperm and drawn separately into a fine catheter, then immediately transferred into the fimbriated end of the Fallopian tube. Fertilization therefore occurs in the Fallopian tubes as with normal conception, rather than in the laboratory. The fertilized egg then travels through the tube to the uterus for implantation, as in normal reproduction.

Gametes will be transferred only if the Fallopian tubes appear healthy; if they are not, IVF will be attempted instead of GIFT.

Although GIFT has the advantages of fertilization and early embryo development occurring in the normal environment, in the absence of a successful outcome, the fertilizing capacity of gametes remains unknown. To overcome this deficiency, the surplus oocytes may be fertilized *in vitro* and then cryopreserved. This 'back-up' IVF has a diagnostic value of confirming fertilization, and also has a therapeutic role which allows transfer of cryopreserved embryos at a later date.

As the results of IVF are increasingly more successful, it is becoming less common to recommend GIFT as the first line of treatment. It may be recommended, however, in special circumstances, such as repeated failure with IVF.

Zygote intrafallopian transfer

This procedure involves the transfer of embryos into the Fallopian tubes. It is carried out through the laparoscope and is used when it is necessary to confirm that fertilization has occurred. Until recently it was extensively used in ovum donation programmes as many clinics reported higher success rates. However, like GIFT, it is being replaced with the increasingly successful IVF technique.

Micromanipulation

Micromanipulation is a technique which allows the embryologist to perform very precise surgical procedures upon eggs and embryos with the use of a micromanipulator. This is a very high-powered microscope with robotic arms, which enables the operator to perform extremely delicate manoeuvres using eggs and sperm which are normally not even visible to the naked eye. This facility is also capable of allowing the embryologist to withdraw as little as one cell from an embryo for research purposes and to look for the presence of genetic diseases such as cystic fibrosis – such research is not widely available at the present time, but it must be regarded as the way forward holding, as it does, vast scope for knowledge within the field of genetic engineering.

Several micromanipulation techniques have been devised to help the sperm pass through the zona pellucida – the tough outer coating of the egg, which is thought to be the main barrier to the penetration of sperm. In cases of male factor subfertility, the ability of sperm to penetrate the zona may be reduced. At present, these methods are used in cases of severe male subfertility and when conventional IVF has failed.

Two main groups of patients suitable for micromanipulation are those couples who have either very poor or no fertilization with a good number of eggs (i.e. four or more), or those couples whose semen contains very low numbers of sperm.

These procedures can also be used to help men who have obstruction of the vas (the tube that connects the testicle to the base of the penis). Sperm can be surgically removed from the epididymis (the area on top of the testes in which sperm are maturing) or directly from the testicle itself.

Intracytoplasmic sperm injection (ICSI)

ICSI has revolutionized the treatment of male infertility, offering assistance to couples who previously had to rely on the use of donor sperm. Until recently the limiting factor in treating male infertility has been the difficulty in isolating sufficient numbers of active sperm to mix with the female partner's eggs in the laboratory. With ICSI very few sperm are required and the ability of the sperm to penetrate the egg is no longer important as this penetration is bypassed by the ICSI procedure. Although ICSI will greatly improve the chances of fertilization occurring, it does not guarantee it.

Couples undergoing ICSI treatment undergo the same ovulation induction regime and egg retrieval as in IVF. The difference is the laboratory process from there on.

In this method, a single sperm is injected into the centre of an egg (Figure 10.4). The sperm that is selected for injection is ideally one of normal shape, morphology and motility, and it is immobilized by having its tail touched with the

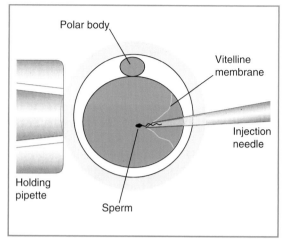

Figure 10.4 Intracytoplasmic sperm injection. The holding pipette keeps the egg in place. The injection needle is loaded with one sperm which is injected directly into the centre of the egg. The needle is then withdrawn, leaving the sperm behind.

microneedle before being picked up. The egg is held in place whilst the needle is passed through its outer layer, and the needle is then brought into contact with the egg's membrane. The membrane is carefully penetrated and the centre of the egg reached, then the sperm is injected and the needle is gently withdrawn, care being taken to leave the sperm within the egg.

The piercing of the egg during the procedure may occasionally lead to damage and this will be evident during or after the procedure. These eggs cannot be used for treatment and 15% of eggs are lost in this way.

The risk of fetal abnormality

Concern has been expressed about the potential risks of fetal abnormality associated with ICSI treatments. To date, there is mixed evidence of an increased risk of birth defects, but the Brussels Free University in Belgium, which has the largest number of babies born from ICSI, consistently reports no increased risk of major abnormalities. It is, however, possible that the genetic disorder that led to a low sperm count in the father may be passed on to the son. It is therefore recommended that couples seek pre-treatment counselling before embarking on an ICSI programme.

All centres performing micromanipulative procedures have a responsibility to their patients and to the medical profession as a whole to record the progress and ultimate development of all children from this treatment. A study at the Royal Free Hospital of children aged 1–2 indicated that to date these children are developing normally (Sutcliffe *et al.*, 1999). Indeed, many of the early anxieties about the health and normalities of babies born as a result of these techniques have been allayed by detailed follow up studies (Sutcliffe, 2002).

Assisted hatching

Before implantation the embryo must hatch from its shell to attach to the womb. In some cases the shell is unusually hard, thus reducing the chance of implantation. Assisted hatching is a procedure in which the outer layers of the embryo (zona pellucida) are either thinned or opened with the assistance of the micromanipulator to facilitate hatching. It is generally recommended for women above the age of 40 years and for women who have had repeated unsuccessful IVF attempts. Whilst in some cases assisted hatching may enhance pregnancy rate, some embryos can be damaged as a result of these interventions. Therefore it is not recommended as a first line of treatment.

Chances of success with assisted reproductive techniques

Human beings, as a species, are not very fertile, and even young couples with normal fertility have only a 25–30% chance of establishing a pregnancy each month (Zinaman *et al.*, 1996). After a woman reaches her mid-thirties, this monthly chance drops to 10–15% and by her early forties is less than 5% per month. If there are other factors influencing the couple's chances of success such as irregular ovulation or poor sperm parameters the chance is even lower.

Whilst IVF has enabled many couples to have children, the treatment is more likely to be unsuccessful than successful in any individual cycle. Perhaps the best measures of success in IVF are therefore the cumulative conception and the cumulative live birth rates – these describe the likelihood of a woman becoming pregnant or having a live birth after a specific number of cycles of treatment.

Similar to nature, the same factors affect IVF pregnancy rates. For example, a 30-year-old woman whose only indication for subfertility is a tubal factor will have a higher probability of achieving a pregnancy than a 40-year-old woman who has extensive endometriosis and whose husband has a male factor.

The current trend towards delayed child bearing due to career or financial pressures, together with a high rate of divorce which results in many women seeking to conceive in a new partnership and at an older age, combine to produce an apparent epidemic of infertility in women over the age of 35. Good nutrition and healthy lifestyles mean that many women in their late thirties and early forties feel and look much younger than they actually are. Their chances of conceiving a pregnancy spontaneously are, unfortunately, low whereas their expectations of fertility treatment are very high. It is therefore the responsibility of the clinician to counsel couples appropriately in order to manage their expectations, and to ensure they understand the meaning of reported statistics, and to know how these apply to their individual circumstances.

Generally speaking, although the chances of success per cycle are only approximately 30%, repeated attempts at treatment are more likely to result in a pregnancy. Figure 10.5 shows a general overview of the IVF pregnancy rates for the Assisted Conception Unit at the Lister Hospital, and Figure 10.6 shows the cumulative live birth rates for IVF.

Ovum donation

The use of donor eggs is a natural extension of the IVF process and recent advances have given hope to many women who are unable to produce eggs, or who fail to achieve a pregnancy using their own eggs. The first successful pregnancy following egg donation was reported by Lutjen *et al.*

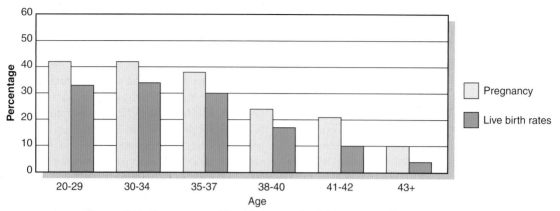

Figure 10.5 Pregnancy and live birth rates (LBR) for IVF according to age, at the Lister Hospital (January 1997–December 2002). *Source*: The Lister Hospital.

in 1984 and since then egg donation has become an increasingly established part of assisted conception programmes around the world. It is used primarily in women who have suffered premature ovarian failure, and for older women who fail to conceive following IVF (Box 10.5).

Couples undergoing treatment with egg donation require extensive counselling prior to commencing treatment, particularly in cases where the

donor is known to the recipients. Close attention must be paid to the long-term attitude towards the child, as well as the proposed definition of future interaction and their relationship with the child.

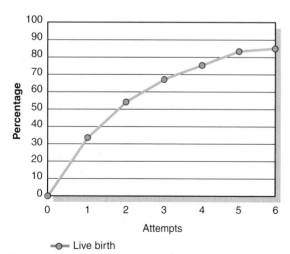

Figure 10.6 Cumulative live birth rates for women under 35 years IVF at the Lister Hospital (January 1997–December 2002). *Source*: The Lister Hospital.

Box 10.5 Conditions treated by ovum donation

Women with ovarian function

These include women:

◆ Carrying an inheritable genetic disorder such as haemophilia

◆ Who repeatedly fail to respond to ovarian stimulation in IVF programmes

◆ Whose apparently normal eggs repeatedly fail to fertilize in IVF programmes

◆ Who may be carriers of disorders such as Tay–Sachs disease, Huntingdon's disease, cystic fibrosis, thalassaemia or sickle cell disease

◆ Who have a history of recurrent miscarriage.

Women without ovarian function

These include women:

◆ Suffering from Turner's syndrome

◆ Suffering from premature menopause

◆ With ovarian damage following surgery, radiation or oophorectomy.

Source of egg donors

Egg donors were originally recruited from women receiving assisted conception treatment, who wished to donate extra eggs for altruistic reasons (Trounson and Mohr, 1983). This source of donors decreased with the introduction of embryo freezing, as most couples opt to store their embryos for a future attempt at treatment. Since then the trend is to encourage all recipients joining an ovum donation programme to help in recruiting their own donor. A study by Kan *et al.* (1998) demonstrated that 44% of the women who donated eggs did so in response to an advertisement placed by the couple requesting donated eggs The payment of egg donors is prohibited by the HFEA and many studies (Kirkland *et al.*, 1992; Kazem *et al.*, 1995) found that the majority of donors wanted no form of payment. A survey of donors was performed to try to ascertain exactly why women donate eggs, and it was found that over 90% of them made the donations simply because they felt the need to help other women (Power *et al.*, 1990).

There is a tremendous demand for egg donation treatment and most centres have a waiting list, as it is not easy to maintain a large pool of egg donors. Also, with the present state of technology, eggs cannot be easily cryopreserved, therefore 'egg banks' do not exist in the same way as 'sperm banks'. The recruitment of egg donors raises many ethical, moral and emotional issues; however, the increasing demand for oocytes requires that this controversial issue be discussed and possible solutions be found (Burton *et al.*, 1990).

Donor anonymity – how the situation has changed

Previously those donating sperm, eggs or embryos have remained anonymous. However, a recent change in the law means that children born as a result of sperm, eggs or embryos donated from April 2005 will be able to access the identity of their donor when they reach the age of 18. Donor anonymity has been removed because many individuals and organizations believe that children born from donated sperm, eggs or embryos should be able to have access to information about their genetic origins. This will not affect existing donors as the new regulations surrounding information on donors will not be retrospective. It is acknowledged that ending donor anonymity does involve some risk to the future availability of donors. However, it is believed that this practical consideration should not outweigh the more fundamental principle that donor offspring should have knowledge about their genetic origins. Children born as a result of donations made before April 2005 are able to ask the HFEA to confirm whether they were born as a result of donated sperm, eggs or embryos. Those intending to marry, including those who plan to do so before their 18th birthday, may also ask whether the HFEA Register shows that they are related to the person they intend to marry.

Donor criteria

The potential donor must be under the age of 36 and have preferably completed her family, although this is not essential. She will be screened for HIV, hepatitis and sexually transmitted infections, and a full medical and family history taken to ensure that there are no known genetically inheritable diseases or defects present.

Physical characteristics are recorded such as nationality, skin, hair and eye colour, height and build to ensure that every care can be taken to find the most suitable donor for each recipient. Recipients of donor eggs frequently enquire about the donor's interests, pastimes, religion and educational qualifications, the answers obtained helping to alleviate their curiosities and fantasies about the potential child. As much information as possible should be made available to them. Frequent questions asked are: 'Is the donor an animal lover?' 'Is she artistic or sporty?' 'Is she intelligent?' 'Does the donor have children and are they healthy?' Currently the clinic is able to provide information about the physical characteristics, background, interests and occupation of the donor. There may also be a pen portrait which the donor is encouraged to write.

Donors are counselled to ensure that they understand all of the implications and issues involved with egg donation. The donor relinquishes all rights to the egg, and has no responsibility towards any resulting children. The Human Fertilization and Embryology Act states that the mother of a child is the woman who actually gives birth to it (HFEA, 1990).

The difficulty and challenge of egg donation revolves around matching the ovulatory cycle of the donor with the appropriate endometrial maturation of the recipient, as a fresh embryo replacement with donor/recipient synchronization is the ideal situation for achieving a pregnancy. The recipient is commenced on hormone replacement therapy in order to synchronize her cycle with that of her donor, as well as for optimal endometrial development. In women with normal ovarian function, the LHRH analogue can be used to suppress the natural cycle. If cycles cannot be synchronized, the eggs can be fertilized and frozen for use in a future cycle.

The donor undergoes a similar stimulation protocol to that described in an IVF cycle, with egg recovery usually being performed vaginally. Following fertilization of the donor eggs, the embryos are transferred to the uterus or the Fallopian tubes.

Egg donation can be an extremely successful method of treating infertility, with a mean pregnancy rate of 27% (as in IVF, the success rate depends upon the cause of subfertility). Patients with primary ovarian failure tend to have a better outcome than those with secondary ovarian failure, and the pregnancy rate in patients with Turner's syndrome is almost 50% (Abdalla et al., 1990).

Egg sharing

The most recent and most controversial source of egg donors is egg sharing. In an effort to resolve the shortage of donors, many IVF units have introduced egg sharing schemes where women undergoing IVF treatment donate some of their eggs to another woman, in return for free treatment. Egg sharing is seen by many as the solution to two difficult problems, one for women who can afford IVF treatment, but require donor eggs, and the other for women who produced good eggs, but cannot afford the cost of IVF treatment. There are others, however, who feel egg sharing is unethical as it places a burden on fertile women to trade their eggs to enable them to receive the treatment they need. Following a five-year debate the HFEA has concluded that under certain circumstances egg sharing can be beneficial to both donors and recipients and have issued guidelines to ensure that both groups are not compromised in any way.

All egg sharers should be counselled to ensure their commitment to and understanding of egg sharing. They have the right to withdraw from the egg sharing programme at any time before the recipient has her embryo transfer. In the event of an egg sharer not producing enough eggs to share, she has the option of not sharing and keeping all the eggs for her own treatment.

A good egg sharing programme should also provide an equal opportunity for both recipients and egg sharing donors to achieve a live birth.

A large retrospective study (Thum et al., 2003) demonstrated that egg sharing does not compromise the chance of donors and recipients achieving a live birth. This study compared the outcome of couples participating in an egg sharing programme with couples undergoing standard IVF treatment, and showed similar pregnancy and live birth rates in both groups.

Whilst the evidence provided in this study promotes a very positive outcome for egg sharers, it does not address the psychological aspect of such a treatment programme. It may be emotionally traumatic for an egg sharer, desperate for a child, to consider that although her treatment has been unsuccessful, recipients could be pregnant with her eggs. She may not reveal her true feelings or share her motivation for wishing to egg share. These issues require further study and a more detailed evaluation of the psychological and emotional impact of participating in an egg sharing programme is currently in progress.

Voluntary register for donor offspring

Due to the planned removal of donor anonymity a voluntary register was set up to enable people conceived by donated eggs, sperm or embryos before 1991 to contact their donors and biological half-siblings. The registry, called UK DonorLink will be available to anyone affected by donor conception, over the age of 18, their half-siblings and their donors. It will offer genetic testing to match offspring with donors and other biologically related offspring who are also registered with the service. It will also offer information, counselling and support.

Since the Human Fertilisation and Embryology Act was passed in 1990, which required that such births are registered, over 18,000 people have been born in the UK following the use of donated embryos or gametes. An estimated 12,000 people were conceived with donor egg or sperm before then. The new register is being established as a pilot by the charity After Adoption Yorkshire. The team at UK DonorLink is committed to ensuring this register is shaped by the needs of donor-conceived people and their families, as well as by donors and their relatives.

Surrogacy

Surrogate parenthood is a highly controversial and emotive issue, and very few fertility centres in the UK currently provide this facility.

Surrogacy involves a fertile woman having a baby, whom she consents to hand over to an infertile couple at birth, and this requires one of two procedures to be performed. In the first, the surrogate mother is artificially inseminated with the sperm of the husband of the infertile woman. In the second, the infertile woman undergoes an IVF procedure whereby an egg is removed from her ovary, fertilized with her husband's sperm and the resulting embryo is then placed in the uterus of the surrogate mother, who carries the baby throughout pregnancy, gives birth and then hands the baby over to the commissioning couple, i.e. a husband and wife who have arranged for a surrogate mother to carry a child for them using their eggs and/or sperm. This latter procedure is called 'host surrogacy'.

Surrogacy is fraught with all kinds of problems, and commercial surrogacy is illegal in most countries. The difficulties include those of a legal nature, such as who determines the pregnancy outcome if fetal abnormalities are detected early on, who bears the responsibility of caring for the surrogate mother and her family if she has medical problems as a result of the pregnancy, who looks after the child if it is born with a defect, and what happens if the surrogate mother forms a strong bond with the baby and refuses to hand it over to the infertile couple.

Previously, the commissioning couple were required to go through an adoption procedure to ensure the legality of the child, but in December 1994 the HFEA introduced new regulations which make it much easier to transfer legal parenthood to the commissioning couple. These parents will therefore no longer need to go through the full adoption procedure.

Adoption

Adoption means to become the legal parents of a child whose biological parents have decided to give up all legal rights over that child.

As a result of improved methods of contraception and the availability of abortion, the numbers of children available for adoption are considerably fewer than the number of prospective parents. Therefore realistically, only a small number of couples are successful in adopting a child and it often means they have to accept an older child rather than a baby.

The child-free option

One of the most common fears that women express when considering a child-free life is that they may regret this decision when they are older, and that they may end up lonely and frustrated. However, there is a difference between choosing to remain child-free and having childlessness forced upon you.

After many years of fertility investigations and treatment, it is very difficult to accept childlessness and focus upon the positive aspects of life without children and some couples might need the help and support of a counsellor to enable them to 'let go' of their quest for a baby and accept their infertility. Initially they may be overwhelmed with feelings of bereavement (as in the death of a relative) which are not visible to others around them, and consequently they do not receive the support and empathy they require.

Couples who perhaps initially postponed trying to conceive or who felt ambivalent about becoming parents often find that once they have taken the decision to cease treatment it is possible to pick up their lives again, and may well be able to rediscover the values which once took priority over having children. There are real advantages in leading a life without children – more personal freedom and more time and energy to invest in one another and in shared interests. Acceptance of subfertility should therefore mark the beginning of a new lifestyle, with new goals and ambitions to strive towards.

Subfertility and sexuality

Subfertility brings about many changes in a couple's relationship. It may bond them closer together in a mutual show of support and understanding for one another, but it may on the other hand bring out feelings of guilt, resentment and despair. Couples must expose the most intimate aspect of their lives – their sexual relationship – in their desire to have children.

In many cases, failure to conceive destroys self-esteem and self-worth. Sex often becomes a chore with a single-minded purpose, and it loses its association with fun and pleasure. It may be useful to seek counselling at this stage to help the couple to separate sex from reproduction.

It is also not uncommon, when faced with the diagnosis of subfertility, for a woman to feel 'less of a woman' and that she has failed to fulfil her role as a woman. These feelings of inadequacy are enhanced during the investigation and diagnosis of her condition.

Procedures such as the post-coital test, although painless, intrude greatly on a couple's intimate relationship. They are required to 'perform' at a specific time, arrive at the clinic at the appointed time and face fear of failure if they do not 'pass the test'.

Men, too, feel that their masculinity is being questioned when asked to produce a semen sample, and it is not uncommon for a man to become impotent for a short period whilst undergoing investigation. It is important for all health professionals concerned in the couple's treatment to be aware of and to identify the emotional problems which their condition may well create, and offer as much support, sensitivity and understanding as possible.

Support groups

A support group provides a safe, comfortable environment in which couples can share their experiences with people who truly understand them – nobody understands subfertility as clearly as those who have been affected by it. Meeting and talking to other couples in a similar situation is a good way of breaking down the barriers of isolation which often accompany this problem, and can help couples to realize that they are not alone in their dilemma. It is also a useful forum in which to exchange ideas and obtain information.

Many couples are reluctant to join such groups as they fear that these gatherings may encourage them to dwell even more on their fertility; but, in reality, subfertility can affect every aspect of their lives, and trying to shut out painful feelings will only make them worse. In many cases, frank discussion with non-medical people is often a tonic in itself, a place in which fear, pain and distress can be released, experiences both happy and sad can be shared, and where empathy and support will always be forthcoming.

Most fertility units will have their own support group but in the absence of this, they will certainly have details of appropriate bodies. A national support network, Infertility Network, exists for this exact purpose and provides practical information, care and support for subfertile couples (see Resources).

Ethical issues

Infertility practitioners are faced with numerous ethical dilemmas and find themselves making ethical judgements on behalf of their patients in their everyday practice. It is impossible to cover all of these issues in this chapter, but no book on infertility is complete without reference to the ethical aspect of the treatment provided. (See Chapter 2 for further discussion on ethico-legal issues.)

A few examples of the issues commonly encountered are: 'Should women be inseminated with their dead husband's sperm?', 'Should homosexual men be provided with a surrogate to enable them to carry a child?' and 'Should we treat couples where one or both partners are HIV positive?'

The management of an infertile woman with HIV is fraught with ethical dilemmas (Smith *et al.*, 1990). The prevalence of HIV in women is rising and as most of these women are in their reproductive years, they naturally want to have children. The desire for pregnancy among women with HIV may be due to the increasing better survival for the HIV-infected individual: earlier diagnosis and the use of antiviral drugs has led to a prolonged AIDS-free survival period. Couples where one or both partners are infected present an especially difficult challenge for staff working in infertility clinics as they are required by law to consider the welfare of the child. With the use of prenatal antiviral treatment, delivery by caesarean section and avoidance of breast-feeding, the vertical transmission rate has been reduced to 1%. This factor has led to a more positive approach towards the treatment of couples with HIV. Do medical staff have the right to deny infertility treatment to well-informed couples who decide to embark on a pregnancy? If one argues that all HIV women should be denied infertility treatment, then all women requesting fertility treatment should be tested for HIV at the point of referral.

Does everyone have a right to treatment? A married heterosexual couple in a stable relationship is considered to be the most appropriate for rearing children. A legal marriage, however, does not guarantee a stable environment and indeed single individuals may not only assert a moral right to be a parent, but may provide a more satisfactory environment in which to bring up a child.

Should we treat single women? Generally speaking, lesbian women have been refused treatment on the grounds that they would not provide an appropriate family environment, as the child would have two mothers and no father. For single, heterosexual mothers it has been argued that the absence of a father might lead to psychological difficulties for the child. Many studies have been carried out concerning the matter and there is very good evidence that these children are not psychologically damaged (Golombok and Tasker, 1994). It is, after all, most likely that it is the quality of parenting that is important.

Should we treat older women? Now that egg donation offers women the opportunity to have a child later in life, many women are seeking treatment well after they have reached the menopause. It has been argued that it is wrong for a woman in her fifties to consider bringing a child into the world when her own life expectancy may be shorter than what would be considered ideal from a child's point of view. Yet no one questions the right of a man to father a child at the age of 50 or even 60; indeed, it is sometimes considered laudable.

We do, however, have to consider the welfare of the child. The question that should be asked is 'is it in the child's best interest for him or her to be born to an older woman, or would they be better served if that child was not born at all?' In reality, it is in very rare circumstances that society would deem that it would be better for a child not to be born.

Another current dilemma is the decision to withdraw donors' rights to anonymity. At present it is a donor's legal right to expect their anonymity to be respected. This is perceived by many as an infringement of the child's right to knowledge of their genetic origins. Clinics, already struggling to provide a service, have major anxieties that such a change in policy would have profound effects on their ability to continue to recruit donors.

With the speed of development in reproductive technology these questions will surface more frequently and will need to be answered by society in general and not left to be resolved by the practitioners alone.

When to stop treatment

The most difficult part of fertility treatment is knowing when to stop. If there is a definite cause of infertility, e.g. premature menopause, when there is no possibility of achieving a pregnancy without treatment, stopping treatment is final. It is much more difficult for couples to stop infertility treatment when the cause of their infertility is unexplained. There are two reasons for this. First, there is a possibility the next cycle of treatment might be the one in which a pregnancy occurs and, second, there is always a chance that pregnancy may occur spontaneously.

It is therefore important that couples are advised to set themselves a target before they commence treatment. To do this they need to understand what the treatment has to offer and have realistic expectations of the outcome. In reality many couples have a poor grasp of statistics and cumulative pregnancy rate and fail to understand that cumulative conception statistics apply to groups of patients rather than individuals, and can only be used as a rough guide to the success of the treatment. It is therefore our role to evaluate each couple following an unsuccessful treatment cycle and if the outlook is not looking positive, prepare them to cease treatment. We find the most successful way of achieving this is by suggesting how many further cycles they should undertake with an agreement to stop after the agreed limit. To advise couples to stop without any prior discussion should be avoided. All couples require sympathy and support during the process of stopping treatment and accepting their infertility.

The future

It has been nearly three decades since the birth of Louise Brown, the world's first 'test tube' baby and since then over a million babies have been born worldwide as a result of this UK-pioneered technique. IVF and ICSI are now regarded as acceptable and successful solutions to the problems of infertility.

Assisted conception techniques have opened up an exciting new world for both patients and medical practitioners. Whilst success rates have not improved dramatically over the past decade, major advances have been made in the field of research. At present research is mainly focusing on pre-implantation diagnosis.

Pre-implantation genetic diagnosis

Pre-implantation genetic diagnosis (PGD) is a technique whereby embryos created outside the body can be tested to see whether they carry a genetic disorder before being transferred to the uterus. It was developed in response to requests for help from families at risk of passing on a serious genetic disorder to their children. It is a two-stage process in which IVF is used to create embryos; these are then tested for a particular genetic disorder or to establish their sex, where the disorder is sex-linked. Embryos that do not carry the genetic disorder or are not of the potentially affected sex can then be transferred to the uterus in the hope that a normal pregnancy will develop. The technique was first successfully used in 1990 to produce two sets of twin girls where families were at higher risk of passing on a serious X-linked disorder. Sexing an embryo to avoid X-linked disorders and testing for age-related aneuploidy (abnormal number of chromosomes) are the most common reasons for pre-implantation diagnosis worldwide. Testing for cystic fibrosis remains the most common use of PGD for a single gene defect. The HFEA prohibits the use of PGD for sex selection for social reasons.

Families known to be suffering from genetic disorders are faced with difficult decisions when considering having children and until recently only three options have been available:

◆ Decide not to have a child
◆ To opt to have pregnancy without genetic testing and so risk passing the disorder on to the child
◆ To proceed with the pregnancy and have the fetus tested using pre-natal diagnosis. If the fetus is found to be carrying a disorder or abnormality the mother then faces the decision whether or not to request a termination (within the provision of current abortion legislation).

For some people termination is not an acceptable option. The prospect of repeating the process of pregnancy and termination one or more times in an attempt to achieve an unaffected pregnancy will be unacceptable to many more.

PGD may offer a fourth option to certain families.

It is also now possible to screen embryos for chromosome abnormalities. This is called pre-implantation aneuploidy screening and is recommended in cases of advanced maternal age where there is a high miscarriage rate due to chromosome abnormalities. It is also recommended for women who have experienced recurrent miscarriages. In this procedure the cells are removed during an embryo biopsy procedure. These cells are then analysed for chromosome abnormalities and only embryos that are chromosomally normal are transferred to the uterus.

Controversy about the application of PGD has arisen because it permits the 'selection' of embryos for transfer with 'desired' genetic characteristics. It is sometimes referred to as the 'designer baby' technique. The complexity and expense of these techniques will, however, ensure that they are rightly restricted for justifiable medical purposes.

Cryopreservation of eggs

Another exciting development has been the successful freezing and thawing of unfertilized eggs. The freezing and thawing of both sperm and embryos has been possible for a number of years – sperm since 1960 and embryos since 1983. The freezing of eggs, however, has proved more difficult. Eggs are large cells and their outer layers are fairly water resistant. When water is trapped inside the egg during freezing, ice crystals may form and damage the egg. It has taken many years of research to provide reassurance that there is no damage to the gene control mechanism which may result in a birth defect.

Egg cryopreservation would be of major benefit to women about to undergo chemotherapy treatment, which may render them infertile. The option of freezing embryos prior to cancer treatment is currently available to women with partners, but for young women and women without partners this is not possible. Egg freezing is therefore a crucial alternative for cancer patients, who may wish to have children after their cancer is cured. There are, however, some concerns that there will be a demand for this service from women wishing to delay their childbearing years in favour of a career. The success of this procedure is currently very low and it is feared many women will have unrealistic expectations and possibly delay motherhood even further.

The thawing and transfer of frozen eggs was, until recently, banned in the UK, because of uncertainty of the risks involved. This ban was lifted by the HFEA in 2000, as the most recent evidence has shown that the procedure is sufficiently safe. To date, more than 100 babies worldwide have resulted from this procedure and all are reported as being normal healthy infants.

Cryopreservation of ovarian tissue

Cryopreservation of ovarian tissue is currently offered to some cancer patients before their chemotherapy or radiotherapy treatment. In time, we will be able to effectively mature eggs from frozen tissue and restore patients' fertility, and cryopreservation of ovarian tissue will be an efficient way to preserve more eggs without the need for ovarian stimulation.

As with all new developments in the field of assisted conception, these remarkable possibilities stimulate wide-ranging discussion of the ethical and social implications of these new techniques.

Conclusion

In summary, the incredible advances in the treatment of subfertility over the last few years have dramatically altered the lives of many couples who had hitherto been regarded as having untreatable problems, and have opened the doors of medicine to a world full of recently unimagined possibilities. Those couples who have lived with subfertility and its associated pain, applaud the advent of these treatments and the medical staff who work so hard to improve them. Staff who work within fertility units and watch the progress of medical science at close range are privileged to be able to witness these advances, and bring the many benefits to those who need them.

Ideas for personal and professional development

- Find out what facilities your local NHS and private fertility clinics have and arrange a visit to both. Does your NHS clinic have a limit on the age of the woman, or how long they have been trying for a pregnancy?

- Collect as much detailed information on infertility and its treatment as possible, e.g. websites, medical journals. Make a leaflet to give to patients

- Contact the HFEA for a list of licensed clinics and the treatments that they offer

- Consider attending a menopause clinic to find out the types of HRT available for those having ovum donation.

Patient education points

- Do not delay. If you have been trying unsuccessfully to conceive for 1 year, ask your GP to refer you for investigations

- Healthy lifestyle. Try to reduce your alcohol intake, cut down smoking and watch your weight

- Reduce external stress. Try not to take on additional stress during treatment and find alternative ways to reduce stress during treatment, e.g. reflexology, acupuncture

- Gather as much information as possible before embarking on treatment regarding success rates, costs, etc., from different clinics

- Do not give up. If the first attempt at IVF is unsuccessful, do not assume that IVF is not the right treatment for you. It may take a few attempts.

Resources

After Adoption Yorkshire
31 Moor Road, Headingley,
   Leeds LS6 4BG
Tel: 0113 230 2100
www.afteradoptionyorkshire.org.uk

British Agencies for Adoption and Fostering (BAAF)
Sky-Line House, 200 Union Street,
   London SE1 0LX
Tel: 020 7593 2000
www.baaf.org.uk

British Infertility Counselling Association
69 Division Street, Sheffield S1 4GE
Tel: 01142 631 448

COTS (Childlessness Overcome Through Surrogacy)
Lairg, Sutherland IV27 4EF
Tel: 0844 414 0181

Daisy Network (Premature Menopause Support Group)
The Daisy Network, PO Box 183,
   Rossendale BB4 6W2
www.daisynetwork.org.uk

Donor Conception Network
PO Box 7471, Nottingham NG3 62R
www.issue.co.uk

Human Fertilization and Embryology Authority
21 Bloomsbury Street, London
   WC1B 3HF
Tel: 020 7291 8200
www.hfea.gov.uk

Infertility Network UK
Charter House, 43 St Leonards Road,
   Bexhill on Sea, East Sussex, TN40 1JA
Tel: 01424 732361
www.infertilitynetworkuk.com

Miscarriage Association
C/o Clayton Hospital, Northgate, Wakefield,
   West Yorkshire, WF1 3JS
Tel: 01924 200 799

**National Infertility Awareness
  Campaign (NIAC)**
PO Box 2106, London W1A 3DZ
Tel: 0800 716 345

National Gamete Donation Trust
PO Box 137, Manchester M13 0YX
Tel: 0161 276 6000
www.NGDT.co.uk

TAMBA (Twins & Multiple Births Association)
Harnott House, 309 Chester Road, Little Sutton,
  Ellesmere Port L66 1QQ
www.tamba.org.uk

UK DonorLink
31 Moor Road, Headingley, Leeds LS6 4BG
www.ukdonorlink.org.uk

Further reading

BALEN, A. and JACOBS, H. (1997) *Infertility in Practice.*
  London: Churchill Livingstone.
BLYTH, E., CRAWSHAW, M. and SPEIRS, J. (1998) *Truth and
  the Child 10 Years on: Information Exchange in Donor Assisted
  Conception.* British Association of Social Workers.
BRIAN, K. (1998) *In Pursuit of Parenthood: Real Life
  Experiences of IVF.* London: Bloomsbury.
CHAMBERS, R. (1999) *Fertility Problems: A Simple Guide.*
  Oxford: Radcliffe Medical Press.
Dr Foster Fertility Guide (2002). London: Vermillion.
FURSE, A (2001) *Your Essential Infertility Companion: A User's
  Guide to Tests, Technology and Therapies.* Thorsons.
HAYNES, J., MILLER, J. (2003) *Inconceivable Conceptions:
  Psychological Aspects of Infertility and Reproductive
  Technology.* Brunner-Routledge.
HFEA (Human Fertilization and Embryology Authority)
  (2003/04). *Your Guide to Infertility.* London: HFEA.
LEE, R.G. and MORGAN, D. (2001) *Human Fertilisation and
  Embryology: Regulating the Reproductive Revolution.*
  Blackstone Press.
McWHINNIE, A. (1996) *Families Following Assisted
  Conception – What Do We Tell Our Child?* Dundee:
  University of Dundee.
PETTLE, S. and BURNS, J. (2002) *Choosing To Be Open About
  Donor Conception: The Experiences of Parents.*
REGAN, L. (2001) *Miscarriage: What Every Woman Needs to
  Know.* Orion Publishing Group.
SINGER, D. and HUNTER, M. (2003) *Assisted Human
  Reproduction: Psychological and Ethical Dilemmas.* Whurr
  Publishers.
SNOWDEN, R. and SNOWDEN, E. (1993) *The Gift of a Child.*
  Exeter: University of Exeter Press.
SUTCLIFFE, A.G (2002). *IVF Children. The First Generation:
  Assisted Reproduction and Child Development.* London:
  Parthenon.
WINSTON, R. (1996) *Infertility – A Sympathetic Approach.*
  London: Vermilion.

References

ABDALLA, H., BABER, R., KIRKLAND, A., LEONARD, T.,
  POWER, M. and STUDD, J. (1990) A report on 100 cycles
  of oocyte donation: factors affecting the outcome. *Human
  Reproduction* 5:1018.
BURTON, G., ABDALLA, H. and STUDD, J. (1990) Ethical
  problems of recruiting oocyte donors. Editorial. *British
  Journal of Hospital Medicine* 44:239.
COOKE, I.D., SULAIMAN, R.A., LENTON, E.A. and
  PARSONS, R.J. (1981) Fertility and infertility statistics:
  their importance and application. In Hull, M.G.R. (ed.)
  Clinics and Obstetrics and Gynaecology. London:
  W.B. Saunders, pp. 531–48.
GARDNER, D.K. and LANE, M. (1997) Culture and
  selection of viable blastocysts: a feasible proposition for
  human IVF. *Human Reproduction Update* 3:367–82.
GOLOMBOK., S. and COOK, R. (1994) A survey of semen
  donation: Phase I – The view of UK licensed centres.
  Human Reproduction 9:882–8.
GOLOMBOK, S. and TASKER, F. (1994) Donor insemination
  for single heterosexual and lesbian women: issues
  concerning the welfare of the child. *Human Reproduction*
  9:1972–6.
HFEA (1990) *Human Fertilization and Embryology Authority
  Code of Practice.* London: Human Fertilization and
  Embryology Authority.
HUGHES E.G., YUNG LAI E.V. and WARD S.M. (1992)
  Cigarette smoking and outcomes of IVF-ET: a prospective
  cohort study. I. *Human Reproduction* 7:358–61.
HULL, M.G.R., GLAZENER, C.M.A., KELLY, N.J. *et al.*
  (1985) Population study of causes, treatment and outcome
  of infertility. *British Medical Journal* 291:1693–7.
KAN, A.K.S., ABDALLA, H.I. and OGUNYEMI, B.O. (1998)
  A study of anonymous oocyte donors: domographics.
  Human Reproduction 13:2762–6.
KAZEM, R., THOMPSON, L.A., HAMILTON, M.P. and
  TEMPLETON, A. (1995) Current attitudes towards egg
  donation among men and women. *Human Reproduction*
  10:1543–8.
KIRKLAND, A., POWER, M., BURTON, R. *et al.* (1992)
  Comparisons of attitudes of donors and recipients to
  oocyte donation. *Human Reproduction* 7:355–7.
LUTJEN, P., TROUSON, A., LEETON, S. *et al.* (1984)
  Establishment and maintenance of pregnancy using IVF
  and embryo failure. *Nature* 307:174–5.
MAREK, D. (1999) Introduction of blastocyst culture and
  transfer for all patients in an in vitro fertilisation
  programme. *Fertility and Sterility* 72:1035–40.
NATIONAL INSTITUTE FOR CLINICAL EXCELLENCE
  (2004). New NHS guidelines on fertility treatment.
  www.nice.org.uk.
POWER, M., BABER, R., KIRKLAND, A., LEONARD, T. and
  STUDD, J.W. (1990) A comparison of the attitudes of
  volunteer donors and infertile patient donors on an ovum
  donation programme. *Human Reproduction* 5:352–5.
RANDALL, J.M. and TEMPLETON, A. (1991) Infertility: the
  experience of a tertiary referral centre. *Health Bulletin
  (Edinburgh)* 49:48–53.
SMITH, J.R., FORSTER, G.E., KITCHEN, V.S. *et al.* (1990)
  Infertility management in HIV positive couples: a
  dilemma. *British Medical Journal* 302:1447–50.

SUTCLIFFE, A.C., TAYLOR, B., LI, J., THORNTON, S., GRUDZINSIKAS, J.G. and LIEBERMAN, B.A. (1999) United Kingdom study of children born after intracytoplasmic sperm injection: population control study. *British Medical Journal* **318**:704–5.

SUTCLIFFE, A.G (2002). *IVF Children. The First Generation: Assisted Reproduction and Child Development.* London: Parthenon.

THUM, M.Y., GAFAR, A., WREN, M., FARIS, R., OGUNYEMI, B., KOREA, L., SCOTT, L. and ABDALLA, H.I. (2003) Does egg sharing compromise the chance of donors or recipients achieving a live birth? *Human Reproduction* **18**(11):2363–7.

TROUNSON, A. and MOHR, L. (1983) Human pregnancy following cryopreservation, thawing and transfer of an 8 cell embryo. *Nature* **305**:707–9.

VESSEY, M.P., SMITH, M.A. and YEATES, D. (1986) Return of fertility after stopping oral contraceptives: influence of age and parity. *British Journal of Family Planning* **11**:120–4.

ZINAMAN, M.J., O'CONNOR, J., CLEGG E.D. *et al.* (1996) Estimates of human fertility and pregnancy loss. *Fertility and Sterility* **65**:503–9.

11: Contraception

Suzanne Everett

OBJECTIVES

This chapter should help you understand:

◆ The different types of contraception and how they work ◆

◆ The problems encountered by clients in trying to choose a method of contraception and the possible solutions ◆

◆ The sexual anxieties encountered with clients ◆

◆ How to identify and correct the misconceptions often held by clients. ◆

Introduction

For thousands of years women and men have attempted to control their fertility using a variety of methods. Few people realize that the name of the condom originated from the Earl of Condom, personal physician to King Charles II, who tried to protect the king from syphilis in the seventeenth century. In the past, women have used oiled rags and halved lemons as diaphragms and men have used condoms made of linen, silk and animal gut. A famous exponent of the condom was Casanova who called it his 'English riding coat' (Durex, 1993). Other methods for preventing pregnancy have been the consumption of mercury by Chinese women and the use of elephant faeces as a vaginal pessary by Arab women.

In the twentieth century we have developed these ideas into more consumer-friendly methods, but there are still many traditional homeopathic remedies in use. For example, women in Sri Lanka eat green papayas to prevent pregnancy, as they contain an enzyme that disables progestogen. Perhaps information such as this will help us with the development of new contraceptive methods for the future.

In the UK, contraception is easily and widely available. Barrier methods can be bought at many retail outlets including chemists, supermarkets, petrol stations and public toilets, or are provided free of charge at family planning clinics, youth advisory services, genitourinary medicine clinics and some GP surgeries. Other methods of contraception are available from the latter sources and there are no prescription charges for contraception in the UK. A woman is entitled to obtain contraception from any GP who is on the contraceptive list; this GP does not need to be the GP with whom she is registered.

In this chapter we discuss all the methods available in detail and outline their advantages and disadvantages.

Safer sex

When discussing the issues of safer sex with clients, it is important to distinguish between 'safe sex' – i.e. sexual activities that carry minimal or no risk of acquiring or spreading HIV – and 'safer sex' – i.e. sexual activities that reduce the risk of transmitting HIV but are not completely safe.

Any sexual activity that includes penetrative sex carries the risk of acquiring or spreading HIV. 'Safe sex' involves activities other than penetrative sex to provide satisfaction and enjoyment, and can include kissing, massaging, masturbation, using sex toys and watching or reading erotic material.

If there is penetrative sex, whether oral, vaginal or anal, then clients should be encouraged to practise 'safer sex', by using condoms to protect themselves from HIV and other sexually transmitted infections. A wide variety of types of condom are easily available and genitourinary medicine clinics can provide a wider selection for certain uses, including dental dams for protection during oral vaginal intercourse. Extra strong condoms are the only type suitable for anal intercourse.

It is recommended, and is becoming increasingly common, to use the 'double Dutch' method, i.e. a condom for protection against HIV and sexually transmitted infections and an additional method such as the pill or an IUD to provide contraception. Nevertheless, comments such as 'it will never happen to me' or 'I can trust him' are not uncommon and in these situations it can be difficult for you to persuade your client that there is a risk in her sexual behaviour. Women should be encouraged for their personal protection to:

◆ Be determined to resist the desire to have penetrative intercourse and to practise safe sex instead

◆ Inform a new partner as early as possible in the relationship that intercourse will not be allowed without a condom

◆ Be prepared and always carry condoms

◆ Discuss the need for screening for sexually transmitted infections with partners at the beginning of a sexual relationship.

Avoiding the issues of safer sex can be dangerous and it is important that you raise the subject with your clients, as they are frequently unable to voice their anxieties with you for fear of being labelled promiscuous.

Barrier methods of contraception

Barrier methods of contraception used to be thought of as 'old fashioned' but due to the advent of HIV and AIDS and with substantial government funding to promote their importance they are now used more extensively.

Barrier methods include the male condom, the female condom, the diaphragm and cervical caps. They are called barrier methods because they not only provide a physical barrier, preventing the sperm from meeting the ovum, but they also give some protection (particularly the condom) from sexually transmitted infections. All users of barrier methods of contraception should be given information about emergency contraception in case of failure in use.

Condoms

Often referred to as 'johnnies', 'rubbers', 'French letters', sheaths, condoms. Condoms are a barrier form of contraception. They prevent pregnancy by stopping the sperm from being released into the vagina, and thus prevent fertilization. Condoms are 85–98% effective in stopping pregnancy and they are also effective in protecting against sexually transmitted infections and HIV (Box 11.1).

Types of condoms

There is a large and bewildering choice of condoms available. They may have different textures (ribbed) to heighten sensitivity, and different colours ranging from gold, black, coral, red, blue to luminous. Unlubricated flavoured condoms are available for oral intercourse. There is a wide range of strengths, the thicker condoms will decrease sensitivity and help the man maintain his erection longer, and also give greater safety against breaking. Extra strong condoms are the only condoms suitable for anal intercourse.

Clients can choose lubricated or unlubricated condoms, the lubricated condoms can contain either a non-spermicidal lubricant or a spermicide and this will be advertised on the packet.

> **Box 11.1** Condoms: advantages, disadvantages and contraindications
>
> **Advantages**
>
> ◆ Easy to use
> ◆ Easily obtained
> ◆ No systemic effects
> ◆ Protects against most sexually transmitted infections and HIV
> ◆ Used by male
> ◆ Possible protection against cervical neoplasia
> ◆ Very effective form of contraception
> ◆ Can be incorporated into foreplay.
>
> **Disadvantages**
>
> ◆ May be perceived as disrupting sexual intercourse
> ◆ Requires motivation to be highly effective
> ◆ Some men report reduced sensitivity
> ◆ Do not allow use of oil-based lubricants.
>
> **Contraindications**
>
> ◆ Failure to maintain an erection
> ◆ Allergic reaction.

Occasionally men or women are allergic to spermicides; in this case a non-spermicidal lubricant should be used. Polyurethane condoms such as Avanti are thinner but are stronger than latex condoms, and are not affected by fat-soluble products like latex condoms. They are also bigger and baggier resulting in less restriction around the glans of the penis and increased sensitivity. It was hoped that with polyurethane condoms there would be reduced accidents; however, controlled clinical trials found that the breakage and slippage rate for polyurethane condoms was 8.5% compared to 1.6% for latex condoms (Frezieres *et al.*, 1999). Spermicides such as nonoxynol 9 have been shown to have microbicidal activity but offer no protection against chlamydia, gonorrhoea or trichomoniasis (Wilkinson and Szarewski, 2003).

You should recommend that your clients use condoms that have the British standards kitemark or the European CE marking which means that they have been tested and fulfil certain regulations.

Teaching clients how to use condoms

Many female clients need and appreciate specific factual advice about how to use condoms so that they can teach their partner and integrate condom use effectively into sex. When discussing the wide variety of condoms available you should also explain about expiry dates, BSI kitemarks, and storage at normal room temperature. Women and men may feel embarrassed and inhibited when purchasing condoms so may be very grateful for advice you can give them.

If a model is available for teaching the application of condoms then this will aid learning, otherwise fingers can be used as a replacement. The client should be shown how to open a condom packet (using an actual packet) by teaching them to push the condom inside the packet away from the edge that will be opened to avoid tearing the condom. The condom should be squeezed out of the packet, taking care not to tear it with long finger nails or rings.

The condom should be unrolled over the demonstration model or your fingers holding the teat with the other hand. Any air should be squeezed out, and the condom should look smooth. Your client may now have gained enough confidence to try applying the condom herself on to the model. A condom should be applied to an erect penis, but it is important that the penis does not come into contact with the vagina before the condom is applied, as semen containing small amounts of sperm is present before ejaculation occurs. Once the man has ejaculated he should hold on to the end of the condom when withdrawing. Clients should only use condoms for one episode of intercourse and should dispose of them carefully after use.

Common problems

◆ '*It came off*'. Condoms usually only fall off when the man loses his erection and withdraws without holding on to the condom, leaving the condom in the vagina. The man should be advised to hold on to the condom when he withdraws.

◆ *'It burst'*. Condoms burst if they are put on incorrectly, for example if there is an air bubble in the teat or if they have been put on inside out. They also burst if oil-based lubricants are used: baby oil, Vaseline, body oil, massage oil, ice cream, butter and margarine, etc. (Durex, 1988). Certain vaginal and rectal preparations also cause condoms to burst: e.g. Nystan cream®, Premarin®, Nizoral®, Gyno-daktarin®, Gyno-pevaryl®, Cyclogest®, etc. You should always advise your clients about products which cause condoms to break.

◆ *'He says he can't feel anything'*. Clients who complain of loss of sensitivity can try ribbed or thinner makes of condoms. 'Gel-charging' – using a non oil-based lubricant inside the condom – can heighten sensitivity for the man.

◆ *'The condoms are too small for him'*. *'He's too big'*. Condoms can accommodate any penis size and different varieties may be more comfortable, e.g. flared, contoured or made of polyurethane.

Condoms and sexuality

Clients use condoms for a variety of reasons; they can be used for a 'one-night stand' and in long-term relationships. Many couples have used nothing else for years, and use the application of the condom as part of foreplay with either partner applying it. Increasingly more clients are using the 'double Dutch' method, using one form of contraception, such as the combined pill, to give contraception and using a condom for protection against sexually transmitted infections and HIV.

The condom is one of the few forms of contraception which gives the man an active part in preventing pregnancy. It also gives both men and women the opportunity to discuss their relationship and contraception. Couples often progress on to other methods after initially starting with the condom. Condoms can be seen as giving a woman permission to touch her partner's genital area, and the idea of helping to apply the condom may feel a 'safer' form of foreplay at first.

Myths and the media

With the advent of AIDS and HIV, condoms have had considerable media coverage. 'Safer sex' is promoted and condom use is an integral part of this message. Condoms are easily available, and are successfully marketed at both men and women. The design of discreet packaging aimed at women has enabled many women to feel comfortable about purchasing and carrying condoms.

The media has created a new image for the condom which shows the condom user to be a sensible and caring individual. This has also advanced the variety of choice available, from flavoured condoms to blue condoms, and all in easy reach of the buyer!

The diaphragm

Women can be influenced tremendously by the nurse who is teaching her about the diaphragm. All your personal feelings can be conveyed at the initial consultation and if these are helpful and positive they will certainly influence her decision. Conversely if you convey negative messages then your client picks these up and her commitment to the method may be less than ideal.

The first consultation can be very time consuming, but it can help to educate women not only about this form of contraception but also about their bodies. Many women do not realize where their cervix is, and find that the fitting of a diaphragm can help to give them permission to understand and examine their bodies.

The diaphragm (Figure 11.1) is a barrier method that many women find simple and easy to use. Often referred to as 'the cap' or the 'Dutch cap', it offers effective contraception without any hormonal effects. It works by acting as a barrier to the cervix, stopping the sperm and ovum from meeting and therefore preventing fertilization. Box 11.2 summarizes the advantages, disadvantages and contraindications of using the diaphragm.

When used with a spermicide, the diaphragm is between 82% and 90% safe or effective in preventing pregnancy; this figure increases to between 92% and 96% safe with careful and consistent use (Bounds, 1994). It is thought that the lower safety

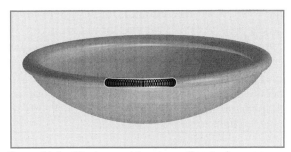

Figure 11.1 Diaphragm (showing coil spring).

Box 11.2 The diaphragm: advantages, disadvantages and contraindications

Advantages

- Under the control of the woman
- Has no systemic or unwanted side effects on the body
- May help to protect the cervix against sexually transmitted infections and cancer by acting as a barrier, and the spermicides may help by killing bacteria
- Can be inserted in advance of sexual intercourse
- Can be used when a woman is menstruating
- When used correctly, an effective method of contraception.

Disadvantages

- Needs to be inserted prior to sexual intercourse and requires forethought
- Sometimes can cause increased cystitis and urinary tract infections, as it may irritate the bladder and urethra through pressure
- Needs to be used with a spermicide to be fully effective and this can be perceived as messy
- May cause vaginal irritation.

Contraindications

- Congenital abnormalities, e.g. septal wall defects (where a woman has an extra vaginal wall separating the vagina into two), two cervices
- Poor muscle tone
- Allergy to rubber
- Inability to touch the genital area through personal choice or religious reason
- An already present infection (either vaginal, cervical, or pelvic should be treated first)
- Undiagnosed genital tract bleeding should be investigated prior to diaphragm fitting
- Past history of toxic shock syndrome. This is rare but has been noted in women who left their diaphragms in for longer than 30 hours
- Lack of personal hygiene
- Vaginal prolapse
- Virgo intacta. This is a term used for a woman who has not had sexual intercourse and has an intact hymen. A diaphragm may be fitted after intercourse has taken place.

rate may be due to the lack of experience of the woman in the first year. As women under the age of 25 years are more fertile they should be advised of their increased risk of pregnancy if they require this method and of the need for careful use. However, for the conscientious woman it can be a very safe and effective form of contraception without any hormonal effects.

Types of diaphragm

A diaphragm should be fitted by a family planning-trained nurse or doctor and it can take up to 30 minutes to instruct a woman how to insert and use one. The session should be held in a warm, private room, free from interruptions where the woman will feel comfortable. The diaphragm is made of latex rubber and there are three types:

- Coil spring
- Flat spring
- Arcing spring.

All three diaphragms are made in sizes 55–95 mm (rising by 5 mm each size). The coil spring diaphragm may be suitable for women with a shallow symphysis pubis, while the flat spring diaphragm is ideal for women with an anterior or mid-plane positioned cervix. The arcing spring diaphragm is ideal for women whose cervix is in a posterior position and who find it difficult to feel their cervix and therefore check that it is covered by the diaphragm.

Fitting the diaphragm

When a woman has chosen to use a diaphragm, a vaginal examination needs to be performed to check the position of the cervix. It may be anterior and near the bladder and easy to feel, or posterior near the rectum, or between the two in a mid-plane position. From this examination it is also possible to check vaginal muscle tone to exclude vaginal wall prolapse and note the retro pubic ridge.

This examination is important for assessing the size of diaphragm required and which type of diaphragm is most suitable. Once the correct size is fitted (Figure 11.2) the client should be unable to feel the diaphragm *in situ*. If she bears down and you can feel the diaphragm protruding forwards into the introitus, then the diaphragm is too big. The client should be shown how to remove and insert the diaphragm, and taught how to locate her cervix, so that she is able to ascertain whether the diaphragm properly covers her cervix.

When the client can fit and remove the diaphragm correctly under supervision she should practise at home over the next week. This practice should include insertion and removal, as well as use during sexual intercourse, sleeping, passing urine and having her bowels open. It is important that the client uses another form of contraception until then. A little spermicide on the rim of the diaphragm helps insertion at this stage, but the full use of spermicide is best left until the diaphragm can be handled with dexterity.

After a week of practising with the diaphragm, whilst using another form of contraception,

the woman returns with her diaphragm *in situ* to be checked. At this visit she should be given the opportunity to discuss any problems she has encountered.

There is a great deal of information that you need to give your client about the use of the diaphragm and it is vital that you back this up with leaflets.

Using spermicides

There is little research on the effectiveness of diaphragms used without spermicides, so you should advise your clients always to use a spermicide. Two 2-cm strips of a spermicidal cream or gel should be squeezed on to each side of the diaphragm before it is inserted. This will give protection for up to 3 hours. If sexual intercourse takes place after 3 hours, a spermicidal pessary should be inserted 5–10 minutes beforehand.

How long to leave the diaphragm in

The diaphragm should be left in for a minimum of 6 hours after sexual intercourse but no longer than 24 hours. If sexual intercourse occurs again before six hours have elapsed, a spermicidal pessary should be inserted to provide additional spermicidal cover.

Care of the diaphragm

The diaphragm should be washed after use with warm water and mild soap, dried carefully with a soft towel and bent back into shape. This is also a good time to check it for holes. Diaphragms should be stored in their cases in a cool, dry place. They should not be stored on radiators or sunny windowsills as they can perish in such conditions. Disinfectants, detergents and talcum powder should not be used on diaphragms.

Follow-up visits

Diaphragms should be checked every 6 months, or annually in those women who are long-term users. Additional checks are advisable in the following circumstances:

◆ If the woman's weight alters by 3 kg

◆ Following any pregnancy

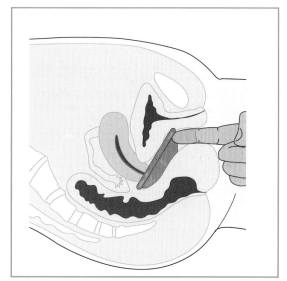

Figure 11.2 Diaphragm fitted correctly. (Reproduced with permission from Louden *et al.*, 1995.)

- If the woman contracts a vaginal infection (this is necessary to prevent re-infection once the infection has been treated)
- If the diaphragm shows signs of deterioration or has a hole in it.

Common problems

- '*I can't find my cervix*'. If your client cannot feel her cervix, suggest that she bears down, which pushes the cervix downwards. If this does not help, try fitting her with an arcing spring diaphragm, which will automatically cover the cervix if inserted correctly. Alternatively, teach the woman's partner to check that her cervix is covered.
- '*It doesn't cover my cervix*'. This may mean that the diaphragm is too small or that the cervix is in a very posterior position and that an arcing spring diaphragm might be more suitable.
- '*It's too messy*'. There may be many reasons for this complaint and changing the spermicide used may help. Some women find cream spermicides easier to use than a clear gel, which tends to be more runny. You could recommend she uses gel or cream spermicide on the side which will be next to her cervix and the use of a foam which comes in an aerosol container with an applicator and is applied once the diaphragm is in place. Bear in mind that a complaint about messiness may indicate underlying feelings about sexual intercourse being messy and dirty. It is important to deal with the problem with understanding and to come up with some solutions. Ask your client how she and her partner feel about using the diaphragm and whether she is having any problems with sexual intercourse in general. Given time, she may be able to express some of her anxieties. A woman may well feel more comfortable complaining about her diaphragm than looking at more personal problems.
- '*My partner can feel the diaphragm*'. This may indicate that the diaphragm is too big or that it has been incorrectly fitted. If the problem remains after changing the size, it may be worth trying a different type of cap.
- '*I find it difficult to remove*'. Remind your client that the diaphragm cannot get lost and that it is important to try not to panic. If she feels upset, she should leave it in and wait until she feels relaxed. Sometimes it helps to take it out in the bath or she could ask her partner to remove it.
- '*I keep getting cystitis*'. Recurrent cystitis indicates that a different type of cap should be fitted that is less likely to press on the bladder and urethra. Encourage your client to empty her bladder completely before and after sexual intercourse.

Disabled clients

If a disabled woman finds difficulty in fitting her diaphragm, you may like to suggest that her partner should be taught how to insert it.

Diaphragms and sexuality

The diaphragm can give women permission to touch and explore their bodies. Women have often used other methods of contraception before, and will choose the diaphragm because they feel it is free from side effects and remains under their own control.

A barrier for many women in choosing and using the diaphragm is ignorance of their body and their fear of expressing this. In a clinical setting it is important for you to allow time for these feelings to be expressed and it may also allow any sexual anxieties to be discussed and any sexual barriers to be dismantled. Comments from clients such as 'does it get lost?' and on seeing their new diaphragm 'am I that big?' are frequently heard.

Choosing the diaphragm as a method of contraception can signify a woman's ease with her own body and with her sexuality.

The cap

Although this type of cap has been used for decades it is often referred to as 'the new cap'.

The cap is smaller than the diaphragm and only covers the cervix itself, being held there by suction. It is made of rubber and works in the same way as the diaphragm in that it stops the sperm from meeting the ova and thus prevents fertilization. It is vital that the client is able to locate her cervix if she is to be able to use a cap. In order to optimize its effectiveness, the cap should be used in conjunction with a spermicide. This should fill one-third of the cap but should not be used on the rim as this would affect the suction. The same care and precautions apply to the cap as the diaphragm, and its advantages and disadvantages are listed in Box 11.3.

There are three types of cap in common use today. These are the cervical cap (prentif cavity rim), the vault cap (Dumas cap) and the vimule cap (Figure 11.3). All caps are fitted in the same way as the diaphragm.

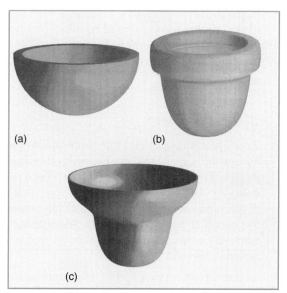

Figure 11.3   (a) Vault cap; (b) cervical cap; (c) vimule cap.

Cervical cap

The cervical cap is thimble-shaped with a wide rim. It comes in sizes from 22 to 31 mm in 3-mm steps. The size to use is determined by measuring the base of the cervix. This type of cap is best for women with a long, parallel-sided cervix as it fits snugly around the base of the cervix (Figure 11.4). It is not suitable for a flat or short cervix.

Box 11.3   The cap: advantages and disadvantages

Advantages

◆ All the advantages listed for the diaphragm in Box 11.2

◆ Suitable for women with poor pelvic muscle control

◆ Less pressure on the urethra and so less tendency to cause cystitis

◆ Less spermicide used so perceived as 'less messy'.

Disadvantages

◆ All the disadvantages listed for the diaphragm in Box 11.2

◆ More difficult to fit and remove

◆ Not suitable for women unable to locate their cervix.

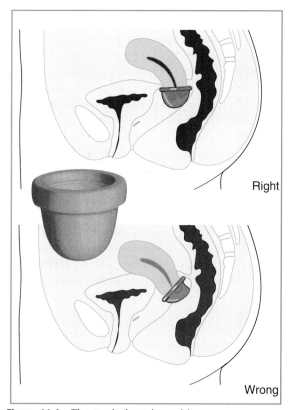

Figure 11.4   The cervical cap in position.

Dumas cap

The Dumas or vault cap is shaped like an upside-down bowl and comes in sizes from 50 to 75 mm in 5-mm steps. It is suitable for women with healthy, short cervices which allow the rim of the cap to adhere to the vaginal wall.

Vimule

The vimule is somewhere between the Dumas and the cervical cap in shape and comes in sizes 45, 48 and 51 mm. It clings by suction to the vaginal wall and is suitable for women who have problems using other types of cap or diaphragm because of poor vaginal muscle tone.

New innovations in cervical caps

New innovations in cervical caps include FemCap, Lea's shield and the Oves Cap.

◆ The FemCap is a reusable cervical cap made of silicone rubber and is available in three sizes. It should be used with spermicide and can be worn for 48 hours. It should remain *in situ* for 8 hours following sexual intercourse. The FemCap is associated with fewer urinary tract infections and although generally acceptable, problems with insertion, dislodgement and removal have been reported (Mauck *et al.*, 1999). Availability is limited in the UK.

◆ Lea's shield is also a reusable cervical cap made of silicone rubber which can be left *in situ* for 48 hours. It should be used with a spermicide and has a one-way valve that prevents the trapping of air and cervical secretions between the cervix and the device. As one size fits all women no fitting is required, making it suitable for over-the-counter use (Bounds, 1999). It is currently not available in the UK.

◆ The Oves cap is the only *disposable* cap (Figure 11.5). It is made from thinner silicone and is available in three sizes. Spermicide use is recommended. The cap can remain *in situ* for 72 hours, and should not be removed until 6 hours after intercourse. After an initial examination to determine which size is

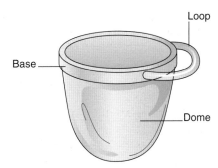

Figure 11.5 Oves™ contraceptive cap.

required, the Oves cap is available as an over-the-counter product. Availability is limited in the UK.

All three caps offer new choices for women, but have only undergone limited clinical trials so true efficacy rates are awaited. As with all barrier methods, the failure rate will increase if not used according to instructions.

The sponge

The contraceptive vaginal sponge was developed as an alternative to the diaphragm. It is made of polyurethane, impregnated with nonoxynol-9 and does not require fitting by a health professional. It can remain *in situ* for 24 hours and can be used for more than one act of intercourse without additional spermicide. The sponge is less effective than the diaphragm in preventing pregnancy (Kuyoh *et al.*, 2002).

The female condom

The female condom is a polyurethane condom with a non-spermicidal lubricant and is the only female condom available in the UK. It has two small rings, one which aids insertion into the vagina like a tampon, and the second to keep it in place on the outside of the genital area (Figure 11.6).

The female condom acts as a barrier preventing sperm from fertilizing the ovum and is as effective as the male condom, which is between 85%

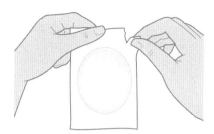

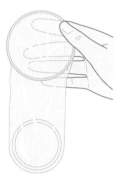

1

Open the package carefully; tear at the notch on the top right of the package. Do not use scissors or a knife to open.

2

The outer ring covers the area around the vagina. The inner ring is used to help hold the sheath in place during sex.

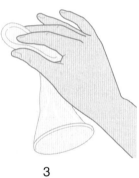

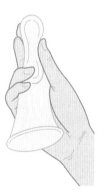

3

While holding the sheath at the closed end, grasp the flexible inner ring and squeeze it with the second or middle finger so it becomes long and narrow.

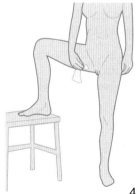

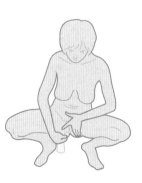

4

Choose a position that is comfortable for insertion – squat, raise one leg, sit or lie down.

Figure 11.6 Guide to inserting the female condom. *Source*: Everett (2004).

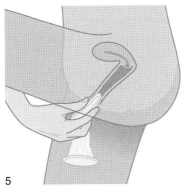

5

Gently insert the inner ring into the vagina. Feel the inner ring go up and move into place.

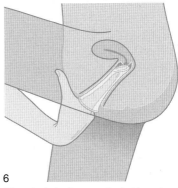

6

Place the index finger on the inside and push the inner ring up as far as it will go. Ensure the sheath is not twisted. The outer ring on the outside of the vagina.

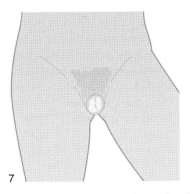

7

The female condom is now in place and ready for use with your partner.

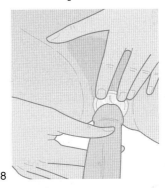

8

When you are ready, gently guide your partner's penis into the sheath's opening with care to make sure that it enters properly – be careful the penis is not entering on the side, between the sheath and the vaginal wall.

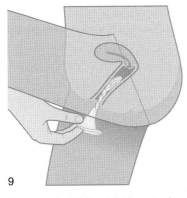

9

To remove the condom, twist the outer ring and gently pull the condom out.

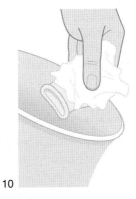

10

Wrap the condom in the package or tissue and throw it in the garbage. Do not put it into the toilet.

Figure 11.6 (Continued)

> **Box 11.4** The female condom: advantages and disadvantages
>
> **Advantages**
>
> ◆ Easily obtained and used
> ◆ Not damaged by oil-based lubricants
> ◆ Protects against most sexually transmitted infections and HIV
> ◆ Possible protection against cervical neoplasia
> ◆ Use can be alternated with male condom, thereby enabling both partners to take responsibility for contraception.
>
> **Disadvantages**
>
> ◆ May be perceived as disrupting sexual intercourse
> ◆ Needs to be inserted prior to sexual intercourse
> ◆ Can only be used once
> ◆ Expensive
> ◆ 'Hangs down' outside the vagina.

> **Box 11.5** Spermicides: advantages and disadvantages
>
> **Advantages**
>
> ◆ Increase efficacy of other methods
> ◆ No systemic effects
> ◆ Easy to obtain and use
> ◆ Provide lubrication
> ◆ May give some protection against sexually transmitted infections and HIV.
>
> **Disadvantages**
>
> ◆ Low efficacy rate
> ◆ Local allergic reaction
> ◆ May be perceived as messy.

and 98% effective in preventing pregnancy. Its advantages and disadvantages are summarized in Box 11.4. Trussel *et al.* (1994) found that the use of the female condom appears to have the potential to reduce the risk of a woman acquiring HIV.

Problems with the female condom

It is possible for the man to insert his penis between the vaginal wall and the female condom, so you should advise your clients to be aware of this possibility and help their partner with insertion.

Female condoms are made of polyurethane, which is stronger than condoms and can make a 'rustling sound'. You can advise women that using extra lubrication eases this problem.

Spermicides

Spermicides prevent pregnancy by killing sperm and by changing the pH in the vagina so that the environment is unfavourable for sperm. It is difficult to assess how effective spermicides, if used on their own, are in preventing pregnancy as research is limited. Usually spermicides are used in conjunction with another method like the diaphragm or condom. Some advantages and disadvantages are listed in Box 11.5.

Spermicides are available in a variety of forms: pessaries, gels, creams and foams. Creams are thicker and white in colour, whereas gels are clear and slightly runnier and personal choice will determine the type used. Pessaries take ten minutes to dissolve; creams, foams and gels can be inserted into the vagina using an applicator similar to a tampon applicator. Most spermicides contain nonoxynol 9 which has been shown to be active against HIV *in vitro* (Bird, 1991). Complaints of 'messiness' can be combated by changing to creams or foam instead of gels.

The combined oral contraceptive pill

Often referred to as 'the pill', the combined oral contraceptive pill (COC) contains the two hormones oestrogen and progestogen. It works in three ways by:

◆ Stopping ovulation
◆ Thickening cervical mucus to stop sperm from entering the uterus
◆ Helping to prevent implantation by alteration of the endometrium.

It is between 97% and 99% effective in preventing pregnancy, although the failure rate can be higher

Box 11.6 The COC: advantages and disadvantages
Advantages
◆ High efficacy
◆ Easy to take, convenient and easily reversed
◆ Reduces dysmenorrhoea and menorrhagia
◆ Less risk of anaemia because of lighter periods
◆ Pelvic inflammatory disease reduced
◆ Protection against osteoporosis
◆ Less benign breast disease
◆ Reduces pain from endometriosis
◆ Fewer ovarian cysts
◆ Protects against cancer of the ovary and endometrium
◆ ? Reduced risk of underactive and overactive thyroid disease.
Disadvantages
◆ Needs to be taken regularly
◆ Does not protect against sexually transmitted infections and HIV
◆ Increased risk of circulatory problems, including migraines, hypertension, deep vein thrombosis, pulmonary embolism and myocardial infarction
◆ Increased risk of liver disorders, such as cholestatic jaundice, gallstones and liver adenoma.

Box 11.7 The COC: absolute contraindications
◆ Pregnancy
◆ Breastfeeding – the combined pill will inhibit milk production
◆ Undiagnosed genital tract bleeding
◆ Focal or crescendo migraines or migraines with aura
◆ Blood lipid disorder with family history of parent with heart disease below 45 years of age
◆ Hypertension
◆ Previous or present circulatory problems (particularly deep vein thrombosis, pulmonary emboli, transient ischaemic attacks)
◆ Prothrombotic abnormalities of coagulation including congenital thrombophilias, acquired thrombophilia, antiphospholipid syndrome
◆ Major surgery or leg surgery
◆ Conditions which predispose to thrombosis including polycythaemia, polyarteritis nodosa
◆ Past cerebral haemorrhage
◆ Liver disorders or impaired liver function tests (the combined pill may be started three months after liver function tests have returned to normal), including gallstones and porphyrias.
◆ Aged 35 or over and a smoker
◆ With a BMI over 40
◆ Diabetes mellitus with severe complications, e.g. renal impairment
◆ Oestrogen-dependent cancers, e.g. breast cancer
◆ Previous serious illness when taking the combined pill, including: hypertension, otosclerosis, pemphigoid gestationis and trophoblastic disease.

with poor compliance. The advantages and disadvantages of using the pill are listed in Box 11.6.

Absolute contraindications

See Box 11.7.

Relative contraindications

With certain women extra care needs to be taken when prescribing the combined oral contraceptive pill. Women with any of the conditions listed below may be prescribed the combined pill, but will require further counselling and increased supervision.

◆ Diabetes mellitus with no complications

◆ Chronic systemic disease

◆ Long-term immobilization

◆ Severe depression

◆ Using enzyme-inducing drugs to treat epilepsy and tuberculosis. These can reduce the safety of the combined pill. Another form of contraception may need to be considered or they can use a higher dose of combined pill

◆ Sickle cell anaemia

◆ Chronic renal disease

◆ Crohn's disease

◆ Hyperprolactinaemia

◆ Treatment for cervical intraepithelial neoplasia (CIN)

◆ Young first-degree relative with breast cancer.

Types of combined oral contraceptives

These days, most women take a monophasic pill which contains the same dose for 21 days. The monophasic pill is less complicated to take, particularly if a pill is forgotten or if wanting to postpone a withdrawal bleed.

Biphasic pills which include two types of pill with different doses of oestrogen and progestogen and triphasic pills which include three types of pills with different dosages were introduced in an effort to mimic the varying hormone levels in the normal menstrual cycle. It is important to take these pills in the correct order.

Every day (ED) combined pills are rarely used in Britain but are used widely in Europe and Australia. An ED packet contains 28 pills and includes 7 inactive pills. ED pills are useful for women who find it difficult to remember to restart their pill after the 7-day break.

Which pill?

There are many different types of combined pill available (see Table 11.1).

The oestrogen in combined pills is ethinylo-estradiol and they contain different types of progestogen. Pills containing the progestogens desogestrel or gestodene are called 'third generation pills'. A new 30 μg pill called Yasmin was launched in 2002. Yasmin is neither a second nor third generation pill, and contains drospirenone (a derivative of spironolactone) and is believed to help to reduce water retention and weight gain (Drugs and Therapeutic Bulletin, 2002). Further research is needed to ascertain the risk of venous thromboembolism in comparison to other combined pills.

It is good practice to start a client on a low-dose pill when they are first given this method of contraception; 30 μg or less of oestrogen is considered low dose. If a woman is started on a low-dose combined pill and this does not suit her, then she can be changed to another low-dose pill from another group or she can be prescribed a slightly higher dose pill.

Venous thromboembolism (VTE)

Three studies in 1995 (Jick *et al.*, 1995; WHO, 1995; Spitzer *et al.*, 1996) showed that women taking pills containing the newer progestogens, desogestrel and gestodene (commonly called third generation progestogens), have an increased risk of VTE when compared with women taking pills containing the older progestogens, levo-norgestrel or norethisterone (second generation progestogens). There was insufficient evidence about pills containing norgestimate.

Following these studies the Committee on Safety of Medicines (CSM) ruled that women with risk factors for VTE should not use third generation progestogens (Committee on Safety of Medicines, 1995). After a lengthy review of the evidence (showing that the difference in VTE risk was smaller than previously thought and that the original studies did not account for biases in prescribing), the CSM in 1999 reversed their earlier advice and third generation pills can now be prescribed from the outset in women with no risk factors for VTE.

The issue remains confusing, however, as a population study from Denmark (Mellemkjaer *et al.*, 1999) found that a 16% increase in admission rate for venous thromboembolism correlates with the increase in prescription of third generation contraceptives.

The Department of Health in 1999 (Guillebaud, 1999) recommended that a woman could jointly decide with the doctor or family planning professional which pill to take as long as she is fully informed in the light of her medical history of the small risks of the combined pill. There has been some disagreement about this view, and the debate continues. However, it is important to explain the risks and take a comprehensive medical history so that the decision is based on all the information available. The adverse publicity surrounding the pill has meant that many women remain anxious and are reluctant to take oral contraception.

Risk factors for VTE include:

◆ Family history of VTE

◆ Varicose veins

◆ Obesity – this is considered if the body mass index (BMI) is over 30 kg/m^2

Table 11.1 Combined oral contraceptives available in the UK

Pill type	Preparation	Manufacturer	Oestrogen (μg)	Progestogen (mg)	
Combined					
Ethinylestrodiol/desogestrel	Marvelon	Organon	30	0.15	
	Mercilon	Organon	20	0.15	
Ethinylestradiol/drospirenone	Yasmin	Schering HC	30	3	
Ethinylestradiol/gestodene	Femodene (also ED)	Schering HC	30	0.075	
	Femodette	Schering HC	20	0.075	
	Minulet	Wyeth	30	0.075	
Ethinylestradiol/levonorgestrel	Eugynon 30	Schering HC	30	0.25	
	Microgynon 30 (also ED)	Schering HC	30	0.15	
	Ovranette	Wyeth	30	0.15	
Ethinylestradiol/norelgestromin	Evra (patches)	Janssen-Cilag	20/24 hours	0.15/24 hours	norelgestromin[a]
Ethinylestradiol/norethisterone type	Brevinor	Pharmacia	35	0.5	norethisterone
	Loestrin 20	Parke-Davis	20	1	norethisterone acetate
	Loestrin 30	Parke-Davis	30	1.5	norethisterone acetate
	Norimin	Pharmacia	35	1	norethisterone
	Ovysmen	Janssen-Cilag	35	0.5	norethisterone
Ethinylestradiol/norgestimate	Cilest	Janssen-Cilag	35	0.25	
Mestranol/norethisterone	Norinyl-1	Pharmacia	50	1	
Biphasic and triphasic					
Ethinylestradiol/gestodene	Tri-Minulet	Wyeth	30	0.05	(6 tabs)
			40	0.07	(5 tabs)
			30	0.1	(10 tabs)
	Triadene	Schering HC	30	0.05	(6 tabs)
			4	0.07	(5 tabs)
			30	0.1	(10 tabs)
Ethinylestradiol/levonorgestrel	Logynon (also ED)	Schering HC	30	0.05	(6 tabs)
			40	0.075	(5 tabs)
			30	0.125	(10 tabs)
	Trinordiol	Wyeth	30	0.05	(6 tabs)
			40	0.075	(5 tabs)
			30	0.125	(10 tabs)
Ethinylestradiol/norethisterone	BiNovum	Janssen-Cilag	35	0.5	(7 tabs)
			35	1	(14 tabs)
	Synphase	Pharmacia	35	0.5	(7 tabs)
			35	1	(9 tabs)
			35	0.5	(5 tabs)
	TriNovum	Janssen-Cilag	35	0.5	(7 tabs)
			35	0.75	(7 tabs)
			35	1	(7 tabs)

[a]Primary active metabolite of norgestimate.
Source: Reproduced with permission from *MIMS: Monthly Index of Medical Specialities*. London: Haymarket Publishing Services, July 2004. Updated monthly.

◆ Immobility

◆ NB: A previous history of VTE is an absolute contraindication to any combined pill.

Gestodene-, desogestrel- and norgestimate-containing pills have been shown to have a 'slightly more beneficial effect on lipid metabolism' (Robinson, 1994) compared to other combined pills. The clinical significance of this is uncertain; however, research (O'Brien, 1999a) has shown that there is a tendency towards a lower risk of myocardial infarction in women taking second generation pills compared to those taking third generation (Dunn *et al.*, 1999a, 1999b; O'Brien, 1999b; Lewis *et al.*, 1997).

A thrombophilia screen is recommended if a woman has a family history of a first degree relative under the age of 45 years old who has had a VTE. With today's wide range of oestrogen-free contraceptive methods it is good practice to discuss other methods which do not have an increased risk. If after discussion a woman with a family history of VTE still wants to try an oestrogen-containing method like the combined pill or patch then it is recommended that the thrombophilia screen should be performed in consultation with the haematologist (FFPRHC, 2003a).

Women are often unaware that pregnancy has a higher incidence of VTE, 6 per 10,000 per year in full-term pregnancy (DoH, 1995), and this information can help to balance the risks of the combined pill. When counselling women it is important that you discuss current research and give updated literature so that they are able to make an informed choice.

A first visit

Often women will have decided that they want to start taking the combined pill before coming to see you. It is useful to find out how much they already know and you can then build upon this information.

Topics to be covered on a first visit include:

◆ Past and present medical history to discover any absolute or relative contraindications

◆ Any current medication that may interfere with the effectiveness of the combined pill

◆ Blood pressure, weight, height and body mass index (BMI)

◆ Smoking history: what, how many and for how long?

◆ Previous contraceptive history: what methods previously used and problems encountered? This could indicate a relative contraindication, and may help in deciding which combined pill to prescribe

◆ Methods of contraception used recently. Does she need emergency contraception?

◆ Date of last menstrual period. Was it a normal period? This will eliminate pregnancy

◆ Date of last cervical smear, if she has had one. What was the result? Have previous smear results been normal? If the client does not know or has had a previous abnormal smear (and there is no smear result available), or it is now 3 years since the last smear then a smear will need to be performed at a convenient date

◆ Any bleeding after sexual intercourse – known as post-coital bleeding (PCB). If there is, a cervical smear will need to be performed with bimanual examination. PCB has a number of causes including cervical ectopy, polyps, infection and malignancy

◆ Any change in normal vaginal discharge. Does it smell? What does it look like? If there are any doubts it is worth screening for infection

◆ Breast awareness. Does she check her breasts regularly for lumps or changes?

◆ Sexual anxieties and problems. Towards the end of the consultation the client is hopefully feeling more relaxed and able to share any anxieties or problems. Is intercourse painful? If it is can she tell you more about the pain?

Having found out about your client's medical history and discussed any problems, you should go on to give clear information about the advantages and disadvantages of the combined pill and about how to take the pill, when to start, and when to use extra precautions, for example after forgetting a pill, after diarrhoea and vomiting or whilst taking other drugs.

Box 11.8 Minor problems encountered when starting the pill

- *Nausea* This normally settles after three packets. It can be avoided by taking the pills with food, after a meal or at bedtime
- *Forgetting to take the pills* Many women find it difficult to remember to take their pills until they get into a regular routine. Helpful tips include:
  - Take the pill on waking or going to bed
  - Take the pill when cleaning teeth
  - Keep the packet in your handbag or by your alarm clock
  - Set your digital watch or mobile phone as a reminder
  - Keep the packet in your coffee jar or tea caddy
- *Breakthrough bleeding* This may occur in the first couple of months. If the pills have been taken correctly, your client's contraception will remain effective
- *Breast tenderness or bloating* Normally these symptoms disappear after three packets.

Box 11.9 Reasons for changing the combined pill

- *Continuing breakthrough bleeding* First check the client is taking her pills correctly and has had no diarrhoea, vomiting or drugs that may interfere with the pill. If it is a new problem then get the client to keep a diary and review the bleeding in a couple of months. Check that a recent smear and vaginal examination have been performed to exclude infection and disease. If necessary, change to a higher dose pill or try a different progestogen
- *Breast tenderness* The client may find that taking evening primrose oil or vitamin B6 one week before the symptoms start is helpful. If necessary, change pill to a lower dose of oestrogen or a different progestogen
- *Vaginal dryness* Is there an underlying sexual anxiety or problem? Try changing pill
- *Nausea* Advise your client to avoid taking the pill on an empty stomach. Change pill
- *Spots and acne* Try changing pill to a different progestogen
- *Weight gain* A small weight gain may be noticed initially. If weight gain continues and a woman's diet is healthy, try changing pill.

Minor problems a woman may encounter when starting the pill are outlined in Box 11.8. You should discuss these thoroughly so that she is prepared for them and to prevent unnecessary worry. It is not advisable to change to a different pill within the first 3 months as a response to any of these minor symptoms. Changing pills may perpetuate the symptoms, and the initial problems normally settle on their own after the first three packets. If, after the first 3 months, problems persist, it will be worth considering a change to a different pill (Box 11.9).

It is important to point out to your client that problems sometimes occur for which she should seek medical attention. These include:

- Pain or swelling in the calf
- Chest pain
- Shortness of breath
- Increasing headaches
- Episodes of loss or disturbance of vision
- Pain, tingling or weakness of an arm
- Jaundice
- Prolonged bleeding or post-coital bleeding.

You should also advise her to return to you if, despite taking the pills correctly, she does not have a withdrawal bleed. It is unlikely that she is pregnant but this should be excluded.

Always discuss how the risks of the pill (e.g. cardiovascular disease) are increased by smoking. If a smoker gives up, these will reduce to the same as those for a non-smoker.

Remind your client that the pill does not protect against HIV or other sexually transmitted infections. To reduce this risk her partner will need to use a condom.

Leaflets containing all this information should be given to back-up your discussion. You should also hand out the telephone numbers of your clinic and emergency advice centres in case she needs further information, and where and when to obtain emergency contraception information.

Follow-up and subsequent visits

It is important to find out how your client has got on with the combined pill and if she has experienced any problems including increased headaches or migraines. It is a good idea to start by asking an open ended question such as 'how have you got on?' and encourage her to talk about anxieties she may have.

Always check blood pressure and weight at each visit to make sure these are within normal limits. If a client smokes it is good practice to check this is not increasing and encourage cessation. At each visit you should check whether there is any new relevant medical history for your client or her immediate family, e.g. any new medication, or mother with a deep vein thrombosis. Check whether a cervical smear test is due, and that the client knows when this needs to be repeated. This is also a good time to check when her last menstrual period was, and whether she has any bleeding at any other time. Does she have any problems with her periods?

The first follow-up visit is an important time to check that your patient is taking the pill correctly and knows what to do if she forgets a pill. Information should be given about emergency contraception.

If there are no problems your client will be given a prescription for 6 months' supply of the combined pill, encouraged to use condoms if necessary, and given another appointment. It is a good idea to encourage women to return before they run out of supplies, and if possible to keep a spare packet of pills for emergencies.

A woman who is happy with the combined pill and has no complications or contraindications can continue using this method until she is aged 50 years.

How to take the combined pill

These instructions are the same for all combined 21-day pills (whether they are monophasics, biphasics or triphasic pills). When starting for the first time, if the pill is started on the first day of the period, no additional contraception is required. If started at any other time in the cycle then additional contraception should be used for 7 days. Take the pill every day at roughly the same time for 21 days following the arrows on the packets. This 21 days of pill taking is followed by a 7-day break during which a period or withdrawal bleed will be experienced. The next

packet of pills after the 7-day break should be started on day 8. Some women get confused trying to remember when to start a new packet. It is always helpful to remind them that all new packets should be started on the same day of the week as when they first started the pill.

When the combined pill is not effective

The pill has reduced effectiveness when:

◆ A client has forgotten to take a pill and is more than 12 hours late
◆ Vomiting occurs within 3 hours of taking the pill
◆ Severe diarrhoea occurs
◆ Certain drugs are taken (Table 11.2).

Instructions for a missed pill (see Figure 11.7)
If a forgotten pill is remembered within 12 hours of when the woman normally takes the pill, then she should take the pill and no other extra precautions are necessary.

Table 11.2 Drugs that affect the efficacy of the combined pill

Group	Drug
Anticonvulsants[a]	Phenytoin
	Primidone
	Carbamazepine
	Barbiturates
Antitubercle[a]	Rifampicin
Diuretics[a]	Spironolactone
Hypnotics[a]	Dichloralphenazone
Tranquilizers[a]	Meprobamate
Antifungal treatments[a]	Griseofulvin
Broad-spectrum antibiotics[b]	Ampicillin
	Tetracycline
	Cephalosporins
Protease inhibitors[a]	Ritonavir
	Nelfinavir
Herbal medicine[a]	St John's Wort

[a]These are all liver enzyme-inducing drugs which increase the metabolism of the combined pill and, as a result, decrease the contraceptive effectiveness.
[b]These affect the bowel flora and consequently the absorption of the combined pill.

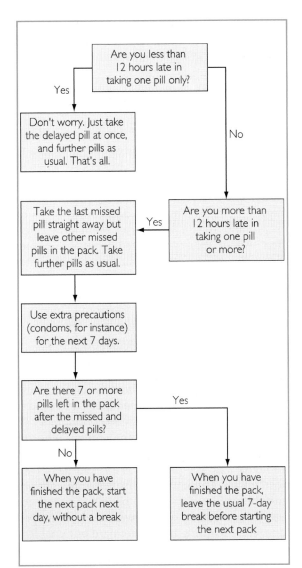

Figure 11.7 Instruction for missed pills (21-day packaging).

having a withdrawal bleed. If the client is taking biphasic or triphasic pills and does not have 7 days' worth of pills left in the packet then she will need to take enough pills from the end of another packet to make 7 days, but they must be of the same colour and same dose.

Women are safe to have sexual intercourse in the 7-day break as long as they do not lengthen this gap any longer than 7 days. If a client forgets the last pill of the packet and then continues to have a 7-day break then she is at risk of ovulating and becoming pregnant. So if a client forgets the last pill of the packet she should be advised to then only have a further 6-day break of the pill so that in total she only has a 7-day gap.

If she forgets the first pill of a new packet then she will have had a total of 8 days break from the pill. She should be advised to take 7 days of consecutive pills before considering her contraception safe. In the meantime she should be advised to use a condom.

Diarrhoea and vomiting

When a client has severe diarrhoea and/or vomiting then her contraception will not be effective. In this situation the client needs to use another form of contraception (e.g. condoms) until the diarrhoea has finished; meanwhile she should continue taking her pills. Once the diarrhoea or vomiting has finished then she should be advised to continue using condoms until she has taken a further 7 days of consecutive pills after which she will be safe to use the combined pill on its own.

Drugs

The drugs that affect the efficiency of the combined pill are summarized in Table 11.2. Some of these, such as spironolactone (a potassium-sparing diuretic), dichloralphenazone (used for insomnia), meprobamate (an anti-anxiety drug), and protease inhibitors, should be avoided altogether with combined oral contraceptive use. Others, such as long-term antibiotics, should be used in conjunction with extra precautions for the first 2 weeks to avoid conception.

If anticonvulsants or liver enzyme inducers are being taken, a woman will need to be given a pill

If, however, it is more than 12 hours from when the pill is normally taken, then the pill should be taken and another contraceptive method used (e.g. condoms) for the next 7 days. Meanwhile the woman should continue taking her pills and once she has taken for 7 consecutive days then the pill will be effective. If there are not enough pills in the packet and the client is taking a monophasic pill then she will need to continue on to another packet without a break and avoid with an increased level of oestrogen of 50 μg and/or to be instructed to tricycle her pill.

Long-term use of anticonvulsants or liver enzyme inducers will mean that the client should be encouraged to consider another form of contraception, such as an IUD or Depo-Provera at a shortened 8-week interval. When enzyme inducers are discussed with the woman, she should be advised that it can take many weeks for liver metabolism to return to normal, and she must wait at least 4–8 weeks before returning to a standard low-dose combined oral contraceptive (COC).

In 2000 the Committee on Safety of Medicines reviewed new evidence about important interactions between St John's wort preparations and certain prescribed medicines, including the oral contraceptive pill. They concluded that the efficacy of the COC is reduced whilst taking St John's wort (Committee on Safety of Medicines, 2000).

Tricycling

In tricycling, three or four packets of monophasic pills are taken without a gap and the woman has her pill-free week at the end of the 3 months instead of monthly. Tricycling may be recommended for problems that occur in the pill-free week; by reducing the number of pill-free weeks in a year the amount of suffering is reduced. It is important to check that the problem only occurs in the pill-free week. This can be done by asking the client to keep a diary of her symptoms and when they occur.

The main reasons for tricycling are as follows:

◆ Headaches during the pill-free week sometimes occur due to a decrease in hormone level. So long as these headaches do not cause focal disturbances – an absolute contraindication to the combined pill – then tricycling will reduce the number of headaches

◆ Premenstrual symptoms may occur during the pill-free week and tricycling can be effective

◆ Recurring vaginal thrush often happens when a period is due and the vaginal pH balance is changed. Tricycling pills may reduce the episodes of thrush

◆ Enzyme-inducing drugs (e.g. anticonvulsants, antifungal, antitubercle) will reduce

the efficacy of the combined pill. Tricycling is used to increase safety and the pill-free week is reduced to 4 or 5 days

◆ At the woman's choice to avoid bleeding.

The combined pill and sexuality

The combined pill is one of the safest, most reliable and easily reversible forms of contraception. It gives women the power to choose when to become pregnant. For some women this control has become difficult to handle; the pill is in some ways too effective and the decision to come off the pill and start a family can seem very calculated. All of this contributed to many women postponing pregnancy and starting families later. Women sometimes feel confused and ask for your advice as they feel guilty about avoiding pregnancy but enjoy their freedom. They may also be anxious about whether their fertility is in jeopardy for taking the pill for many years.

Conversely, women who have been on the pill for a number of years and then discontinue in order to become pregnant become very anxious if this does not happen immediately, and tend to blame the pill for their failure to conceive.

Alternatively there are some women who frequently forget their pill or continually find new problems with the pill and as a result have tried most brands. These women are not only unhappy with their pill but may also be trying to tell you there is something wrong with their lives, perhaps really wanting to get pregnant but unable to admit it to herself or her partner. The client who constantly finds problems with her pills may have other underlying problems not directly related to contraception but having an effect on her sexuality which you may be able to uncover with sympathetic questioning.

Myths and the media

There are many myths surrounding the combined pill. It is often felt that it is not natural to suppress ovulation, yet it is forgotten that in many countries women spend most of their fertile years suppressing ovulation through pregnancy and breastfeeding. It could be argued that it is not natural to ovulate every month.

Another myth is that the pill causes breast cancer which is regularly reinforced by the media and new 'scare' stories. The incidence of breast cancer is high and inevitably will develop in women whether or not they take the COC. However a major reanalysis of epidemiological studies (Collaborative Group on Hormonal Factors in Breast Cancer, 1996) has shown that the relative risk of having a breast cancer diagnosed is 1.24 for current users of the COC compared to non-users. The risk is the same regardless of the level of dosage or duration of use, but decreases after stopping the COC and disappears after 10 years. They also found that the cancers found in women taking the combined pill were less clinically advanced. What the media do not mention is how much the pill protects women from getting cancer of the endometrium and ovaries.

That the pill is dangerous is a misconception held by many people. In fact it is a very safe form of contraception that is highly acceptable to large numbers of women. Perhaps it should be put another way: that smoking can be dangerous, but if you smoke and take the combined pill it is the smoking and not the pill that is dangerous. Smoking is considered a risk to your health because of the damage it causes to your circulatory system. If you do not smoke and there are no other contraindications then there is no reason why you cannot take the combined pill indefinitely.

The combined contraceptive patch

There is only one contraceptive patch, known as Evra. Evra is a 20 cm self-adhesive transdermal patch delivering 150 µg of norelgestromin and 20 µg of ethinyoestradiol into the bloodstream daily. Evra is 99% effective in preventing pregnancy; however, efficacy may be reduced in women whose weight is over 90 kg (Janssen-Cilag, 2003). Compliance with the patch regime has been shown to be better than the contraceptive pill, particularly in young women. Only 68% of women under the age of 20 took their pills correctly, compared with 88% of those using a patch (Archer *et al.*, 2002).

The patch is changed weekly for three weeks with the fourth week being the patch-free week when a withdrawal bleed is experienced. A new

contraceptive patch is applied after 7 patch-free days. Evra prevents pregnancy by inhibiting ovulation, altering cervical mucus by making it impenetrable to sperm, and by making the endometrium unfavourable for implantation. At the moment there is limited research on the risk of VTE, cervical and breast cancer with Evra (FFPRHC, 2003b).

Absolute and relative contraindications
The absolute and relative contraindications are the same as for the combined contraceptive pill.

How to use the contraceptive patch
Evra is applied on the first day of a period and remains there for 7 days, It is then removed on day 8 when a new patch is applied. On day 15 the second patch is removed and the third patch applied which will need to be removed on day 22 when the 7-day patch-free interval begins. A new patch is applied on the 8th day following the patch-free week. It can be seen therefore that patches should usually be changed on the same day of the week.

What to do if the contraceptive patch comes off?
If Evra detaches for less than 24 hours then the patch should be reapplied or replaced with a new patch and no extra contraception will be required; the patch-change day will remain the same. If Evra detaches for more than 24 hours then a new patch should be applied and a new cycle commenced; additional contraception should be used for 7 days.

What if the patch is not changed on the correct day?
If the patch is forgotten at the beginning of a new cycle the woman my not have adequate contraception. She should apply the first patch as soon as possible and use additional contraception (non-hormonal) for the next 7 days. There will now be a new patch-change day.

If she forgets to change a patch in the middle of the cycle, but remembers within 48 hours, she should change the patch immediately and no additional contraceptive use is required providing the patch was worn correctly in the previous 7 days. If more than 48 hours have elapsed then she should stop the current patch cycle and start a new four-week cycle immediately. There is now a new day 1 and patch-change day. Additional contraception (non-hormonal) should be used for the next 7 days.

What reduces the effectiveness of the contraceptive patch?

Drugs that reduce the effectiveness of Evra are enzyme-inducing drugs, broad-spectrum antibiotics and St John's wort.

The combined contraceptive patch and sexuality

The contraceptive patch increases the choices available to women, giving women an effective method of contraception which does not need to be remembered every day. It appeals to young women who may be forgetful about taking a daily pill and who see it as fashionable and more convenient.

Progestogen-only pill

The progestogen-only pill, commonly known as the 'mini pill', is not to be confused with low-dose combined pills. Often abbreviated to the POP, the progestogen-only pill prevents pregnancy in four ways:

◆ By making the cervical mucus impenetrable to sperm

◆ By making the endometrium less favourable for implantation

◆ By occasionally suppressing ovulation in some women

◆ By reducing Fallopian tube function.

A new progestogen-only pill, Cerazette, containing 75 μg of desogestrel, prevents pregnancy by the ways above, but inhibits ovulation in 97% of cycles making it a highly effective contraceptive (FFPRHC, 2003c). Women should be warned that they are more likely to have amenorrhoea with Cerazette.

The progestogen-only pill is 96–99% effective in preventing pregnancy. Its advantages, disadvantages, and absolute and relative contraindications are outlined in Box 11.10.

Box 11.10 The progestogen-only pill: advantages, disadvantages and contraindications

Advantages

◆ Does not inhibit lactation, therefore suitable for breastfeeding women

◆ No evidence of increased circulatory disease or malignancy

◆ Can be given to women who have side effects with the combined pill, e.g. headaches, weight gain, reduced libido

◆ Can be given to women over 35 who smoke

◆ Can be given to hypertensive women.

Disadvantages

◆ Needs to be taken reliably and regularly

◆ Not as effective as the combined pill

◆ Irregular bleeding pattern

◆ Small number of women may develop symptomatic functional ovarian cysts

◆ Slight increase in ectopic pregnancy if the pill fails to be effective.

Absolute contraindications

◆ Past or present severe arterial disease

◆ Liver adenoma, cholestatic jaundice, or present liver disease

◆ Pregnancy

◆ Undiagnosed genital tract bleeding

◆ Serious side effects with the combined pill, not linked to oestrogen

◆ Trophoblastic disease

◆ Past history of an ectopic pregnancy in a nulliparous woman.

Relative contraindications

The POP may be given to women with relative contraindications but will need extra monitoring.

◆ Functional ovarian cysts

◆ Sex steroid cancers

◆ Focal migraines, hypertension, lipid abnormalities

◆ Relevant interacting drugs and severe malabsorption.

Types of progestogen-only pill

There are seven progestogen-only pills on the market (Table 11.3).

What reduces the effectiveness of the progestogen pill?

The effectiveness of the progestogen-only pill will be reduced if:

◆ A woman has severe diarrhoea

◆ Vomiting occurs within 3 hours of taking the pill and the woman fails to retake it

◆ A woman takes drugs which are enzyme inducers, like rifampicin, griseofulvin or anti-convulsants. In this situation an injectable form of contraception is preferable. If this is unsuitable she may need to increase the dose of progestogen she takes to 3–4 pills a day. The efficacy of this regime is unknown

◆ There is some evidence to suggest a trend in reduced efficacy if a woman weighs more than 70 kg. Taking two pills a day would increase efficacy as would changing to Cerazette.

Teaching a client how to take the POP

The client should start the progestogen-only pill on the first day of her period, and will need no extra precautions. She should take it every day at around the same time. If the client takes her pill more than 3 hours late then the pill's efficacy will be reduced and she will need to use another form of contraception for the next 2 days whilst continuing to take her pill. With Cerazette it is different as this pill mainly works by inhibiting ovulation. Additional precautions need only be used if the pill is taken over 12 hours late (rather than 3 hours). These precautions need to be used for 2 days.

The POP is taken continuously; there is no gap between packets. Periods will usually be similar to her previous cycle, but occasionally they can be irregular with spotting and sometimes stop altogether.

As the POP mainly stops pregnancy through thickening cervical mucus its effectiveness will be greatest a few hours after ingesting the pill, and lowest when a new pill is due to be taken. You should advise your clients to take the POP a few hours before the time when regular sexual intercourse takes place, so that the effect on cervical mucus is at its optimum, e.g. early evening on the assumption that most couples have intercourse late evening.

When should the POP be started after pregnancy?

If a woman is not breastfeeding she may start the POP on day 21 after birth; no extra precautions are needed. If a woman is breastfeeding she can start the POP 4 weeks after delivery with no extra precautions. The POP does not affect lactation nor does it affect the baby.

Table 11.3 Progestogen-only pills available in the UK

Pill type	Preparation	Manufacturer	Oestrogen (µg)	Progestogen (mg)	
Desogestrel	Cerazette	Organon	–	0.075	
Levonorgestrel	Microval	Wyeth	–	0.03	
	Norgeston	Schering HC	–	0.03	
Norethisterone type	Femulen	Pharmacia	–	0.5	ethynodiol diacetate[a]
	Micronor	Janssen-Celig	–	0.35	norethisterone
	Noriday	Pharmacia	–	0.35	norethisterone
Norgestrel	Neogest	Schering HC	–	0.075	

[a]Converted (>90%) to norethisterone as the active metabolite.
Source: Reproduced with permission from *MIMS: Monthly Index of Medical Specialities*. London: Haymarket Publishing Services, July 2004. Updated monthly.

Problems encountered

No menstrual bleed

Irregular bleeding is common with the POP, but some women find that their menses cease altogether, especially with Cerazette. As long as pregnancy has been excluded, then she can be reassured that in fact the POP is working even more effectively and stopping ovulation as well as thickening cervical mucus.

Breakthrough bleeding

If a woman complains of breakthrough bleeding with the POP it is important to check that she is taking her pills correctly and not taking pills late, thereby reducing efficacy. If this is not the problem it may be a good idea to change her to a different progestogen pill (Table 11.3), ask her to keep a diary of the bleeding, and review in three months.

Care of a client taking the progestogen pill

Initial visit

- Explain how to take the POP, its advantages and disadvantages
- Check the client is not taking any drugs that will reduce the effectiveness of the POP
- Take a full case history so that any contra-indications can be ascertained
- Check blood pressure and weight
- Discuss smoking cessation if she smokes – although smoking is not contraindicated in the POP at any age
- Check that her cervical smears are up to date
- Discuss safer sex
- Discuss emergency contraception
- Back-up verbal information with leaflets and relevant telephone numbers
- Give the client three packets of pills and arrange a review before the end of the third packet.

Follow-up visits

These sessions are to ascertain whether a client has any problems with the POP. It is important to find out if she is having a regular bleeding pattern, with no breakthrough bleeding or amenorrhoea, and investigate accordingly. Blood pressure and weight should be checked, and cervical smears should be performed as required. If a client has no problems and there is no new relevant medical or family history, then she can be prescribed further supplies of the progestogen-only pill and reviewed at 6-monthly intervals.

Myths and the media

The media always seems to focus its interest towards the combined pill, and as a result the POP is largely a forgotten method of contraception. Many women still refer to the POP as the 'mini pill', resulting in the belief that it is not very safe. In fact, if taken correctly it is a very effective form of contraception.

POP and sexuality

Women may be prescribed the POP because they have contraindications to the combined pill. This may mean that the POP is not their first choice of contraception, and they may be more easily dissatisfied with it. As the POP is not as effective as the combined pill there can be anxiety over unwanted pregnancies: and some women may choose to use spermicides or condoms as well as the POP to increase efficacy.

Women who frequently say 'I can't remember to take my pill' may subconsciously be hoping to become pregnant, but not ready yet to admit this to themselves. If given time, they may be able to discuss what makes it difficult for them to remember to take it, and how they feel about becoming pregnant. The acceptability of the POP depends very largely on your attitude and the confidence with which you talk to your clients about the method.

Injectables

Depo-Provera is the most widely used injectable contraceptive in the UK. It is often shortened by clients to 'Depo'. Injectables prevent pregnancy primarily by stopping ovulation. As with other hormonal methods they thicken cervical mucus preventing sperm penetration, and cause the endometrium to become less favourable to implantation.

Depo-Provera and Noristerat are 99–100% effective at preventing pregnancy and are the most effective reversible methods of contraception. Their advantages, disadvantages and contraindications are listed in Box 11.11. It is important to keep up to date with changes in recommended clinical practice, particularly if a woman is late for her injection, and the best source of current information for this is www.ffprhc.org.uk.

Types available

Depo-Provera

This is a 150 mg injection of depot medroxyprogesterone acetate, which is given every 12 weeks by deep intramuscular injection into the buttock. The ampoule should be shaken thoroughly before use. The injection site should not be massaged afterwards as this shortens its duration of effectiveness.

Noristerat

This is a 200 mg injection containing norethisterone oenanthate, which is given every 8 weeks by deep intramuscular injection into the buttock. The ampoule should be warmed to body temperature before administration as the solution is thick and oily, and the injection site should not be massaged afterwards.

Care of a woman having injectables

Initial visit

It is important that the woman is aware of the advantages and disadvantages of injectables. Once the injection has been given it cannot be removed, so the client should be especially aware of possible menstrual irregularity, amenorrhoea, and delay in return of fertility.

Routine blood pressure and weight should be recorded. Weight measurement is important and can be useful at a later date when clients may feel they have increased in weight and tend to blame the injection.

A full past and present medical history should be taken to exclude any contraindications. A cervical smear test should be performed if necessary.

Box 11.11 Injectables: advantages, disadvantages and contraindications

Advantages

◆ Effective, does not require the client to remember to take daily pills, so has a very low user failure rate
◆ Less premenstrual tension in some women
◆ Reduced dysmenorrhoea and menorrhagia
◆ Suitable for breastfeeding women
◆ Free of oestrogen-related side effects
◆ Beneficial in endometriosis
◆ Method of choice in sickle cell disease.

Disadvantages

◆ Delay in return of fertility for up to a year
◆ Irregular bleeding and spotting
◆ Amenorrhoea
◆ Increase in weight due to increased appetite
◆ Galactorrhoea
◆ Depression and loss of libido have been reported but it is difficult to know whether they are due to the injection or other circumstances
◆ ? Possible increased risk of osteoporosis.

Absolute contraindications

◆ Present or past severe arterial disease, or high blood lipid levels
◆ Pregnancy
◆ Undiagnosed genital tract bleeding
◆ Trophoblastic disease
◆ Serious side effects with the combined pill which are not oestrogen related.

Relative contraindications

Injectables may be given to women who have the following problems, but only under specialist supervision and close observation.

◆ Liver disease
◆ Sex steroid-dependent cancers
◆ Past history of severe depression
◆ Obesity.

Smoking cessation and breast awareness should be discussed where applicable. Leaflets backing up verbal information and emergency telephone numbers should be given.

The first injection should be given within the first five days of the menstrual cycle. If it is given at this time then contraception is immediate. If given at any other time then additional contraception (non-hormonal) should be used for the next seven days. Women who wish to have the injection following birth should wait 5–6 weeks after delivery, to reduce the risk of menorrhagia.

Subsequent injections and visits

Noristerat should be given every 8 weeks, and the client should be warned of the importance of not delaying her injection.

Depo-Provera should be given every 12 weeks and again it is important to stress the necessity of not being late with repeat injections. These injections can be given earlier if holidays, etc., are planned to coincide with appointment dates. At each visit blood pressure and weight measurements should be taken and it should be checked that there is no new relevant medical or family history. Time should be given to the client so that any anxieties or problems, e.g. about irregular bleeding, may be discussed. Clients should be aware when future injections are due.

If a woman wishes to become pregnant she should be advised that it may take up to a year from the last injection for her periods to return to a regular cycle and to conceive.

Drugs that reduce the efficacy of the injectable

Enzyme-inducing drugs may reduce the efficacy of the injectable so the frequency should be increased. Depo-Provera should be given every 10 weeks or earlier at 8 weeks if rifampicin is prescribed. Noristerat should be given at 6-week intervals.

Depo-Provera and osteoporosis

There has been considerable discussion over the possible risks of osteoporosis with long-term use of Depo-Provera, although current research has not confirmed the initial anxieties. It may be that women who choose to use Depo-Provera are more at risk of osteoporosis because of pre-existing risk factors. You should discuss with women the risk factors for osteoporosis (smoking, family history of osteoporosis in a first degree relative, personal history of fractures, anorexia nervosa,

amenorrhoea and use of steroids) and assess her risk. Peak bone mass is attained by the age of 18 in women so it may be a good idea to avoid Depo-Provera until peak bone mass is achieved (Wilkinson and Szarewski, 2003). If a woman has a predisposing factor for osteoporosis then measurement of bone mass density should be considered. If she is approaching the menopause and has risk factors for osteoporosis then these should be discussed with her, along with her choice of contraception with an experienced doctor in this area.

Some common problems

Irregular bleeding

The injections can cause irregular bleeding, although any undiagnosed genital tract bleeding should be investigated before starting injections. If there is excessive bleeding, injections can be given earlier, but not less than four weeks from the last injection. Oestrogen may be prescribed to treat bleeding if not contraindicated.

Myths and the media

Many women are concerned about the effect the injections have on their menses. 'What happens to the blood?' 'Doesn't it all build up?' and 'Isn't it harmful not to have a period?' are questions that are frequently asked. At the moment the long-term implications of amenorrhoea are not fully understood, and research into the possible risk of osteoporosis is being undertaken.

Sexuality and injectables

For many women the injectable is the answer to a prayer. They may be unable to take the combined pill because of contraindications, be anxious about the reduced effectiveness of the progestogen-only pill, and be unhappy with other methods. The injectable is very effective, and if a woman is not planning to become pregnant in the near future, and is happy with the possibility of irregular bleeding, this may be an anxiety-free method that is exactly what she needs and wants.

Many women, once established on the injection, are very reluctant to change their method as they are happy with amenorrhoea and the increased freedom that they feel this method gives them.

Other women may choose the injectable so that they do not have to think about contraception. It is easy, quick and only has to be given four to six times per year and is almost 100% effective. It may help postpone or avoid the decision of permanent contraception like sterilization. 'I can never decide whether I want to be sterilized or not, because then I have to decide if I definitely don't want more children'. So by continuing with the injection the decision can be delayed, sometimes indefinitely!

Implants

Implanon is the only available implant in the UK following the withdrawal of Norplant in 1999. Implanon is a single-rod implant containing the progestogen etonogestrel. The implant is flexible and is 4 cm in length and 2 mm in diameter (see Figure 11.8) and lasts for 3 years (Edwards and Moore, 1999). Implanon is nearly 100% effective at preventing pregnancy, first by inhibiting ovulation and second by thickening cervical

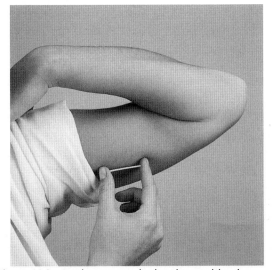

Figure 11.8 Implanon capsule showing position in arm. (Reproduced with kind permission of Organon Laboratories Ltd.)

mucus. No pregnancies occurred in clinical trials (Croxatto, 1998).

What you need to tell your client

Your client must use contraception up to the time of fitting to exclude pregnancy. If possible she should have her Implanon injected on the first day of her menstrual period, as it is effective immediately and no extra precautions will be required. Otherwise Implanon should be inserted during the first 5 days of a period. If it is inserted at any other time in her cycle, pregnancy must first be excluded and an additional contraceptive method used for 7 days.

It is important that your client is fully aware of the disadvantages of the implant, such as irregular bleeding (see Box 11.12), and is prepared to accept this. This menstrual irregularity is similar to that of the progestogen-only pill, i.e. irregular periods, prolonged bleeding, spotting or amenorrhoea, but this should settle after the first year. Research has found that women who receive implant counselling are more likely to continue with this form of contraception despite menstrual irregularities (Mascarenhas *et al.*, 1994).

Implanon should be inserted into the upper arm (non-dominant) about 6–8 cm above the elbow crease. Local anaesthetic should be injected initially. The implant is contained in the cannula of a disposable sterile applicator and the injection is simple, taking about 2 minutes. A compression bandage should be applied to reduce any bruising: this can be removed after 24 hours. Implanon should not be visible unless the woman is very thin; however it should be possible to feel Implanon beneath the skin.

Unlike the oral contraceptive pill there is no reduced effectiveness of Implanon with severe diarrhoea, as it is absorbed directly into the bloodstream.

Drugs that reduce the efficacy of Implanon

The effectiveness of Implanon is reduced by certain anticonvulsants (phenytoin, primidone, carbamazepine, barbiturates), and also by the

> **Box 11.12** Implants: advantages, disadvantages and contraindications
>
> **Advantages**
>
> ◆ Very effective and lasts 3 years
> ◆ Once removed, fertility rapidly returns
> ◆ Free from oestrogen-related side effects
> ◆ Once in place, nothing to remember.
>
> **Disadvantages**
>
> ◆ Has to be inserted under local anaesthetic by trained professional
> ◆ Irregular bleeding ranging from amenorrhoea to persistent bleeding
> ◆ Possible difficulty removing capsule
> ◆ Occasional problems with headaches, acne, weight gain, nausea, mastalgia, hair loss and abdominal pain.
>
> **Absolute contraindications**
>
> ◆ Pregnancy
> ◆ Undiagnosed genital tract bleeding
> ◆ Hypersensitivity to components of Implanon
> ◆ Sex hormone-related neoplasia (including trophoblastic disease)
> ◆ Active thromboembolic disease
> ◆ Acute porphyria
> ◆ Present severe hepatic disease
> ◆ Present or past history of severe arterial disease or raised lipid profile.
>
> **Relative contraindications**
>
> These clients may need more careful monitoring in first few months.
> ◆ Hypertension
> ◆ Diabetes
> ◆ Depression
> ◆ Risk factors for arterial disease
> ◆ Chronic systemic disease
> ◆ Previous chloasma.

antibiotics rifampicin and griseofulvin and hydantoins.

Follow-up of a client with an implant

As with any hormonal method of contraception, the client should be seen 3 months after insertion for routine blood pressure, weight check and to check her bleeding pattern is satisfactory. If there are no problems they should be seen at yearly intervals or sooner if a problem develops.

Women should be informed about when their Implanon will need to be renewed.

Removal procedure

The removal of Implanon takes 3–5 minutes. It is carried out under local anaesthetic, and a small incision is made at the previous insertion site. A new Implanon can be inserted after removal through the same incision.

Myths and the media

It was originally felt that implants would be suitable for women who had completed their families. However, from current usage in the UK and experience from abroad it seems that younger women are choosing this method if they definitely want to postpone a pregnancy, because of its convenience, efficacy and easy reversibility.

Implants and sexuality

This method gives women freedom from taking pills, using condoms, etc., yet is very effective and easily reversible. 'What's the catch?' clients ask, as for many this appears to be an ideal method of contraception and is just what they have been waiting for. It helps give women who are unable to take the combined pill another choice, and also gives women time to decide on a more permanent form of contraception.

Emergency contraception

Emergency contraception, or post-coital contraception, is often referred to as the 'morning after pill', which is an unfortunate misnomer as it can be taken up to 72 hours after unprotected intercourse.

Research has revealed that hormonal emergency contraception is most effective if given within the first 24 hours following unprotected sexual intercourse, and if possible should be commenced within this time. However, it is still effective within 72 hours of unprotected sexual intercourse (Task Force on Postovulatory Methods of Fertility Regulation, 1998).

It is unclear precisely how emergency contraception works but it is thought to prevent implantation of the ovum (which occurs 5 days after ovulation if fertilization has occurred). Implantation is prevented by making the endometrium unsuitable to support a developing blastocyst. If emergency contraception is given prior to ovulation it may postpone or prevent ovulation. If it is given after ovulation it may prevent pregnancy by blocking progesterone and oestrogen receptors, and interfere with the ovum transport mechanism.

The hormonal method of emergency contraception is about 97–99% effective whilst the intrauterine device is almost 100% effective at preventing pregnancy.

The advantages, disadvantages and contraindications of emergency contraception are outlined in Box 11.13.

Emergency contraception is available free from:

◆ Any GP who provides contraceptive services
◆ Any family planning clinic
◆ A young persons' clinic or Brook Advisory Centre
◆ Some hospital accident and emergency departments
◆ Some genitourinary medicine (GUM) clinics.

Hormonal emergency contraception is also available over the counter from pharmacists under the name Levonelle priced at approximately £24.

Types of emergency contraception

The two main types of emergency contraception are:

◆ Insertion of an intrauterine device
◆ Hormonal method.

Intrauterine device

A copper-bearing IUD is fitted up to 5 days after the calculated date of ovulation. Almost 100% effective in preventing pregnancy even in cases of multiple exposure, the IUD works primarily by blocking implantation.

Hormonal method

Progestogen-only emergency contraception (POEC) marketed in the UK as Levonelle 2, contains two tablets of 750 µg of levonorgestrel each.

They should be taken together within 72 hours of unprotected sexual intercourse. Previously this method was given as two separate doses 12 hours apart; however research has shown that one dose of 150 mg is as effective as the two separate doses and reduces the risk of forgetting the second pill at the correct time. Randomized trials have researched the use of Levonelle 2 beyond 72 hours. They showed that if given between 73 and 120 hours it prevented 60–63%

> **Box 11.13** Emergency contraception: advantages, disadvantages and contraindications
>
> **Advantages of the IUD and hormonal methods**
> ◆ Effective in preventing pregnancy
> ◆ IUD may be kept *in situ* and provide continuing contraception
> ◆ Extended time span (up to 5 days for an IUD) allows women the opportunity to obtain emergency contraception; e.g. weekends
> ◆ Unrelated to partner.
>
> **Disadvantages**
>
> The IUD:
> ◆ Increased risk of pelvic infection
> ◆ Minor 'surgical' procedure
> ◆ Complications related to IUD insertion, e.g. pain, expulsion, perforation and infection.
>
> Hormonal methods:
> ◆ Does not provide future contraception
> ◆ Nausea
> ◆ Next menstrual period may be delayed
> ◆ Failure rate approximately 1–3%.
>
> **Contraindications**
>
> The IUD:
> ◆ Pregnancy
> ◆ Active pelvic or sexually transmitted infection
> ◆ Undiagnosed genital tract bleeding
> ◆ Past history of an ectopic pregnancy, although an IUD may be inserted but removed following the next menstrual period.
>
> Hormonal methods:
> ◆ Pregnancy
> ◆ More than 72 hours has elapsed since unprotected sexual intercourse
> ◆ Active acute porphyria
> ◆ Severe liver disease
> ◆ Allergy to levonorgestrel.

of pregnancies; however, few women used this method beyond 72 hours (FFPRHC, 2003d). If Levonelle 2 is given beyond 72 hours the responsibility will be the prescriber's as Levonelle 2 is not licensed for use beyond 72 hours.

History taking

It is important when clients attend for emergency contraception that you are able to put them at their ease, as information about their sexual activity is very personal and the situation can feel threatening and embarrassing. Clients will often remember and talk about the most recent act of sexual intercourse, but may forget about unprotected sexual intercourse earlier in the month, thinking they would have been 'safe' then. Earlier unprotected sexual intercourse beyond 72 hours could contraindicate the hormonal method, but it may be possible for the woman to have an IUD inserted within 5 days of the calculated date of ovulation, thereby preventing pregnancy from previous exposures. It is helpful to chart the first day of the last menstrual period and episodes of unprotected sexual intercourse on a menstrual calendar, as this will make it easier to calculate when ovulation may occur. A full medical history should be taken to eliminate any contraindications and weight and blood pressure measured.

Often women will tell you they either did not use contraception or that there was an accident with the method they used. Common statements about the condom are: 'It came off!', 'It burst!', and about the oral contraceptive 'I ran out of pills', 'I forgot to take them' or about the diaphragm 'I forgot to put it in', 'I found it had a hole when I took it out afterwards', etc. If the client does not volunteer whether she used contraception or not, it is important to ask as this is an ideal time to discuss and advise on future contraception.

With increased incidences of sexually transmitted infections (STIs) being reported in the UK it is extremely important to discuss the issue of screening following an episode of unprotected sexual intercourse. Many women do not realize that an STI may be symptomless. To highlight risks you may like to ask how long a woman has been with her partner, has either of them been screened before, and does she know where to go for screening. Discussing these issues often encourages women to think about the risks and attend for screening. Women should attend for screening 14 days after an episode of unprotected sexual intercourse so that any infections can be incubated.

Information the client needs to know about hormonal emergency contraception

If possible, clients should be encouraged to commence POEC within the first 24 hours of unprotected intercourse. It will still be effective if taken within 72 hours although the efficacy is decreased.

Very rarely the tablets may cause nausea so you should advise your client to avoid taking them on an empty stomach, and either take them with or after food or else with a medication which prevents travel sickness. If she vomits within 2 hours of taking the pills she should return for more pills. The hormonal method will not protect the client from becoming pregnant for the rest of the month so she will need to abstain from sexual intercourse or use a condom. If her period does not come when she expects it, then she should return for a pregnancy test, providing it is more than two weeks since the episode of unprotected intercourse.

If a client wishes to start the combined oral contraceptive pill she could be given a packet to commence on the first day of her next menstrual period providing it is normal.

The advantages and disadvantages should be discussed and this information should be backed up with suitable leaflets.

Information the client needs to know about the IUD for emergency contraception

The IUD will give the woman contraception for the rest of the month. If she wishes, the IUD can be left *in situ* after her next period or she may wish to have it removed at that time.

You should show your client how to check her IUD threads, and warn her that she may get period-like pains after it is fitted. If she experiences persistent pain she should seek medical attention to exclude an ectopic pregnancy.

The advantages, disadvantages and insertion procedure should be discussed and relevant leaflets given.

IUD insertion

Prior to fitting an IUD, chlamydia screening should be performed. The results will not be known before fitting the IUD in cases of post-coital contraception and some doctors may pre-scribe prophylactic antibiotics. Analgesia (e.g. mefenamic acid) may be given prior to fitting the IUD if the client prefers. Follow-up is essential.

Follow-up visit

Your client should return 3–4 weeks later with details of her first period after having emergency contraception. If she has not had a period a pregnancy test can be performed. The first period after emergency contraception may be earlier or slightly later than expected and should seem like a normal period to the woman. If the period seems shorter or lighter than normal, a pregnancy test should be performed. It is important to find out whether the client had any problems with her emergency contraception, e.g. vomiting, abdominal pain, etc., to exclude any reduced efficacy. You should also check at this visit if she is happy with her chosen method of contraception and, if she has decided to take hormonal contraception (COC or POP), that this is being taken correctly.

Myths and the media

Originally emergency hormonal contraception was advertised as the 'morning after pill'. This gave the impression that it could only be taken the morning following unprotected sexual inter-course, and prevented many women from seek-ing advice and help. As a result of this, the name was changed to emergency contraception but many women are still unaware of the two main types of emergency contraception or the length of time available.

The effectiveness and easy availability of postcoital contraception should be more widely advertised. Many women are unsure where to obtain it, and are unaware of how it works, wrongly believing that it induces an abortion. Levonelle 2 is now widely available to purchase at pharmacists without a prescription although it does mean missing out on other sexual health advice given by a GP or other clinic.

Emergency contraception and sexuality

The request for emergency contraception may be the first time a woman consults you for contracep-tive advice, so the impression you give can encour-age or discourage her attendance in the future. Often women attend expecting to be chastised for their failure to use contraception correctly and will relax visibly in the chair when they realize some-one is going to help and support them. After all we are all human! Clients who frequently attend for emergency contraception may need time to dis-cuss problems they have with their chosen method of contraception. If they choose to use no contra-ception but attend for emergency contraception only, this may illustrate poor self-esteem and their feelings of powerlessness over their lives.

The intrauterine device

The intrauterine device (IUD) or intrauterine con-traceptive device (IUCD) is often referred to as 'the loop' or 'the coil'. It is a device that is inserted into the uterus through the cervical canal. It may have copper wrapped around the body (Figure 11.9) or it may contain the hormone levonorgestrel. The GyneFix is a frameless intrauterine device with an anchoring mechanism designed to reduce the risk of expulsion and symptoms of dysmenorrhoea (Masters and Guillebaud, 1999). The IUD has threads which hang down into the vagina, so that women are able to reassure themselves and check it is still *in situ*.

The IUD prevents pregnancy by:

◆ preventing implantation – this is the main mode of action;

◆ altering uterine and Fallopian tube fluids, thereby impeding the meeting between

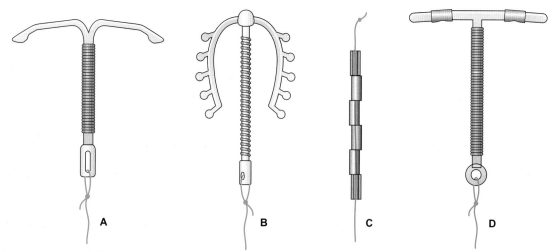

Figure 11.9 Four different intrauterine devices. (a) Nova T380; (b) Multiload Cu 375; (c) GyneFix; (d) T-Safe Cu 380A.

sperm and ovum and preventing fertilization; and

◆ causing a foreign body reaction, with increased leucocytes and phagocytosis.

The IUD is between 98% and 100% effective in preventing pregnancy; after the first year of use it is almost 100% effective. The advantages, disadvantages and contraindications are listed in Box 11.14.

When should an IUD be inserted?

The IUD is usually inserted at the end of a menstrual period as the cervix is fractionally more dilated, therefore making insertion easier. However, an IUD can be inserted any time up to day 19 of a 28-day cycle, which is particularly useful for post-coital insertion.

Before insertion of IUD

Prior to insertion of an IUD a full explanation of the advantages and disadvantages should be discussed, with a leaflet backing up the verbal information. The insertion procedure should be explained.

Analgesia, e.g. mefenamic acid, may be prescribed and given 20–30 minutes before insertion to help reduce pain from period-like cramps. It is a good idea to encourage clients to

eat something an hour or so before insertion, as it has been found that clients who miss meals are more likely to faint. Prior to IUD insertion the woman should be encouraged to empty her bladder, as a full bladder can prevent the uterus being felt abdominally and makes the procedure more uncomfortable.

All women should be screened for chlamydia prior to IUD insertion. Ideally this should be performed 1 week before insertion, so that treatment may be given. If this is not possible then chlamydia screening may be performed at insertion with treatment given as a prophylaxis. A review (Farley *et al.*, 1992) of the incidence of pelvic inflammatory disease and IUDs showed that it was strongly related to the insertion process and sexually transmitted infection history. It showed that the risk of pelvic infection was six times higher during the first 20 days – indicating how important it is to screen for infection prior to insertion. Because of the increased risk of pelvic infection at insertion it is important that IUDs are left *in situ* for their recommended time rather than changed at the whim of the client.

Care of client and insertion procedure

During insertion of an IUD the client will need support; she may want someone to hold her hand or want someone to talk to her and tell her

---

Box 11.14 The IUD: advantages, disadvantages and contraindications

Advantages

◆ Safe and immediately effective, no extra contraception required
◆ No drug interactions
◆ Long lasting
◆ Once inserted the woman does not have to remember to do anything else
◆ Not related to sexual intercourse.

Disadvantages

◆ Menorrhagia and dysmenorrhoea
◆ Slight increased risk of ectopic pregnancy
◆ Increased risk of pelvic infection
◆ Expulsion of the IUD
◆ Perforation of the uterus
◆ Malposition of the IUD
◆ Pregnancy caused by expulsion, perforation or malposition of the IUD.

Absolute contraindications

◆ Previous ectopic pregnancy in a nulliparous woman
◆ Abnormalities of the uterus, e.g. bicornuate uterus
◆ Pelvic or vaginal infection; once treated an IUD may be fitted
◆ Pregnancy
◆ Undiagnosed genital tract bleeding; once the cause has been diagnosed and treated an IUD may be inserted
◆ Allergy to components of IUD, e.g. copper
◆ Wilson's disease
◆ Heart valve replacement because of the increased risk of infection
◆ HIV and AIDS because of the reduced immune system and increased risk of infection from the IUD.

Relative contraindications

◆ History of pelvic infection
◆ Fibroids, endometriosis
◆ Nulliparity
◆ Diabetes
◆ Dysmenorrhoea and or menorrhagia
◆ Penicillamine treatment may reduce the effectiveness of copper.

---

what is happening. This can be by far the most important part of an IUD insertion; it can make the procedure easier for the client by reducing anxiety and as a result pain, and also can be supportive to the person inserting the IUD.

The skill and expertise of the inserter will help to reduce insertion problems and side effects. An audit (Andrews *et al.*, 1999) concluded that appropriately trained nurses were as successful as doctors at inserting IUDs in both multiparous and nulliparous women. If a client has had problems with IUD insertions in the past or feels she would like stronger analgesia, then local anaesthetic may be used to reduce pain. This can be with lignocaine cream, Instillagel or a paracervical lignocaine block and referral may be necessary to a hospital clinic which specializes in difficult insertions and removals.

Prior to insertion a bimanual examination is carried out to ascertain the size, position and direction of the uterus and that there is no tenderness. The inserter will choose an IUD that is most suitable for the length and size of uterus, whilst at the same time choosing an IUD with a long lifespan and high efficacy. IUDs with a long lifespan mean that the IUD will need not be changed so frequently and will therefore reduce the risks of perforation and infection associated with insertion.

Insertion is by a 'no-touch' technique, so a clean (not sterile) pair of gloves are needed after the bimanual examination. A sterile speculum is inserted into the vagina and the cervix located and cleaned with antiseptic solution. A uterine sound is inserted through the cervical canal into the uterus to ascertain the patency of the cervical canal and the length and direction of the uterus. The cervix may be stabilized with Allis forceps or a tenaculum so that the IUD can be inserted more easily, although these can cause some discomfort as the cervix can be very sensitive. The IUD is inserted and IUD threads shortened so that they can be tucked up behind the cervix. If there are any problems with insertion of an IUD then the client should be referred to a doctor experienced in IUD difficulties.

Once the IUD is inserted the client may need to rest for a few minutes; analgesia may be given for period-like cramps. It is recommended that the client's pulse rate is checked following insertion (FFPRHC, 2004) because of the risk of bradycardia. If a client gets up too quickly she may feel faint. A sanitary pad may be required as she may bleed slightly. It is advisable not to use tampons for any bleeding following insertion. This is because the cervical os has been dilated and the IUD could inadvertently be removed when removing a tampon. This is a good time to remind her of any initial problems she may have with period pains and bleeding. If a client has persistent pain or change in her normal vaginal discharge she should be advised to telephone for advice and return for an examination. The woman should be shown what the threads feel like by showing her those that have been trimmed earlier, and should be encouraged to feel her IUD threads at the top of the vagina once a month after a period in case the device has been expelled during heavy menstruation. No extra contraception is required as the IUD is effective immediately. The actual IUD insertion procedure takes about 10 minutes.

Vasovagal attacks and anaphylaxis

Although vasovagal attacks and anaphylaxis following IUD insertion are rare, equipment should be readily available for an emergency and should include clear guidelines on how to manage such a crisis. The woman may become pale, sweaty and complain of feeling faint or sick and have a slow pulse. If not completed, the insertion procedure should be stopped and the client laid in the supine position, the head lowered and the feet raised. If bradycardia persists then slow intravenous atropine 0.3–0.6 mg may be required. If she has difficulty breathing and there is loss of consciousness and absence of a carotid pulse, her airway should be maintained with a pocket mask and one-way valve, and emergency help sought. The client should be laid in the left lateral position; if there is no central pulse then 1/1000 of adrenaline 0.5–1.0 ml may be given by deep intramuscular injection. If there is no improvement, this may be repeated at 10-minute intervals to the maximum of three doses. If required, cardiopulmonary resuscitation should be commenced. The IUD may need to be removed.

Follow-up

A follow-up visit should take place 4–6 weeks after insertion so that the IUD can be checked and any problems discussed. At this session you should check that the woman is happy with her method of contraception, her bleeding pattern has been satisfactory, she can feel the threads and they do not cause any problems to her partner. The woman should be examined using a speculum so that the IUD threads can be observed, any signs of infection can be assessed, and a cervical smear can be taken if required. Following a speculum examination a bimanual examination should be performed. Occasionally the tip of the IUD can be felt at the cervical os which might not have been seen on speculum examination. If the tip is felt then the IUD is too low in the uterine cavity and should be removed and a new IUD inserted. This is also a good opportunity to check for any cervical excitation, by moving the cervix gently from side to side. If any pain or discomfort is felt then the woman may have an infection or an ectopic pregnancy.

If there are no problems then the IUD should be checked every 6 months.

Lifespan of an IUD

The officially approved lifespan of an IUD varies from 3 to 8 years. Any device inserted after the age of 40 years may be left in place until the menopause but should be removed 1 year postmenopause (Szarewski and Guillebaud, 1991).

Removal of the IUD

The IUD can be removed at any time but if a client does not wish to become pregnant then another form of contraception should be provided first. This may mean starting an oral contraceptive pill or learning how to use a diaphragm before removal. The IUD is removed by inserting a speculum into the vagina. Spencer Wells forceps are applied to the IUD threads and gentle traction is applied. The IUD should slowly begin to descend into the vagina. If the IUD does not descend then it may have become embedded inside the uterus and the woman may need referral to a doctor who is skilled in difficult removal procedures. Sometimes the IUD removed is an old device, which has long since ceased manufacture and has not been in use for many years in the UK. If the IUD has been inserted abroad it can be very interesting to compare the different shapes, sizes and materials used!

Problems with IUDs

Lost threads

If you or your client are unable to locate the IUD threads then you should advise that she uses an alternative form of contraception as she is at risk of becoming pregnant. Lost threads can indicate that the IUD has been expelled or that the IUD has moved within the uterus or perforated the uterus, taking the threads with it. She may already be pregnant so it is important to exclude this possibility. Details of last menstrual period and symptoms of pregnancy should be obtained, and a bimanual examination and pregnancy test performed. If a client is pregnant and wishes to continue, the IUD may be left *in situ*, as it would be difficult to remove with absent threads, but she should be advised of the increased rate of spontaneous abortion, antepartum haemorrhage, premature labour and stillbirth, and the IUD should be located after the birth if there are no complications.

If the client is not pregnant, the threads may be retrieved with Spencer Wells forceps or thread retrievers by an experienced nurse or doctor. If this is unsuccessful then the woman should have an ultrasound performed to locate the exact position of the IUD. If this shows the IUD to be correctly positioned in the uterus then no further action will be necessary. If, however, no IUD is seen in the uterus then a straight abdominal X-ray will need to be performed to exclude perforation.

Perforation

This usually occurs at insertion or shortly afterwards and is extremely rare. It most commonly happens when an IUD is inserted postpartum in a lactating woman. For this reason a client should always be advised to return if she is suffering from persistent abdominal pain.

The IUD will need to be located by ultrasound and X-ray and removed by laparoscopy. The risk of perforation of the uterus occurs in less than 1 in 1000 insertions (FFPRHC, 2004).

Infection

A client should return to see you if she has an increased vaginal discharge, which may be of a different colour or odour, or cause itching and pain. If full screening for *Chlamydia* and other sexually transmitted infections is unavailable then she should be referred to her local genitourinary medicine clinic.

To reduce the risk of infection and increase the efficacy of the IUD, particularly mid-cycle, a client may wish to use spermicides. The spermicides will act as a germicide, killing bacteria.

Ectopic pregnancy

If a client complains of persistent localized abdominal pain then an ectopic pregnancy may be the cause. A pregnancy test and bimanual examination will be performed to confirm diagnosis. If the client has a positive pregnancy test and pain she should be referred to her local hospital for prompt emergency treatment. If the pregnancy test is negative then an ultrasound may be performed to further exclude any likelihood of an ectopic pregnancy.

Pain or bleeding

If a woman complains of continuing pain or bleeding then she should be examined to exclude infection, perforation and an ectopic pregnancy. A full history of the pain and pattern of bleeding needs to be taken and the relevant tests performed such as ultrasound, infection screening, pregnancy test, bimanual examination and cervical smear test. If the pain continues and there is no evidence of infection, perforation and ectopic pregnancy then appropriate analgesia should be given. Sometimes removal of the existing IUD and then refitting with another type of IUD after a few weeks is an appropriate solution.

Actinomyces

Actinomyces is a bacterium found occasionally in women with IUDs *in situ*, and is usually diagnosed by cytologists when a cervical smear test is performed. If pelvic infection is suspected the IUD should be removed and sent for culture (minus the threads) and appropriate antibiotic therapy commenced. If, after a thorough history and full counselling, pelvic infection is not suspected, then the IUD can remain *in situ* and the woman has repeat smears at intervals stipulated by the National Screening Programme (FFPRHC, 2004).

Levonorgestrel Intrauterine System (IUS)

The levonorgestrel IUS is a T-shaped IUD containing the progestogen levonorgestrel in a sleeve around its stem (Figure 11.10). It is inserted and removed by the same method as other IUDs, and is marketed in the UK under the name Mirena.

The levonorgestrel IUS prevents pregnancy in the same way as a standard IUD but has the added benefit of the levonorgestrel, which is released at 20 µg a day. This helps to make the cervical mucus impenetrable to sperm, the endometrium less favourable for implantation and causes a reduction in Fallopian tube function. In some women it may also prevent ovulation.

The levonorgestrel IUS is 99.5% effective in protecting against pregnancy. It provides most of the benefits of both hormonal and intrauterine contraception without the disadvantages of

> **Box 11.15** Levonorgestrel IUS: advantages and disadvantages
>
> **Advantages**
> ◆ High safety rate
> ◆ Reduced risk of infection
> ◆ Reduced dysmenorrhoea
> ◆ Oligomenorrhoea and amenorrhoea.
>
> **Disadvantages**
> ◆ Intermenstrual bleeding
> ◆ Amenorrhoea
> ◆ Expensive
> ◆ Body of IUS is wider than other IUDs, therefore the cervix may need some dilatation.

either and is becoming a popular form of contraception. It is licensed for 5 years. The advantages and disadvantages are listed in Box 11.15.

The levonorgestrel IUS is currently licensed in the UK for contraception and for treatment of primary menorrhagia. It is ideal for the older perimenopausal woman who wants to start hormone replacement therapy (HRT) but still requires contraception. In the future, women who are already established on HRT may find this method of administering progestogen more convenient than having to take regular systemic progestogen to protect the endometrium from hyperplasia. Although the IUS is widely used for this purpose in Scandinavia, it does not yet have such a licence in the UK. The levonorgestrel IUS is particularly suitable for women with menorrhagia and may reduce iron deficiency anaemia and the need for a hysterectomy.

Sexuality and IUDs

Many women chose the IUD because 'once in, it can be forgotten'. Although an IUD may cause some problems, many women see these as minor when compared to the convenience of the IUD. Once an IUD is inserted no additional contraception is required, and in effect it can be forgotten, it cannot be felt *in situ*, and there is nothing to remember prior to intercourse which would interrupt spontaneity.

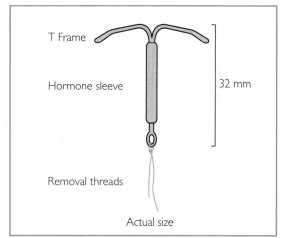

Figure 11.10 Levonorgestrel IUS. (Reproduced with permission of IPPF, London.)

Myths and the media

The IUD is frequently portrayed as an abortifacient by the media, nursing and medical professions. This mistaken and ignorant view unfortunately prevents many women from choosing this method. Women are often given the impression that the IUD is 'bad news' with a painful insertion, painful heavy periods, and a high risk of infection. Unfortunately women have only heard bad news about an IUD from one source and may need reminding of the many thousands of women who are delighted with this method of contraception. With the development of new improved IUDs, and the opportunity of pre-insertion analgesia and local anaesthetic, a painful insertion and menorrhagia are less likely to occur.

Fertility awareness

Common names

Fertility awareness is also known as natural family planning, the 'rhythm method' or 'the safe period'. There are four main methods (summarized in Figure 11.11) that a woman should be taught so that she can more accurately calculate when to avoid intercourse. These are:

◆ The calendar method
◆ The temperature method
◆ The cervical mucus method or Billings method
◆ The sympto-thermal method or double check method.

Fertility awareness is a way of predicting ovulation and the information can be used by the client as a way of either *preventing* or *achieving* pregnancy. Ovulation usually takes place 14 days before the first day of the next menstrual period and not 14 days after the last menstrual period as many women think. So, for example, a woman with a regular 28-day cycle would be likely to ovulate around day 14 and a woman with a regular 30-day cycle would ovulate on day 16. An ovum can live for up to 24 hours, whereas sperm can live in the female body for up to 7 days. It is this estimation of ovulation and sperm survival time which indicates the fertile time (Figure 11.11).

The efficacy of fertility awareness varies from 80% to 98%. The sympto-thermal method is considered the safest of the four methods. The advantages and disadvantages are summarized in Box 11.16.

The calendar method

A woman is taught to calculate when she ovulates by looking at, retrospectively, at least six menstrual cycles, and calculating ovulation as 14 days before the first day of when her next menstrual period is due. As stress and illness can cause cycle irregularity this is considered the least safe of the methods, but is useful to teach clients when they are fertile if they are trying to become pregnant.

The temperature method

A woman can calculate her day of ovulation by taking her temperature daily either vaginally or orally, but it must be the same route each day. Her temperature is taken for a minimum of 3 minutes on waking and should be done before getting out of bed and before having a drink or cigarette as this will affect the accuracy of the result. After she ovulates her basal body temperature (BBT) will go down slightly and then rise by 0.2°C and stay up until the next period. A special thermometer needs to be used for this measurement, and the results are plotted on a chart. Basal body temperature can increase with infections, making it harder to estimate ovulation.

Cervical mucus method

A woman is taught to observe her cervical mucus by looking at the texture, colour and amount. Prior to ovulation, under the influence of oestrogen, cervical mucus looks like raw egg white and is stretchy, transparent and glossy – this is called spinnbarkeit mucus. After ovulation, cervical mucus becomes thick and dry under the influence of progesterone. This method of looking at cervical mucus is affected by vaginal infections, arousal and sexual intercourse. The increase of vaginal mucus that occurs at arousal can look similar to ovulatory mucus.

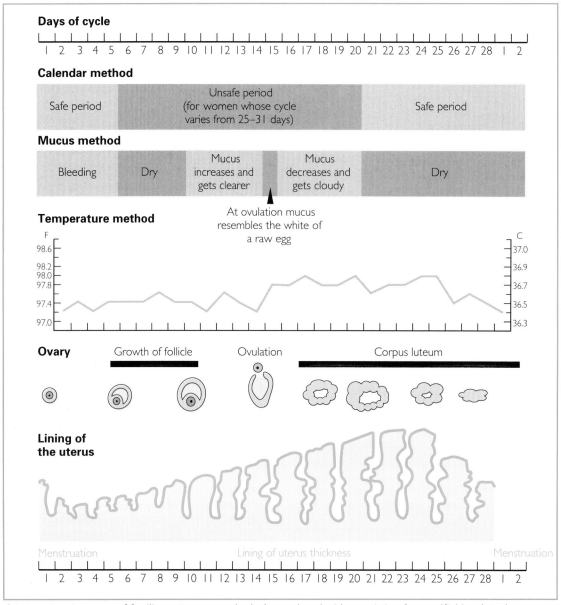

Figure 11.11 Summary of fertility awareness methods. (Reproduced with permission from Belfield, T. (1993) FPA Contraceptive Handbook: The Essential Reference Guide for Family Planning and Other Health Professionals, 2nd edn. London: FPA.)

Sympto-thermal method

This is a combination of the above methods and is considered the safest. A woman may use some or all of the above methods to estimate her fertile period, plus the measurement and consistency of the cervix, the observation of *mittelschmerz* (ovulation pain) and cyclic changes such as breast tenderness, etc. A woman is taught how to locate her cervix and measure its position every day, and to assess the softness and opening of the cervical os. When a client is about to ovulate the cervix rises in the vagina and is almost out of

> **Box 11.16** Fertility awareness: advantages and disadvantages
>
> **Advantages**
> - No side effects
> - Under the control of the couple
> - Acceptable to certain religious beliefs, e.g. Roman Catholics
> - Once taught, no further expense or follow-up required
> - Can help couples plan a pregnancy.
>
> **Disadvantages**
> - Requires motivation
> - Requires commitment
> - Requires daily observation and record keeping.

reach of her finger, becoming soft with the cervical os opening slightly.

Teaching fertility awareness

A woman will need careful explanation of how these methods can be used, with the aid of diagrams and appropriate leaflets. Learning how to use and interpret this method takes place over a period of time under supervision, where women record details of their cycle, vaginal mucus, cervical position and temperature. See Resources for training in natural family planning.

Personal contraceptive system

Persona, a small handheld computerized monitor which can be bought from chemists, is between 93% and 97% effective in preventing pregnancy with careful and consistent use. Through a database, Persona monitors luteinizing hormone and oestrone-3-gluronide, a metabolite of oestradiol. Persona tells a woman through testing her urine when she is in her fertile period through a series of lights. A green light indicates that she is in her infertile period and therefore safe to have sexual intercourse; a red light indicates that it is the fertile period and abstinence or a barrier method should be used. A yellow light indicates that a further urine test is required to give the database more information.

Persona is not suitable for:

- Women with cycles outside 23–35 days
- Breastfeeding women
- Menopausal women
- Women taking hormone treatments
- Women with polycystic ovarian syndrome
- Women with kidney and liver disease
- If hormonal emergency contraception has been used, two normal cycles must have passed before Persona can be restarted.

Lactational amenorrhoea method

Lactational amenorrhoea method (LAM) is the use of breast feeding to inhibit ovulation and act as a contraceptive.

For LAM to be effective as a method of contraception three criteria have to be met:

- The baby is less than 6 months old
- The woman must be fully breastfeeding with no additional supplements
- The woman must be amenorrhoeic.

If all these are met then LAM is 98% effective in preventing pregnancy (Pyper and Knight, 2001). However, if a woman is not fully breastfeeding or not amenorrhoeic then efficacy will be reduced.

Fertility awareness and sexuality

Women who use fertility awareness as a way of preventing or achieving pregnancy find their increased knowledge encourages them to listen to their bodies and interpret its signals. Women are often unaware of how much their cervical mucus changes in their cycle, mistaking any changes for infections. Fertility awareness can help to inform them and alleviate anxiety.

Coitus interruptus

Coitus interruptus, or withdrawal, where a man controls his ejaculation during sexual intercourse and ejaculates outside the vagina, is often referred to by clients as 'being careful' and some women may say that their partners 'look after things'. Many euphemisms are used, such as 'getting off a stop too early'. Coitus interruptus is about 90% effective at preventing pregnancy. Failure of this method tends to arise as small amounts of semen are leaked before ejaculation takes place. The advantages and disadvantages are listed in Box 11.17.

Myths and the media

Coitus interruptus is more widely used than is generally thought and is the oldest form of contraception. It is referred to in the Bible, and is used widely throughout the world by different cultures.

Female sterilization

Female sterilization involves the blocking or excision of the Fallopian tubes, thereby preventing the ovum from meeting the sperm and fertilization taking place. Women often refer to being sterilized by saying 'I've had my tubes tied'. Findings from the US Collaborative Review of Sterilization (CREST) study in 1996 (Peterson *et al.*, 1996) demonstrated that although tubal sterilization is highly effective, the risk of failure is higher than originally thought. It is estimated that the risk of failure is 1 in 200, depending on the method of sterilization used, and that this risk persists for many years following the procedure.

These lower efficacy rates, combined with the advent of new highly effective reversible contraception, are likely to lead to a decrease in requests for sterilization.

The advantages, disadvantages and contraindications are listed in Box 11.18.

Procedure

Female sterilization can either be performed under local or general anaesthetic and it can be performed abdominally by laparoscopy or minilaparotomy. The Fallopian tubes can be excised or blocked by: (1) applying a Hulka or Filshie clip which flattens and occludes the Fallopian tube; (2) drawing up and applying a Falope ring to a section of the Fallopian tube; (3) cauterization and diathermy; (4) excising and ligating the Fallopian tube (Figure 11.12).

Postoperative care and advice is similar to laparoscopic procedures mentioned in Chapter 19.

Counselling a client

Guidelines issued by the Royal College of Obstetricians and Gynaecologists (RCOG, 2004) advise that women should be counselled, that vasectomy carries a lower failure rate in terms of post-procedure pregnancies, and that there are fewer risks related to the male procedure.

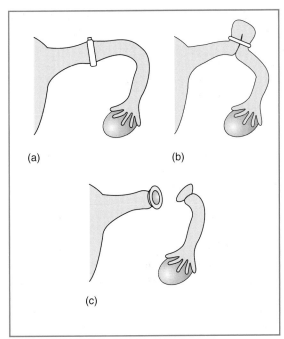

Figure 11.12 Female sterilization techniques. (a) Filshie clip; (b) Falope ring; (c) tying the ends after the tubes have been cut.

As this procedure is permanent and has to be considered irreversible, it can take women some time to decide whether or not to proceed. They also need time to discuss sterilization with their partner. It is important that they think about how they would feel if they lost their present partner, and met someone new – would they like to have children with a new partner or would they feel too old? Many women are certain that they would not want more children, but how would they feel if they lost a child? If a woman has not had children is she sure that she might not change her mind in the future? These are occasionally difficult areas to discuss and there are no set answers for all the questions, but it is important that the client and her partner think through the issues involved. It is easy to influence clients with your own views about these situations, but it is important that women and their partners are given unbiased counselling, as sterilization should be looked upon as irreversible.

Many women request sterilization thinking that it is 100% effective. On learning about the small failure rate, and after discussion about other highly effective contraceptive options they may well decide on postponing a sterilization whilst they try another method which they had not previously considered.

It is useful to discuss with the client whether she suffers from menorrhagia or dysmenorrhoea as these will continue following sterilization, and a hysterectomy may be a more appropriate option. In the past many women complained that being sterilized increased menorrhagia and dysmenorrhoea, but it is more likely this was due to the fact they had used a method of contraception like the COC which caused light and pain-free periods and they reverted to their true cycle following sterilization. The woman should be advised to continue to use her method of contraception until after the procedure, so that she is not pregnant that cycle. If a woman has an IUD then she should also use condoms for the menstrual cycle prior to surgery to ensure that no sperm are in the Fallopian tubes which could fertilize an ovum that is released shortly after surgery thereby causing an ectopic pregnancy.

Side effects

Female sterilization is relatively free of side effects. Pregnancy is very rare but if it does occur there is a higher risk of an ectopic pregnancy. Occasionally women regret their decision and loss of fertility, although counselling prior to the operation should reduce this. Women should be offered postoperative counselling if they are encountering problems. Sterilization should not be performed at a termination of pregnancy or following childbirth as the failure rate is higher due to increased vascularity of the tissues involved.

Reversal of female sterilization

Although female sterilization should be considered irreversible, it can occasionally be successfully reversed. Two factors are important at determining the success of the reversal. First, the type of surgical procedure originally used and, second, the skill of the individual surgeon at delicate reversal techniques. The most easily reversible methods are the Hulka and Filshie clips as these flatten the Fallopian tube which can then be reinflated. Cautery and diathermy are used less often these days as it is easy to damage other organs and they are hardest to reverse. The Falope ring can cause a section of the Fallopian tube to necrose. There is an increased risk of an ectopic pregnancy following a sterilization reversal. The success of the operation in achieving a pregnancy can be between 50% and 90%, depending on the original method used.

Sexuality and female sterilization

Many women feel liberated once they have been sterilized. They no longer have anxieties about having to rely on a method of contraception that they may not have been particularly happy with, and concerns about pregnancy become remote. This new found freedom from anxiety enables many women to explore their own sexuality and enjoy sex in a way they have not previously been able.

Male sterilization

Male sterilization, or vasectomy, is often referred to as 'having the chop' or 'having the snip'. It involves the excision or removal of part of the vas deferens which is the tube which transports sperm from the testes to the penis (Figure 11.13).

Male sterilization is 99.9% effective in preventing pregnancy. Its advantages, disadvantages and contraindications are listed in Box 11.19.

Procedure

A vasectomy can be performed under local or general anaesthetic. An incision is made on either side of the scrotum and the vas deferens located, excised and ligated. Men should wear a scrotal support and be encouraged to take things gently for the first week following a vasectomy by avoiding strenuous exercise, heavy lifting and sexual intercourse.

It takes about 3 months for a man's ejaculate to be clear of sperm, and he cannot consider it safe to have sexual intercourse without contraception until he has had two consecutive clear sperm counts.

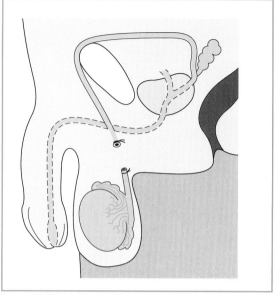

Figure 11.13   Male sterilization.

Counselling a client

When counselling men who are considering a vasectomy, it is important that they are given unbiased advice and information. Men should be encouraged to consider how they would feel if their present relationship ended and they found a new partner, or if one of their children died – would

---

Box 11.19   Male sterilization: advantages, disadvantages and contraindications

Advantages

◆ Permanent
◆ Highly effective.

Disadvantages

◆ Not effective immediately – can take up to 3 months
◆ Not easily reversed
◆ Minor surgical procedure.

Contraindications

◆ Indecision about operation by either partner
◆ Relationship problems
◆ Psychiatric illness
◆ Present urological problems.

they want more children? Men are often anxious about vasectomy and keen to know if they will notice any change in their libido, or whether they will still be able to ejaculate properly. You should advise them that everything will remain the same, the ejaculate will look the same but will not contain sperm but this is not detectable to the human eye.

While discussing a vasectomy many men will ask about the risk of testicular and prostate cancer and whether there is any increase in incidence. It may be that men who have had vasectomies are more aware of their testicles and seek advice more quickly if they find a problem. At the moment there is no definite proof of a link between prostate cancer and vasectomies, and if there is it is very small. It is not known what the cause of prostate cancer is, but clients should be advised that smoking increases all forms of cancer.

Side effects

A vasectomy is a very safe form of contraception with relatively few side effects: infection, haematoma and sperm granuloma. Infection should be treated with antibiotics, and a haematoma with analgesia and support. Haematoma usually occurs if the client has not given himself time to rest and recuperate. A sperm granuloma occurs when sperm leaks into the surrounding tissue from where the vas deferens has been incised. This can be asymptomatic but can also cause pain and localized swelling and may need excision.

A small number of vasectomies fail, even after negative sperm counts. This is thought to be due to re-canalization of the vas deferens and all men should be warned about the small failure rate.

Reversal of a vasectomy

Reversal of a vasectomy is easier than reversal of a female sterilization, but may be only 50% successful in achieving a pregnancy. The main problem in reversing a vasectomy is due to the development of anti-sperm antibodies in some men. Re-anastomosis of the vas may be successful but antibody production may mean that the sperm count is very low and a pregnancy difficult to achieve.

Sexuality and male sterilization

For many clients this decision has taken a great deal of time and thought. It may cause arguments between a couple – 'I feel it's his turn to do something' – and sex can be used as a weapon to influence emotionally the decision – 'we're not doing anything until he does something'. There can be an element of self-sacrifice and martyrdom about the decision which may continue to cause conflict in the future.

Many couples may postpone the final decision of sterilization, but a pregnancy 'scare' will suddenly make both partners seek a more permanent method of contraception.

Many men feel only too happy to have a vasectomy – 'It's my chance to do something' – especially if their partner has had a difficult time with finding a satisfactory method of contraception. Some men, however, feel that a vasectomy will affect their ability to function as a man and see it as tantamount to castration.

After a vasectomy, a man may subconsciously suffer from grief – of loss of fertility, of opportunity and of sexuality. On the other hand sterilization can also help cement the relationship if it is a shared decision, and can give the couple freedom to enjoy sexual intercourse without the anxiety of pregnancy.

Myths and the media

Sterilization has become a more popular choice of contraception in recent years. More men are choosing to have a vasectomy; not only has it become fashionable but it coincides with the 'new sharing/caring male image' created by the media. However, misconceptions still exist and it is still commonly believed that male sterilization causes impotence and sexual dysfunction.

Contraceptive problems

The younger client

By the time many young women consult you requesting contraception they will usually have started having sexual intercourse with or without a condom. Their first visit to discuss contraception will often coincide with a condom failure or having had unprotected sexual intercourse and requesting emergency contraception. The young woman often expects to be reprimanded for her mistake, and may come to the consultation 'quaking in her shoes'. If given time and non-judgemental counselling, it is likely that she will continue to consult in the future. Many young women feel that the confidentiality they are entitled to will be betrayed, but this should be respected unless the health, safety or welfare of someone other than the woman is at serious risk (BMA *et al.*, 1993).

Occasionally young clients are being physically abused, although this may not come out on an initial consultation. If a rapport is allowed to develop and the young woman trusts you she will return and may begin to confide in you. You will then have to decide what to do with the information with which you have been trusted, and refer on for further counselling or advise the child protection agencies if necessary. Individual Trusts usually run child protection courses at level 1 and level 2 which help to highlight these situations. You may like to investigate and see what is available to you in your local area.

However young the woman is, it is surely preferable that she has an effective method of contraception rather than an unplanned pregnancy. It is also important to discuss the issues surrounding HIV and safer sex, and two methods of contraception may be required: one to help prevent pregnancy, like the COC, and a second method to protect against HIV, like condoms. Such a method is known as the 'double Dutch method' as it is widely practised in the Netherlands. It is important to give young women highly effective contraception if they do not wish to become pregnant as this age group is very fertile. The combined pill may be the method of choice and they should be commenced on a low-dose pill. Many young women are anxious that their parents remain unaware of the fact that they are sexually active. The pill in such cases may be difficult for them to keep secret in case the packet is noticed. In such cases an injectable method may be chosen. For further information see Chapter 7.

Contraception following pregnancy

Women who have had a baby are often anxious to avoid becoming pregnant again too soon. They may remember the delivery vividly and be unwilling to repeat such an event – this is frequently the time when clients say 'never again'.

Breastfeeding alone does not give complete protection against pregnancy although many new mothers mistakenly believe this to be the case and do not use a form of contraception whilst lactating (see also page 289). They assume their amenorrhoea is due to breastfeeding and are unaware that it might be due to another pregnancy. Such women who have had unprotected intercourse need careful questioning about other symptoms of pregnancy and a pregnancy test performed if necessary. Ovulation may occur by about day 28 after delivery, so early contraception is vital for the postnatal woman who does not want to become pregnant.

If the woman is breastfeeding, the COC should not be used as it inhibits lactation and enters the milk in small quantities. The progestogen-only pill, however, is perfectly safe in breastfeeding women as it does not affect the supply of breast milk and only an insignificant amount enters the milk. If the POP is used it should be started 4 weeks after delivery in breastfeeding women. In women who are not breastfeeding, the COC or POP should be started 3 weeks after delivery. If the woman wishes to use an injectable form of contraception this should be given 6 weeks following delivery to reduce the risk of irregular bleeding, whether she is breastfeeding or not.

An IUD may be inserted at 6 weeks postpartum and extra care is needed to avoid perforation as the uterus is still soft following delivery – particularly so in a woman who is breastfeeding. Caps and diaphragms need refitting 5–6 weeks following delivery (even after a Caesarean section) as a different size may be required. Fertility awareness methods are difficult at this time due to the fluctuating hormone levels and lack of a regular cycle. Condoms should be used until other methods are established.

Ovulation may occur as early as 10 days following an abortion. Hormonal methods of contraception can be commenced on the same day as the abortion or an IUD may be inserted at the end of the surgical procedure. Sterilization is not usually recommended to be performed at the same time as an abortion due to the extra operative risks and the emotional trauma that may be involved.

The older woman

In the past, sexuality was a subject often avoided, but with wider media coverage both men and women now expect to be having and enjoying sexual relationships regardless of their age. This is often a time when women have a 'stronger sense of themselves', their children are growing up and they now have greater freedom to do what they want.

There is also an increasing number of women who are delaying their first pregnancy until they are in their forties, unaware that their fertility reduces as they get older. They see famous women (of a similar age) in the media and assume they will get pregnant easily but unfortunately this may not be the case. You will need to be aware of all the issues women in this age group face and counsel accordingly.

Women are sometimes unaware that contraception is still required in their forties and fifties. It is recommended that contraception is continued for 2 years after her last menstrual period if this occurs when a woman is under 50 years old, and for 1 year after her last menstrual period if this occurs when she is over 50 years old.

When discussing contraception with the older woman it is important that you assess her individual needs and health. If she is over 35 years old and smokes then the combined oral contraceptive pill will be contraindicated. Many women who are non-smokers will want to continue with the COC, particularly if they have been happy with this method in the past. It is possible for a woman with no contraindications to stay on this until the menopause providing she is regularly and carefully monitored. Longer lasting methods like injectables, IUDs, implants may be preferred by clients as they take away the anxiety of pregnancy, and may give greater freedom.

With the increasing divorce rate some older women might be starting on a new relationship after many years of celibacy. They may be unaware of the many advances in contraception over recent years and that emergency contraception is just as suitable for them as for their adolescent children. It is equally important that they do not miss out on safe sex advice – STIs are no respecter of age.

Those perimenopausal women who have already started HRT must be advised on the continuing need for contraception. Barrier methods, an IUD or an IUS are ideal. The POP appears to be effective in conjunction with HRT and women simply take both preparations daily. Although this combination is quite widely prescribed, and there have been no reports of failure, it must be emphasized that there are no clinical data to support such use (Gebbie, 1996). See also Chapter 16.

Disabled clients

It is important that each client is treated as an individual, as an absolute contraindication to a method of contraception may become a relative contraindication if pregnancy is considered detrimental to the woman's health. If a client wishes to use a diaphragm or a cervical cap but is unable to fit it herself, then her partner can be taught this simple procedure. Involvement of the partner can not only increase the choices available to your client, but may also give you the opportunity to counsel the couple about any problems they may be experiencing in their sexual relationship. They may well appreciate advice you can give them about different sexual positions and that sex need not be penetrative for both of them to gain pleasure. Partners of clients who have become disabled through illness, e.g. myocardial infarction, prostate problems, etc., may feel angry, guilty and even suffer grief. They may find it difficult to discuss their emotional and sexual needs with their partner, and as a result may be unaware of what is possible sexually, and how they can initiate it. Sensitive counselling by you will enable them to explore these other possibilities.

Clients who have mental disabilities may have had little opportunity in the past to discuss sexual intercourse and contraception, and may require more frequent consultations with you, particularly if their memory is poor. Always try and involve the partner if there is one.

If a woman is wheelchair-bound then the COC is not suitable due to increased risk of deep vein thrombosis. However the injectable method may be very convenient, as this will produce amenorrhoea and may be very acceptable to the woman.

For further information, see Chapter 6.

The future

What does the future hold for the professional working in the contraceptive field? The introduction of patient group directions which allow for first-time and repeat issuing of hormonal contraception, along with increased provision for screening for sexually transmitted infections within family planning clinics, has widened the role of the nurse. For clients this has made services more flexible which is becoming increasingly important with rising numbers of men and women accessing genitourinary medicine clinics.

What does the future hold for developments in contraception? Research is being carried out into biodegradable implants and different formulations of oral contraceptive pills. The hormonal

---

Ideas for personal and professional development

To extend and develop your skills in this area why not:

- Visit your local reproductive sexual health services/family planning clinics so that you are up to date with the services available

- Visit sexual health/genitourinary medicine services so that you are able to advise clients on the clinics, their opening times and whether appointments are needed

- Compile a list of services available specifically for young people

- Research local services for teaching fertility awareness

- Compile a folder with relevant journal articles, e.g. about new contraceptive methods, factors affecting client choice, etc.

Patient education points

Clients should be aware of:

- The need to protect against sexually transmitted infections as well as pregnancy

- Understand the benefits and risks of their chosen method of contraception and when to seek advice

- How to use different methods of contraception and the action to take if the method fails

- What to do and where to go when everything goes wrong, e.g. emergency contraception

- There are many methods of contraception that are equally as effective as female sterilization.

IUS may be developed to contain different hormones. Trials are still taking place on a vaginal ring which will release progesterone, and with the advent of HIV it is likely that improvements in male and female condoms will be made. We may start taking our hormonal contraception via a nasal spray or perhaps the combined oral contraceptive will become available in the form of an injectable. Men may also have an increased choice as a subdermal implant alongside three-monthly injections is currently undergoing phase three trials. One thing is for certain: women are choosing to have children later in life and are having smaller families, therefore the need for new research into highly effective methods of contraception is increasing.

Resources

Brook Advisory Centres
National Office Tel: 0800 0185023
www.brook.org.uk
Will provide details of local clinics nationwide.

Faculty of Family Planning
RCOG, 27 Sussex Place, Regent's Park, London NW1 4RG
www.ffprhc.org.uk
Publishes the *Journal of Faculty of Family Planning and Reproductive Health Care.*

Family Planning Association
2–12 Pentonville Road, London N1 9FP
Tel: 020 7837 5432 (switchboard)
www.fpa.org.uk
Helpline: 020 7837 4044

Family Planning Association Scotland
Unit 10, Firhill Business Centre,
 Glasgow G20 7BA
Helpline and Admin Tel: 0141 676 5088

Family Planning Association Wales
Graces Phillips House, 4 Museum Street,
 Cardiff CB1 3BG
Helpline Tel: 01222 342766
Admin. Tel: 01222 644034

Fertility UK
Bury Knowle Health Centre, 207 London Road,
 Headington, Oxford OX3 9JA
www.fertilityuk.org
Information on fertility awareness and natural
 family planning services.

**International Planned Parenthood Federation
(IPPF)**
PO Box 759, Inner Circle, Regent's Park,
 London NW1 4NS
Tel: 020 7487 7900
www.ippf.org.uk
Gives access to the directory of hormonal
 contraception. Promotes sexuality awareness
 and sexual health among the family
 planning associations who form the IPPF.

Margaret Pyke Centre
73–75 Charlotte Street, London W1T 1LB
Tel: 020 7530 3600
www.margaretpyke.org

Marie Stopes
153–157 Cleveland Street, London W1P 5PG
Central booking (local rate): 0845 3001212
Freephone: 0800 716 390
www.mariestopes.org.uk

**National Association of Nurses in
 Contraception and Sexual Health (NANCSH)**
9 Church Close, Drayton Bassett, Nr. Tamworth,
 Staffordshire B78 3UJ
Tel: 01827 260117
www.nancsh.org.uk

Further reading

BELFIELD, T. (1999) *FPA Contraceptive Handbook. The
 Essential Reference Guide for Family Planning and other
 Health Professionals*, 3rd edn. London: FPA.
BLACKBURN, M. (2002) *Sexuality and Disability*.
 Butterworth Heinemann.
CURTIS, H., HOOLAGHAN, T. and JEWITT, C. (1995)
 Sexual Health Promotion in General Practice. Oxford:
 Radcliffe Medical Press.
EVERETT, S. (2004) *Handbook of Contraception and
 Reproductive Sexual Health*, 2nd edn. Edinburgh:
 Baillière Tindall.
GLASIER, A. and GEBBIE, A. (eds) (2002) *Handbook of Family
 Planning and Reproductive Health Care*, 4th edn. London:
 Churchill Livingstone.
GUILLEBAUD, J. (2003) *Contraception: Your Questions
 Answered*, 4th edn. Edinburgh: Churchill Livingstone.
KUBBA, A., SANFILIPPO, J. and HAMPTON, N. (1999)
 *Contraception and Office Gynaecology: Choices in Reproductive
 Healthcare*. London: W.B. Saunders.
MONTFORD, H. and SKRINE, R. (eds) (1993) *Contraceptive
 Care: Meeting Individual Needs*. London: Chapman and
 Hall.
ROWLANDS, S. (1997) *Managing Family Planning in General
 Practice*. Oxford, Radcliffe Medical Press.
SZAREWSKI, A. and GUILLEBAUD, J. (2000)
 Contraception: A User's Guide, 3rd edn. Oxford: Oxford
 University Press.
WHITE, S. (1998) *Supporting Effective Contraceptive Use:
 A Resource for Practice Nurses*. London: Contraceptive
 Education Service.
WILKINSON, C. and SZAREWSKI, A. (2003). *Contraceptive
 Dilemmas*. St Albans: Altman.

References

ANDREWS, G.D., FRENCH, K. and WILKINSON, C.L.
 (1999) Appropriately trained nurses are competent at
 inserting intrauterine devices. *European Journal of
 Contraception and Reproductive Health Care* 4:41–4.
ARCHER, D.F., BIGRIGG, A., SMALLWOOD, G.H.,
 SHANGOL, G.A., CREASY, G.W. and FISHER, A.C.
 (2002). Assessment of compliance with a weekly
 contraceptive patch (OrthoEVRA/EVRA) among
 North American women. *Fertility and Sterility*
 77(2, Suppl 2):S27–31.
BIRD, K.D. (1991) The use of spermicides containing
 nonoxynol 9 in the prevention of HIV infection. *AIDS*
 5:791–6.
BMA, GMSC, HEA, BAC, FPA and RCGP (British Medical
 Association, General Medical Science Committee, Health
 Education Authority, Brook Advisory Centres, Family
 Planning Association and Royal College of General
 Practitioners) (1993) Joint guidance note. *Confidentiality
 and People Under 16*.
BOUNDS, W. (1994) Contraceptive efficacy of the
 diaphragm and cervical caps used in conjunction with a
 spermicide – a fresh look at the evidence. *British Journal of
 Family Planning* **20**:84–7.

BOUNDS, W. and GUILLEBAUD, J. (1999) Lea's shield contraceptive device: pilot study of its short-term patient acceptability and aspects of use. *British Journal of Family Planning* **24**:117–20.

COLLABORATIVE GROUP ON HORMONAL FACTORS IN BREAST CANCER (1996) Breast cancer and hormonal contraceptives: collaborative reanalysis of individual data on 53297 women with breast cancer and 100239 women without breast cancer from 54 epidemiological studies. *Lancet* **347**:1713–27.

COMMITTEE ON SAFETY OF MEDICINES (1995) Combined oral contraceptives and thromboembolism. Letter. London: CSM.

COMMITTEE ON SAFETY OF MEDICINES (2000) Important interactions between St John's wort (*Hypericum perforatum*) preparations and prescribed medicines. Open letter to doctors and pharmacists. London: CSM.

CROXATTO, H.B. and MAKARAINEN, L. (1998) The pharmacodynamics and efficacy of Implanon. An overview of the data. *Contraception* **58**(6, Suppl):91S–97S.

DoH (Department of Health) (1995) The response for doctors to the committee on safety of medicines. Letter. FPA and Faculty of Family Planning and Reproductive Health Care of the Royal College of Obstetricians and Gynaecologists. London: HMSO.

DRUGS AND THERAPEUTICS BULLETIN (2002). Is Yasmin a 'truly different' pill? *Drug and Therapeutics Bulletin* **40**(8):57–9.

DUNN, N., THOROGOOD, M., FARAGHER, B. *et al.* (1999a) Oral contraceptives and myocardial infarction: results of the MICA case-control study. *British Medical Journal* **318**:1579–84.

DUNN, N., THOROGOOD, M., FARAGHER, B. *et al.* (1999b) Oral contraceptives and myocardial infarction: results of the MICA case-control study. Correction. *British Medical Journal* **318**:1739.

DUREX (1988) *Oil-based Lubricants and Ointments can Damage Condoms and Diaphragms.* London: Durex Information Service for Sexual Health.

DUREX (1993) *History of the Condom.* London: Durex Information Service For Sexual Health.

DUREX (1994) *The Durex Report. A Summary of Consumer Research into Contraception.* London: London Rubber Co.

EDWARDS, J.E. and MOORE, A. (1999) Implanon. A review of clinical studies. *British Journal of Family Planning* **24**(Suppl 4).

FACULTY OF FAMILY PLANNING AND REPRODUCTIVE HEALTH CARE (1998) *Recommendations for Clinical Practice: Actinomyces like Organisms and Intrauterine Contraceptives.* CSC 1/98.

FACULTY OF FAMILY PLANNING AND REPRODUCTIVE HEALTH CARE (2003a) FFPRHC Guidance (October 2003). First prescription of combined oral contraception. *Journal of Family Planning and Reproductive Health Care* **29**(4):209–22.

FACULTY OF FAMILY PLANNING AND REPRODUCTIVE HEALTH CARE (2003b) New Product Review (September 2003). Norelgestromin/ethinyl oestradiol transdermal contraceptive system (Evra). *Journal of Family Planning and Reproductive Health Care* **30**(1):43–5.

FACULTY OF FAMILY PLANNING AND REPRODUCCTIVE HEALTH CARE (2003c) New Product Review (April 2003). Desogestrel only pill (Cerazette). *Journal of Family Planning and Reproductive Health Care* **29**(3):162–4.

FACULTY OF FAMILY PLANNING AND REPRODUCTIVE HEALTH CARE (2003d) FFPRHC Guidance Emergency Contraception. *Journal of Family Planning and Reproductive Health Care* **29**(2):9–16.

FACULTY OF FAMILY PLANNING AND REPRODUCTIVE HEALTH CARE (2004) FFPRHC Guidance. The copper intrauterine device as long-term contraception. *Journal of Family Planning and Reproductive Health Care* **30**(1):29–42.

FARLEY, T., ROSENBERG, M., ROWE, P., CHEN, J.-H. and MEIRIK, O. (1992) Intrauterine devices and pelvic inflammatory disease: an international perspective. *Lancet* **39**:785–8.

FREZIERES, R.G., WALSH, T.L., NELSON, A.L., CLARK, V.A. and COULSON, A.H. (1999). Evaluation of the efficacy of a polyurethane condom: results from a randomised, controlled clinical trial. *Family Planning Perspectives* **31**(2):81–7.

GEBBIE, A. (1996) Contraception for the over forties. In Studd, J.W.W. (ed.) *Progress in Obstetrics and Gynaecology*, Vol. 12. New York: Churchill Livingstone.

GUILLEBAUD, J. (1999) *Contraception: Your Questions Answered.* London: Churchill Livingstone.

JANSSEN-CILAG INTERNATIONAL NV (2003). Summary of product characteristics. Belgium: Janssen-Cilag International NV.

JICK, H., JICK, S.S., GUREWICH, V., MYERS, M.W. and VASILAKIS, C. (1995) Risk of idiopathic cardiovascular death and nonfatal venous thromboembolism in women using oral contraceptives with differing progestogen components. *Lancet* **346**:1589–92.

KUYOH, M.A., TOROITICH-RUTO, C., GRIMES, D.A., SCHULZ, K.F. and GALLO, M.G. (2002) Sponge versus diaphragm for contraception (Cochrane Review). In *The Cochrane Library*, Issue 1, 2004. Chichester: John Wiley.

LEWIS, M.A., LOTHAR, A.J., HEINEMANN, W.O., SPITZER, K.D., MacRAE, S. and BRUPPACHER, R. (for the Transnational Research Group on Oral Contraceptives and the Health of Young Women) (1997) The use of oral contraceptives and the occurrence of acute myocardial infarction in young women. *Contraception* **56**:1–12.

LOUDEN, N., GLASIER, A. and GEBBIE, A. (eds) (1995) *Handbook of Family Planning and Reproductive Health Care*, 3rd edn. London: Churchill Livingstone.

MASCARENHAS, L., NEWTON, P. and NEWTON, J. (1994) First clinical experience with contraceptive implants in the UK. *British Journal of Family Planning* **20**:60.

MASTERS, T. and GUILLEBAUD, J. (1999) GyneFix. *Contemporary Reviews in Obstetrics and Gynaecology*, 213–17.

MAUCK, C., CALLAHAN, M., WEINER, D.H., DOMINIK, R. and FemCap Investigators' Group (1999) A comparative study of the safety and efficacy of FemCap, a new vaginal barrier contraceptive, and the Ortho All-Flex diaphragm. *Contraception* **60**:71–80.

MELLEMKJAER, L., SORENSEN, H.T., DREYER, L., OLSEN, J. and OLSEN, J.H. (1999) Admission for and mortality from primary venous thromboembolism in women of fertile age in Denmark, 1977–95. *British Medical Journal* **319**:820–1.

O'BRIEN, P.A. (1999a) The third generation oral contraceptive controversy. The evidence shows they are less safe than second generation. Editorial. *British Medical Journal* **319**:795–6.

O'BRIEN, P.A. (1999b) Study confirms tendency towards lower risk of myocardial infarction with second generation oral contraceptives in UK. Letter. *British Medical Journal* **319**:1195.

PETERSON, H.B., XIA, Z., HUGHES, J.M., WILCOX, L.S., TAYLOR, L.R. and TRUSSELL, J. (1996) The risk of pregnancy after tubal sterilization: findings from the US Collaborative Review of Sterilization. *American Journal of Obstetrics and Gynecology* **174**(4):1161–8.

PYPER, C.M.M. and KNIGHT, J. (2001). Fertility awareness methods of family planning: the physiological background, methodology and effectiveness of fertility awareness methods. *Journal of Family Planning and Reproductive Health Care* **27**(2)103–10.

ROBINSON, G.E. (1994) Low dose combined oral contraceptives. *British Journal of Obstetrics and Gynaecology* **101**:1036–41.

ROYAL COLLEGE OF OBSTETRICIANS AND GYNAE-COLOGISTS (2004) Male and female sterilisation. Evidence-based Clinical Guideline Number 4. London: RCOG. www.rcog.org.uk.

SPITZER, W.O., LEWIS, M.A., HEINEMANN, L.A.J., THOROGOOD, M. and MACRAE, K.D. (1996) Third generation oral contraceptives and risk of venous thromboembolic disorders: an international case-control study. *British Medical Journal* **312**:83–8.

SZAREWSKI, A. and GUILLEBAUD, J. (1991) Regular review: contraception: current state of the art. *British Medical Journal* **302**:1224–6.

TASK FORCE ON POSTOVULATORY METHODS OF FERTILITY REGULATION; WORLD HEALTH ORGANIZATION (1998) Randomised controlled trial of levonorgestrel versus the Yuzpe regimen of combined oral contraceptives for emergency contraception. *Lancet* **352**:428–33.

TRUSSEL, J., STRICKLER, J. and VAUGHAN, B. (1993) Contraceptive efficacy of the diaphragm, the sponge and the cervical cap. *Family Planning Perspectives* **25**(3):100–5, 135.

TRUSSEL, J., STURGEN, K., STRICKLER, J. and DOMINIK, R. (1994) Comparative contraceptive efficacy of the female condom and other barrier methods. *Family Planning Perspectives* **25**(2):66–72.

WHO (1995) World Health Organization Collaborative Study of Cardiovascular Disease and Steroid Hormone Contraception. Venous thromboembolic disease and combined oral contraceptives: results of international multicentre case control study. *Lancet* **346**:1575–81.

WILKINSON, C. and SZAREWSKI, A. (2003). *Contraceptive Dilemmas*. St Albans: Altman.

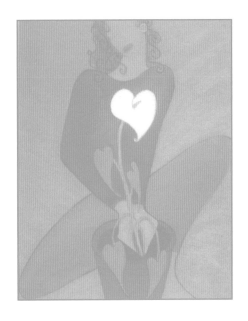

Women's Health Issues

12: Breast Screening and Breast Disorders

Karen Burnet ◆

OBJECTIVES

This chapter should help you understand:

◆ The importance of promoting breast health awareness for women ◆

◆ The structure and function of the healthy breast ◆

◆ The epidemiology and risk factors for breast cancer ◆

◆ What happens in a breast screening unit, covering clinical examination, breast awareness and diagnostic investigations ◆

◆ The role of surgery, radiotherapy and chemotherapy in the treatment of breast cancer ◆

◆ The need for psychological and social care for the woman with breast cancer ◆

◆ The need for symptom control in the palliation of metastatic disease. ◆

Introduction

Breasts are an obvious indication of femininity and are seen by both men and women as symbols of womanhood, fertility and motherhood. In Western society the breast is associated with sexual attractiveness and sexual stimulation, whereas in many other cultures the breasts' purpose is purely functional and utilitarian – feeding babies.

Women tend to be very conscious of their breasts. Breast problems and anxieties account for a large number of consultations in GP surgeries, family planning and well-woman clinics. Nurses are in the 'front line' in many of these consultations and so it is important that they have up-to-date information and are aware of the psychological aspects of breast disease.

This chapter focuses on some of the problems associated with benign breast disease and breast cancer and provides an insight into all aspects of breast care. There is so much to learn about breast screening and breast disorders that it is impossible to cover the subject in finite detail in a chapter of this nature. It is therefore suggested that the reader should refer to the further reading list and references at the end of the chapter if they need more information.

Anatomy and physiology of the breast

The breast is a glandular organ which lies over the 2nd to 6th ribs on the chest wall. During fetal development an ectodermal ridge (milk line) extends from the axilla to the groin bilaterally; in time this disappears, leaving a pair of breasts in the position described above. During puberty, due to the influence of the female sex hormones oestrogen and progesterone, breasts begin to develop, their connective tissue increases, the milk ducts lengthen and breast lobules are formed.

The ductal system of the breast extends from the nipple to the lobule (Figure 12.1). There are approximately 15–20 ducts which open on to the nipple. From the lobule, which ends in 100 or so tiny bulbs called acini – where milk is produced – the ducts extend towards the nipple and enlarge, where they are called the lactiferous sinuses. It is these that open on to the nipple for the secretion of milk. The nipple is surrounded by the areola, which may vary in colour from pinkish to dark brown. The areola contains small nodules known as the tubercles of Montgomery which produce lubrication to facilitate breastfeeding.

Apart from lobules and ducts, the breast contains fat and blood vessels, predominantly from branches of the internal mammary artery and of the lateral thoracic artery. Major lymph drainage is to the axilla, which is anatomically divided into three levels up to the clavicle, and internal mammary lymph node chain. The lymph drainage system is thought to be important in relation to the spread of malignant disease. The breast tissue is held in position by Cooper's ligaments – fibrous bands which run from the muscle fascia to the skin. Breast tissue extends up towards the armpit, forming the axillary tail. Two muscles lie beneath the breast – the pectoralis major and pectoralis minor.

Breast structure varies considerably. At the time of menarche the breasts begin to grow rapidly under the influence of sex hormones. Each month, when a woman approaches menstruation, the size of the breasts may increase. This is in preparation for a possible pregnancy. If a pregnancy does occur, the breast continues to enlarge and the acini multiply. By the end of pregnancy the breast is almost entirely a glandular structure for the purpose of milk production.

Following pregnancy these changes subside and the breast becomes less glandular.

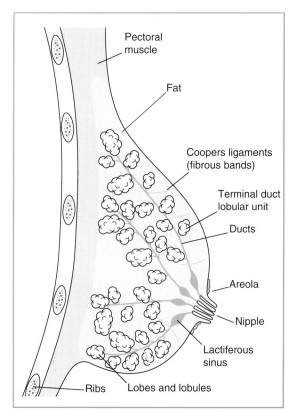

Figure 12.1 Sagittal section of the breast.

As the woman grows older the lobules and acini begin to decrease and the proportion of fatty tissue increases. This is accelerated with the onset of the menopause.

Oestrogen and progesterone produced by the ovaries influence the initial growth and subsequent development of the breast. The proliferation and development of the mammary tissue during pregnancy is stimulated by oestrogen and progesterone produced by the corpus luteum and the placenta. Other hormones believed to be involved are prolactin and the adrenal corticosteroids. It has been surmised that the high levels of sex steroids present during pregnancy inhibit the action of prolactin on breast tissue. After the separation of the placenta at delivery there is rapid fall of oestrogen and progesterone production, the inhibitory effect is lifted, and milk production is stimulated. Prolactin levels rise rapidly during breastfeeding, thus stimulating additional milk production. In the absence of breastfeeding, prolactin levels drop to a normal non-pregnant state within seven days after delivery (Di Saia, 1993).

Epidemiology and risk factors for breast cancer

Epidemiology is the study of the distribution of diseases in a population. Breast cancer is the commonest malignancy in the female population in the UK and is the commonest cause of death in women between the ages of 44 and 50. It is estimated that 1 in 9 women develop breast cancer in the UK (Breast Cancer Care, 2003). In most countries breast cancer is increasing in frequency and represents 18% of all female cancers (McPherson *et al.*, 2000).

Risk factors

Age
Age is a very important factor, with older women being at a much greater risk than younger women. The increase of risk rises steadily from the age of 40. Breast cancer is most common in women between 45 and 75 years (Cancer Research UK, 1997).

Family history
The most common risk factor is a history of breast cancer in a first-degree relative on the maternal side. This risk nearly doubles if the relative was pre-menopausal and almost trebles if the cancer was bilateral, or there was more than one first-degree relative who was pre-menopausal.

Women with a family history of breast cancer may be fortunate enough to be referred to one of the diagnostic or screening units in the UK. In many areas GPs are given guidelines on what family history details constitute a low- or high-risk patient and, as a result, are being more specific about the patients they are referring to a geneticist for counselling.

Genetic predisposition
All breast cancer can be termed 'genetic' as cancer is caused by genetic mutations (alterations in the DNA code) which result in abnormal cellular growth and/or proliferation but only a small proportion of breast cancer cases (approximately 5–10%) are due to the inheritance of a cancer predisposing gene. This gene alteration will be present in every somatic cell and, on average, half the eggs or sperm (each egg/sperm only contains half of the total genes) and therefore can be passed on to a proportion of the offspring. Currently we know of two genes in which mutations are associated with an increased risk of breast and ovarian cancer, *BRCA*1 (Miki *et al.*, 1994) and *BRCA*2 (Wooster *et al.*, 1995) which together account for almost all families affected by both breast and ovarian cancer and about 60% of breast-cancer-only families. The familial risk of having a *BRCA*1/2 mutation is partly dependent on ethnic origin with an increased risk associated with Jewish (particularly Ashkenazi and Sephardic Jews) (Struewing *et al.*, 1995), Icelandic (Thorlacius *et al.*, 1997), Norwegian and Dutch origins. It is likely that other breast cancer genes will be identified in the future.

Approximately, a further 20% of breast cancer cases can be described as familial, i.e. there is a clustering of cancer cases within the family but they do not show a well-defined pattern of inheritance. These cases may be due to the chance clustering of common cancers, the inheritance of genes that are associated with only a slightly increased cancer risk, the sharing of common environmental influences or may be of multifactorial origin, possibly as a result of the inheritance of genes which render an individual more susceptible to environmental influences.

Women suspected to have a familial risk of breast cancer could be referred to a cancer family clinic by their GP. As a quick guideline, taking a history of all first-degree relatives and then asking if there are any other cancers in the family will detect 95% of family cancer syndromes. At the clinic an assessment is made as to the personal risk of breast cancer and the likelihood of the presence of an inherited genetic mutation in the family. Breast and/or ovarian cancer screening is offered depending upon individual cancer risks, and genetic testing for *BRCA*1/2 mutations may also be possible. The search for a genetic mutation in a family starts with genetic material (blood) taken from a family member who has already developed cancer, so genetic testing cannot be undertaken in a family when all affected relatives have died. When the familial mutation has been identified, testing for this specific mutation can then be performed on any other relative, providing consent is granted, affected or not.

Menstrual history

An early menarche before 12 years and a late menopause after the age of 55 years increase risk. Women who have had a pre-menopausal oophorectomy have a substantially reduced risk of developing breast cancer.

Reproductive history

Nulliparous women are at greater risk than those who have had children, but another important risk factor is a woman's age at her first full-term pregnancy. The risk of breast cancer in women who have their first child after the age of 30 is about twice that of women who have their first child before the age of 20. Women who have their first child after the age of 35 appear to be at even higher risk than nulliparous women (Dixon and Sainsbury, 2000).

Breastfeeding

Results of studies on lactation and breast cancer are confusing although breastfeeding appears to be protective against the development of breast cancer, particularly in young women (Chilvers et al., 1993). This study also demonstrated that the risk decreases with increasing duration of breastfeeding, with breastfeeding each baby for 3 months or longer giving greatest protection.

Oral contraception

Numerous case-controlled studies have been done comparing use of the contraceptive pill in breast cancer cases and age-matched controls. In 1996 a major reanalysis of nearly all of the available epidemiological studies on hormonal contraceptives and breast cancer clarified some of the issues. Their findings indicated a small increased risk of having a breast cancer diagnosed with current users of the combined oral contraceptive pill (COC) compared to non-users. The risk is the same regardless of the level of dosage or duration of use, but decreases after stopping the COC and disappears after 10 years. Cancers diagnosed in women who had used COCs at any time were less advanced than cancers diagnosed in women who had never used COCs, although it is not known whether this also leads to improved survival (Collaborative Group on Hormonal Factors in Breast Cancer, 1996). Oral contraception, however, seems to have a protective effect against benign breast disease (Chamberlain, 1993).

Hormone replacement therapy (HRT)

The benefits of HRT are well known, i.e. control of menopausal symptoms and protection against osteoporosis as well as an increased quality of life. With regards to breast cancer risk most studies have shown a slightly increased risk in long duration of use (see page 468). However, it appears that if breast cancer is diagnosed in women who are already taking HRT then it will be picked up at an earlier stage, it tends to be of a lower grade and with a relatively good prognosis (Marsden and A'Hern, 2003; Daling et al., 2003).

Exposure to radiation

Follow-up of survivors of the nuclear bombings in Japan has demonstrated an increased risk of breast cancer. A number of other studies of women who received large doses of ionizing radiation for medical reasons have also shown an increased risk and this is particularly relevant for young women who have previously been treated with mantle radiotherapy and chemotherapy for Hodgkin's disease (Chamberlain, 1993; Deniz et al., 2003).

Diet, weight and alcohol

Fat consumption has been investigated, but no definite conclusion can be drawn from available data although it has been shown that obese women are at a greater risk than slim women. Alcohol has been associated with a moderately increased risk of breast cancer, particularly in thin, pre-menopausal women (IARC, 1988).

Geographic variations

There is marked variation in the incidence and mortality of breast cancer between different countries (Figure 12.2). In families migrating from Japan (a low-incidence country) to the USA (a high-incidence country), studies show that

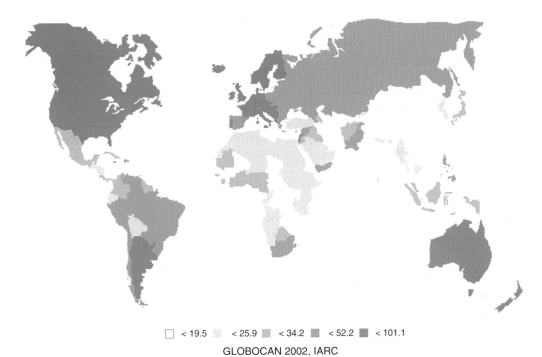

< 19.5 ☐   < 25.9 ▨   < 34.2 ▨   < 52.2 ▨   < 101.1 ▨

GLOBOCAN 2002, IARC

Figure 12.2 Age-standardized breast cancer incidence rates per 100,000 women (Ferlay *et al.*, 2002; data on mortality from WHO database which can be accessed via www-dep.iarc.fr).

second-generation women acquire the same incidence as the host country. England and Wales have the highest age-standardized mortality figures for breast cancer in the world (McPherson *et al.*, 2000).

Other risk factors

Factors associated with breast cancer are constantly being reviewed, the latest example being the association between antiperspirants and the active ingredient, parabens, and breast cancer. Studies continue in this area but, to date, the evidence is either based on small sample sizes or has not shown an association (Mirick *et al.*, 2002). No national recommendations have been made telling women to avoid using anti-perspirants at present.

Clinical examination

When undertaking a clinical examination of the breasts it is very important to take a detailed history before starting. If any of the risk factors mentioned earlier are present then these are taken into account. It is important, if the woman is pre-menopausal, to determine the start of her last period because this may necessitate bringing her back for a further examination at a different time in her cycle as breasts are frequently tender and lumpy premenstrually.

Obviously symptoms noted by the woman herself are important:

◆ If the patient has found a lump in her breast, has it changed in size, become larger or smaller? Is it tender?

◆ Has one breast increased or decreased in size? Most women have one breast slightly larger than the other and this sometimes becomes more obvious if the patient has put on weight. Many women, however, are unaware of this asymmetry and 'my husband has never noticed' is a frequently heard comment.

◆ Has there been any nipple discharge? This is particularly significant if it occurs sponta-neously. Was the discharge blood-stained? Has there been any nipple change? Has the nipple started to retract, or does it appear to be pointing in a different direction?

◆ Is there any nodularity or thickening in one area? This can be just as important as a lump.

◆ Has the woman noticed a dimple or crease, and what position was she in when she noticed this? For instance, was she looking down on her breasts or was she looking in the mirror, and what position were her arms in at the time? If she was looking down, then the examiner should look at the breasts in the same position, i.e. from behind the patient and looking down.

◆ Any other symptoms, e.g. pain that is unilateral? Many patients do not have a definite symptom but state that they have an 'increased awareness' of one breast.

Examination of the breasts should always be performed in two parts: either *looking* and then *feeling* or vice versa. If you are looking first then the patient should sit on the side of the couch, facing you and you should stand back to see if there is any difference in size or shape. As mentioned earlier, it is very common to have one breast slightly larger than the other and the woman may be unaware of this and ask if it means something is wrong. She needs to be reassured and it must be stressed that this is a common occurrence. Asking if her bra seems to have always been slightly tighter on one side can sometimes confirm this. If not, then particular attention should be paid when examining this breast. The woman should then be asked to raise her arms above her head for you to observe any dimples or creases, then she should place her hands on her hips, push in and bring the elbows forward. At this point, it may be necessary to bend down and look at the breasts from beneath – there are not many breast sizes that you can see the lower part of the breast without bending down. The woman should then put her hands on the side of the couch keeping the arms straight and pushing down and then lean forward. Again you must bend down to observe the lower part of the breast. Women feel reassured if you always explain what you are doing and what you are looking for.

These three positions that the woman is asked to adopt – with hands raised, with hands on hips, and leaning forward – are very important when looking for a dimple or crease because they may only appear in one of these positions. When documenting findings it is essential that if a dimple or crease has been observed, then the position the woman was in must be stated, i.e. dimple only seen with hands on hips. If an abnormality has been noted, it is sometimes helpful to mark the area so that when physically examining the patient attention can be paid to this area with regards to identifying any nodularity, thickening or lump which may be associated with the dimple or crease which has previously been observed.

Whilst the woman is in the sitting position, the supraclavicular fossa can be palpated, either standing in front of the patient or from behind. The infraclavicular area can also be felt by running the hands down from the clavicle to the breast. Then the axilla should be palpated by feeling high up into the axilla with the flats of the fingers and bringing them down towards the axillary tail.

On completion of this part of the examination, the woman should then be asked to lie down.

 SCENARIO

Doreen, aged 66, had been routinely screened at a diagnostic unit for many years. She had no family history of breast cancer. At one routine screening appointment, when a detailed history was taken, she reported that her left nipple was becoming more retracted than had previously been noted. There were no problems with her right breast. Before starting a clinical examination, it was noted that Doreen had a slight crease in the inner central area of the right breast which she had not noticed. On examination, an area of discrete nodularity was noted. The left breast, which Doreen was more concerned about, was normal. On sitting, the crease was again observed in the right breast. No actual clinical mass was left.

Because of these findings Doreen was sent for a mammogram. The report stated that there was a carcinoma in the right breast and that Doreen's left breast was normal.

This was an impalpable cancer in a large breast – 42D – that was detected only because of the observed crease.

The arm should be raised above the head on the side of the breast that is to be examined first. The clinical examination should be performed with the flat of the fingers and a systematic examination should be carried out. If an abnormality is detected then the fingertips are used to determine consistency, size and mobility. The clinical examination must cover the whole breast and not miss the axillary tail and beneath the nipple. After examining both breasts individually, then the patient should be turned on her side in the oblique position, with her arm raised above her head. This positioning allows for a more thorough examination of the outer quadrant of the breast, particularly in the larger-breasted patient, and quite often a lump which was not felt with the patient lying on her back can be very obvious in this position.

If a suspected abnormality is found, then all the characteristics must be noted and documented and the position of the abnormality accurately stated. Figure 12.3 shows the most common sites for breast cancer.

Many nurses undertake breast examination as part of their role. However, the Royal College of Nursing has issued guidelines recommending that nurses should not undertake the practice of

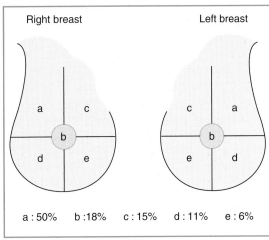

Figure 12.3   Most common sites for breast cancer.

breast palpation unless they have had specialist training and are attached to a specialist unit with access to breast mammography and ultrasound (RCN, 1995).

Breast awareness and breast care advice

There has, and probably always will be, controversy surrounding the issue of breast self-examination. It has been stated that self-examination causes unnecessary anxiety, and that finding a cancer in the breast will not necessarily alter the course of the disease. On the other hand, it could be argued that even if it does not alter the course of the disease, perhaps the initial treatment need not be so aggressive.

Many women have made statements to the effect that it was nursing a close relative with breast cancer that made them anxious in the first place. Whatever the reasons, if a woman is going to perform self-examination then she needs some guidance about how and when to perform it. It can be helpful to explain the basic anatomy and physiology of the breasts, so that women understand why their breasts might feel lumpy premenstrually – particularly in the upper outer quadrants.

SCENARIO

Annie, aged 61, had been routinely screened at a diagnostic unit for 12 years. Her maternal aunt had breast cancer. Annie presented for a routine screening appointment. She was asymptomatic and had been taking HRT for four years. On clinical examination, she was found to have a cystic-feeling nodule adjacent to the areola in the right breast. She was sent for an ultrasound which reported a highly suspicious 0.9-cm nodule in the right breast. Because of this report, she was sent for a mammogram which stated that she had no radiologically sinister features on either side.

Aspiration cytology was performed on the lump, which felt gritty to the needle. Cytology report was C4, suspicious of cancer and this was confirmed by biopsy.

Nowadays breast self-examination has been overtaken by the concept of 'breast awareness' which is what all health care professionals should be promoting in their advice to women. The difference between the two is subtle as women are still being asked to look at and feel their breasts but not in such a ritualistic way as with breast self-examination. Women should be encouraged to become familiar with how their breasts normally look and feel and how this can vary at different times of the month. They are not being asked to look specifically for lumps but just to notice any *change* from their norm. Helpful guidance can include such tips as:

◆ Don't feel the breasts before a period

◆ Use the flat of the fingers and not the fingertips

◆ Don't feel the breasts between the thumb and forefinger

◆ Remember that 9 out of 10 breast lumps are *not* cancer.

There are two distinct parts to being breast aware: *looking* and *feeling*.

Looking

◆ Note any change in the shape of the breast looking down and looking in the mirror

◆ Note any puckering or dimpling of the skin. A crease in the skin can also be important

◆ Note any change in the nipple, i.e. if the nipple starts to go in, or points in a different direction; if the nipple becomes reddened, and perhaps moist.

Feeling

The most important aspect of feeling is for women to get to know what is normal for them, and then to notice if there is any change from this normality. A lump in the breast should never be ignored, and any change in the way the breast normally feels should be followed up – that is why being breast aware just before a period is due is not sensible, and can give rise to unnecessary anxieties. However, women who are breast aware will appreciate that such changes are normal for

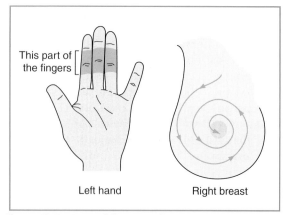

Figure 12.4 Area of fingers to be used in breast awareness and circular method of self-examination.

them and not be alarmed at pre-menstrual lumpiness and tenderness.

The flat of the fingers should be used when checking the breasts, either in the bath/shower with a soapy hand or lying on the bed using talcum powder. Starting at the 12 o'clock position, move the fingers, pressing gently down around the outer circumference of the breast, and then in ever decreasing circles towards the nipple – making sure that all areas of the breast have been examined. Finally gently press down on the nipple (Figure 12.4).

If a woman finds anything that is different (i.e. a lump, puckering, nipple change, etc.) or is anxious or worried about her breasts then she should be advised to see her doctor (Box 12.1).

Breast care advice

Brassieres

Women often complain of breast discomfort, particularly premenstrually, and one of the reasons for this can often be an ill-fitting bra. Women should be advised to be correctly fitted – most large department stores have experienced staff who can measure and give advice on this. Underwired bras that are not fitting properly can often cause discomfort in the outer quadrant of the breast; if this only happens premenstrually, then wearing a bra without a wire at this time should resolve the situation. Underwired bras are unsuitable for pregnant women.

> **Box 12.1** Breast awareness: a summary
>
> Women should be aware of:
> - Change in breast shape or size
> - Any dimpling/puckering or creases in the skin
> - Any lump or thickening in the breast
> - Any alteration in the nipple, whether it starts to go in, or starts pointing in a different direction
> - Any discharge from the nipple
> - Pain

SCENARIO

Annette is a regular attender at a diagnostic unit. For years she has had multiple cysts and she was breast aware. She returned between appointments because she had felt a lump in the breast that felt different to her more usual cysts – this was, in fact, a carcinoma.

Intertrigo

A rash in the inframammary fold is common in women with large breasts and is usually due to not drying the area thoroughly after a shower/bath. Excessive perspiration can also cause a rash and advice about wearing a cotton bra can be helpful. Talcum powder should not be applied. Calamine cream or lotion may be soothing, but if the area becomes inflamed then hydrocortisone cream, obtainable from a chemist, should be applied sparingly.

Hairs

Hairs may be removed from the areola with tweezers. These can be removed permanently by electrolysis but only by a trained professional. Depilation creams should not be used on the breast.

Inverted nipples

Inverted nipples can often be normal and may be bilateral or unilateral. They should be kept clean by gently using a cotton wool bud. If a woman notices a new inversion or any change in a pre-existing nipple inversion, she should consult her doctor.

Spots

Spots should not be squeezed as this may lead to an infection.

Breast pain (mastalgia)

Breast discomfort can be distressing and affect the quality of life for some women. GPs can do a lot to help, but some women may need referral to a specialist breast clinic for more specific advice. A detailed history of the breast pain should be taken from the woman, particularly to ascertain if she is pre- or postmenopausal. Sometimes women are asked to fill out a breast pain diary to assist both themselves and the clinician in understanding the pattern of their breast pain.

Breast discomfort can often be helped by taking evening primrose or starflower oil (both containing gamolenic acid) which should be tried for a minimum of three months. Although evening primrose oil has lost its licence for treating mastalgia, it is still available 'over the counter'. Vitamin B6 is still prescribed in the UK for mastalgia although there is no evidence that this is helpful (Purushotham *et al.*, 2000).

Reducing or abstaining from caffeine can also be helpful, as can reducing fat and salt intake although some women find this easier to do than others.

The manipulation of the female hormones can help with breast pain.

Hormonal treatments that may be prescribed include:

- Danazol, a synthetic steroid that blocks the action of oestrogen and progesterone on the breast tissue
- Tamoxifen, an oestrogen receptor blocker
- Luteinizing hormone-releasing hormone (LHRH) agonist.

These last two work by inhibiting the action of the sex hormones on breast tissue so reducing pain (Purushotham *et al.*, 2000).

Occasionally, if there is fluid retention, a diuretic may be prescribed.

Breast pain, of any type, is a rare symptom of breast cancer, and it is estimated that only 7% of patients with breast cancer have mastalgia as their only symptom.

Diagnostic investigations

Mammography (breast X-ray)

Mammography is an X-ray technique used to visualize the internal structures of the breast. The National Health Service Breast Screening Programme (NHSBSP) has been phased in since 1986 by the Department of Health following the Forrest Report (DHSS, 1986) and aims to screen asymptomatic women between the ages of 50 and 70 years by inviting them to attend for mammography every three years. The aim of the NHSBSP is to reduce mortality from breast cancer by 25% in the population of women invited to be screened.

The recommended view chosen for mammography screening is the mediolateral oblique as this single view demonstrates the maximum amount of breast tissue. The axillary tail, pectoral muscle and inferior portion of the breast are visualized. Most abnormalities are found in the upper outer quadrant and such a mammogram clearly demonstrates this area (Yeowell, 1993). It is now normal that a cranio-caudal view should also be performed on the first screening visit. This view demonstrates whether abnormalities are medial, central or lateral to the nipple. Both these mammograms are obtained by the breast being compressed between two plates whilst the exposure is made. The procedure may be uncomfortable but should not be painful. Suspicious mammograms will prompt a recall to the screening unit, inevitably causing anxiety to the woman, but further investigations may show nothing abnormal. It is hoped that taking two mammograms as a routine will reduce the number of recall visits and minimize stress and needless worry. The mammograms are then read by two consultant radiologists. Radiographers are now being trained to read mammograms as well as take them.

The practice nurse, by being a member of the primary care team, is in an ideal setting for encouraging women in this age group to attend for screening by providing information and counselling related to all aspects of the programme. It must be stressed that women should not be made to feel guilty if they are reluctant to attend for screening. In an ideal world there should be 100% uptake but the actual uptake for screening is slightly more than 70% in most centres. A woman may not want to attend because a previous mammogram was painful or because a relative's or a friend's breast cancer was detected on a screening test. There is also the common underlying fear of all women that they may have breast cancer themselves and they do not want to know about it.

There is no current evidence to support screening in women under the age of 50 years. This is due to the poorer sensitivity of X-rays in the more dense breasts of a pre-menopausal woman, and the fact that breast cancer incidence is less common in younger women. At present there is a two-centre trial being conducted in women from 40 to 47, but to date the screening programme is still from 50 years. Women over the age of 70 will not be routinely screened but can be given a mammogram on request, but not more than once every three years (NHSBSP, 2001).

Mammographic screening of asymptomatic women can pick up small impalpable tumours and microcalcification which may be the only indication of early disease such as ductal carcinoma *in situ* (DCIS). In symptomatic women it is a technique used for problem-solving, although it must be remembered that 5–10% of cancers are not detected by mammography due to the density of the cancer being less than the glandular tissue (Yeowell, 1993). This can usually be resolved by clinical examination, ultrasound and fine needle aspiration. In the case of an impalpable lesion or suspicious grouped microcalcification where surgery has been recommended then the woman will go to the X-ray department for needle localization before she goes to theatre or may undergo a very accurate X-ray controlled biopsy called a mammotome (see below).

Ultrasound (sonomammography)

Breast ultrasound is now widely accepted as a valuable adjunct to mammography and is more useful in the younger woman. High-frequency sound waves are beamed through the breast using a handheld 7.5 MHz transducer. Images are built on a screen which are then frozen and a picture can be printed. The use of ultrasound in the clinical area can be very helpful for distinguishing between cystic and solid lesions. If there is any doubt with regards to the interpretation of any abnormality then the woman would be referred for detailed ultrasound in a diagnostic imaging unit.

Ultrasound can also be used for obtaining cells from an impalpable lesion by helping with guided needle aspiration or core biopsy. The lesion is visualized on the screen and a needle is introduced into the breast and guided into the lesion by watching the screen. Cells or cores of tissue are withdrawn and sent for cytological examination. This is not unduly painful and takes only a few minutes.

Cytological and pathological investigations (Box 12.2)

Fine needle aspiration cytology

Fine needle aspiration cytology (FNAC) has become an accepted diagnostic procedure in out-patient departments and specialist centres (although trucut or core biopsies are becoming increasingly used as a diagnostic tool). The test should only be performed by professionals trained in the procedure. The advantages of the test are that it is simple, quick and relatively painless, and in a rapid diagnostic unit results are obtained whilst the woman is in the clinic, thereby making further visits to obtain results unnecessary. If a cancer diagnosis has been made then staging investigations and treatment can be discussed at that visit. If the woman is to have a mammogram then this should be undertaken before FNAC or cyst aspiration is performed as the oedema or small haematoma caused will obscure detail and give rise to a false positive diagnosis. Ideally, mammograms should be left for two weeks after FNAC if this procedure has been performed first (Tucker, 1993).

The thought of having a needle inserted into the breast is frightening for most women. It should be explained that it is very rarely painful and the majority of women admit afterwards that it was nothing like they thought it was going to be. Most women appreciate a hand to hold whilst the test is being performed. This may sound simplistic but put yourself in their position and maybe you will understand.

Stereotactic core biopsy or mammotome

This is a diagnostic technique used in some breast clinics and X-ray departments. A needle is guided into an impalpable lesion or an area of grouped microcalcification under X-ray control and cells are obtained for cytological examination. Core biopsies are often taken for a more detailed histological diagnosis. The advantage of this test is that it usually obtains enough tissue to make a definitive diagnosis, and may, in some circumstances, avoid surgery for the patient if the lesion is benign and 'cored' out. This procedure is not available in all breast cancer centres as it requires special X-ray equipment. For further details the reader is referred to the paper by Heywang-Köbrunner *et al.* (1998).

Core biopsy

This test is now more commonly being performed as it can give a lot of pathological information on

---

Box 12.2   Cytological investigations

Cytological investigations are carried out on the following:

◆ *Nipple discharge* If a discharge is elicited by gently squeezing the nipple then it should be tested to see if it is bloodstained. A slide should be gently drawn across the nipple to obtain a smear. If two slides are obtained then one is wet-fixed with cytofixative and one is air-dried. This is because of the different staining techniques used by the cytologist. The slides must be clearly marked with the woman's name, hospital number (if applicable), which breast side and whether wet-fixed or air-dried

◆ *Cyst aspiration* The fluid obtained from the cyst is discarded, but if the aspiration is bloodstained then the contents in the syringe should be emptied into a universal container and sent for cytological examination

◆ *Solid nodule or nodular area* Fine needle aspiration is performed to obtain cells from the appropriate site for diagnostic purposes. It is now becoming an accepted practice in younger women to leave fibroadenomas *in situ* once a diagnosis has been established.

the breast lesion, i.e. type and grade. Local anaesthetic is infiltrated into the skin and the breast where the core of tissue is to be removed. A small incision is made in the skin and a narrow-bore cutting needle which has been inserted into a mechanical biopsy gun is then inserted through the incision and guided to the area to be sampled. A core of tissue is obtained which is then fixed in formalin. The test should not be painful, but the slight noise of the needle action should be demonstrated first so that the woman is prepared. Firm pressure should be applied over the area for a few minutes afterwards to prevent bleeding, then an occlusive dressing is applied.

Problems

Complications which may occur after fine needle aspiration or core biopsy, although rare, may include the following:

◆ *Haematoma or bruise* This can occur if a large vessel is punctured during aspiration or core and the procedure may have to be abandoned and pressure applied; or it may occur if pressure is not applied correctly after completion of aspiration. An explanation to the woman that bruising may appear which will resolve in time will relieve the anxiety if this does happen. Occasionally a mild analgesic may be appropriate.

◆ *Pneumothorax* This is a rare complication and may go undetected if the pneumothorax is small. Subtle clues such as sharp pain, coughing or a hiss of air on withdrawing the needle without evidence of air in the syringe, may occur (NHSBSP, 1993).

A woman should be advised to see her GP if she is concerned about unexpected pain, bruising or oedema after any of the above procedures.

Benign breast disorders

Cysts

Breast cysts are basically fluid-filled sacs and are found most commonly in the 40–60-year age group. They can vary enormously in size,

depending upon the amount of fluid in the sac. On clinical examination cysts can feel soft and mobile and may be described as a lax cyst. A tense/tension cyst can feel round and hard, and can clinically resemble a carcinoma. Cysts are frequently multiple in nature, and can also be bilateral.

Symptoms of tension cysts include pain and tenderness. Cysts can fill rapidly, which may be very frightening to a patient and this is something that you should explain when discussing breast awareness with your patient.

Cysts usually subside or disappear with the menopause unless the woman is taking HRT when they may persist.

Treatment

A mammogram may be performed to rule out an incidental carcinoma. Ultrasound, if available, should be performed, although occasionally some cysts can create echoes that are produced by the turbid contents of the cyst.

Needle aspiration of a cyst should be performed if the cyst is causing pain, is very large, or if it is worrying the patient. The fluid from a cyst can vary in colour – clear, green, straw-coloured, milky, chocolate-coloured or bloodstained. The fluid is not usually sent for cytology, unless it is evenly bloodstained.

After aspiration of the cyst the patient should be re-examined to determine whether there is any residual mass. If there is, then repeat needle aspiration should be performed and the cells sent for cytology to check for an underlying cancer.

Fibroadenomas

Fibroadenomas are the most common benign lumps in younger women and usually occur between the ages of 20 and 30 years. A fibroadenoma is a solid, fibrous nodule which is histologically composed of glandular elements and connective tissue found in the breast. It is now considered to be an aberration of normal development. On clinical examination a fibroadenoma is usually well circumscribed, firm and mobile, and is often referred to as a 'breast mouse' because of its mobility. Methods of diagnosis are clinical examination, ultrasound and FNAC or core biopsy.

Fibroadenomas may increase in size, may stay the same, or disappear. If ultrasound is performed then a measurement can be taken, and when the patient is reassessed at a later date the ultrasound and measurement may be performed again to see if there is any change in size. If the above tests have been performed and it has been established that the lump is a fibroadenoma then the patient is usually discharged from the clinic unless, in extreme cases, she wishes to have the fibroadenoma removed. Fibroadenomas regress with age, and coarse nodular calcification due to necrosis may appear on mammography as the woman gets older. This is known as a degenerating fibroadenoma and no treatment is necessary.

Juvenile and giant fibroadenomas

When a fibroadenoma grows rapidly and exceeds 5–6 cm in size in the breast of an adolescent it is referred to as a juvenile fibroadenoma. The usual course of treatment is surgical removal for cosmetic reasons. Giant fibroadenomas attain a similar size but are usually found in the breasts of pregnant or lactating women. They usually shrink in size when the hormonal influences diminish but if they remain large they can be removed surgically. These two lesions do not have malignant potential (Purushotham *et al.*, 2000).

Phyllodes tumour

Phyllodes tumours are rare and can range from benign to malignant. On clinical examination they often seem like a fibroadenoma but microscopically they are distinct neoplastic lesions. They are removed surgically by wide local excision for a complete pathological diagnosis and further treatment if required (Purushotham *et al.*, 2000).

Mondor's disease

Caused by superficial thrombosis of a vein in the breast. Mondor's disease can present as a pain with a crease in the skin. Malignancy should always be excluded, but apart from this

no treatment is necessary as the condition usually resolves within 6 months.

Tietze's syndrome

Tietze's syndrome is not common, but occurs when the costal cartilages become enlarged, painful and tender. If it is persistent then treatment with local anaesthetic and steroid injections is effective.

Gynaecomastia

Gynaecomastia is an abnormal development of male breast tissue and is therefore outside the scope of this book on women's health.

Galactocoele

A galactocoele is a cystic lesion in women which can occur during or after pregnancy or during breastfeeding. Treatment is by aspiration. This may have to be performed on several occasions in order to allow the walls of the cyst to adhere to one another, thus obliterating the space (McKinna, 1983).

Fat necrosis

Fat necrosis was originally thought to be caused by trauma. However, Haagensen (1986) described only 32% of patients who gave a history of previous trauma. Fat necrosis presents as a painless mass which is ill-defined, and can often be mistaken for a carcinoma. Diagnosis is by clinical examination, mammography and FNAC or core biopsy. If malignancy cannot be excluded, then biopsy is indicated. Otherwise management should be by observation.

Duct papilloma

Duct papillomas are very common and may be single or multiple. They are caused by solitary papillary benign lesions growing in one of the main ducts close to the nipple. Presentation will be with nipple discharge which may be serous or bloodstained. Occasionally a palpable mass may be felt at the areolar margin. Treatment is usually excision of the offending duct through a circumareolar excision (Purushotham *et al.*, 2000).

Duct ectasia

Duct ectasia is a benign condition that mostly affects older women and is caused by a loss of elastin within the walls of the milk duct leading to dilatation of these ducts and an associated chronic cell infiltrate.

Symptoms include nipple discharge, nipple retraction and/or a palpable mass. Investigations performed are mammography, ultrasound and clinical examination. If the diagnosis is confirmed the woman may be reassured, but if the discharge is troublesome, then total duct excision would be suggested. Sometimes there is an associated infection in the dilated ducts called periductal mastitis. Smoking is an important contributory factor. Antibiotics would be given as the first-line treatment but repeated episodes of infection need complete duct excision with further antibiotic cover (Purushotham *et al.*, 2000).

Mammary duct fistula

These fistulae occur in the subareolar duct and the skin usually following an episode of periductal mastitis. Again this condition is more common in smokers. Treatment would be complete duct excision with removal of the fistula. The rare but important side effects of loss of nipple sensation, necrosis and loss of the nipple should be discussed with the woman when the complete duct excision is proposed. There would need to be antibiotic cover with this procedure.

Lipoma

Lipomas, or fatty growths, may be found in the breast and can be mistaken for cysts because on physical examination they are mobile and smooth. Ultrasound and FNAC or core biopsy will establish a diagnosis.

Intramammary lymph nodes

Occasionally intramammary lymph nodes can be felt in the outer quadrant of the breast. On clinical examination they can feel firm and mobile. Fine needle aspiration will usually establish a diagnosis.

Breast infections

Lactating breast infections

Women who are breastfeeding can develop cellulitis, lactating mastitis or an abscess in their breast. The cause of the infection is usually *Staphylococcus aureus* and arises from a cracked nipple. The symptoms are similar to any other infection, i.e. pain, swelling and erythema of the overlying skin. Antibiotics are needed, and if the infection does not resolve then drainage of the pus may be required. The woman is usually encouraged to continue breastfeeding if she can, as emptying the breast of milk can relieve the symptoms and improve the outcome of the treatment.

Non-lactating breast infections

Breast abscesses occur in women with other underlying conditions such as diabetes, steroid therapy and rheumatoid arthritis. The clinical presentation and treatment are similar to lactational abscesses.

Breast cancer

Breast cancer is a serious problem in Britain. There are 40,000 new cases of breast cancer each year and, unfortunately, 13,000 deaths annually from the disease (Breast Cancer Care, 2003). Much can be done to help women, particularly in the early stages of their diagnosis and treatment. As mentioned before, women 'at risk' can be identified and screened earlier than ever. For those women who have a positive diagnosis there is a bewildering range of available treatments which can cause confusion for her, her family and other health professionals with whom she may wish to discuss the issues.

It was felt appropriate to include a substantial section on the medical treatment of breast cancer in this chapter as a significant number of women will undergo this treatment. These women will often seek physical and psychological care and advice from those not directly involved in their immediate treatment. This section is written as a guide to what is currently available so that you, as a nurse, will be able to understand the range of treatment options your patients are faced with when coping with a diagnosis of breast cancer.

Types of breast cancer

Most breast cancers develop from the epithelial lining cells of the terminal duct lobular unit (see Figure 12.1). The cancer cells that remain within this structure are termed as non-invasive or *in situ*. Cancer cells that have the ability to disseminate outside the basement membrane of the ducts and lobules are described as invasive (Sainsbury *et al.*, 2000).

It is important to define the type of cancer as this will determine the future treatment for the woman. Types of breast cancer are now defined by their growth patterns and other cellular characteristics.

Carcinoma in situ

Carcinoma *in situ* is characterized by a proliferation of malignant epithelial cells that remain confined to the terminal duct lobular unit. There are two types of *in situ* disease which are described as ductal or lobular. Ductal carcinoma *in situ* (DCIS) is more prevalent than lobular carcinoma *in situ* (Crowe and Lampejo, 1996). Until recently, the standard treatment for DCIS was the removal of the affected breast by mastectomy. Now, mastectomy is usually only considered if the disease extends over a wide area of the breast. Other treatments include less invasive surgery, the use of radiotherapy and the anti-oestrogen tablet Tamoxifen (Hwang and Esserman, 1999).

Infiltrating breast cancer

Infiltrating carcinoma has the ability to escape from the structures of the breast. The two main infiltrating breast cancers are lobular and ductal. These cancers have the potential to metastasize, or spread through the body, although they do not do so in every case. Other variants of breast cancer include Paget's disease of the breast and inflammatory breast cancer. There are rarer breast cancers and more information about these can be obtained from the reading list at the end of the chapter.

Paget's disease

The incidence of this breast cancer is low, representing 0.5–3.2% of all breast cancers (Fowble *et al.*, 1991). It usually involves the nipple epidermis and the woman often presents to her GP with a nipple discharge, eczema-like skin changes, nipple retraction and sometimes an underlying thickening of the breast tissue. Treatment depends on what the woman will accept and the particular surgeon's choice. Either excision of the nipple and underlying tissue with postoperative radiotherapy, or a mastectomy is usual. If treated correctly the woman has a good chance of being cured of the disease, but the extent of the breast surgery will mean that she requires similar support to women who have the more common types of breast cancer.

Inflammatory breast cancer

About 4% of all breast cancers are diagnosed as inflammatory. The woman presents with a breast that is swollen and red, and has skin oedema with induration of the underlying breast tissue (peau d'orange). The overall survival of these patients is particularly poor (Rodger *et al.*, 2000). Radiotherapy and chemotherapy are the mainstays of treatment but if a woman's tumour responds particularly well then surgery may be added, to give the woman the best possible chance of local control and survival.

Clinical staging

Before the surgeon and the woman decide on the most acceptable surgical intervention for breast cancer the disease should be staged as accurately as possible. With information from pathology, mammography, ultrasound imaging and a full clinical examination the surgeon, as a part of the multidisciplinary team of clinicians caring for the woman, will be able to choose the best operation for the size of lump and its location in the breast. Because breast cancer has the ability to spread via the blood vessels and the lymphatic system supplying the breast, further staging investigations can be performed if there is clinical indication of metastatic spread and according to the treatment policy of the unit.

Clinical staging tests include:

◆ Blood tests (full blood count and liver function biochemistry)

◆ Bone scan

◆ Chest X-ray

◆ Liver ultrasound.

Whilst the staging investigations are taking place, the woman can be under extreme stress. It is essential that the nursing and medical staff recognize this. Support should be offered by contact with a specialist breast care nurse, giving telephone numbers of various support agencies, and by listening to the woman's hopes and fears. No assumptions should be made about how the woman is feeling at such a time. Because of initial shock she may have little opinion about what is happening to her, or she may have previous experience of cancer which could be positive or negative. Some breast cancers have a genetic basis and the woman may have already nursed a mother or sister through the disease. For this reason it must be emphasized that each cancer experience is different and that treatments are constantly changing for the better. Some women will wish to discuss the elements of their treatment slowly, with careful thought, before considering what comes next, while others are keen to know straight away what could be ahead of them.

Waiting for the outcome of bone scan or liver ultrasound tests can be an excruciating time for these women: 'It's the waiting for results I can't stand. I want to know what I'll be dealing with and get on with it', is a frequently heard comment.

Surgery

Once all the necessary information about the woman's breast disease has been collected, a date will be set for surgery. There is some controversy surrounding surgical options for breast cancer and there has been a considerable change of opinion over the past few years. A survey carried out in 1983 showed that mastectomy was the most commonly performed operation for breast cancer with only 18% of surgeons undertaking conservative treatment (Gazet et al., 1985). By 1989, 64% of surgeons were performing conservative surgery (Morris et al., 1989). Work carried out in Milan between 1973 and 1980 comparing radical mastectomy for breast cancer with wide local excision of the disease plus an axillary lymph node dissection and radiotherapy showed clearly that there was no difference in survival between the two groups receiving the different treatments, thus providing solid evidence for the effectiveness of breast conserving surgery (Veronesi et al., 1990).

The surgeon will recommend the type of surgery offering the best chance of successful treatment, depending on the size and location of the lump. Mastectomy is usually required if the tumour:

◆ Is more than or equal to 4 cm in size

◆ Has invaded the underlying muscle of the chest wall

◆ Is directly beneath the nipple

◆ Is multi-focal

◆ Is locally relapsed disease previously treated by breast conservation

◆ If the breast is small.

However, if the tumour can be excised without major disfigurement, which principally relates to the size of the tumour relative to the breast, the surgeon should recommend wide local excision. Surgeons may feel that by offering to preserve a woman's breast they are lessening her trauma. Offering the woman choice has been shown not to reduce the psychological morbidity (Fallowfield et al., 1990). In fact, when women are given the choice of surgery some do not automatically choose to retain their breast, and feel that they are better off without the affected part (Wilson et al., 1988).

Assumptions about what the woman wants should not be made. She should be at the centre of the team involved in her care, and her needs taken into account at every stage of the decision-making process. For some women, however, this responsibility and choice proves too much and they ask the team to make the decision for them.

The timing of surgery during the menstrual cycle

Pre-menopausal women have circulating unopposed oestrogen (i.e. not opposed by progesterone) between days 3 and 12 after their last menstrual period (LMP). For the rest of the cycle these hormones are low (0–2 days) or high (13–28 days). There is a small body of evidence to suggest that unopposed oestrogen at the time of surgical intervention may encourage dissemination of micrometastases (the shedding of cancer cells). Studies are continuing in this area to refute or to confirm the findings but there is no firm conclusion as yet (Badwe, 1993).

Mastectomy

A mastectomy is the surgical removal of the breast. This can mean several different operations, ranging from those that remove the breast, chest muscles and axillary lymph nodes, to an operation that only removes the breast itself.

Mastectomy may be radical, modified radical or simple (Figure 12.5).

◆ *Radical mastectomy* Not often performed today, this operation removes the breast, the pectoralis major and minor muscles, all the axillary lymph nodes, and some additional fat and skin. This procedure is also known as a Halsted mastectomy. It is an extensive operation which leaves a long scar on the chest wall and a hollow chest area. The removal of all the lymph nodes may lead to arm swelling or lymphoedema, some loss of muscle power in the arm and restricted shoulder movement. Intensive physiotherapy may be needed after surgery.

◆ *Modified radical or Patey mastectomy* Rarely performed today unless there is extensive local tumour spread. This operation removes the breast, the axillary lymph nodes and the lining of the chest wall muscles. Sometimes the pectoralis minor muscle is removed or divided, to allow access to the axilla. Because the pectoralis major muscle is maintained, the strength of the arm is also maintained, and swelling of the arm is less likely. Breast reconstruction will be easier to achieve because more skin is left compared with a radical mastectomy.

In either of the above procedures, where the axilla is dissected to remove nodes, numbness in the inner aspect of the upper arm results from

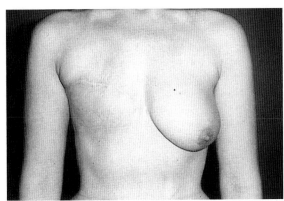

Figure 12.5   Mastectomy scar.

division of a nerve (the intercostobrachial) which traverses the axilla.

◆ *Simple or total mastectomy* This removes only the breast and is the procedure used most often today if the woman needs and/or wants a mastectomy. If the woman has an invasive cancer then the axillary lymph nodes will be removed to anatomical level two (into the axilla but not as far as the supraclavicular fossa) unless there is considerable local spread, in which case the lymph nodes will be removed to level three. Axillary lymph nodes are removed to give an indication of whether the cancer has spread beyond the breast to the lymphatics. The advantage is that the chest muscles are not removed and arm strength is not diminished.

Reconstructive surgery

If a woman's breast(s) have to be removed because of cancer or because the woman herself wishes her breast(s) to be removed because she has a genetic predisposition to breast cancer, she should be offered the option of immediate breast reconstruction (National Institute for Clinical Excellence, 2002). If a woman has already undergone a mastectomy she can be offered reconstructive surgery at a later date. Reconstructive surgery is not a skill that all breast surgeons have, but can be explained to the woman as a treatment choice even if referral to an oncoplastic surgeon or more specialized unit is needed.

Women need to be told about their surgical options as the loss of the breast can be a very emotive event causing a fear of disfigurement and worry about rejection (Kasper, 1995; Kissane *et al.*, 1998). By giving the woman information about the disease and choices about her treatment she may feel she has more control over a frightening situation. A breast care nurse with specialist knowledge about breast reconstruction could prove invaluable as the woman's advocate, presenting her needs and expectations regarding her treatment to the doctor concerned.

There are some contraindications to reconstructive surgery:

◆ If the woman has a large, aggressive tumour

◆ If there are chest wall metastases

◆ If there is extensive disease involvement of other body systems (distant metastases)

◆ If the woman has significant cardiopulmonary or other systemic disease.

When discussing reconstructive surgery it must be made clear that breast and nipple sensation will not be restored. The aim of surgery will be to retain the shape and form of the breast mound but the reconstructed breast will not be the same as the breast that has been lost.

There are several methods of reconstructing a breast. The method chosen will be after consideration and recommendation from the plastic surgeon who should also take into account the woman's wishes for her appearance and the type of operation she is prepared to undergo.

The simplest form of breast reconstruction is when the surgeon, working at the site of the mastectomy scar, lifts muscle and fascia away from the chest wall to create a pocket for an implant. The surgeon then inserts the implant into the formed pocket and stabilizes the pocket with sutures to prevent upward or lateral movement (Solomon, 1986; Mulata *et al.*, 2000). The implant can be silicone, or a silicone capsule filled with silicone gel (Figure 12.6). There has been considerable controversy recently concerning silicone and its possible leakage causing connective tissue autoimmune diseases and cancer. A recent meta-study of 20 research papers showed that

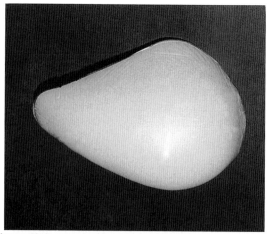

Figure 12.6 External breast prosthesis.

there is no statistical evidence that silicone implants are associated with such diseases (Janowsky *et al.*, 2000). Implants containing saline in a silicone envelope can be used instead of solid silicone. These implants are filled with saline injected through a device attached to the implant, the filling port. The advantage of this type of implant is that it consists largely of saline rather than the silicone gel (see Figure 12.7). These implants can be filled over a period of time, from a few weeks to a couple of months, slowly stretching the skin that overlaps the implant. The implant can be overfilled and then deflated slightly, stretching the skin to achieve the droop or ptosis of a normal breast. Once the final shape and volume are attained, the filling port attached to the implant is removed as a day-case procedure under a light general anaesthetic.

For women with larger breasts, the more complex latissimus dorsi (LD) flap procedure can be used. The LD muscle, which runs from the broad origin on the back to insert in the upper arm, is partially dissected to fill the space of the missing pectoralis muscle. The surgeon takes a flap of skin from the back to reconstruct the new breast. The skin and muscle has an intact blood supply and is rotated from the back to the front of the chest at the incision of the mastectomy scar. The surgeon can then place an implant under the muscle, shaping the rotated flap around it (Mulata *et al.*, 2000). Occasionally, if the woman's

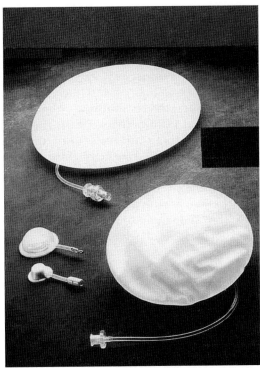

Figure 12.7 Silicone implant with filling port for saline.

the perforator blood vessels of the deep epigastric blood supply. The advantage of this is that there is no muscle sacrifice and so the avoidance of hernias and bulges, ideal for the younger woman who lives an active life or who may wish to get pregnant in the future (Mulata *et al.*, 2000; West, 2003).

For the LD, TRAM and DIEP reconstructions there are scars on the part of the body from where the flaps are raised. The woman should be counselled carefully before consenting to such an operation so she understands what is involved. Photographs of the surgeon's previous work are useful to explain the surgery, and information booklets or leaflets are helpful to reinforce what has been explained. The decision for such surgery needs considerable thought, as there are drawbacks with these types of breast reconstruction. These include capsular contraction around the implant, flap necrosis and silicone gel 'bleed'. There may be disparity between the colour of the transplanted skin and the woman's other breast, and the new breast may not have the same shape as the original breast (Mitchell and Gamble, 2001).

There is much to be understood about breast reconstruction particularly as more women are being offered this option at the time of their initial breast surgery for breast cancer and for women who have prophylactic mastectomies because of genetic risk. It is not within the remit of this chapter to describe extensively the techniques and nursing care but the reader is referred to West (2003) and Mulata *et al.* (2000) for greater detail.

Breast conservation

Breast conservation, also known as a wide local excision, removes the tumour plus a margin of normal tissue surrounding it, usually 0.5–1 cm in every direction. The axillary lymph nodes are removed to anatomical level two in the axilla and does not include the supraclavicular nodes. This procedure should be followed by radiation therapy of the breast to ensure equal local control of the disease compared to mastectomy and better survival (Veronesi *et al.*, 1990; Overgaard *et al.*, 1997). A wide local excision has the advantage of breast conservation. However, if the woman has medium- or small-sized breasts, this procedure

breasts are small, this method of breast reconstruction can be performed without a silicone implant.

The more complex types of breast reconstruction use autologous tissue and avoid the use of silicone implants. There are several ways of reconstructing the breast using the woman's own tissue. A widely used autologous breast reconstruction is the transverse rectus abdominis flap (TRAM) (Mulata *et al.*, 2000). An ellipse of skin and muscle is raised from the upper abdomen or the suprapubic region. The flap raised is the whole width of the rectus muscle; the distal end of the muscle flap is transected and the flap is rotated up into the mastectomy defect (Ward, 1987; Watson *et al.*, 1995; Mulata *et al.*, 2000). There are several variations of this procedure each used to suit the physical needs and wishes of the woman concerned.

Finally, the deep epigastric perforator flap (DIEP) is the latest and most complicated method of reconstruction. This procedure preserves the whole of the rectus muscle and sheath and uses can noticeably change the breast shape. If radio-therapy is then given to both the breast and axilla the risk of lymphoedema is increased significantly (Kissin *et al.*, 1986).

Excision biopsy

Sometimes a breast lesion cannot be biopsied as an outpatient procedure and the patient has to undergo an excision biopsy. This procedure means that only the breast lump is removed with little or no normal tissue margin. The tissue removed will be examined to ensure that the full pathology is known. The breast is unlikely to be greatly altered in shape unless the lump was large and the breast small. There would be some scar tissue from this procedure which might make it difficult to examine the breast at a later date.

Axillary surgery

If the initial pathology shows an invasive breast cancer an axillary node sampling or clearance is usually performed. The British Association of Surgical Oncologists (BASO, 1998) recommends that all patients with breast cancer, irrespective of age, should have some form of axillary surgery as it provides invaluable information for the future management of the woman's disease and will also help to prevent the recurrence of breast cancer in the axilla. It is usual for patients to undergo an axillary dissection to the anatomical level two in the axilla.

Sentinel lymph node surgery

There is ongoing important research aimed at detecting whether the cancer has spread to the lymphatic system at the time of primary surgery without removing the majority of the axillary lymph nodes. Axillary surgery has the associated morbidity of the risk of lymphoedema and arm stiffness and if the cancer cells have not spread to the lymph nodes then it would be advantageous to the patient to spare the axilla. Using conventional methods of surgery there is no way of knowing if the lymph nodes are involved with the tumour prior to operation and pathological analysis of the lymph nodes. A new technique of identifying the sentinel, or first draining lymph node from the breast and analysing this for cancer

cells has been developed as it is believed that cancer cells spread systematically through the lymph nodes. During the operation the main lymphatic drainage system is identified by the injection of a radioactive tracer around the tumour about two hours before the surgery and dye intra-operatively into the tumour bed (McIntosh and Purushotham, 1998). The area is X-rayed at regular intervals until the main drainage lymph node(s) are highlighted. The node or nodes (there may be several sentinel lymph nodes) are removed and sent to pathology as a frozen section, or with the whole breast specimen for paraffin slide mounting and extensive pathological analysis. If the lymph node(s) contains tumour cells, more extensive lymph node surgery is undertaken (Mitchell and Gamble, 2001). If this research continues to show positive results, this technique will have the advantage of sparing the patient the potential morbidity of an extensive axillary node clearance if there is no evidence of cancer spread to the lymph nodes.

Needle localization

Sometimes a breast lesion is seen on mammogram but is so small that it cannot be felt by palpation. Often areas of microcalcification can be seen on the X-ray film indicating disease. This area needs to be removed for diagnostic reasons to exclude the likelihood of malignancy. The radiologist will be involved to locate the area for the surgeon. Using local anaesthetic, a fine guidewire is inserted into the woman's breast indicating the suspicious area. The area is also located with a mammogram. The woman is then sent to theatre with the needle in place, taped to her skin. The surgeon, using the needle and the mammograms as guidance, excises the area. The removed tissue is X-rayed whilst the woman is under the anaesthetic to check that the affected area is totally removed. Further excision will be needed if any residual disease is left behind.

Nursing care following surgery

Unless really extensive, or involving reconstructive surgery, breast surgery needs careful but limited postoperative care. Drains from the breast or chest wound site are removed 24–48 hours post-surgery according to the local policy and the surgeon's preference. Drains inserted into the axillary wound stay in for a few days, or until the sero-sanguinous fluid reduces significantly. There has been some research about letting the patient home after surgery with their axillary drain *in situ*. With back-up care provided by community nurses and the breast care nurse and clear instructions about what to do and who to contact should something go wrong, some breast units and their patients have found this a satisfactory way of going home early (Chapman, 2001).

Physiotherapy can start 24 hours postoperatively and the woman will be taught a selection of exercises to improve her arm movement. Often an information booklet is provided to encourage the woman to continue the exercises whilst at home. Additional exercises are taught according to the operation and individual requirements.

Dressings should be light and non-occlusive and replaced only if soiled. The woman's sensitivities should be taken into account when considering the type of dressing used. She may prefer that the wound is covered up securely until she is ready to look for herself.

Immediate postoperative complications may include the formation of a haematoma if there has been insufficient cautery of the smaller blood vessels at the time of surgery. The woman may have to return to the operating theatre for drainage of the haematoma and re-cautery of blood vessels. Seroma formation is always a risk after axillary and breast surgery. Sero-sanguinous fluid collects beneath the wound and can be aspirated with a needle and syringe as a simple outpatient procedure. These aspirations can continue until the fluid stops collecting although if the woman is comfortable and the fluid is not infected small seromas can be left to re-absorb naturally.

The woman should be encouraged to look at her scar whilst in hospital if she has had a wide local excision but particularly if she has undergone a mastectomy. The first time she looks can be an extremely traumatic moment for her but the shock can be lessened with an understanding and supportive approach to her care. A nurse should be present when a woman looks at her scar for the first time and should encourage the

woman to discuss what she is feeling about the way she looks. The woman may wish for her partner to be present although she may want to come to terms with the scar herself before exposing herself to another person. This 'coming to terms' with her body image can be a slow and painful process, which will be helped by continuing support from the nursing team and the woman's family and friends. This is a time when the provision of telephone support numbers, details of support groups, and contact with a specialist breast care nurse is especially important. The woman should be encouraged to ask for help from whichever agency she feels is appropriate for her needs.

If the woman has had a mastectomy she should be fitted with a soft breast form into a supportive bra or 'crop top' before she leaves hospital. This soft breast form or 'comfie' will not irritate the stitch line but will give the woman some equality of shape before she faces the outside world. An arrangement for a more permanent breast prosthesis should be made for 6–8 weeks after surgery unless the woman is undergoing radiotherapy, in which case the fitting should take place about 4–6 weeks after the radiotherapy has finished to allow the treated skin to heal. The restoration of the woman's external body image can be associated with her ability to cope and adjust to her diagnosis of cancer (Denton and Baum, 1983).

Lymphoedema

Lymphoedema is caused by an excessive collection of lymph in the tissues, and when it occurs can cause discomfort and pain, altered body image and a lack of mobility. There are two main categories of lymphoedema:

◆ *Primary:* is a congenital problem when the structure of the lymphatic system has not developed properly

◆ *Secondary:* when the lymphatic system is damaged by surgery, radiotherapy or by disease infiltration and is the category associated with treatment for breast cancer.

The breast is particularly well supplied with lymphatic channels which drain largely into the axillary lymph nodes. From there, lymph drains into the supraclavicular fossa and lower neck.

Surgical intervention for a malignant breast lump may involve an axillary dissection. This may remove a large number of the lymph nodes, depending on the level of dissection undertaken, thereby compromising the lymphatic system. Research by Kissin *et al.* (1986) showed that about 15% of women will be at risk of developing arm swelling after an axillary dissection has been performed, and this risk increases to 25% if the axilla is then treated with radiotherapy. However, Keeley (2000) comments that it is difficult to draw conclusions from the studies undertaken on lymphoedema because of the different variables used in the data collection. For practical purposes, though, any woman who has undergone axillary surgery should be considered at some risk of developing lymphoedema. Women can develop lymphoedema of the arm soon after surgery, but it is more likely to develop after several months and it is known that infection or trauma of the arm can precipitate swelling (Mozes, 1982; Keeley, 2000).

Advice about reducing the risk of lymphoedema can start whilst the woman is still in hospital (Box 12.3).

Box 12.3   Advice to give on reducing the risk of lymphoedema

◆ Avoid injections in the affected arm
◆ Continue the exercises taught by the physiotherapist
◆ Use gloves when gardening to avoid cuts and abrasions and the risk of local infection
◆ Do not have blood pressure taken on the affected arm
◆ Do not lift heavy weights
◆ Keep the skin on the arm in as good condition as possible
◆ Use depilatory cream instead of a razor to remove under-arm hair
◆ Treat cuts on the affected arm immediately by washing and applying an antiseptic cream
◆ Take care when cutting nails
◆ Seek medical attention promptly if the arm starts to feel tight or look swollen.

Treatment of lymphoedema

Treatment for lymphoedema should follow the well-established guidelines of the British Lymphology Society (Woods, 2003). The recommendations include re-education about skin care and an explanation of why the lymph fluid is accumulating. Prompt referral to a specialist will ensure that the woman gets the right advice and education about her condition. Measurement of the limb provides a baseline for any future interventions and when compared to the measurements of the unaffected arm will give an indication of how swollen the arm has become. Exercises for the swollen limb to help mobilize lymph fluid will be taught and the fitting of an appropriate compression sleeve will further assist the drainage of fluid. Simple self-massage of the remaining lymphatic system can also be taught. Enabling the woman to take some control of her condition can help to lessen the distress from this unfortunate side effect of breast cancer and its treatment. For a chronically swollen arm, bandaging carried out daily for a prolonged period can help to reshape the limb prior to fitting a compression sleeve. Community nurses can take over this treatment successfully.

Useful information about lymphoedema can be found by contacting the British Lymphology Society or the Lymphoedema Support Network (see Resources).

Management of inoperable breast cancer

If the patient presents with a locally advanced breast cancer, surgery is not the best option and primary medical treatment is considered. A locally advanced breast cancer is defined as having the following characteristics:

◆ Overlying, widespread oedema, and/or ulceration
◆ Chest wall fixation
◆ Skin nodules
◆ Disease-infiltrated axillary nodes
◆ An inflammatory component
◆ Supraclavicular nodal spread.

The treatment of choice depends on the menopausal status of the woman, the extent of the disease, and the woman's wishes. Treatment will normally involve radiotherapy plus hormone manipulation, with or without chemotherapy.

Nursing care of fungating breast cancer

Some women present with locally advanced disease which has ulcerated due to infiltration of the skin of the breast. Care of lesions of this sort will involve careful assessment and skilful choice of dressing.

Ulcerated lesions always grow some organisms, usually skin commensals, but sometimes pathogenic organisms can colonize the wound. Swabs should be sent for microbiological culture, and systemic or topical antibiotics given as necessary. It is usual to clean the wound with normal saline or, if it is large, it can be cleaned gently with a shower attachment. Useful topical applications, depending on the exact nature of the ulcer, can debride and deslough the wound. Cleaning agents would include those with enzymatic activity to deslough the wound, and the hydrocolloids and hydrogel which are effective debridants.

For wounds that smell particularly offensive, live yoghurt applied and left for 30 minutes and then washed off can be beneficial. This method of wound cleansing has not been researched in depth and should be used carefully. When planning care it is important to ensure that dressings are not too bulky, that they are comfortable, and will remain in place. Every effort should also be made to preserve the woman's dignity. For further information the reader is referred to Mallett *et al.* (1999) and King (2003) for expert detail.

Pathological staging

Clinical staging of the breast cancer takes place prior to surgery and is based on the size of the tumour, any palpable lymph nodes and any evidence of metastatic disease. A preliminary TNM (tumour, node, metastases) classification would have been assigned to the woman's disease. The pathological staging follows surgery and uses the histological details from the excised tissue (see Box 12.4).

Breast cancer cells are graded from I to III, where I is a well-differentiated cell which looks very similar to the tissue from which it originated, and III is undifferentiated, retaining few of the characteristics of the cell of origin. The higher the grade, the more likely the cells are to have spread through the body, either through the lymphatic system or via the bloodstream (Fowble *et al.*, 1991). Systemic adjuvant (additional) treatment will be based on the Nottingham Prognostic Index, which further clarifies the TNM classification system and includes the size of the tumour, the histological grade, menopausal status, age and the axillary nodal status (i.e. the number of nodes positive to cancer cells) of the patient (Sainsbury *et al.*, 2000). This adjuvant treatment must be explained and discussed carefully with the woman in order to lead her gently on to the next phase of her treatment.

The woman is likely to receive her definitive diagnosis and plans for future treatment after her surgery at her first follow-up visit. The wait can be a trying and nerve-wracking time both for her and also for her partner and family. The extent to which the axillary lymph nodes are invaded is a prognostic factor and the details of cell type will also show if the cancer is aggressive. The woman will have her cancer 'staged' according to the size of the breast cancer, the involvement of the axillary nodes and the presence of distant metastases.

During her first follow-up clinic appointment the movement of the arm will be assessed and arm exercises reinforced. If the woman is not able to move her arm with ease then further physiotherapy should be arranged. Women often develop 'cording', thought to be axillary wound scarring causing tightening of the lymphatic vessels. These cords can sometimes be felt running down the length of the arm. The physiotherapist will concentrate on trying to break these cords with gentle exercise and massage.

Chemotherapy

Breast cancer not only has the ability to spread to the axillary nodes but also to distant sites throughout the body via the lymphatics and the bloodstream. Some women who present with breast

---

Box 12.4 TNM classification (UICC, 1997)

TX   Primary tumour cannot be assessed

T0   No evidence of primary tumour

Tis Carcinoma *in situ*: intraductal carcinoma, or lobular carcinoma *in situ*, or Paget's disease of the nipple with no tumour

Note: Paget's disease associated with a tumour is classified according to the size of the tumour.

T1   Tumour 2 cm or less in greatest dimension
     T1a 0.5 cm or less in greatest dimension
     T1b More than 0.5 cm but not more than 1 cm in greatest dimension
     T1c More than 1 cm but not more than 2 cm in greatest dimension
T2   Tumour more than 2 cm but not more than 5 cm in greatest dimension
T3   Tumour more than 5 cm in greatest dimension
T4   Tumour of any size with direct extension to chest wall or skin

Note: Chest wall includes ribs, intercostal muscles and serratus anterior muscle but not pectoral muscle.

     T4a Extension to chest wall
     T4b Oedema (including peau d'orange), or ulceration of the skin of the breast, or satellite skin nodules
         confined to the same breast
     T4c Both 4a and 4b, above
     T4d Inflammatory carcinoma

Note: Inflammatory carcinoma of the breast is characterized by diffuse, brawny induration of the skin with an erysipeloid edge, usually with no underlying palpable mass. If the skin biopsy is negative and there is no localized, measurable primary cancer, the T category is pTX when pathologically staging a clinical inflammatory carcinoma (T4d).

   When classifying the primary tumour (pT) the tumour size is a measurement of the *invasive* component. If there is a large *in situ* component (e.g. 4 cm) and a small invasive component (e.g. 0.5 cm) the tumour is coded pT1a. Dimpling of the skin, nipple retraction or other skin changes, except those in T4, may occur in T1, T2 or T3 without affecting the classification. Regional lymph nodes are termed as pN and distant metastases as pM.

N – Regional lymph nodes

NX Regional lymph nodes cannot be assessed (e.g. previously removed)
N0 No regional lymph node metastasis
N1 Metastasis to movable ipsilateral axillary node(s)
N2 Metastasis to ipsilateral axillary node(s) fixed to one another or to other structures
N3 Metastasis to ipsilateral internal mammary lymph node(s)

M – Distant metastasis

MX Presence of distant metastasis cannot be assessed
M0 No distant metastasis
M1 Distant metastasis (includes metastasis to supraclavicular lymph nodes)

The category M1 may be further specified according to the following notation:

Pulmonary	PUL	Bone marrow	MAR
Osseous	OSS	Pleura	PLE
Hepatic	HEP	Peritoneum	PER
Brain	BRA	Skin	SKI
Lymph nodes	LYM	Other	OTH

---

cancer will already have microscopic cancer cells in other parts of their body. If left untreated these cells would almost certainly grow into metastases despite the original breast cancer being excised. Adjuvant chemotherapy or hormone therapy will be offered to these women to prevent or delay the development of this metastatic disease. A 'meta-analysis' published in the *Lancet* looked at a large number of adjuvant chemotherapy trials and showed that chemotherapy given to a woman with early breast cancer meant a longer (statistically significant) time to recurrence and a small but significant increase in time of survival. This overview also showed that women whose biopsied lymph nodes were negative, 30% of whom develop metastases, would also benefit from adjuvant, systemic therapy (EBCTCG, 1992, 1998a). This is compelling evidence for offering

SCENARIO

Elizabeth, a 40-year-old, had accepted and understood the reasons for surgery. She needed a wide local excision and follow-up radiotherapy treatment. After the surgery the histology showed a grade III, high-grade tumour, and 4 out of 20 lymph nodes were positive to cancer cells. Elizabeth was pre-menopausal and was advised to have adjuvant chemotherapy (in addition to the surgery). She was initially very upset by the suggestion of an additional 6 months of chemotherapy. She felt she had 'paid the price' of her breast cancer already and now wanted to recover physically and mentally from the surgery and radiotherapy. With careful explanation and supportive counselling Elizabeth gradually accepted the need for systemic treatment as the cancer had already demonstrated the ability to spread (metastasize). Elizabeth was introduced to other women who had undergone similar treatment and found their support invaluable.

G_1 – During this phase, cells carry out their routine functions; the centrioles replicate.

S – This starts with synthesis of DNA and ends when the DNA has been replicated. This is also known as interphase.

G_2 – This is a short phase during which materials needed for cell division are synthesized.

M – The mitotic phase, when the cell physically divides.

The length of the cell cycle varies with different cell types, G_1 phase being the longest and most variable phase. Most chemotherapy agents prevent the cell from dividing in one of these phases and are grouped accordingly (Table 12.1). Adjuvant regimes given for breast cancer are usually a combination of several types of chemotherapy agents that act in different ways to effect greater cell kill (Harris *et al.*, 1993; DeVita *et al.*, 1993). Some common regimes are shown in Table 12.2.

Depending on the treatment centre, other regimens may include Cyclophosphamide, Doxorubicin or Epirubicin, maybe a Taxane (usually as part of a trial) and now Capecitabine. The optimal drug combination, treatment frequency and how long the chemotherapy should be given have not been firmly established yet, but it does seem that a regimen containing an anthracycline drug will become standard (Poole *et al.*, 2003).

Adjuvant chemotherapy is usually given as an intravenous injection in an outpatient oncology clinic every three to four weeks. The implications of receiving chemotherapy should be carefully

some systemic treatment following surgery to most women with breast cancer and there is gathering evidence to support *all* premenopausal women with breast cancer receiving adjuvant chemotherapy (EBCTCG, 1998b; Kroman *et al.*, 2000). A combination of chemotherapy drugs is usually given. Chemotherapy is started a few weeks after surgery and is usually given in divided doses over a 6–8-month period depending on the drug regimen.

In order to understand how chemotherapy works it is necessary to understand how the cell grows and divides. This is defined as follows:

Table 12.1 Groups of chemotherapy agents

Group	Mode of working	Examples
Anthracyclines and antibiotics	Intercalate with DNA and prevent the DNA from untangling prior to replication	Doxorubicin, Epirubicin, Mitozantrone and Bleomycin
Antifolates and antimetabolites	Prevent the constituents of DNA being synthesized	Methotrexate, 5-flurouracil
Alkylating agents and vinca alkaloids	Prevent the cell from being replicated	Cyclophosphamide, Vincristine
Antimitotic agents	Prevent the cell from physically dividing, i.e. mitosis	Vincristine, Actinomycin D
Miscellaneous	Prevent the cell from growing and dividing	Taxanes

Table 12.2 Two common chemotherapy regimens for breast cancer

Drug	Dose	Route	Days	Frequency
Epirubicin	90 mg/m²	IV bolus	1	21 days × 4
Cyclosphosphamide	600 mg/m²	IV bolus	1	21 days × 4
Docetaxel	100 mg/m²	IV infusion	1	21 days × 4
Epirubicin	100 mg/m²	IV bolus	1	3 weekly Cycles 1–4
Cyclosphosphamide	600 mg/m²	IV bolus	1 + 8	4 weekly from day 1 Cycles 5–8
Methotrexate	40 mg/m²	IV bolus	1 + 8	4 weekly from day 1 Cycles 5–8
5-flurouracil	600 mg/m²	IV bolus	1 + 8	4 weekly from day 1 Cycles 5–8

explained to the woman. The necessity for chemotherapy and its effect on a woman's life can cause a range of feelings. Fear and anxiety about whether the cancer has spread further than the breast are common emotions. Every woman must evaluate the known side effects of the chemotherapy and discuss this with the medical and nursing team before making a decision about her treatment. Because research in this area is ongoing the woman may be asked to enter a trial which could include randomization to different treatment regimens. Again details of the trial and its consequences should be made clear to the woman before she gives consent. Several visits to the medical oncologist and input from nurse specialists and research nurses may be necessary before the woman feels confident to make a decision. Information leaflets can be useful to facilitate this decision-making process and these are often available from the oncology unit. The woman's lifestyle may have to change dramatically to fit in with the administration of the treatment and its side effects, especially if she has children or other dependents.

High-dose chemotherapy

For women who are found to have a high number of axillary lymph nodes involved with cancer cells or who have developed widespread metastatic disease, high-dose chemotherapy has been proposed as an alternative treatment. The treatment usually involves a pre-treatment of

outpatient chemotherapy, before the peripheral blood stem cells are collected from the patient's own blood. The woman is then treated with the high-dose chemotherapy. The dose is large enough to ablate the patient's bone marrow and necessitates in-patient hospital care before the blood stem cells are replaced and the white cell count reaches safe levels. This hospital admission enables the oncology team to treat any infections that may develop while the white cell count is low and to administer supportive platelet and blood transfusions. Results for this treatment are not encouraging and further randomized studies will be necessary to demonstrate whether this treatment provides a real survival advantage (Rodenhuis *et al.*, 1998; Berger, 1999). This method of giving chemotherapy is not routinely used in the UK at present.

Primary medical therapy

Some women will present with large breast tumours which are inoperable because of the extent of disease, or because the size and location of the breast lump make a mastectomy inevitable. By giving these women chemotherapy or endocrine treatment first it may be possible to shrink the tumour to make surgical intervention less invasive and to treat the rest of the body for the likely spread of metastases (Mansi *et al.*, 1989; Smith and DeBoer, 2000).

Primary medical therapy is an area of current research and so women may undergo this treatment even if their tumour is considered operable. Several chemotherapy regimens have been used, often using an anthracycline-based drug. Usually six cycles are given before further surgery or radiotherapy is given. If the tumour does not shrink at all in response to two cycles of treatment the woman will probably be considered for surgery.

 SCENARIO

Patricia presented with a large inoperable tumour in her right breast. She had a mammogram whilst she was working abroad the previous year and the result was clear, so the positive diagnosis from a biopsy performed on the lump in her right breast was a great shock. The medical team caring for Patricia suggested that she undergo primary medical therapy to shrink the tumour and then receive a course of radiotherapy if the tumour had regressed sufficiently. Patricia needed a lot of time with the medical and nursing teams before she felt able to accept the need for treatment. She was quite surprised that the treatment was not conventional surgery although the need for medical treatment was explained. Formalized counselling was commenced with the nurse counsellor and Patricia asked if her partner could be present at these sessions. After some considerable thought and consideration Patricia decided that she felt able to agree to the chemotherapy and felt she understood the implications of her treatment. She was introduced to another woman undergoing the same treatment and they were able to offer each other mutual support. Because the tumour shrank successfully Patricia underwent a course of radiotherapy to the breast and was commenced on the anti-hormone drug tamoxifen.

Administration of chemotherapy

The delivery of vesicant (vein-damaging) chemotherapy over a six- to eight-month period can cause considerable damage to the veins. For this reason many women are offered a permanent venous access line to make the administration of chemotherapy easier. Two types of central venous lines are commonly used for the delivery of chemotherapy:

◆ The skin-tunnelled lines of the 'Hickman' type are catheters which are inserted through

the skin along the chest wall into a large vein leading to the heart (see Figure 12.8)

◆ The peripherally inserted central catheter or PICC line which has become very popular for the administration of adjuvant chemotherapy. Insertion involves a minor surgical procedure and venous access is obtained through a vein in the antecubital fossa. PICC lines can be inserted by specially trained nurses (Oakley, 1997) and allow easy venous access for blood sampling but also ensure that prolonged (usually 6–8 months) administration of chemotherapy does not damage peripheral veins.

The woman will have been taught how to care for her central or PICC line by the hospital. General practice and community staff back-up is essential to continue this support and there needs to be excellent communication between these teams and the woman for the continued care of her central line. Infection of the exit site is fairly common and the woman should have written instructions about what to do and contact numbers of the hospital team should this occur.

Some women find it disturbing to have a central line protruding from the skin of their chest. In addition, primary chemotherapy and adjuvant chemotherapy usually includes an anthracycline, taxane or platinum-based drug which will mean some side effects and hair loss. However, if appropriate support and careful explanation are given, and the treatment works at shrinking the tumour, most women cope very well.

Nursing care during chemotherapy

In some areas across the UK women are benefiting from their chemotherapy being delivered at home by specially trained domiciliary chemotherapy nurses. This avoids the inevitable delays whilst waiting to be treated and the repeated journeys to the oncology centre.

Side effects

Side effects from the chemotherapy are related to the types of drugs given and are usually limited to

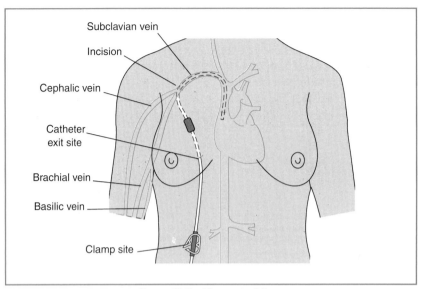

Figure 12.8 The central line.

the parts of the body that have actively dividing cells (Goodman, 1989).

Lowered blood count. The bone marrow is constantly developing cells that make up blood, i.e. white cells (neutrophils), red cells and platelets. The numbers of these circulating cells are reduced by chemotherapy. Depending on the chemotherapy given, the number of blood cells will reach a trough or nadir usually 8–12 days after the treatment has been administered. The numbers of white cells and platelets will start to recover after this point and should be at an acceptable level before the next treatment is given. The woman should be advised to contact her GP or the oncology clinic if she experiences bleeding gums or a tendency to bruise, the symptoms of a low platelet count. Infection, feverish chills and a high temperature could indicate a lowered white cell count and the woman must be aware of the significance of such symptoms. If the chemotherapy is particularly strong, blood levels will be taken at the predicted nadir and prophylactic antibiotics given if the white cell count is particularly low, i.e. below 2.0×10^9 per litre. For women receiving adjuvant

chemotherapy a lowered white cell count is short and recovery is predictable (Judson, 1993).

Hair loss or alopecia. Most breast chemotherapy regimens tend to include a Taxane or an anthracycline causing complete hair loss and this can be devastating for the woman who has already lost part of or all of her breast. She is probably struggling to maintain her self-esteem and body image anyway so hair loss can take on an even greater significance. Support and practical advice can be invaluable to the woman at this time. Information on hair care, use of scarves and hats and how to obtain an NHS wig, if required, can ease the woman's distress and should be arranged before chemotherapy is started. Hair usually starts to regrow 4–6 weeks after chemotherapy has finished and can be softer and curlier than before.

Scalp cooling, by applying ice packs, cold caps or other methods to supercool the scalp, can help to reduce loss. By reducing the temperature of the scalp the blood supply to the hair follicles is depleted, thus depriving the hair follicle of the chemotherapy. The scalp cooling is usually left on the head for 20 minutes after the chemotherapy has been given, by which time the level of the circulating chemotherapy has dropped sufficiently not to have an effect on the hair. Scalp cooling does not always work but should be tried for any woman receiving an anthracycline as a bolus dose (Tierney, 1987; Judson, 1993).

Sore eyes. Antifolate and anthracycline chemotherapy often affect the conjunctiva of the eyes, causing stickiness and sometimes a dry soreness. Folinic acid given as an oral tablet can reduce the effects of an antifolate and the use of artificial tears can provide some comfort (Goodman, 1989).

Sore mouth. The mucous membrane of the mouth normally replaces itself quickly and is readily affected by chemotherapy. The woman should be advised to use a softer toothbrush to prevent unnecessary scratching. Mouth hygiene should be encouraged and fluid input should be at least 2–2.5 litres per day. Any dental work should be completed before treatment starts or just before the next course of treatment when the blood count has recovered. Any fungal infections should be treated with fluconazole, nystatin or amphotericin. The woman may develop herpes simplex which must be treated promptly with Zovirax. Methotrexate often causes mucositis. This can be largely prevented by the administration of folinic acid 15 mg tablets for six doses at 24 hours post-chemotherapy.

Any crusting on the lips should be gently removed with warm water, and petroleum jelly applied. If stomatitis is detected in the mouth it is advisable to clean gently with swab sticks soaked in warm water, or a thin layer of chlorhexidine gel or chlorhexidine mouth wash (0.2%) (Jones, 1998). Mouth ulcers can be treated with sucralfate mouthwash. Saliva substitutes are available for the relief of a dry mouth (Oakley and Burnet, 2001).

Mouth washes containing a local anaesthetic such as Difflam® may be soothing if mouth ulcers develop. A chlorhexidine-based mouth wash may be appropriate if there is evidence of oral infection. The woman's diet should be well balanced, containing high proportions of vitamins and proteins to promote healing.

Nausea and vomiting. Because the body recognizes the chemotherapy as a toxic substance and because of increased gastric acidity, nausea and vomiting may occur. The woman is usually given anti-emetic to take whilst at home but these may not be sufficient or appropriate. She should be encouraged to report her experiences of nausea prior to her next treatment so adjustments can be made to her anti-emetic control. Anti-emetics that are 5-HT$_3$ antagonists can significantly reduce nausea and should be prescribed as appropriate. Because the side effects of chemotherapy can be so traumatic, some women begin to associate attending the department with feeling sick. This anticipatory nausea can be treated prophylactically with conventional anti-emetics and sometimes anxiolytics may be useful. Women will receive their chemotherapy as an outpatient and will then be encouraged to continue their normal routine. It is essential that care and support for symptoms should be shared and continued by their primary care team.

Nausea can be eased by taking a prescribed antacid, drinking flat or fizzy drinks such as soda water, coke or lemonade, drinking ginger tea, or eating dry biscuits. It also helps to take small, frequent meals and to eat bland food. Prolonged nausea can severely affect quality of life and considerable efforts should be made to reduce this unfortunate side effect.

Diarrhoea. This can be caused by chemotherapy damaging the gastrointestinal mucosa. Anti-diarrhoeal agents may be effective. If the problem becomes prolonged, management may require the use of parenteral nutrition in addition to fluid replacement. This would be unlikely with most chemotherapy regimens for breast cancer and would, of course, mean hospital admission.

Fatigue. The insidious tiredness, which is not eased by sleep, affects most women who receive chemotherapy and increases towards the end of the usual 6 months of treatment. Some women manage to continue with their working lives, perhaps with more flexible working hours, whilst others require considerable rest and could not possibly work. No predictions should be made about how a woman might feel. She should be supported through this time and be reassured that her 'lethargy' is a normal response to the treatment although excessive tiredness could be an indication that the woman is not coping with her treatment or diagnosis and this needs to be addressed. She should be allowed to rest when tired, and family and friends should be involved to help them understand this side effect of chemotherapy.

Fertility. Many women who are premenopausal and receive chemotherapy will experience an early menopause, therefore becoming infertile (McCoy, 2003). Such women should be counselled of the risks of infertility and given appropriate support and advice if this is an issue for them. In one case there has been successful preservation of ovarian tissue. Substantial research is ongoing in this area to make this a more widely offered treatment.

Immunotherapy

Immunotherapy offers another choice of treatment for women with breast cancer, particularly for those women with metastatic disease. The most widely used drug, Herceptin, a monoclonal antibody, has been developed to specifically bind to the HER-2 (human epidermal growth factor receptor 2) which is over-expressed in some breast cancer cells. Women who are diagnosed with breast cancer are now having their tumours tested for the HER-2 routinely as part of their histopathological assessment. HER-2 plays a significant role in cell growth and division and Herceptin works by binding to HER-2 cell surface receptors, blocking their action as cell growth promoters. For patients who may benefit, Herceptin is given as a weekly short intravenous infusion. As the drug affects the immune system the side effects can be chills, transient fever and pain (Hadden, 1999). There is also some evidence that Herceptin may cause cardiac dysfunction but this was thought to be related to its administration with an anthracycline chemotherapy drug and they are no longer given together. If given with chemotherapy Herceptin is given with a Taxane, usually as part of a clinical trial. Theratope and other experimental vaccines are also being developed to help the immune system recognize breast cancer cells. By provoking the immune system to recognize the abnormal cancer cells the body produces antibodies to fight the breast cancer (Hadden, 1999).

Hormone therapy

The effectiveness of endocrine manipulation on breast cancers has long been known. Many newly diagnosed breast cancers and about one-third of metastatic breast cancers are responsive to hormone manipulation. The primary hormones involved are oestrogen and progesterone. Hormones are steroids which can be involved in stimulating tumour cell proliferation. They can affect tumour cells by interacting with the relevant hormone receptor within the cell's stroma and nucleus. The number of hormone receptors can be measured by histopathologists once some breast cancer tissue has been removed from the tumour *in vitro* and a percentage value assigned. The presence of oestrogen and progesterone receptors, ER and PR respectively, usually correlates with the clinical behaviour of the disease. The more oestrogen receptors the more likely the woman's breast disease will respond to hormone therapy. There are several types of hormone therapy; presently, the most widely used is the drug tamoxifen.

Tamoxifen

Tamoxifen is a steroid antagonist which acts by inhibiting the action of hormones on their target tissues. Tamoxifen has evolved from being a treatment for advanced metastatic disease, to being an effective adjuvant and primary therapy, and has been scrutinized as a chemo-preventative agent for asymptomatic women with a high risk of breast cancer with differing conclusions being drawn (Fenlon, 2003). In America tamoxifen is being used as a preventative drug for women with a higher risk of developing breast cancer but in Europe the research is still continuing. The tamoxifen tablet is taken daily at a dose of 20 mg and it is recommended that the drug is taken at a similar time each day. Side effects include transient nausea, increased vaginal secretions, and hot flushes associated with an induced menopause (Fenlon, 2003). Unusual vaginal bleeding should be reported to the GP and investigated if it persists. There is no consensus for how long the drug should be taken but it is usual that tamoxifen is prescribed for at least five years (Harris *et al.*, 1993).

Tumour regression can occur when a hormone drug is stopped, although 6 weeks should elapse before another hormone therapy is tried.

Aromatase inhibitors

Post-menopausal women still have a small level of circulating oestrogen despite their ovaries not working. Their oestrogen is synthesized from androstenedione (released by the adrenal glands) by the action of the enzyme aromatase and is released into the bloodstream (Fenlon, 2003). In the past, an adrenalectomy was the treatment for a woman with post-menopausal breast cancer and aminoglutethamide, an aromatase inhibitor, was a drug designed to supersede the adrenalectomy.

Aminoglutethimide. This drug works by blocking the conversion of androgens (produced by the adrenal glands) to oestrogens in the peripheral tissues. The tablets used to be given with hydrocortisone because one of the side effects is that it inhibits normal glucocorticoid production (the body's normal steroid hormones), although this does not occur at the lower daily dose of 250 mg. Other side effects include transient lethargy, nausea and muscle cramps. Some patients develop a widespread macular rash which generally disappears spontaneously and rarely requires cessation of treatment.

Because of these significant side effects and the need for more effective treatments for breast cancer, a new generation of aromatase inhibitors has been developed. These are anastrazole (Arimidex®) letrozole (Femara®), formestane (Lentaron®) and exemestane (Aromasin®). The side effects of these drugs are tolerated well by women. Long-term use of these aromatatse inhibitors may be associated with loss in bone density and a possible increase in the incidence of osteoporosis so research is ongoing to define how long they can be taken for, but initial results as to their effectiveness are looking very promising (Harvey, 1998; Baum, 2001).

Progestogens

Medroxyprogesterone acetate (MPA) is similar to the hormone progesterone, and is designed to inhibit the circulating levels of oestrogen and block progesterone receptors. The drug is taken daily in tablet form. The particular side effects of this drug can include acne, fluid retention, an irregular menstrual cycle and changes in libido. It is often given to post-menopausal women as a second-line treatment for metastatic disease.

Ovarian ablation

In pre-menopausal women the ovaries are the main source of circulating oestrogen. Three methods are used to reduce the amounts of this circulating hormone. The ovaries

◆ Can be removed surgically
◆ Can have their function permanently ablated by radiotherapy
◆ Can be suppressed by chemical means.

A chemical way of suppressing the ovaries is the administration of an LHRH agonist. There are several LHRH analogues in use at the moment and these include goserelin (e.g. Zoladex®), leuprorelin (e.g. Prostap®) and buserelin (e.g. Suprefact®). Both goserelin and leuprorelin are administered as a depot injection into the abdominal wall on a monthly basis. Sometimes local anaesthetic is used to make the procedure more comfortable. The drug is then slowly released over the next month. The advantage of a chemical castration is that once the drug is stopped the effect will be reversed, which is especially pertinent to women who wish to try for a family later if their treatment is successful. These LHRH antagonists can be used as adjuvant therapy and also for the treatment of advanced disease.

Nursing care

All hormone treatments work by blocking or manipulating the normal hormone levels and so can cause many symptoms associated with the menopause. These can include hot flushes, vaginal dryness, tiredness, weight gain and night sweats. Clonidine has been given with limited effect to reduce some of these symptoms.

Vitamin and mineral supplements such as vitamin E and oil of evening primrose, zinc and magnesium have been reported as helping with menopausal symptoms but there is no definitive research to support these claims. Women wishing to try these supplements would be advised to check with their clinician.

There has been a great deal of interest in the use of plant-derived phytoestrogens for the relief of menopausal symptoms (Nestel *et al.*, 1999). Phytoestrogens can be found in soya, red clover and most legumes. Research is being conducted that is studying the effect of these compounds on women who have had breast cancer but no conclusive evidence has been found so far that supports a woman taking them over any period of time.

Menopausal symptoms need to be given as much credence as those caused by other treatments for breast cancer. The woman should be told what to expect and be allowed to discuss her feelings about such symptoms. The prospect of an early menopause can be yet another assault on a woman's body image and sexuality. Infertility can be a distressing side effect for the woman who was planning a late pregnancy or for someone who has had problems conceiving. However, some younger women continue to menstruate whilst taking tamoxifen (Nolvadex), albeit irregularly, and contraceptive advice should be given.

Radiotherapy

Radiotherapy is the delivery of high-energy ionizing radiation which destroys the cancer cells' ability to grow and multiply. Most radiotherapy departments use a linear accelerator or cobalt machine to deliver this high energy.

Radiotherapy can be used in three main situations for the treatment of breast cancer:

◆ As an addition to surgery
◆ As a primary treatment for a large invasive tumour

◆ For recurrent disease at the original site or for systemic metastatic disease, particularly bone or brain metastases.

As an addition to surgery

Usually radiotherapy treatment fractions (as an adjunct to surgery) are given as 2.0 grays per day in 25 fractions, over 5 weeks, or as 2.67 grays per day in 15 fractions over 3 weeks. Because of the disparity between the treatment regimes in different radiotherapy centres a national trial has been implemented to discover which treatment regime is the optimal. Called START, the trial randomized women requiring radiotherapy between regimes of differing dose and fractions (Standardization of Breast Radiotherapy Protocol, 1998). The START trial has finished but the results are still being analysed. Radiotherapy has been proven to help prevent local recurrence of disease (Fisher *et al.*, 1995) and to increase survival (Overgaard *et al.*, 1997) in women with breast cancer.

Radiotherapy treatment should aim to start about four weeks after the surgery or chemotherapy but this is not the case in many UK treatment centres due to increasing workloads and lack of machinery. Once started, the treatment is given every weekday with weekends off. It takes 10–15 minutes to set up the treatment machine for the individual patient, and then only 2–3 minutes for each 'fraction' to be given. The radiotherapist takes care to avoid delicate structures such as the lungs and heart by planning the treatment field very clearly. In order to align the radiotherapy machine, markings are drawn on the skin and a small tattoo is usually made with Indian ink to ensure that the treatment is accurately reproduced every day. The woman should be warned about the permanency of these marks during the course of radiotherapy and the small tattoo will always remain. Following a wide local excision, typical radiotherapy involves treatment to the whole breast followed by a 'boost' to the bed of the tumour. Women who undergo a mastectomy would not necessarily have radiotherapy, unless their tumour was poorly differentiated, was classified as a T3 (or greater) tumour, was close the chest wall or had involved axillary lymph nodes.

Brachytherapy. Some radiotherapy centres use radioactive implants to give follow-up radiotherapy treatment. Under anaesthetic, between 4 and 25 wide-gauge hollow needles are passed through the breast tissue to where the tumour was excised. Iridium-192 wire, a radioactive source, is then inserted or 'afterloaded' into the tubes and secured firmly at each end. The wires stay in long enough to deliver the required dose of radiation, usually 2–5 days. The woman is nursed in a single lead-lined room to protect other patients, and also the nursing and medical staff from excessive radiation exposure.

Nursing care

Some women have a marked radiation reaction on the treated area, with skin eythema, soreness, swelling of the breast and, rarely, moist desquamation or breakdown of the skin. Topical applications are to be avoided unless necessary and then only aqueous cream and hydrocortisone 1% ointment is the treatment of choice. Moist desquamation may mean that radiotherapy is stopped until the skin recovers. Even without a marked skin reaction, general advice about skin care will be given by the local treatment centre. There may be several reasons for variation in skin reactions to radiotherapy, including differences in intrinsic sensitivity (Turesson and Thames, 1989; Burnet *et al.*, 1992). General advice on skin care should be given according to the College of Radiographers guidelines (Glean *et al.*, 2001) (Box 12.5).

Some physical support needs to be given to the treated breast but a conventional bra may not be suitable. Cotton vests, 'crop tops' and sports bras can all give gentle support to the treated breast and will be better than an ill-fitting nylon bra (Oliver, 1988). It must be stressed that only the area being treated will be affected by the radiotherapy.

Some women find radiotherapy a depressing experience. Some of this is due to tiredness which can continue for up to 7 weeks after the radiotherapy finishes (Graydon, 1994; Faithfull, 1998).

> **Box 12.5** Advice to give on skin care following radiotherapy
>
> ◆ Wear cotton or natural material next to the skin
> ◆ Do not use perfumed soaps or deodorants on the areas being treated
> ◆ Wash the area with water only and pat dry with a soft towel
> ◆ Use aqueous cream or hydrocortisone cream 1%
> ◆ If talc has to be used, baby powder is the best option.

Women can find the daily travelling to the radiotherapy centre quite a strain. Support at home with provision of home help and childcare as appropriate can be vital to ensure that the woman receives her full treatment. Involvement of the GP, practice and community nurses will also facilitate this treatment.

Side effects from breast radiotherapy are purely local and it must be stressed that nausea and hair loss do not usually occur. The skin may darken further, changing a breast that has already had shape-altering surgery. Long-term effects may include the fibrosis of small blood vessels, causing further discoloration. The rarer complication of rib weakness, pneumonitis and cardiotoxicity are now largely avoided because of better planning techniques.

Primary radiotherapy for a large invasive tumour

Women with large lesions that are inoperable by virtue of tumour extent or because of the woman's general health can be managed with radiotherapy. Most radiotherapists will treat the whole breast and axilla, and the supraclavicular fossa. Intensive radiotherapy can cause long-term side effects such as fibrosis of the breast and lymphoedema. The prognosis for such women is particularly poor but the short-term benefits of local control are thought to outweigh the morbidity of the long-term effects.

The role of radiotherapy in metastatic disease is discussed later in this chapter.

Psychological care

For the woman with newly diagnosed breast cancer her whole world can appear to be falling apart. She may well feel relatively fit and healthy but will have to face up to treatment for a disease that will at some point alter her body shape, make her feel unwell, and will not carry a certainty of cure.

There can be a great disparity between what we as health professionals think the woman wishes to know or is experiencing and what she actually feels about her diagnosis. Becoming a recipient of care takes control away from the woman and this lack of control is one factor that can lead to psychological morbidity (Morris, 1983; Macarthy and Loren, 1997). Other factors that can predispose to psychological morbidity include:

◆ Lack of social support

◆ Not having a regular partner

◆ Additional concurrent stress

◆ An adverse experience of cancer in the family

◆ Previous psychiatric history

◆ Marital problems

◆ A change in body shape, especially if the woman's breasts were an important part of her self-image

◆ The physical effects of having treatment

◆ Doubts about her future.

(Watson, 1991)

Much can be done to recognize, ameliorate or prevent this psychological morbidity, starting from the time the woman is diagnosed with cancer. Morris *et al.* (1977) observed that newly diagnosed women with breast cancer display five different ways of coping with their diagnosis:

1. *Denial* The woman actively rejects her diagnosis. She 'blocks' any information given about her disease and cannot actively be involved with decisions about her treatment

2. *Fighting spirit* The woman has the ability to display a hopeful, questioning attitude to her disease. She appears to want to make the best of what has happened

3. *Stoical acceptance* Such women acknowledge their diagnosis but do not enquire any further about details. These women seem to carry on with their life without much concern for their illness

4. *Anxious/depressed acceptance* Such women react to knowledge of their diagnosis with excessive anxiety or depression. They ask for large amounts of information but this information does not reassure them

5. *Helpless/hopelessness* These women are completely overcome by their diagnosis. Their lives are disrupted by their anxieties so they can no longer function effectively.

It is not unusual for women who have been given their diagnosis to display one or several of these behaviours. As nurses caring for such women it is important to recognize these coping strategies and to suggest therapeutic intervention or referral for counselling when appropriate.

The breast care nurse, nurse counsellor, psychologist and specialist counsellor can all contribute to a woman's psychological care and their help should be offered as appropriate; but why is psychological care so important for the woman with breast cancer? In the late 1970s Maguire, a clinical psychologist, studied the psychological morbidity of women who were diagnosed and treated for breast cancer. One study concluded that as much as one-third of the women who had been diagnosed with breast cancer developed severe anxiety or a depressive illness within 12 months (Maguire, 2000).

Physically, psychologically, socially and financially it makes sense to reduce or prevent the woman's psychological morbidity. This allows the woman to re-establish herself as a functioning member of society by returning to work and/or caring for her family more quickly, as well as freeing up other care agencies (Maguire *et al.*, 1982). A further controlled study carried out by Maguire and colleagues showed that when women had the services of a specialist breast care nurse their physical and social recovery following mastectomy improved (Maguire *et al.*, 1983).

Work by Fallowfield questioned the concept that it was just the disfiguring surgery that caused psychological problems, and suggested that having breast cancer, with all its implications, was also a contributing factor. She concluded that specialist support should be available to all women who undergo treatment for breast cancer and not just those who undergo mastectomy (Fallowfield *et al.*, 1990). It is now accepted that the breast care nurse is an essential and integral part of the breast care team (NICE, 2002). Watson and her colleagues suggested from their studies in the 1980s that a nurse specialist might offer more effective support if counselling were to begin as soon as the woman was diagnosed (Watson *et al.*, 1988). Their suggested framework for counselling concentrated on three different areas:

◆ Emotional support and facilitation of adjustment

◆ Information about the woman's physical state

◆ Practical advice on prostheses.

Emotional support and facilitation of adjustment

To strengthen a woman's coping mechanisms she should be encouraged to ask for support. The spouse, family and friends can give practical help and emotional support although this would involve permission from the woman herself, since not all women want their family and friends involved. Using helpline numbers, support groups, the GP, practice nurses, community nurses, Macmillan and Marie Curie nurses (if appropriate) and the breast care nurse can reinforce the woman's support network. This support should help the woman regain some control over her life.

Information about her physical state

Most women need to understand something about their treatment. Gauging how much they want to know is difficult and requires skill. Because there is so much to know about breast cancer, and some of it is quite complex, time and

sensitivity must be employed when explaining details. When first diagnosed, the woman will not be able to take in most of what she is hearing. The shock of being told she has breast cancer will be all that most women can immediately absorb. The role of the nursing team, including the breast care nurse, in reiterating what she has already been told is crucial in helping her to come to terms with her diagnosis.

Treatment may not only be new to the woman but she may also be asked if she wishes to take part in a medical trial. Perhaps surprisingly, this does not appear to cause excessive stress. Providing adequate information is given, women who allow themselves to be randomized do not suffer from any greater psychological, sexual or social problems than those treated outside a clinical trial (Fallowfield *et al.*, 1990). Later research by Fallowfield showed that the woman's need for choice is less important than her need for clear and accurate information (Fallowfield *et al.*, 1994).

Practical advice on prostheses

Recognition and acknowledgement of a woman's potential for experiencing psychological problems associated with her body-altering surgery and the subsequent restoration of a woman's external body image is linked with her ability to cope and adjust to her breast cancer (Denton and Baum, 1983; Salter, 1997). Helping to restore the woman's shape by giving advice on the right bras to wear, the fitting of the initial cumfie (soft breast form) and the fitting of the more permanent prosthesis can help the woman's return to normality. Advice on other clothing and swimwear can also facilitate recovery and the Breast Cancer Care association can be very helpful.

Many help agencies (see Resources) can be contacted by health professionals, or the woman and her family themselves, and can offer a wealth of advice and information to help psychological adjustment.

Female sexuality

A very important aspect of psychological care to consider when caring for the woman with breast cancer is her sexuality. Body image and sexual function are represented as a central, intellectual component of the way the woman feels about herself. Derogatis (1986) wrote that a positive body image is essential to effective sexual functioning. The self-esteem and therefore sexuality of the woman can be severely threatened by the loss or disfigurement of the breast and changes in her body as a whole. If the woman already feels insecure about herself and her body image prior to treatment for breast cancer, the problem can be amplified into a serious psychological disorder (Derogatis, 1986).

Although sex is an important aspect of life for most women, for some their sexuality is a central part of their life, and for these women the effects of treatment for breast cancer can be devastating. Baldwin (1990) writes that society's view of the perfect woman is constantly presented through the media as usually tall, thin and with two perfectly formed breasts. The breast is a symbol of many things about a woman:

◆ A symbol of womanhood
◆ A symbol of motherhood
◆ A symbol of sexuality.

For a woman who has undergone treatment for breast cancer that is disfiguring, the difference between the reality and the 'ideal' can be a cause of great stress (Baldwin, 1990). Sexuality is much more than the sexual act; it is about the quality of the human being. Individuals with a positive self-concept respect themselves and consider themselves worthwhile in a sexual sense, whilst those with a negative self-concept are often not satisfied with themselves sexually. A woman being treated for breast cancer may feel she is no longer sexually attractive even when her partner is trying to tell her otherwise. She may fear rejection by her partner and may withdraw from a physical and close relationship. Her partner, in turn, may view this as a sign that she no longer wishes a physical relationship, and so misunderstanding can be perpetuated.

Many research papers look at the sexual effects of losing a breast and there is sometimes a misconception that if a woman has breast conservation her psychological trauma will be less. However, work by Rutherford, who studied women undergoing a lumpectomy, highlighted the physical changes that occur. These include deformity, which may be substantial, thickening of skin and subcutaneous tissue, enlarged and pronounced pores, changes in breast contour, erythema and pain over the scar (Rutherford, 1988). Apart from the visual changes, the sensitivity of the breast can diminish because of radiotherapy or surgery.

Chemotherapy can cause fatigue, malaise, depression, alopecia and amenorrhoea, which are yet another assault on the woman's sexuality. A husband or partner can experience as much distress as the woman herself over the course of her treatment. Their feelings need to be taken into account and provision should be made for them to express their concerns.

Sexuality as an issue is rarely explored by nurses. Better education and more openness might encourage discussion and allow the woman to work through this very important issue. Women who tend to cope better with changes in their sexuality are those who have been able to resolve past life crises. Good sexual functioning prior to the illness tends to predict a return to a satisfactory sexual adjustment (Derogatis, 1986). The nature and quality of the woman's relationship with her primary partner and the size and nature of her support network are also important when reaffirming personal value and contributing to psychological adjustment. A woman's sexuality and her body image are about herself and the way she relates to the outside world. Such an important area of care should not be ignored by health care professionals when looking after the woman with breast cancer.

For more detail on this subject the reader is referred to the reading list at the end of this chapter.

Metastatic disease

Breast cancer can spread to the bones, lungs, liver, brain, and almost any other soft tissue. Recurrence is sometimes detected by the woman herself, with the development of pain, another lump, breathlessness or feeling unwell. It may also be detected at routine follow-up visits. Investigations for metastatic disease include routine blood tests, X-rays, liver and bone scans, and perhaps the use of computerized tomography (CT) or nuclear magnetic resonance imaging (MRI) to determine the nature and extent of the metastatic disease.

The aims of management of metastatic disease are first to palliate symptoms and second to reduce the tempo of the disease. There is no longer an expectation of cure. The timing of recurrence in relation to first presentation and the site of relapse may predict the survival of the woman. Those women who have hormone-sensitive tumours and who have had a long interval between diagnosis and relapse are likely to do better than women who develop secondaries, especially in visceral sites, shortly after initial treatment (Leonard *et al.*, 2000). Some women, particularly post-menopausal patients with bone disease, may survive for many years with metastatic disease. The treatments for metastatic breast cancer are the same modalities as for primary disease.

Radiotherapy

Radiotherapy has a very large part to play in the palliation of metastatic disease. Painful bone disease is the most common manifestation of metastatic disease, and this can be treated very effectively with radiotherapy. Radiotherapy may also give considerable relief from disease in other organs, e.g. the brain, with a minimum of side effects. Treatment may require several fractions of radiotherapy, but bony metastases in particular often respond well to a single treatment.

Hormone treatment

As described previously, there is a variety of hormone drugs available. Overall, the likely response rate for the first hormone treatment is about 30%. If the woman has disease that has responded to first-line hormone treatment, then it is more likely that a second line of hormone treatment will be effective. With each successive hormone treatment the probability of response diminishes.

Chemotherapy

Chemotherapy given for advanced disease has a disease response rate of between 40% and 60%, with a median disease relapse rate of 6–10 months (Leonard *et al.*, 2000). When treating the woman with chemotherapy the intent should be symptom control without paying the price of excessive toxicity. The drug regimens used in metastatic disease are similar to combinations used for adjuvant therapy. Multi-agent combinations including anthracyclines have the highest response rates, but also the highest toxicity. The choice of regime will depend on many factors.

Currently there is considerable work looking at the effectiveness of new drugs, and new combinations of existing drugs. High-dose chemotherapy has been used, mostly in the USA, but more studies are required to compare this treatment with conventional drug regimes. Careful symptom control is of paramount importance when women with metastatic disease are receiving such therapy.

Pain

Pain can be controlled with effective analgesia as well as by treatment of the underlying disease with either chemotherapy or radiotherapy. Pain itself can be a complex problem with many components making up the subjective experience. In a woman who has chronic pain, fear, despair, anger and anxiety can all influence what she is experiencing. When caring for such a woman an accurate measurement of the site and severity of the pain is important to understand her experience and to measure the effectiveness of any interventions. The objective of pain control should be that the woman is pain-free at night, at rest and on movement.

Pharmaceutical intervention will start with mild analgesia, e.g. paracetamol or soluble aspirin or other non-steroidal anti-inflammatory drugs (NSAIDs). Aspirin and the NSAIDs should be used with caution if the woman has any history of gastric problems as they can cause gastric irritation. If the pain does not respond to this, weak opioid analgesia will be tried, e.g. dihydrocodiene or coproxamol (Distalgesic), a dextropropoxyphene/paracetamol combination and Tramadol. If a stronger analgesia is needed then the opioid morphine is the drug of choice. Dose requirements may start at 5–10 mg 4-hourly but can be increased to 2–3 g 4-hourly, although there is no upper limit if the patient is still experiencing pain. Measurement of the woman's pain is important so that drug dosage can be titrated against it.

Morphine can be administered as an elixir or tablet every 4 hours or as a slow-release tablet every 12 or 24 hours. Other opioids include Fentanyl, a synthetic opioid used in anaesthesia. Conversion from one opioid to another must be done with great care to avoid under-dosing or over-dosing the patient. Any increase in the opioid dose should not be fully assessed until 24 hours has passed (Hanks and Mansi, 1988). Constipation is very likely to be a problem if the patient is receiving an opioid drug and regular aperients should be prescribed as well as giving advice about taking plenty of fluid, eating fresh fruit and vegetables and other fibre-containing foods.

Co-analgesics can be used with great effect to control pain and should be used with every category of analgesia. NSAIDs can relieve bony pain or pain related to nerve compression. The use of steroids in advanced disease can also have a beneficial effect by relieving inflammation and by giving the woman a feeling of well-being. Bone pain can be significantly helped with the use of bisphosphonates (pamidronate) which, when administered intravenously, inhibits bone resorption when there is infiltration of the bone by breast cancer. Carbamazepine, gabapentin, sodium valproate and amitriptyline can be useful for nerve pain. The use of anxiolytics such as diazepam can reduce the psychological component of the pain as well as helping with muscle spasm.

Non-drug measures for pain relief can include the use of massage, hot and cold packs, transcutaneous nerve stimulation and relaxation therapy. In an effort to relieve pain these are often more acceptable to the woman than taking more medication. By providing pain relief with non-interventionist measures the woman can feel more in control of her situation. More detail about these methods of pain relief can be found in Regnard and Tempest (1998) and Lomas (2003).

Liver metastases

Liver metastases carry a grave prognosis. Chemotherapy is normally given, though care must be taken with the selection of drugs and dosages if there is significant impairment of liver function.

Lung metastases

Lung metastases typically present with shortness of breath. Management involves excluding other causes of breathlessness, including benign causes such as pulmonary embolus or tuberculosis, and other malignant causes such as pleural effusion. Treatment of pulmonary metastases has to be systemic, either with chemotherapy or hormone manipulation. The prognosis is generally poor.

Pleural effusions

Many women with metastatic disease develop a pleural effusion. This collection of fluid in the pleural cavity is caused by deposits of cancer cells, and has the effect of compressing the lung. The woman usually presents with shortness of breath and possibly pain on inspiration. The usual care is to insert a catheter into the intercostal space, drain the fluid off slowly and then to instil an irritant to adhere the pleural membranes together. Many different agents have been used but intrapleural bleomycin, talc or tetracycline, plus a local anaesthetic, are most popular. Surgical intervention by a partial thoracotomy is sometimes used to drain off fluid and to instil an adhesive substance, and in a fit woman this can be a very effective way of preventing reaccumulation of the fluid (Powles and Smith, 1991; Lomas, 2003).

Pericardial effusion

Rarely, fluid can collect in the pericardium because of tumour infiltration. Diagnosis of this can be confirmed by ultrasound and, if tamponade is present, then drainage must be carried out quickly. If fluid collects again quickly a permanent 'window' can be surgically created in the pericardium for the long-term drainage of the effusion.

Malignant ascites

This is a rare site of secondary disease in women who have breast cancer. Deposits that develop between the peritoneum of the abdomen can cause fluid to accumulate in the peritoneal cavity. The fluid collection can be large in volume and cause discomfort, and breathlessness if pressing on the diaphragm. Drainage or paracentesis is carried out by inserting an indwelling catheter. The peritoneal fluid should drain at a rate of around 1 litre per 4 hours for 24 hours and then be allowed to drain freely. Treatments can be given intraperitoneally but these have not proved to be useful. Systemic therapy as for other sites of metastatic disease is more likely to be the treatment of choice. If the ascites becomes recurrent, a shunt may be inserted which drains fluid from the peritoneal cavity into the right subclavian vein or superior vena cava (Le Veen *et al.*, as cited by Powles and Smith, 1991).

Hypercalcaemia

This is a frequent complication of breast cancer and is caused by increased osteoclastic bone destruction releasing calcium into the bloodstream. Higher than normal calcium levels in the woman's bloodstream may make her feel thirsty, nauseous, disorientated, dehydrated and polyuric, and sometimes may cause an altered conscious state. These symptoms are usually reversible if the condition is diagnosed and treated quickly. Hydrating the woman with intravenous 0.9% saline usually helps, but with the addition of specific agents to help to stabilize the bone, the calcium level can be kept within normal limits for longer. The most likely group of drugs to be used are the bisphosphonates which are very efficient at inhibiting the osteoclastic bone resorption. Pamidronate sodium (APD) at a dose of 30–90 mg is often used for this purpose (Coleman, 1999).

Brain metastases

Presentation may occur in a number of ways. These include symptoms of raised intracranial pressure, namely headache, vomiting, dizziness, visual disturbance and impaired intellectual function; neurological deficits specific to the site of disease, such as weakness or loss of balance; or, less commonly, fits.

The initial treatment would be the administration of steroids and then whole-brain irradiation. For single brain lesions in a woman who has no other evidence of disease, surgical intervention, or higher dose radiotherapy, can be offered. Radiotherapy treatment will be given with steroid cover to reduce excessive brain swelling. The woman may experience the side effects of steroid use, which include weight gain, water retention, proximal myopathy, susceptibility to infection and possible steroid-induced diabetes.

Spinal cord compression

Metastatic deposits of disease within the vertebrae or dura can cause spinal cord compression. A woman developing spinal cord compression can have symptoms of leg or arm weakness, sphincter disturbance, and sensory changes. If any of these symptoms develop the woman should be referred to her oncologist as an emergency. Treatment starts immediately, with dexamethasone 4 mg q.d.s. and emergency radiotherapy. Less commonly, surgical decompression is used. The better the patient's neurological status when treatment begins, the better the long-term outlook. This condition can be extremely frightening for the woman as she is in danger of becoming paralysed.

Carcinomatous meningitis

Metastatic involvement of the meninges can cause headache, confusion, diplopia, cranial nerve palsies and impaired sensation. The clinical diagnosis is usually confirmed with a lumbar puncture, although cancer cells are not necessarily found in the cerebrospinal fluid. The prognosis is poor, but treatment can be whole-brain radiotherapy or chemotherapy, particularly using intrathecal methotrexate.

The future

There has been a lot of political interest and focus on the delivery of cancer care in the UK. Breast cancer has been particularly highlighted probably because of the high number of patients that are treated for this disease. Breast care services have been scrutinized and organized by the Calman-Hine report (Calman and Hine, 1995), peer review, the NHS cancer plan and, recently, the NICE guidance on improving the outcomes in breast cancer (NICE, 2002). As a result of these initiatives the care of a woman with breast cancer is managed by a multidisciplinary team approach using accepted standards and guidelines to deliver the care she requires (Douek and Taylor, 2003). Each of the specialists will be expected to keep up with the latest developments in their field of expertise and there is a move for faster access to care, e.g. two-week referral to a breast unit from the GP and four weeks to first cancer treatment (NICE, 2002). The next few years will be dedicated to further implementing these cancer care initiatives.

In future there will be much more choice of the types of surgery the woman is offered. Many more women will be offered immediate breast reconstruction if they need a mastectomy and there will be more use of the sentinel lymph node procedure preventing unnecessary lymph node surgery. Radiotherapy will be planned and delivered with greater accuracy, possibly using CT scanning for planning the treatment field and shaping the radiation beam using specialized equipment to give a more accurate and equal dose of radiation to the breast. There has been some research into the use of a portable electron beam emitting device (shaped like a lollipop) for delivering radiotherapy intraoperatively to the tumour cavity. Called Targit, this method of radiotherapy delivery is currently being evaluated across the UK and may provide an alternative method of radiation treatment (Burnet, 2003).

It is accepted that breast cancer patients who are diagnosed with the same type of breast cancer can have very different outcomes, some doing much better than others. There has been an active move towards individualizing treatments for particular patients by identifying which patients will do better, or worse, and 'tailoring' their treatment accordingly. The use of gene profiling is one of these methods of identification of an individual's risk of recurrence. The researchers use DNA microarray analysis to highlight those patients who would have a poor prognosis and who would benefit from an aggressive approach to their adjuvant chemotherapy and hormone therapy (van't Veer et al., 2003).

Conclusion

Teamwork and the role of the multidisciplinary team is an important factor in breast screening and caring for women with breast disorders. As we do not live in an ideal world, treatment is often fragmented between hospital, screening unit and home, proving emotionally traumatic for the woman and her family. The research and advances being made into the diagnosis and treatment of breast disorders means that guidelines are constantly changing, requiring all health care professionals to keep up to date. The informed nurse can provide support and information, but most importantly can provide continuity of care for the woman undergoing treatment for a breast problem.

Ideas for personal and professional development

- Ask your breast screening unit if you may observe a woman having a mammogram. It is much easier to encourage women to take part in the breast screening programme if you can advise them about what will happen
- Find out what the 'take up' rate for screening is in your area: you may be surprised at the figures
- Access the Breast Cancer Care website as an education resource
- List some advantages and disadvantages of the national breast screening programme
- Find out where your local breast unit is. Try and spend a session with the specialist breast nurse.

Patient education points

- Breast awareness is getting to know what is normal and then noticing any *change*. It involves looking and feeling
- Mammography is a simple and effective screening tool
- The vast majority of breast lumps are not cancerous
- Breast reconstruction can be offered to most women at the first time of surgery.

Resources

BACUP (British Association for Cancer United Patients)
3 Bath Place, Rivington Street, London EC2A 3JR
Freephone: 0808 800 1234
www.cancerbacup.org.uk
Cancer nurses provide information and emotional support by phone or letter. Booklets on cancer care are available. A one-to-one counselling service is also available.

Break Through Breast Cancer
Weston House, 3rd Floor, 246 High Holborn, London WC1V 7EX
Freephone: 08080 100200
www.breakthrough.org.uk

Breast Cancer Care
Kiln House, 210 New Kings Road, London SW6 4NZ
Tel: 0808 800 6000
www.breastcancercare.org.uk
Scotland: Floor 4, 40 St Enoch Square, Glasgow G1 4DH
Tel: 0141 221 2244
Offers help, information and support to women who have breast cancer or other breast-related problems. Services include free leaflets, a prosthesis-fitting service and one-to-one emotional support from volunteers who have themselves experienced breast cancer.

Breast Care Campaign
Blythe Hall, 100 Blythe Road, London W14 OHB
Tel: 020 7371 1510

British Association for Counselling and Psychotherapy (BACP)
35–37 Albert Street, Rugby, CV21 2SG
Tel: 0870 443 5252
www.bacp.co.uk

British Lymphology Society
www.lymphoedema.org/bls/index.html

Cancer Link
11–21 Northdown Street, London N1 9BN
Helpline: 0808 808 2020

Lymphoedema Support Network
St Luke's Crypt, Sydney Street, London SW3
Tel: 020 7351 4480

Macmillan Cancer Relief
89 Albert Embankment, London SE1 7UQ
Tel: 020 7840 7840
www.macmillan.org.uk

Rigby Peller Corsetry Specialists
2 Hans Road, Knightsbridge, London SW3 1RX
Tel: 020 7589 9293
22A Conduit Street, London W1R 9TB
Tel: 020 7491 2200
Able to advise women who need larger bras or have special requirements, for example after mastectomy.

Royal Marsden NHS Trust
203 Fulham Road, London SW3 6JJ
www.royalmarsden.org
Information leaflets on breast cancer and aspects of breast cancer treatments.

Women's Health
52 Featherstone Street, London EC1Y 8RT
Tel: 020 7251 6580

Women's Health Concern (WHC)
PO Box 2126, Marlow, Bucks SL7 2RY
Helpline: 0845 1232319
www.womens-health-concern.org

Internet sites regarding breast disease

General breast disease sites

www.obgyn.net/bh/bh.asp
www.breastdiseases.com
www.breastcancercare.org.uk

Cancer awareness and oncology-related sites including complementary therapies

www.cancernet.co.uk (good links to other cancer related sites)
www.cancer.gov/cancer_information (NCI link)

www.cancerresearch.org/breastcancer
www.cancerhelp.org.uk
www.cruk.org.uk (Cancer Research UK)
www.ons.org (Oncology Nursing Society, USA)
www.ucl.ac.uk/oncology (University College London, UK)
www.nice.org.uk

Male breast cancer

www.interact.withus.com/interact/mbc

Further reading

BAUM, M., SAUNDERS, C. and MEREDITH, S. (1994) *Breast Cancer: A Guide for Every Woman.* Oxford: Oxford University Press.

BREAST CANCER CARE (2003) Fact sheet. www.breast-cancercare.org.uk.

BURNET, K.L. (ed.) (2001) *Holistic Breast Care.* Edinburgh: Harcourt Health Sciences.

CHAPMAN, D. and GOODMAN, M. (1997) Breast cancer. In Groenwald, S.L., Goodman, M., Frogge, M.H. and Yarbro, C.H. (eds) *Cancer Nursing: Principles and Practice,* 4th edn. Massachusetts: Jones and Bartlett, Chapter 34, pp. 916–79.

DIXON, J.M. (2000) *ABC of Breast Diseases.* London: BMJ Publishing.

DIXON, J.M. and SAINSBURY, R. (1993) *Diseases of the Breast.* Edinburgh: Churchill Livingstone.

FALLOWFIELD, L. and CLARK, A. (1991) *Breast Cancer. The Experience of Illness Series.* London: Tavistock/Routledge.

HARMER, V. (2003) *Breast Cancer: Nursing Care and Management.* London: Whurr Publishers.

POWLES, T.J. and SMITH, I.E. (1991) *Medical Management of Breast Cancer.* London: Martin Dunitz.

References

BADWE, R.A. (1993) Timing of surgery during the menstrual cycle for operable breast cancer. *Cancer Topics* 9(4):42–3.

BALDWIN, E. (1990) Sexuality and breast cancer. *Midwife, Health Visitor and Community Nurse* 26(10).

BASO (British Association of Surgical Oncologists) (1998) *Guidelines for Surgeons in the Management of Symptomatic Breast Disease in the United Kingdom (1998 Revision).* London: BASO Breast Speciality Group.

BAUM, M. (2001) A vision for the future? *British Journal of Cancer* 85(Suppl 2):15–18.

BERGER, A. (1999) High dose chemotherapy offers little benefit in breast cancer. *British Medical Journal* 318:1440.

BREAST CANCER CARE (2003) Fact sheet. www.breast-cancercare.org.uk.

BURNET, K. (2003) Radiotherapy as a treatment for breast cancer. In Harmer V. (ed.) *Breast Cancer: Nursing Care and Management.* London: Whurr Publishers, Chapter 9, pp. 169–88.

BURNET, N.G., NYMAN, J., TURESSON, I. *et al.* (1992) Improving radiotherapy cure rates by predicting normal tissue tolerance from *in vitro* cellular radiation sensitivity. *Lancet* 339:1570–1.

CALMAN, K. and HINE, D. (1995) A policy for commissioning cancer services. A report by the expert advisory group on cancer to the chief medical officers of England and Wales. London: Department of Health.

CANCER RESEARCH UK (1997) *Breast Cancer UK, Fact sheet 6.1–6.5.* London: Cancer Research Campaign.

CHAMBERLAIN, J. (1993) Epidemiology. In Tucker A.K. (ed.) *Textbook of Mammography.* Edinburgh: Churchill Livingstone, Chapter 13, pp. 318–22.

CHAPMAN, D (2001) There's no place like home. *Nursing Standard* 16(11):18–19.

CHILVERS, C.E.D., McPHERSON, K., PETO, J., PIKE, M.C. and VESSEY, M.P. (1993) Breast feeding and risk of breast cancer in young women. *British Medical Journal* 307:17–20.

COLEMAN, R.E. (1999) Medical management of bone metastases. *Continuing Medical Education Bulletin* 1(3):70–5.

COLLABORATIVE GROUP ON HORMONAL FACTORS IN BREAST CANCER (1996) Breast cancer and hormonal contraceptives: collaborative reanalysis of individual data on 53,297 women with breast cancer and 100,239 women without breast cancer from 54 epidemiological studies. *Lancet* 347:1713–27.

COLLABORATIVE GROUP ON HORMONAL FACTORS IN BREAST CANCER (1997) Breast cancer and hormonal replacement therapy: collaborative reanalysis of data from 51 epidemiological studies of 52,705 women with breast cancer and 108,411 women without breast cancer. *Lancet* 350:1047–59.

CROWE, D.R. and LAMPEJO, O.T. (1996) Malignant tumours of the breast. In Blackwell, R.E. and Grotting, J.C. (eds) *Diagnosis and Management of Breast Disease.* Massachusetts: Blackwell Science.

DALING, J.R., MALONE, K.E., DOODY, D.R. *et al.* (2003) Association of hormone replacement therapy to prognostic factors among women diagnosed with breast cancer aged 50–64 years. *Cancer Epidemiology Biomarkers Prev.* 12(11, pt 1):1175–81.

DENIZ, K., O'MAHONY, S., ROSS, G. and PURUSHOTHAM, A. (2003) Breast cancer in women after treatment for Hodgkin's disease. *Lancet Oncology* 4(4):204–14.

DENTON, S. and BAUM, M. (1983) Psychological aspects of breast cancer. In Margolese, R. (ed.) *Breast Care.* Edinburgh: Churchill Livingstone.

DEROGATIS, L. (1986) The unique impact of breast and gynaecologic cancers on body image and sexuality in women – a reassessment. In Vaeth, R. (ed.) *Body Image, Self Image and Sexuality in Cancer Patients,* 2nd edn. Basel: Karger.

DEVITA, S.R., HELLMAN, S. and ROSENBERRG, S.A. (eds) (1993) *Cancer Principles and Practice of Oncology,* 4th edn. Philadelphia: J.P. Lippincott.

DHSS (Department of Health and Social Security) (1986) *The Forrest Report.* London: HMSO.

DiSAIA, P.J. (1993) Hormone replacement in patients with breast cancer. *Cancer Supplement* 71(4):1490–8.

DIXON, M. and SAINSBURY, R. (1993) *Diseases of the Breast.* Edinburgh: Churchill Livingstone.

DOUEK, M. and TAYLOR, I. (2003) Good practice and quality assurance in surgical oncology. *Lancet Oncology* **4**:626–30.

EBCTCG (Early Breast Cancer Trialists' Collaborative Group) (1992) Systemic treatment of early breast cancer by hormonal, cytotoxic, or immune therapy. *Lancet* **339**(8784):1–15, 71–85.

EBCTCG (1998a) Tamoxifen for early breast cancer: an overview of the randomised trials. *Lancet* **351**:1451–67.

EBCTCG (1998b) Polychemotherapy for early breast cancer: an overview of the randomised trials. *Lancet* **352**:930–42.

FAITHFULL, S. (1998) Fatigue in patients receiving radiotherapy. *Professional Nurse* **13**(7):459–61.

FALLOWFIELD, L.J., BAUM, M. and MAGUIRE, G.P. (1986) Effect of breast conservation on psychological morbidity associated with diagnosis and treatment of early breast cancer. *British Medical Journal* **293**:1331–4.

FALLOWFIELD, L.J., HALL, A., MAGUIRE, G.P. and BAUM, M. (1990) Psychological outcomes of different treatment policies in women with early breast cancer outside a clinical trial. *British Medical Journal* **301**:575–80.

FALLOWFIELD, L.J., HALL, A., MAGUIRE, G.P., BAUM, M. and A'HERN, R.P.A. (1994) Psychological effects of being offered choice of surgery for breast cancer. *British Medical Journal* **309**:448–551.

FENLON, D. (2003) Hormones as a treatment for breast cancer. In Harmer V. (ed.) *Breast Cancer: Nursing Care and Management*. London: Whurr Publishers, Chapter 10, pp. 188–214.

FERLAY, J., BRAY, F., PISANI, P. and PARKIN, D.M. (2002) *GLOBOCAN: Cancer Incidence, Mortality and Prevalence Worldwide. IARC CancerBase no.5 version 2.0*. Lyon: IARC Press, 2004.

FISHER, B., ANDERSON, S., REDMOND, C.K., WOLMARK, N., WICKERHAM, D.L. and CRONON, W.M. (1995) Reanalysis and results after 12 years of follow-up in a randomized clinical trial comparing total mastectomy with lumpectomy with or without irradiation in the treatment of breast cancer. *New England Journal of Medicine* **333**(22):1456–61.

FOWBLE, B., GOODMAN, L.R., GLICK, J.H. and ROSATO, E.F. (1991) *Breast Cancer Treatment – A Comprehensive Guide to Management*. St Louis: Mosby.

GAZET, J.C., RAINSBURY, R., FORD, M., POWLES, T. and COOMBES, R. (1985) Survey of treatment of primary breast cancer in Great Britain. *British Medical Journal* **290**:1793–5.

GHALIE, R., RICHMAN, C.M., SOLOMON, S. *et al.* (1994) Treatment of metastatic breast cancer with a split course, high-dose chemotherapy regimen and autologous bone marrow transplantation. *Journal of Clinical Oncology* **12**:342–6.

GLEAN, E., EDWARDS, S., FAITHFULL, S., MEREDITH, C., RICHARDS, C., SMITH, M. and COLYER, H. (2001) Intervention for acute radiotherapy induced skin reactions in cancer patients: the development of a clinical guideline recommended for use by the College of Radiographers. *Journal of Radiotherapy in Practice* **2**:75–84.

GOODMAN, M. (1989) Managing the side effects of chemotherapy. *Seminars in Oncology Nursing* **5**(2 Suppl 1):29–52.

GRAYDON, J.E. (1994) Women with breast cancer: their quality of life following a course of radiation therapy. *Journal of Advanced Nursing* **19**:617–22.

HAAGENSEN. C.D. (1986) *Diseases of the Breast*, 3rd edn. Philadelphia: W.B. Saunders.

HADDEN, J.W. (1999) The immunology and immunotherapy of breast cancer: an update. *International Journal of Immunopharmacology* **21**(2):79–101.

HANKS, G.W. and MANSI, J. (1998) The management of symptoms in advanced cancer: experience in a hospital-based continuing care unit. *Journal of the Society of Medicine* **81**:341–4.

HARRIS, J., MORROW, M. and BONNADONNA, G. (1993) Cancer of the breast. In DeVita, S.F., Hellman, S. and Rosenberg, S.A. (eds) *Cancer: Principles and Practice of Oncology*, 4th edn. Philadelphia: J.B. Lippincott.

HARVEY, H.A. (1998) Emerging role of aromatase inhibitors in the treatment of breast cancer. *Oncology-Huntington* **12**(3 Suppl 5):32–5.

HEYWANG-KÖBRUNNER, S.H., SCHAUMLÖFFEL, U., VIEHWEG, P., HÖFER, H., BUCHMANN, J. and LAMPE, D. (1998) Minimally invasive stereotaxic vacuum core breast biopsy. *European Radiology* **8**:377–85.

HWANG, E.S. and ESSERMAN, L.J. (1999) Management of ductal carcinoma in situ. *Surgical Clinics of North America* **79**(5):1007–30.

IARC (International Agency for Research on Cancer) (1988) *Monographs on the Evaluation of Carcinogenic Risks to Humans: Alcohol Drinking*. IARC Scientific Publication 44. Lyon: IARC, p. 387.

JANOWSKY, E.C., LAWRENCE, K.L. and HULKA, B.S. (2000) Meta-analyses of the relation between silicone breast implants and the risk of connective-tissue diseases. *New England Journal of Medicine* **342**(11):781–90.

JONES, C.V. (1998) The importance of oral hygiene in nutritional support. *British Journal of Nursing* **17**:274–83.

JUDSON, I.R. (1993) Toxicology of chemotherapeutic agents. In Andrews, P. and Sanger, G. (eds) *Emesis in Anticancer Therapy*. London: Chapman and Hall.

KALACHE, A. (1990) Risk factors for breast cancer with special reference to developing countries. *Health Policy and Planning* **5**:1–22.

KASPER, A.S. (1995) The social construction of breast loss and reconstruction. *Women's Health* **1**(3):197–219.

KEELEY, V. (2000) Classification of lymphoedema. In Twycross R., Jenns K. and Todd, J. (eds) *Lymphoedema*. Oxford: Radcliffe Medical Press.

KING, R. (2003) Fungating wounds. In Harmer, V. (ed.) *Breast Cancer: Nursing Care and Management*. London: Whurr Publishers, Chapter 12, pp. 233–50.

KISSANE, D.W., CLARKE, D.M., IKIN, J., BLOCH, S., SMITH, C.G., VITERRA, L. and McKENZIE, D.P. (1998) Psychological morbidity and quality of life in Australian women with early stage breast cancer: a cross sectional survey. *Medical Journal of Australia* **169**(4):192–6.

KISSIN, M., QUERCI DELLA ROVERE, G., EASTON, D. and WESTBURY, G. (1986) Risk of lymphoedema following the treatment of breast cancer. *British Journal of Surgery* **73**:580–4.

KROMAN, N., JENSEN, M., WOHLFHART, J., MOURIDSON, H.T., ANDERSEN, P.K. and MELBYE, M. (2000) Factors influencing the effect of age on prognosis in breast cancer: population based study. *British Medical Journal* **7233**:474–8.

LEONARD, R.C.F., RODGER, A. and DIXON, J.N. (2000) Metastatic breast cancer. In Dixon J.M. (ed.) *ABC of Breast Diseases*. London: BMJ Books, Chapter 12, pp. 65–72.

LOMAS, E. (2003) Advanced disease. In Harmer, V. (ed.) *Breast Cancer: Nursing Care and Management*. London: Whurr Publishers, Chapter 13, pp. 250–85.

MAGUIRE, G.P., BROOKE, M., TAIT, A. *et al.* (1983) The effect of counselling on physical disability and social recovery after mastectomy. *Clinical Oncology* 9:319–24.

MAGUIRE, G.P., PENTOL, A., ALLEN, D. *et al.* (1982) Cost of counselling women who undergo mastectomy. *British Medical Journal* 284:1933–5.

MAGUIRE, P. (2000) Psychological aspects. In Dixon J.M. (ed.) *ABC of Breast Diseases*. London: BMJ Books, Chapter 15, pp. 85–90.

MALLETT, J., MULLHOLLAND, J., LAVERTY, D. *et al.* (1999) An integrated approach to wound management. *International Journal of Palliative Nursing* 5(3):124–32.

MANSEL, R.E. (1994) Breast pain. *British Medical Journal* 309:866–8.

MANSI, J.L., SMITH, I.E., WALSH, G. *et al.* (1989) Primary medical therapy for operable breast cancer. *European Journal of Cancer and Clinical Oncology* 25(11):1623–7.

MARSDEN, J. and A'HERN, R. (2003) Progesterones and breast cancer risk: the role of hormonal contraceptives and hormone replacement therapy. *Journal of Family Planning and Reproductive Health Care* 29(4):185–7.

McCOY, J. (2003) Chemotherapy as a treatment for breast cancer. In Harmer, V. (ed.) *Breast Cancer: Nursing Care and Management*. London: Whurr Publishers, Chapter 8, pp. 150–69.

McINTOSH, S.A. and PURUSHOTHAM, A.D. (1998) Lymphatic mapping and sentinel lymph node biopsy in breast cancer. *British Journal of Surgery* 85(10):1347–56.

McKINNA, J.A. (1983) Clinical features of breast disease. In Parsons, C.A. (ed.) *Diagnosis of Breast Disease*. Baltimore: University Park Press, p. 42.

McPHERSON, K., STEEL, C.M. and DIXON, J.M. (2000) Breast cancer. Epidemiology, risk factors, and genetics. In Dixon, J.M. (ed.) *ABC of Breast Diseases*. London: BMJ Publishing Group.

MIKI, Y., SWENSEN, J., SHATTUCK-EIDENS, D. *et al.* (1994) Isolation of *BRCA1*, the 17q-linked breast and ovarian cancer susceptibility gene. *Science* 266:66–71.

MILLER, W.R. (1995) Prognostic factors. In Dixon, J.M. (ed.) *ABC of Breast Diseases*. London: BMJ Publishing Group.

MIRICK, D.K., DAVIS. S. and THOMAS, D.B. (2002) Antiperspirant use and the risk of breast cancer. *Journal of the National Cancer Institute* 94(20):1578–80.

MITCHELL, J. and GAMBLE, A. (2001) Surgical interventions for disorders of the breast. In Burnet, K.L. (ed.) *Holistic Breast Care*. London: Harcourt Health Sciences.

MORRIS, J., ROYLE, G.T. and TAYLOR, I. (1989) Changes in the surgical management of early breast cancer in England. *Journal of the Royal Society of Medicine* 82:12–15.

MORRIS, T. (1983) Psychosocial aspects of breast cancer: a review. *European Journal of Cancer and Clinical Oncology* 19(12):1725–33.

MORRIS, T., GREER, H. and WHITE, P. (1977) Psychosocial and social adjustment to mastectomy – a 2-year follow-up study. *Cancer* 40:2381–7.

MOZES M. (1982) The role of infection in postmastectomy lymphoedema. *Surgery Annual* 14:73–83.

MULATA, C.M., McINTOSH, S.A. and PURUSHOTHAM, A.D. (2000) Immediate breast reconstruction after mastectomy. *British Journal of Surgery* 87:1455–72.

NATIONAL INSTITUTE FOR CLINICAL EXCELLENCE (2002) NICE guidance on improving the outcomes in breast cancer. www.nice.org.uk.

NESTEL, P.J., POMEROY, S., KAY, S. *et al.* (1999) Isoflavones from red clover improve systemic arterial compliance but not plasma lipids in menopausal women. *Journal of Clinical Endocrinology and Metabolism* 84(3):895–8.

NHSBSP (1993) *Guidelines for Cytology Procedures and Reporting in Breast Cancer Screening*, No. 22, p. 12.

NHSBSP (2001) *Clinical Guidelines for Breast Screening Assessment*, Publication No. 49.

OAKLEY, C. (1997) Home or hospital intravenous therapy for cancer: a pilot instrument to aid professional decision making. Unpublished dissertation, University of Manchester.

OAKLEY, C. and BURNET, K.L. (2001) Medical treatments for breast cancer. In Burnet, K.L. (ed.) *Holistic Breast Care*. London: Harcourt Health Sciences, Chapter 6.

OLIVER, G. (1988) Radiotherapy. In Tschudin, V. (ed.) *Nursing the Patient with Cancer*. Hemel Hempstead: Prentice Hall, Chapter 5.

OVERGAARD, M., HANSEN, P.S., OVERGAARD, J. *et al.* (1997) Post operative radiotherapy in high risk premenopausal woman who receive adjuvant chemotherapy. *New England Journal of Medicine* 337:949–54.

PARKIN, D.M., WHELAN, S.I., FERLAY, J., RAYMOND, L. and YOUNG, J. (eds) (1997) *Cancer Incidence in Five Continents (volume VII)*. IARC Scientific Publication 143. Lyon: International Agency for Research on Cancer.

POOLE, C., EARL, H.M., DUNN, L. *et al.* (2003) NEAT (National Epirubicin Adjuvant Trial) and SCTBG BR 9601 (Scottish Cancer Trials Breast Group) phase III adjuvant trials show a significant relapse free and overall survival advantage for sequential ECMF. *Proceedings of the American Society of Clinical Oncology* 22(4):abstr 3.

POWLES, T.J. and SMITH, I.E. (1991) *Medical Management of Breast Cancer*. London: Martin Dunitz.

POWLES, T.J., HARDY, J.R., ASHLEY, S.E. *et al.* (1989) A pilot trial to evaluate the acute toxicity and feasibility of tamoxifen for prevention of breast cancer. *British Journal of Cancer* 60:126–31.

PURUSHOTHAM, A.D., BRITTON, P. and BOBROW, L. (2000) Benign breast disease. In Borgen, P.I. and Hill, A. (eds) *Breast Diseases*. London: Landes Bioscience.

RCN (Royal College of Nursing) (1995) Breast palpation and breast awareness: guidelines for practice. *Issues in Nursing and Health Series No. 35*. London: RCN.

REGNARD, C. and TEMPEST, S. (1998) *A Guide to Symptom Relief in Advanced Disease*, 4th edn. Cheshire: Hochland and Hochland.

RODENHUIS, S., RICHEL, D., VAN DER WALL, E. *et al.* (1998) Randomised trial of high dose chemotherapy and haemopoietic progenitor cell support in operable breast cancer with extensive axillary lymph node involvement. *Lancet* 352:515–21.

RODGER, A., LEONARD, R.C.F. and DIXON, J.M. (2000) Locally advanced breast cancer. In Dixon, J.M. (ed.) *ABC of Breast Diseases*. London: BMJ Publishing Group, Chapter 11, pp. 61–5.

RUTHERFORD, D. (1988) Assessing psychosexual needs of women experiencing lumpectomy. *Cancer Nursing* 11(4):244–9.

SAINSBURY, J.R., ANDERSON, T.J. and MORGAN, D.A. (2000) Breast cancer. In Dixon, J.M. (ed.) *ABC of Breast Diseases*. London: BMJ Publishing Group, Chapter 7, pp. 38–44.

SALTER, M. (1997) *Altered Body Image: The Nurse's Role*, 2nd edn. London: Baillière Tindall.

SMITH, I.E. and DE BOER, R.H. (2000) Role of systemic therapy for primary operable breast cancer. In Dixon, J.M. (ed.) *ABC of Breast Diseases*. London: BMJ Publishing Group, Chapter 10, pp. 55–61.

SOLOMON, J. (1986) The good news about breast reconstruction. *Registered Nurse* November:47–54.

START (Standardization of Breast Radiotherapy Protocol) (1998) *A randomised Comparison of Fractionation Regimes after Local Excision or Mastectomy in Women with Early Stage Breast Cancer.* START Trials Office: Institute of Cancer Research.

STRUEWING, J.P., ABELIOVICH, D., PERETZ, T. *et al.* (1995). The carrier frequency of the *BRCA*1 185delAG mutation is approximately 1 percent in Ashkenazi Jewish individuals. *Nature Genetics* **11**(2):198–200.

THORLACIUS, S., SIGURDSSON, S., BJARNADOTTIR, H. *et al.* (1997) Study of a single *BRCA*2 mutation with high carrier frequency in a small population. *American Journal of Human Genetics* **60**(5):1079–84.

TIERNEY, A.J. (1987) Preventing chemotherapy induced alopecia in cancer patients. Is scalp cooling worthwhile? *Journal of Advanced Nursing* **12**:303–10.

TUCKER, A.K. (1993) Introduction. In Tucker, A.K. (ed) *Textbook of Mammography*. Edinburgh: Churchill Livingstone, pp. 2–3.

TURESSON, I. and THAMES, H. (1989) Repair capacity and kinetics of human skin during fractionated radiotherapy: erythema, desquamation and telangiectasia after three and five years follow-up. *Radiotherapy and Oncology* **15**:169–88.

UICC (1997) Sobin, L.H. and Wittekind, C.H. (eds) *TNM Classification of Malignant Tumours*, 5th edn. New York: Wiley.

VAN'T VEER, L.J., DAI, H., VAN de VIJVER M.J. *et al.* (2002) Gene expression profiling predicts clinical outcome of breast cancer. *Nature* **415**:530–5.

VERONESI, U., SALVADORI, O., LUINI, A. *et al.* (1990) Conservative treatment of early breast cancer. Long-term results of 1232 cases treated by quadrantectomy and radiotherapy. *Annals of Surgery* **211**:250–9.

WARD, D.J. (1987) Breast reconstruction. *Hospital Update* September:725–34.

WATSON, J.D., SAINSBURY, J.R.C. and DIXON, J.M. (1995) Breast reconstruction after surgery. ABC of breast diseases. *British Journal of Medicine* **310**:117–21.

WATSON, M. (1991) Breast cancer. In Watson, M. (ed.) *Patient Care, Psychosocial Treatment Methods*. Cambridge: British Psychological Society, Cambridge University Press.

WATSON, M., DENTON, S., BAUM, M. and GREER, S. (1988) Counselling breast cancer patients: a specialist nurse service. *Counselling and Psychology Quarterly* **1**(1):23–32.

WEST, N. (2003) Breast reconstruction. In Harmer, V. (ed.) *Breast Cancer Nursing Care and Management*. London: Whurr Publishers, Chapter 7, pp. 122–50.

WILSON, R.G., HART, A. and DAWES, P.J.D.K. (1988) Mastectomy or conservation: the patient's choice. *British Medical Journal* **297**:1167–9.

WOODS, M. (2003) Lymphoedema and breast cancer. In Harmer, V. (ed.) *Breast Cancer: Nursing Care and Management*. London: Whurr Publishers, Chapter 11, pp. 214–33.

WOOSTER, R., BIGNELL, G., LANCASTER, J. *et al.* (1995) Identification of the breast cancer susceptibility gene, *BRCA*2. *Nature* **378**(6559):789–92.

YEOWELL, M. (1993) In Tucker, A.K. (ed) *Textbook of Mammography*. Edinburgh: Churchill Livingstone, Chapter 3, pp. 28–54.

13: Cervical Screening and Abnormalities

Vicky Padbury

OBJECTIVES

This chapter should help you understand:

◆ How to inform and update on the NHS Cervical Screening Programme ◆

◆ The nature of abnormalities of the cervix ◆

◆ The ethics of cervical screening ◆

◆ The relevant anatomy and physiology of the cervix and associated structures and organs ◆

◆ What is entailed in the treatment and management of cervical abnormalities

◆ How to take a cervical smear. ◆

Introduction

Cervical screening has suffered, like no other screening procedure, from considerable adverse publicity in the UK in recent years. This has been due to various factors including:

◆ Inadequately trained professionals taking cervical smears

◆ Under-diagnosis of abnormal smears at laboratory level (NHS Executive, 1998)

◆ Poor levels of understanding amongst press and public regarding screening.

Training smear-takers. There is much the appropriately trained nurse can do to help counter this unfortunate situation. The vast majority of cervical screening takes place in the primary care setting (Table 13.1) and Atkin *et al.* (1993) state that 75% of practice nurses are undertaking the role of cervical smear-taker.

As nurses, we are all accountable for our own actions, and therefore should not take on any tasks that we do not feel competent to undertake, but should seek out further training. The NMC document *Code of Professional Conduct* (NMC, 2002a) is useful to refer to.

Problems in laboratories. Problems within some laboratories have been widely reported by the media, leading to much anxiety for the women concerned, and also for those who regularly attend for smears. This has now led to the compulsory accreditation of all laboratories

Table 13.1 Percentage of smears examined by source, England 2002–2003

Source	Percentage
General practice	87.4%
Community clinics	4.5%
GUM clinics	0.8%
NHS hospitals	6.2%
Private hospitals	0.6%
Other	0.5%

Adapted from DoH Bulletin 2003

involved in cervical cytology, with some staff being retrained and small laboratories being merged or closed (Warden, 1998).

The nature, benefits and limitations of screening in general, and cervical screening in particular, have led to serious misconceptions about the cervical screening programme. The NHS Executive (1998) report recommended four key messages to be used on posters for women:

◆ the smear test aims to prevent cancer and is **not** a test for cancer

◆ 100% accuracy is **not** possible

◆ women should **always** report any abnormal bleeding to their GP

◆ the screening programme prevents up to 3900 cancers a year.

History of the NHS cervical screening programme (NHSCSP)

Organized screening programmes have been in operation in parts of Europe and North America for over 30 years. The Nordic countries – Denmark, Finland, Iceland and Sweden – started screening in the 1960s with highly organized programmes and achieved almost complete coverage of their target populations. As these countries are very small, effective screening was generally easier.

Britain has been screening since 1964, although initially in an uncoordinated way. By the mid-1980s, although many women were having regular smear tests there was concern that those at greatest risk were not being tested, and those that had positive results were not being followed up and treated effectively. Since then new initiatives have been introduced to make screening more effective and in 1988 organized cervical screening really started in England and Wales.

The main points of the Department of Health (DoH) guidelines of 1988 were:

◆ The provision of clear policy guidelines recommending 5-yearly cervical smear tests for women aged between 20 and 64 years of age

◆ Introduction of a computerized call and recall scheme

◆ The production of professional guidelines through the medium of an Intercollegiate Report (RCOG *et al.*, 1987)

◆ The introduction of a number of policy initiatives designed to improve the quality of the service

◆ Clear guidelines on fail-safe systems and identification of one person as being responsible for the coordination of the fail-safe system

◆ Introduction of an external laboratory quality assurance system

◆ The nomination of an individual who could be held to account for the organization and effectiveness of cervical cancer screening (NCN, 1991).

Since the advent of Primary Care Trusts (PCTs) in 2002, each Trust has a nominated person responsible for its cervical screening programme and for implementing the national guidelines. PCTs commission cervical screening from their overall allocation received from the DoH.

Strategic Health Authorities (SHAs) have superseded Regional Health Authorities and undertake performance management of local NHS Trusts and PCTs. Regional directors of quality assurance teams work with the Trusts and also monitor the laboratories. Regional directors of public health oversee the development of local services, and maintain key links to SHAs, particularly relating to quality assurance issues (DoH, 2002).

The National Coordinating Network (NCN)

The NCN was originally set up in the early 1990s, and represented five main interest groups: women, research workers, service providers, policy-makers and professional organizations with the objective of promoting the exchange of good ideas for quality improvement.

Since then the NCN has become the NHS Cancer Screening Programmes and covers both cervical and breast cancer; their headquarters are in Sheffield (see useful addresses). The NHSCSP is responsible for improving the overall performance of the screening programme, with priorities to:

◆ Develop systems and guidelines which will assure a high quality of cervical screening throughout the country

◆ Identify important policy issues and help resolve them, and improve communications both within the programme and to women (NHSCSP, 1999b).

The NHSCSP is an important source of excellent publications, including the Links magazine published quarterly, which are free to those working in the screening programme.

To complete the picture of the history of our cervical screening programme, two more events need mentioning.

The first was the 1990 GPs' Contract which introduced target payments as incentives to GPs to screen 50% (lower payment) and 80% (higher payment) of their target population of women (aged 20–64 years) every five years. This initiative has been very successful (Figure 13.1) and has led to a marked increase in cervical screening activity, but may have raised some problems:

◆ Not all 20-year-olds and upwards will be sexually active, some will be inappropriately screened (see page 362 for update on screening ages)

◆ If a GP has a highly mobile practice population it may be difficult to reach targets, therefore cervical screening might become a low priority within the practice

◆ Coercive tactics have been reported to encourage women to have their smear test at their GP's surgery.

This creates a conflict, in that it goes against the spirit of enabling women to make informed choices about whether or not they wish to be screened and where they wish to go for screening (Austoker and McPherson, 1992).

The second event was the publication in July 1992 of the DoH's *Health of the Nation* document (DoH, 1992). In this document the DoH set targets for the reduction of preventable disease to improve the nation's health. Cancers are the second most common cause of death (25%) in England. In the *Health of the Nation* document, four cancers (breast, cervical, lung and skin) were targeted for action. With cervical cancer the aim was to reduce the number of women with newly detected invasive cervical cancer by at least 20% by the year 2000 which would equal 12.8 per 100,000 women. This target was achieved earlier than expected (see Figure 13.2) (NHSCSP, 1998a).

Screening in itself can cause stress and anxiety. It should be remembered that we are dealing with a seemingly healthy population and if a smear has to be repeated for any reason at all it can be the source of much worry. The belief by some women that the test will be 'painful, embarrassing or unpleasant' is a strong reason for non-attendance (Gillam, 1991). The principles of screening for disease are outlined in Box 13.1. You will see as we go through this chapter how well cervical screening fits in with most of these principles.

What is cervical screening looking for?

Cervical screening is undertaken to detect very early changes in cells from the cervix which,

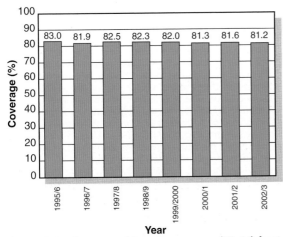

Figure 13.1 Coverage of target age group (25–64) from 1995 to 2003.
(Crown copyright material is reproduced with the permission of the controller of HMSO and the Queen's printer for Scotland. Crown copyright reproduced from Department of Health Statistical Bulletin, Cervical Screening Programme England 2002–2003.)

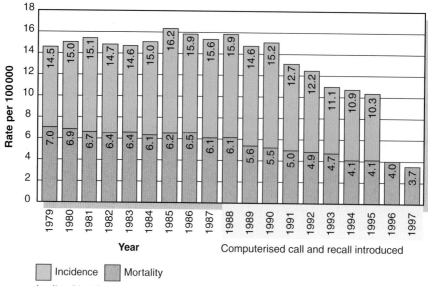

Figure 13.2 Age-standardized incidence of and mortality from cervical cancer, England. (Reproduced with kind permission of the NHSCSP.) Directly age-standardized using the European Standard Population to take account of the changing age structure of the population over time.

Box 13.1	The principles of screening

The *Principles and Practice of Screening for Disease* was a Public Health Paper formulated in 1968 for the World Health Organization by Wilson and Junger and seems just as appropriate three decades later when we are considering cervical screening. The basic principles are as follows:

◆ The condition should pose an important health problem

◆ The natural history of the disease should be well understood

◆ There should be a recognizable early stage

◆ Early treatment should be more beneficial than at a later stage

◆ There should be a suitable test

◆ The test should be acceptable to the population

◆ There should be adequate facilities for the diagnosis and treatment of abnormalities detected

◆ For disease of insidious onset, screening should be repeated at intervals determined by the natural history of the disease

◆ The chance of physical or psychological harm must be less than the benefits

◆ Cost of screening should be balanced against the benefits it provides.

SCENARIO

Gwyneth, a 58-year-old woman, attended for her first ever smear (having ignored all previous invitations). The practice nurse realized that she would have to explain everything carefully to Gwyneth who looked very nervous and said even though she'd given birth to two children, having a smear had always sounded horrific. She had called the test the 'cancer smear'. The practice nurse thought that this was a good area to start giving information and explained that the test was in fact looking for very early changes in the cells from the cervix, that if left undetected and untreated might over a period of years change to cancer. This, along with giving Gwyneth more up-to-date information and spending some time showing her the equipment, helped to make the situation less formidable.

When the nurse took the cervical smear there was some contact bleeding. She informed Gwyneth of this and said that the laboratory might not be able to get such a good look at the cells that they want to see, and in that case they would most likely request a repeat of the smear.

She was 'not to panic' therefore if she was called back to the surgery. All this was understood by the client who went home much better informed than when she had arrived, and because the nurse had spent time explaining things to her, Gwyneth was less likely to worry if called back for a repeat smear.

if left untreated, could lead to squamous cell carcinoma. In other words, cervical screening is a way of interrupting the natural history of the disease at an earlier and more treatable stage.

Other abnormalities may be picked up coincidentally by the cervical smear and these are discussed later in the chapter.

The cervical smear test or the 'Pap' smear

We have the Greek scientist and humanitarian George N. Papanicolaou (1883–1962) to thank for the modern smear test. He began scientific work in Monaco in the field of oceanography and physiology, but moved to New York in 1913 where he joined the department of pathology at Cornell Medical College. Here he demonstrated changes in vaginal epithelium at different phases of the menstrual cycle, and developed a cytological test for malignant change in the squamous epithelial tissue of the cervix uteri.

It took many years for his research to be recognized, but his test for the early detection of cervical cancer has been widely used since the late 1940s and is known as the 'Pap' smear test. ('Smear' refers to the action of smearing the cells within the mucus onto a glass slide.) It is said (Barker, 1987) that Papanicolaou used his wife as a volunteer to obtain cervical cells. He used a pipette to draw fluid from the posterior fornix of the vagina in which can be found cervical cells (as cells from the cervix exfoliate like any other epithelial covering).

While we no longer use this pipette method to obtain the sample of mucus, the principles of the test remain the same.

Epidemiology of cervical cancer

Cervical cancer incidence rates vary greatly throughout the world.

◆ In developing countries cervical cancer is amongst the commonest female cancer

◆ An estimated 471,000 new cases of cervical cancer are diagnosed each year in the world, with approximately 80% of these occurring in the less developed world

◆ In less developed countries such as India, cervical cancer is the most common cancer in women

◆ Cervical cancer is the eleventh most common cancer in women in the UK with incidence rates slightly below the European Union average although the mortality rates are slightly higher

◆ Mortality rates in 2000 were 60% lower (3.3 per 100,000 women) than they were 30 years earlier (8.3 per 100,000 in 1971) (see Figure 13.3).

All statistics from Cancer Research UK (2003).

The natural history of cervical cancer

The majority (around two-thirds) of cancer of the cervix is squamous cell carcinoma. Adenocarcinoma, which originates deep within the glands of the endocervical canal, is very difficult to pick up on a cervical smear. The number of smears reported with a potential glandular abnormality remains a very small proportion of all smears reported at 0.04% for 2002–03 (NHSCSP, 2003). To a certain extent some of the problems at Kent and Canterbury were due to this very subject of adenocarcinoma not being identified from cervical smears (Dyer, 1999). At the secondary screening stage, colposcopy (see page 375), adenocarcinoma is the next most common histology (around 15%) of all invasive cervical cancers. One study (Vizcaino, 1998) reported an increase in adenocarcinoma and a downward trend in squamous cell carcinoma in many countries worldwide. This could be due to increased awareness and referrals for diagnosis of abnormal glandular cells of unknown significance (Cancer Research UK, 2003).

Squamous cell carcinoma

Epidemiological evidence has linked squamous cell carcinoma with sexual habits. One of the

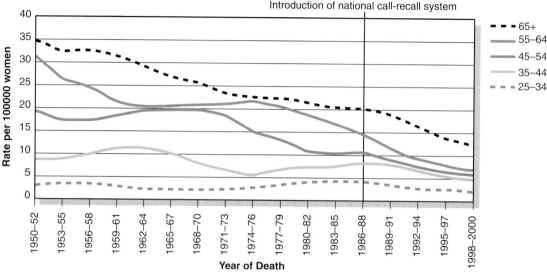

Figure 13.3 Reduction in death rates from cervical cancer in different age groups. (Reproduced with permission of Cancer Research UK.)

first people to take an epidemiological approach to cancer was a doctor called Domenico Rigoni-Stern who was born in 1810 in Italy. He graduated as a medical doctor and surgeon from the University of Padua in 1834 and published numerous papers during the 1830s and 1840s on the incidence and mortality of various cancers. In 1842 he published his most notable study of 'Statistical data relative to the disease of cancer' (Scotto and Bailar, 1969). In this study he noted the higher frequency of breast cancer among unmarried women and nuns, relative to married or widowed women. He also found that uterine cancer (data did not distinguish between uterine cervix and uterine corpus, but it is thought that most of the uterine cancer was primarily in the cervix) was not common in unmarried women and was very rare in nuns. This finding was later confirmed by Gagnon (1950) in a study of nuns in Quebec, Canada.

In the 1960s attention turned to the role of the male in the incidence of cervical cancer. It was found that wives of men whose first wives had died from cervical cancer were more likely to develop the disease; wives of husbands with penile cancer were also found to have a high incidence (Smith et al., 1979). These studies led to the concept of the 'high-risk' male, a category that

can include men who work away from home and consequently have greater opportunity to have more than one sexual partner. Singer and Szarewski (1988) commented in their book that the wives of Colombian businessmen from social class 1 had a high incidence of the disease. The wives were usually faithful to their husbands but it was found that the husbands were accustomed regularly to visiting prostitutes.

In England and Wales, incidence and mortality from cervical cancer (Quinn et al., 2001) has been analysed by Carstairs deprivation category. Women living in the most deprived areas have rates more than three times as high as those in the least deprived areas. In addition a link has been demonstrated between social class and cervical cancer which indicates that cervical cancer incidence is considerably higher among women of working age in manual than in non-manual classes (Brown et al., 1997). There may be many confounding factors within this, such as smoking habits (Simons et al., 1993), early age of sexual intercourse, the likelihood of having more than one partner in a lifetime and the increased probability of having more pregnancies.

The sexually transmitted agent that is strongly linked with cervical cancer is the human papillomavirus (HPV) (Eluf-Neto *et al.*, 1994), which is also known as wart virus.

When a cell is invaded by HPV, characteristic changes can be seen under the cytologist's microscope and the nucleus gives the appearance of having a halo round it. The cells invaded are called koilocytes.

There are over 60 different kinds of wart virus, identified by the type of DNA they contain and they are individually numbered. The association with cervical cancer is verified by the fact that around 90% of women with cervical cancer have antibodies to HPV in blood samples, while antibodies to HPV have also been found in about 95% of people who have genital warts. When a group of women without genital warts, cervical cancer or pre-cancerous changes was studied, virtually none had antibodies to HPV; with this evidence Singer and Szarewski (1988) concluded that the wart virus or HPV is a major cause of cervical cancer.

There are about 13 so-called 'high-risk' HPV types, for example 16 and 18 are known to be associated with cervical cancer, but unfortunately they cannot be specifically identified from a cervical smear test alone. The World Health Organization (WHO) and the International Agency for Research on Cancer (IARC) now officially classify HPV 16 and 18 as carcinogenic agents (Cuzick *et al.*, 2000). To distinguish which HPV was present the DNA would have to be examined. Advances in HPV testing are discussed in more detail on page 380.

Risk factors associated with cervical cancer

Sexual behaviour

It is recognized that certain areas of sexual behaviour are associated with increased risk of cervical cancer. These include:

◆ *Age at first sexual intercourse* The transformation zone (see page 359) is very evident and active in puberty making it more susceptible to possible carcinogens such as HPV

◆ *Number of sexual partners* Because HPV is transmitted through sexual activity, the numbers of sexual partners of both the woman and her partner are risk factors

◆ *Number of pregnancies* During pregnancy the transformation zone is very evident and active and therefore more vulnerable to sexually transmitted agents. Pregnancy also suppresses the immune system.

Suppression of the immune system

A weakened immune system would make the cervix more susceptible to the disease.

◆ Human immunovirus (HIV) and acquired immune deficiency syndrome (AIDS)

◆ Treatments for cancer – chemotherapy

◆ Post-transplant treatment to prevent rejection of the new organ

Smoking habit

There is some controversy as to whether the link is causal, or in some way reflects residual confoundings with other unmeasured aspects of sexual behaviour. Barton *et al.* (1988) showed that nicotine found in high concentrations (smoking over 20 cigarettes a day) in the cervical cells of smokers damages the cells' immune response (Langerhans cells), making them more susceptible to forms of infections such as wart virus. Epidemiological evidence strongly links smoking with squamous cell cervical cancer and high-grade CIN. There appears to be over a two-fold increased risk for cervical cancer in smokers (Szarewski and Cuzick, 1998). Cigarette smoking has been linked to inactivation in cervical tumours of the fragile histidine triad putative tumour suppressor gene (Society for Gynecologic, 2000). Smoking cessation in women with low-grade cervical lesions seen at colposcopy was shown to have a beneficial effect on the size of their lesions: it seems stopping smoking may allow the cervix to heal itself (Szarewski *et al.*, 1996).

It is evident that all the risk factors mentioned above can be interlinked and can have an impact on each other.

Method of contraception

The combined oral contraceptive pill has been implicated in cervical cancer possibly due to the oestrogen in the pill making the ectropion (see Colour plate 3) on the cervix more extensive, therefore offering a larger area where metaplasia can be more vulnerable to HPV.

A review by Smith *et al.* (2003) showed a possible link between extended use of oral contraceptives and an increased risk of cervical cancer. The authors suggest that more research is needed to establish the extent to which women remain at an increased risk after they have stopped using oral contraceptives. Unfortunately the term 'oral contraceptives' is not defined and does not distinguish from pills containing oestrogen or progestogen only.

Professor Martin Vessey, Chair of the Advisory Committee on Cervical Screening, commented in response to the findings of the review by Smith *et al.* (2003) 'While this paper supports the view that long term use of oral contraceptives is associated with an increased risk of cervical cancer, it is important to remember that the benefits of taking oral contraceptives far outweigh the risk for the majority of women. In particular oral contraceptive use markedly reduces the risk of ovarian cancer and cancer of the endometrium'. Julietta Patnick, Director of the NHSCSP, added that 'one of the biggest risk factors could be women who do not have cervical smears'.

A co-factor could be that pill users are less likely to use barrier methods in addition to their pill. A clear message that health professionals should give to clients is that the pill will protect from pregnancy, and the use of condoms will protect from HIV, STIs and in particular reduce the transfer of HPV during sexual intercourse. The use of both methods is known as the double Dutch method.

Alternative sexual practices

So far we have been discussing risks associated with penetrative sexual intercourse. Not all women are in a heterosexual relationship, and lesbian relationships need to be considered.

A lesbian coming for a cervical smear should have sexual intercourse and her own sexual activities discussed in a sensitive manner. Knowing that the high-risk agent is wart virus, sexual practices should be addressed, to decide whether the woman is at risk and whether a smear is relevant. If a cervical smear is decided against, then there are many other well-woman checks that can be undertaken, e.g. breast awareness, and health advice given on other topics such as diet, smoking, etc. Ultimately it is the woman's choice whether she would like a smear test or not.

Anatomy and physiology

The uterus

The uterus is a hollow, pear-shaped muscular organ situated in the pelvic cavity between the bladder and the rectum. In 80% of women it is anteverted (tilted forward) and anteflexed (curved forward on itself) from the level of the internal os (Figures 13.4 and 13.5).

The body or corpus of the uterus is 5 cm long, with the neck or cervix uteri 2.5 cm long; the lower part of the cervix protrudes at approximately 90° into the upper part of the vagina. Because the cervix protrudes into the high vagina it forms a space around it, which is divided into four fornices:

◆ The anterior space or fornix between the cervix and bladder
◆ The posterior space or fornix between the cervix and the rectum
◆ The right and left (or lateral) fornices, taken up by the ovaries and Fallopian tubes. These are called the right and left adnexae.

The inner layer of the body of the uterus is lined with endometrial cells which are constantly changing in thickness and vascularity according to the phases of the menstrual cycle (see page 516). The superficial layers are shed during menstruation and evidence of them can be found up to days 10–12 of the next menstrual cycle if cervical mucus is examined under the microscope. This underlines the need to put the first day of the last

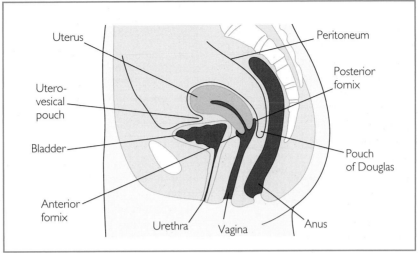

Figure 13.4   The pelvic organs in sagittal section.

menstrual period on the laboratory form. If there are endometrial cells present and your client is more than 10–12 days into her menstrual cycle the laboratory may ask for a repeat smear (your client might have an endometrial tumour).

The importance of informing the laboratory of an intrauterine contraceptive device being *in situ* is also associated with endometrial cells being present later in the cycle (Hopwood, 1995).

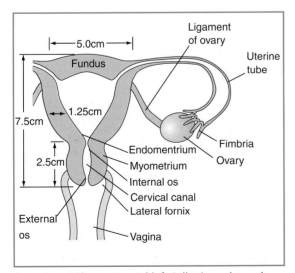

Figure 13.5   The uterus and left Fallopian tube and ovary.

The cervix

The outer part of the cervix, the ectocervix, is covered by thick multilayered stratified (meaning horizontal sheets) squamous epithelium. In healthy women in their reproductive years, this consists of up to 20 layers of cells which arise at the basement membrane and mature in an orderly way, gaining increased amounts of cytoplasm as they approach the surface of the epithelial covering. The blood vessels and glands are contained in the basement membrane under the tough squamous epithelium, giving the ectocervix a dusky pink sheen, which can be a helpful guide to you when endeavouring to locate the cervix during smear taking. It is quite different from the darker pink epithelium of the vaginal walls.

Under the microscope, the surface of the ectocervix is not smooth but rather like the coastline on a map, irregular with many folds. Sometimes these folds become blocked with mucus. When this happens they look like little cysts on the surface of the cervix and are called retention cysts or Nabothian follicles (see Colour plate 2).

Looking at the cervix from the vagina it could be likened to a Victoria plum in shape and size, with the 'stalk' at the cervical hole or os. The cervical os is the opening into the cervical canal. The endocervical canal is lined by epithelium

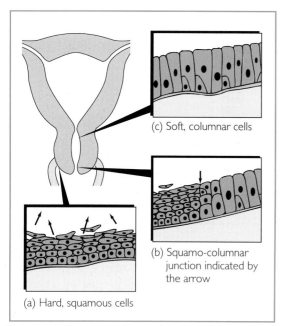

Figure 13.6 Squamo-columnar junction of the cervix.

(c) Soft, columnar cells

(b) Squamo-columnar junction indicated by the arrow

(a) Hard, squamous cells

Box 13.2 Factors that decide the position of the squamo-columnar junction

◆ Individual endogenous hormones during adolescence, puberty, the reproductive years and the climacteric/menopause

◆ Extra exogenous hormones in the form of the oral contraceptive pill and hormone replacement therapy.

only one cell thick, arranged in columns called columnar epithelium (Figure 13.6). Within these cells are found deep branching glands called compound racemose glands, which secrete alkaline mucus. It is within these glands that the uncommon adenocarcinoma can arise. See page 353 for further information on adenocarcinoma.

Separating the endocervical canal from the cavity of the uterus is the internal cervical os, which has a strong muscle surrounding it. This is important for maintaining a pregnancy.

The cervix is a very dynamic organ and changes throughout the different phases of a woman's life. It is under the influence of ovarian and pituitary hormones which are very active at puberty and during pregnancy. These start to decline during the climacteric and cease completely after the menopause. An experienced smear-taker could probably guess the approximate age of a woman by just looking at her cervix.

The squamo-columnar junction (SCJ)

The point at which the squamous cells of the ectocervix meet the columnar cells of the endocervix is known as the squamo-columnar junction (SCJ). Depending on the age and hormonal

state of the woman this junction could be in the lower third of the endocervical canal or out on the ectocervix (Box 13.2). See Colour plate 1.

Within the confines of the alkaline endocervical canal the delicate columnar cells are protected from the acid pH of the vagina and also from the natural friction of the penis pushing against the cervix during sexual intercourse. It is a natural process for the columnar cells to migrate downwards on to the ectocervix, moving the SCJ to a new position. Ectropion, or ectopy, is the appearance of a red area of columnar epithelium around the cervical os by this process (Hopwood, 1990). This is a normal physiological state and the term 'erosion' formerly used should be avoided as it is liable to conjure the impression of something 'wearing away' (see Colour plate 3).

SCENARIO

The nurse was clearing up her room after a busy afternoon in the surgery undertaking 'well-woman' checks which included taking cervical smears. The phone rang. On the line was a very tearful client: Sharon, a 25-year-old woman, who had seen the nurse for a smear that afternoon. The nurse had commented when taking the smear that there was an 'erosion' present on her cervix. Sharon, not wanting to seem ignorant, did not ask for more information, but on arriving home had looked up 'erosion' in the dictionary and was distraught to see it connected with 'wearing away'. The nurse was able to reassure her and admitted to using a term that is no longer in common use and instead talked of an ectopy which now made sense to Sharon. This was a salutary lesson to the nurse to be more careful and sensitive when offering information to clients.

Transformation zone or transitional zone

The migrated columnar cells at the SCJ on the ectocervix will start to break down in the acid environment of the vagina. Squamous cells begin to grow from beneath the columnar epithelium and gradually replace it. This normal replacement of one type of cell by another is called squamous metaplasia and where it takes place is called the transformation or transitional zone (Figure 13.7).

The SCJ and the transformation zone are the most common sites where pre-cancerous changes originate (Chomet and Chomet, 1989) due to these areas being active and vulnerable. It is imperative that the smear-taker understands this concept in order to take the best possible smears. See page 365 for more information on which sampler type to use.

The nurse's role as a smear-taker

It is important for you, the smear-taker, to be up-to-date and well informed regarding all aspects of cervical cytology and this in turn will allow you to give your client advice and information prior to her smear being taken.

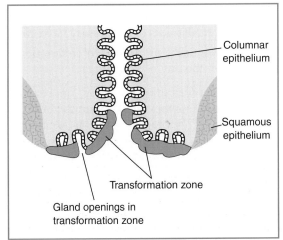

Figure 13.7 Transformation zone. The surface of the everted columnar epithelium gradually changes to squamous epithelium. This altered area, consisting of metaplastic squamous epithelium, is known as the transformation zone. In post-menopausal women there is a reduction in size of the cervix. The squamo-columnar junction and part of the transformation zone come to lie in the endocervix.

Your attitude is very important. Not only is it desirable to have someone who is sensitive to the client's fears, feelings and possible misgivings about having a smear taken, but also someone who is comfortable with undertaking this most intimate of examinations. It is a presumption that all nurses feel able to undertake the role of smear-taker. Nurses may have problems with their own sexuality, which are not necessarily associated with the 'older' or 'younger' nurse. It may not be until the nurse starts learning how to take smears, that she realizes she has such a problem that she may have subconsciously denied or hidden until this time.

As a smear-taker, you will not only need to feel comfortable with your own sexuality, but also be able to discuss any problems or anxieties that your client may reveal at this most sensitive and intimate of times (Tunnadine, 1970).

It is not expected that you will have all the answers to whatever a client reveals, but very often just the fact that the woman has voiced some concern or anxiety to you can be of enormous benefit to her, even though you may have said or done very little, apart from listening.

SCENARIO

An instructing nurse was discussing smear taking with her new family planning student. She had been aware of a distinct feeling of discomfort and embarrassment while observing the student taking a smear. The feeling certainly was not coming from the patient who was a very relaxed and chatty woman who, knowing it was a training session for the student was doing all she could to help the situation. When the instructing nurse enquired of the student how she felt she had done, the nurse became quite emotional and said that she had found it a most embarrassing situation to be in, and that if smear taking was an essential part of the course she wondered if she should continue.

After sitting down together and discussing the matter it transpired that the nurse had an unconsummated marriage of 4 years, and up to then had not admitted this to anyone. The instructing nurse was able to put the student in touch with a local psychosexual counsellor. The nurse did not continue with the course but hoped to do so when she had resolved problems in her life that were having an impact on her work.

Training to become a smear-taker

All nurses who take cervical smears should have undertaken an appropriate course. Various courses are available:

◆ The Family Planning Courses ENB 901 and A08 have now been superseded by courses in reproductive and sexual health that may not necessarily include cervical cytology training; each course will have to be looked at carefully to check that the contents fulfil your specific needs. The 8103 and S103 are such courses and nowadays are linked with universities.

◆ The Marie Curie Cancer Screening Courses for Practice Nurses are run throughout the UK (see Resources).

◆ Many PCTs/organizations are now running basic courses in cervical cytology which include both theory and practice. The NHSCSP has been instrumental in helping produce an excellent aid to training: 'Resource Pack for Training Smear Takers' (NHSCSP, 1998b) that has enabled trainers to offer a common core of learning to all smear-takers. This has helped to introduce consistency within the cervical screening programme and provides learning to a minimum recognized standard. An important part of the course is having a supervisor to work with, and be able to consult at various stages throughout the course. A portfolio is kept by the trainee and all elements of the course have to be completed, including the auditing of at least 20 smears with an overall adequacy rate of 80%, before a certificate of basic competence is given.

The British Society for Clinical Cytology (BSCC) brought out a new video/CD with a booklet and workbook (see Resources for further details). This resource should be used as part of the above mentioned Training Pack.

Smear taking should not be task-orientated. A sound knowledge of relevant anatomy and physiology, the natural history of the disease, associated risk factors, abnormalities and possible treatment would not only be a distinct advantage to you but also to your clients, to whom you can give up-to-date information and advice.

It is quite common for many of the more popular courses to be over-subscribed. There can be problems getting funding to attend courses and it is not always easy to get time away from work. 'In-house' training from doctors and experienced nurses may be an alternative, and can be excellent for practical sessions, but the knowledge gained from a reputable course is invaluable.

Information for women before the smear

Before attending for a cervical smear, women should be provided with information about how to prepare for the procedure. This could be in the form of a leaflet given out in your practice or clinic, or details given over the telephone when appointments might be made.

◆ 'Ideally your smear should be taken half-way between your periods

◆ Avoid having a bath on the day of your smear: a shower or stand-up wash would be better

◆ For about 48 hours before your smear use a condom or abstain from sexual intercourse

◆ If you have recently used a vaginal pessary for treating an infection such as thrush, it is advisable to have a period before your next smear, to make sure all traces of the pessary have gone

◆ If you are using an oestrogen cream, do not apply on the day of your smear.'

This useful information is based on common sense and will enable you to obtain the best possible smear for cytological analysis. Remember these are ideals, and few women can manage all of them. The most important factor is that she is not too near the time of her period.

Informed choice and consent

The woman should be fully informed of the reason for the procedure and the implications for her future health and well-being. To help women make an informed choice about whether or not to have a smear taken, all eligible women now receive a leaflet, 'Cervical Screening – The Facts', with their invitation. The leaflet explains the benefits and limitations of cervical screening.

Consent. The law in England and Wales assumes that every adult (18 years and over) has the capacity (or competence) to consent to treatment unless it can be proved otherwise. The NMC (2002a) states: 'as a registered nurse or midwife, you must obtain consent before you give any treatment or care' and 'when obtaining valid consent, you must be sure that it is:

◆ Given by a legally competent person
◆ Given voluntarily
◆ Informed'.

You do not need written consent to take a smear, but it is useful to reiterate all of the above information before starting the procedure.

Women with learning disabilities registered with GPs are invited to attend for smears, and this can pose problems for the woman herself and for the health professional who is to take the smear. To enable the woman to make an informed choice as to whether she needs a smear, a booklet, *Good Practice in Cervical Screening for Women with Learning Difficulties*, has been produced by the NHSCSP, and is designed to be used alone or with the help of a carer. Additionally other specialist health professionals have formulated their own resources to use with their clients, based on the original work from the NHSCSP. From a smear-taker's perspective it would be helpful if such a resource could be brought along to the consultation with some form of acknowledgement that the woman is making an informed choice.

Taking a cervical smear

A smear test should be taken in such a way as to provide an adequate sample for assessment with the minimum of distress or discomfort to your client.

Environment

Privacy is an essential prerequisite when a smear is taken. Ideally the room should also:

◆ Be warm
◆ Have a screen around the examination couch
◆ Have a good adjustable lamp
◆ Have a trolley or work-surface next to the couch
◆ Have a sink with hot and cold water supply.

The examination should be performed without interruptions.

Equipment

A note from the author: I am continuing to describe equipment needed to undertake the traditional Papanicolaou smear, as this method will continue for some time yet until liquid-based cytology is rolled out throughout the UK by 2008. See page 366.

◆ An autoclave which is regularly serviced and complies with current guidelines (DoH, 1988, 1994) if instruments are sterilized within the clinic
◆ Vaginal speculae (stainless steel or disposable in various sizes)
◆ Cytology slides with frosted ends and a sharp pencil
◆ Fixative containing alcohol and carbo wax (dropper or spray)
◆ Assorted spatulae and cervical brushes currently recommended
◆ Swabs for culture
◆ Latex examination gloves, protein-free or non-latex
◆ Water-based lubricating jelly
◆ Smear request forms and boxes for transporting slides
◆ Container with preservative if liquid-based cytology is used.

Interview and completion of the smear form

It is very important to record a menstrual/obstetric/contraceptive history in the client's notes as these are relevant to cervical cytology. This is also a good opportunity for your client to

---

Box 13.3 Key questions to ask prior to taking a smear

- ◆ Do you understand the purpose of this test?

- ◆ Do you have any bleeding after sexual intercourse (post-coital)?

- ◆ Are you currently using a method of contraception?

- ◆ Do you have any intermenstrual bleeding (if the patient is using oral contraception this may be the reason)?

- ◆ Do you have any pain during or after sexual intercourse (dyspareunia)?

- ◆ Do you have painful or heavy periods? (This would be important if the pattern and severity had altered without any changes in circumstances or lifestyle.)

- ◆ Have you noticed any change in your vaginal discharge?

---

air any anxieties or recent problems she may have had. Key questions are listed in Box 13.3.

With the appropriate range of questions you will have formed a full picture of the woman's menstrual and sexual health. Relevant information should be recorded in her notes. It is very important to allow your client to know what is being recorded, and to check that she does not object to you writing an item down that she may have disclosed which is of a sensitive or confidential nature. Useful reading is the NMC's guidelines for records and record keeping (NMC, 2002b).

It is a good idea at this point (prior to taking the smear) to write in pencil the name and date of birth of the woman on the frosted end of the glass slide, at the same time ensuring (by wiping with a tissue) that the slide is free from dust and grease.

Changes to the national HMR101 test request/report form

A number of amendments to the national HMR101 form are now in place:

- ◆ The four options previously asked in the 'reason for smear' section did not cover all the valid reasons for taking a smear. Not only

that, but 'clinically indicated' was included which is inappropriate for a screening test.

- ◆ Two questions have been added to the 'clinical data' section to support the requirements detailed in NHSCSP publication no. 1 (NHSCSP, 2004). The cervix must be visualized at the time the smear is taken and the full circumference of the cervix must be sampled. The new questions are:

- ◆ 'Cervix visualized – Yes or No?' and

- ◆ '360° sweep – Yes or No?'

- ◆ Other minor amendments include changes to historic references (e.g. 'FHSA') and to improve the layout of the form. A small space labelled 'ID' has been allocated for smear-taker identification. This information is not mandatory but laboratories may find it helpful for reporting smear quality to individual smear-takers, but would only be provided by local agreement where a suitable coding scheme has been established and agreed.

- ◆ Local variations to the form will be allowed, and single-part and multi-part versions will still be available.

Preprinted forms with the woman's full details may be available in the near future for use in primary care, but will not be available in other services (e.g. family planning clinics) where women might chose to attend as an alternative to their GP.

It remains highly important for these forms to be completed clearly and correctly (see checklist in Box 13.4).

Changes to the frequency of cervical screening

New recommendations made by Cancer Research UK scientists have changed the optimal frequency of cervical screening (Sasieni *et al.*, 2003):

- ◆ First invitation age: 25 years
- ◆ 3-yearly: 25–49 years
- ◆ 5-yearly: 50–64 years.

Women over 65 should only be screened if they have not been screened since the age of 50.

> **Box 13.4** Checklist for filling in the laboratory request form
>
> ◆ Client's name (correctly spelt) and maiden name if appropriate
>
> ◆ Address with postcode
>
> ◆ Date of birth
>
> ◆ NHS number is important, it can be found on the invitation letter if the PCA has requested the test
>
> ◆ Today's date
>
> ◆ The first day of the last menstrual period, or bleed if using oral contraception or hormone replacement therapy (see page 356 for relevance of this)
>
> ◆ Date of the last smear
>
> ◆ Contraceptive type: oral contraceptive, injectable contraceptive or implant. HRT type with name. State if intrauterine device (IUD) or intrauterine system (IUS) is present
>
> ◆ Complete reason for smear, e.g. call/recall; previous abnormal
>
> ◆ If early recall, state last test result or if known give the slide serial number from the previous laboratory form.

Women who do not need smears

Women are sent a request for a smear by age alone. This will mean that many women who do not need smears at the present time are sent for. Austoker and McPherson (1992) state that 'all women aged 20–64 who are or ever have been sexually active should be offered screening'.

Never sexually active

During the interview with your client you should be able to sensitively ascertain if she is or ever has been sexually active. This could be by asking 'are you using any contraception at the moment?' If the answer is 'no' it may mean that she is celibate or trying to become pregnant or that she or her partner is sterilized. If this is not the case then the conversation could continue: 'if you don't mind me asking, are you sexually active?' It may be necessary to be even more explicit: 'sexual activity' does not have to include sexual intercourse.

If it is found that a smear is not appropriate at this time, it is worth mentioning that if circumstances change and she becomes sexually active then she can return for a smear. The Primary Care Agency (PCA) should be informed by writing only 'not applicable at this time' on the tear-off portion of the invitation letter; she will be recalled at a suitable interval, depending on national guidelines.

Many nurses have been in the embarrassing position of having prepared a woman for a smear, only to get to the point of looking at her vaginal opening (introitus) to then have doubts as to whether she has ever had sexual intercourse. Unfortunately, the woman has had to go through the ordeal of very nearly having a procedure undertaken that is not appropriate.

The NHSCSP says that in this case the chance of developing cervical cancer is very low. They do not say 'no risk', but leave the decision up to the individual woman.

It need not be a wasted journey for the woman if she finds she does not need a smear, as teaching breast self-awareness (see page 309) and giving health promotion information on other well-woman issues will be useful.

Previous hysterectomy

Women who have had a hysterectomy for benign reasons do not need vault smears.

Women who have had a subtotal hysterectomy for benign reasons such as menorrhagia need regular smears with routine recall (Austoker *et al.*, 2003). A woman may have had a subtotal hysterectomy through personal choice or due to technical difficulties during surgery.

A hysterectomy undertaken for CIN2 or CIN3 with apparent complete excision is different, and vault smears should be performed. Vault smears are not part of the NHSCSP and follow-up should be in accordance with the recommendations of the woman's gynaecologist. Austoker *et al.* (2003) suggest the following frequency:

◆ Vault smear at 6 months

◆ Vault smear at 12 months – if negative result, discontinue all further vault smears

◆ Gynaecological referral if abnormalities are suspected.

Women under the screening age of 25 years

Cervical cancer is rare in women under 20. Teenagers' bodies, particularly the cervix, are still developing, which means young women may get an abnormal smear result when there is nothing wrong. This could lead to unnecessary treatment so screening young women might do more harm than good. Under the age of 25 years, invasive cancer is extremely rare, but changes in the cervix are common. Although lesions treated in very young women may prevent cancers from developing many years later, the evidence (Sasieni *et al.*, 2003) suggests screening could start at age 25. Lesions that are destined to progress will be screen-detectable and those that would regress will no longer be a source of anxiety. Young women therefore will not have to undergo unnecessary investigations and treatments.

We should advise young women under the screening age of 25, who are concerned about risks of developing cervical cancer or their sexual health, to seek up-to-date advice from a health professional in primary care/family planning or GUM services.

The change to the age of commencement for screening may be contentious amongst health professionals who will be at the forefront of explaining the changes to women, and may find it difficult to refuse requests for smears from those between the age of 20 and 24.

Taking the smear

Prior to starting the procedure, run through a checklist of preparations (Box 13.5).

Warm (or cool) the speculum under running water to reach body temperature. (Nowadays good-quality disposable perspex speculae are available as an alternative to metal.) If necessary, lightly smear the sides but not the end of the speculum with a water-based lubricant; usually the warm water is sufficient. Inspect the vulva for any sore areas, genital warts or unusual skin textures or colours. A gentle one-finger examination to locate the cervix can be helpful but care should be taken that the immediate area surrounding the os is not touched roughly. Pass the

---

> **Box 13.5** Checklist prior to taking a smear
>
> ◆ Does your client need to empty her bladder?
>
> ◆ Is all the equipment needed on a trolley/work-surface as close as possible to the examination couch?
>
> ◆ Have you asked her permission to take the smear?
>
> ◆ Is your client in a comfortable position on the couch with underwear removed?
>
> ◆ Have you offered your client a cover, if she is not wearing a petticoat?

---

speculum into the vagina gently, with due regard to the woman's reaction. Locate and visualize the cervix, making sure the cervical os is well in view. It is only after the os has been seen that the appropriate spatula can be chosen. Note the position of the SCJ to ensure that the transformation zone is sampled. The NHSCSP when looking at standards for cytology stated:

> It is the responsibility of the smear-taker to make every effort to sample the whole of the transformation zone (TZ). The cervix must be visualized at the time the smear is taken and the full circumference of the cervix must be sampled. Primary screening should not be carried out with an endocervical brush alone. Evidence of TZ sampling is not firm evidence that the cervix has been adequately sampled. It is only evidence that part of the TZ has been sampled.
>
> (NHSCSP, 2000)

Additionally, advice given to laboratories: 'The smear should be reported as inadequate if the cervix is said by the smear-taker not to have been completely visualized or if the smear is said not to have been taken in an appropriate manner (e.g. "finger smear") unless abnormal cells are seen in which case it should be reported according to the degree of abnormality present'.

Insert the spatula well into the cervical os and rotate it twice (using pencil pressure) through 360°. A cervical brush may be used (if the os is very tight) but first the blunt end of a spatula should be rotated around the ectocervix, then the brush inserted for sampling the endocervix. Due to the horizontal position of the bristles there is no need to twist the brush through 360°, introducing it gently into the cervical canal and twisting through only about 45° is sufficient to sample the endocervical canal without causing too much discomfort and bleeding.

A plastic Cervex brush has the advantage of sampling both the endo- and ectocervix at the same time. Care should be taken, as the Cervex brush should only be rotated clockwise (Waddell, 1994) through five turns. One of the main findings of a systemic review and meta-analysis (Martin-Hirsch, 1999) was that the blunt-ended Ayre's spatula, when used alone, is the least effective device for cervical sampling and should be superseded by extended-tip spatulas for primary screening (Figure 13.8).

Quickly transfer the cells from the spatula on to the slide, using two lengthways strokes, spreading the specimen evenly. If a cervical brush is used, the specimen should be applied using a rolling action. Once the cells are removed from the cervix they are dying and must be preserved without delay. Whichever fixative is used it must be applied immediately, gently flooding the slide, and left to dry horizontally for at least 10–15 minutes. The more experienced smear-taker will remove the speculum at the same time as the sample is taken, having a receptacle at hand to drop the used speculum into. Nurses new to the procedure may find it better to leave the speculum in position until the specimen is fixed. Leaving the speculum in the vagina also has the advantage of your being able to have a second look at the cervix and to note its condition and any contact bleeding that might have occurred.

Bacterial swabs could be taken after the smear if there is a heavy or unusual discharge, if the cervix looks sore or if your client has commented on symptoms arising from her vaginal discharge.

Gently remove the speculum, making sure that it is clear of the cervix before allowing the blades to start closing. This can be achieved by holding the speculum at its hinges and carefully making tiny rotating movements as you move away from the cervix.

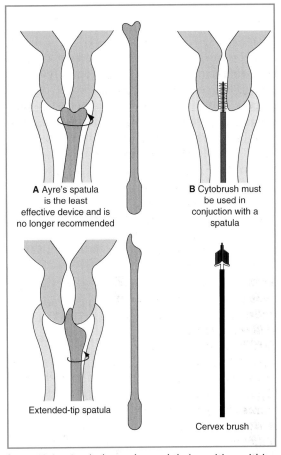

A Ayre's spatula is the least effective device and is no longer recommended

B Cytobrush must be used in conjuction with a spatula

Extended-tip spatula

Cervex brush

Figure 13.8 Cervical spatulae and their position within the external os. (Redrawn with permission from Szarewski, A., 1994.)

Bimanual examination of the pelvis

Bimanual pelvic examination need not be undertaken as a routine procedure on an asymptomatic woman. However, if the woman has any of the following symptoms a bimanual examination of the pelvis should be done (RCN, 1995):

◆ Very painful and/or heavy periods

◆ Intermenstrual bleeding

◆ Urinary symptoms

◆ Abdominal swelling

◆ Lower abdominal pain or discomfort

◆ Pain on sexual intercourse (dyspareunia)

◆ Post-coital bleeding.

(The second, fifth, sixth and seventh symptoms in the above list can also be symptoms of chlamydia infection, see page 398.)

If you are not trained to undertake this, it is advisable to ask for assistance from a relevantly trained nurse or doctor. If this is not possible, discuss with your client whether she could return at her convenience to complete the check.

If she has none of the symptoms mentioned, a simple check for cervical excitation could be performed:

◆ Ask the client's permission to examine her

◆ Apply lubricating jelly to the index and third finger of the examining hand

◆ Gently insert one finger into the vagina, followed by the second finger

◆ The idea is gently to hold the end of the cervix between the tips of the two fingers and move the cervix slightly from side to side (laterally)

◆ This should not cause any sudden pain or discomfort to your client

◆ If this is painful, it could be due to pelvic inflammatory disease (PID) (see page 531), a pregnancy outside of the uterus (ectopic) (see page 533), a deep-seated carcinoma or ovarian cysts

◆ Ask for a second opinion from an experienced nurse or doctor while keeping your client informed.

Completing the HMR101 laboratory form and your responsibilities

The clinical observations of the cervix should now be recorded on the laboratory form. It is not up to you to diagnose what has been observed on the cervix. It is much easier to describe exactly what is seen: 'red cervix, bled on contact', 'large ectropion-like area seen', greenish vaginal discharge at os'. The cyto-screener has only a few cells in front of him or her on which to base their report, therefore the more you can describe what is seen on the cervix the better. It is important for you to sign your own name and possibly print it underneath for clarity.

The cytology slides should dry for at least 15 minutes before they are put into the transport box.

Do not let individual slides come into contact with each other and do not overfill the transport box so that the last slide is touching the side of the box: it may adhere to the box and be overlooked at the laboratory and the specimen may be spoiled. Remember that if a slide is broken or is badly named or sent without its laboratory form it could mean your client having to return for a repeat smear which is both worrying and inconvenient for her.

Receiving results. It is officially your responsibility as the smear-taker to inform your client of how and when she will receive her results and what action to take if no results appear. All women should receive their results in writing. Eighty per cent should receive their results within 4 weeks of having had their smear, and 100% should have received results by 6 weeks (NHSCSP, 1996).

Finally, remember to offer advice and interpretation of smear results, should your client need to contact you.

The responsibilities of the smear-taker are outlined clearly in the *Resource Pack for Training Smear Takers* (NHSCSP, 1998b).

Liquid-based cytology (LBC)

In October 2003 the NHSCSP announced that following recommendations from the National Institute for Clinical Excellence (NICE), LBC will be introduced across the cervical screening programme in England. The decision was based on evidence from the three pilot project sites in Bristol, Newcastle and Norwich. The roll-out of the new system will take 5 years, with cytology training schools being part of the first phase of training for laboratory staff.

LBC is a new way of preparing cervical samples for examination in the laboratory. All laboratories will have new machinery to screen the samples (this part of the new technology will be the most expensive).

How will it be different for smear-takers? The sampling devices will be either the cervex type of plastic brush or in some cases the cervical brush (see Figure 13.8) which all smear-takers will know how to use from their basic training course. Instead of spreading the specimen on a slide, the smear-taker will either shake the brush in a vial which will contain preservative fluid, or break off the head of the brush into the vial which will be specifically labelled with your client's details. Which of the two methods used will depend on which system your laboratory has purchased. It is not thought that proposed future additional training for smear-takers will be lengthy and some of it may include the use of a CD-ROM. Scotland is currently using such a resource as part of their LBC training.

The sample is sent to the laboratory where it is spun and treated to remove obscuring material, e.g. mucus or pus, and a random sample of the remaining cells is taken. A thin layer of the cells is deposited onto a slide where it will be screened.

The benefits of LBC will be:

◆ Reduction in the number of inadequate smears from 9% to 1–2% (as reported by the three pilot sites using LBC). This will reduce the pressure on both smear-takers and cyto-screeners, and importantly reduce the anxiety that women may suffer who are recalled for a repeat smear

◆ Reduces the risk of human error during 'spreading and fixing' of the specimen

◆ Testing for HPV and chlamydia using the remaining specimen in the vial is being considered, (again this would depend on the system used in the laboratory).

The estimated cost of changing from conventional screening to LBC is £10 million, but the reduction in the 'inadequate' rate will reduce the overall costs of screening, as fewer smears will have to be taken, prepared and read (NHSCSP, 2003).

Problems inserting the vaginal speculum

At all times you should be sensitive to the woman's reactions, particularly as you are about to insert the speculum into the vagina. Many things could happen:

◆ Your client clamps her thighs together and says 'I can't go through with this'. You should

cease the procedure and gently ask the woman what is on her mind and would she like to talk about it. Among an almost limitless list of causes, this may reveal such things as sexual abuse; rape; a previous miscarriage or termination of pregnancy; depression; or a previous bad experience of a gynaecological examination. The condition when a woman cannot allow a speculum (or a penis) to enter her vagina is called vaginismus (Valins, 1988) (see page 87). The smear should be delayed until the woman feels able to cope with the procedure; often just the fact that she has revealed an anxiety to someone is an enormous step forward. She also may need referring on to a counsellor before she can progress

◆ The opening to the vagina (introitus) looks small and when a fingertip is put into the entrance to the vagina an intact hymen is present. The woman has not had sexual intercourse (virgo intacta). You should explain that women who have never had sexual intercourse do not need smears, but if her circumstances change, she should return for a smear some time after she becomes sexually active, or if this coincides with a test request

◆ When the outer folds of the vagina (labia majora) are parted, the inner folds (labia minora) look unusual; the whole area looks as though it has been surgically treated; the introitus may be very small and scar tissue may be obvious. If these signs are present in a woman from the east, north-eastern or western parts of Africa, or some parts of the Middle East or South-East Asia, it may well be that she has undergone female genital mutilation (Box 13.6)

◆ Women who have had a caesarean section may have tight vaginal muscles which have never been stretched by the head of the baby in the birth canal. The inserting of the speculum can be quite uncomfortable. You should try to pick a speculum that is not too big; it is useful to have a good assortment of sizes and lengths available

◆ Peri-menopausal and post-menopausal women often present with drying and

> **Box 13.6** Female genital mutilation
>
> This is a collective term used for different degrees of mutilation of the female external genitals (RCN, 1994). As more refugees from Africa arrive in the UK, so more nurses working in primary care will come across women who have been genitally mutilated.
>
> The procedure is illegal in Britain under the Prohibition of Female Circumcision Act 1985, although parents determined to have it carried out may take their children abroad.
>
> It has no benefits to the woman and can cause problems such as painful intercourse (dyspareunia), no orgasms (as the clitoris is removed) and urinary and menstrual problems. Often the first time the mutilation is observed is during pregnancy. Problems commonly occur during labour. There are no easy answers to this problem, but when found, you should be sensitive, non-judgemental and supportive to the woman. It may be impossible to take a smear without surgical intervention. (See also page 134.)

thinning of the vaginal epithelium. Again, a smaller speculum should be chosen and the use of lubricating jelly (sparingly smeared) on the blades will make the procedure more comfortable, as described in the Report of the Intercollegiate Working Party (RCOG *et al.*, 1987).

Doubts when the cervix is visualized

If the cervix is covered with thick mucus, do not clean it: cells that might be abnormal may be present. Take a first sweep of the cervix with the spatula, immediately followed by a second sweep with another spatula; spread them side by side on the slide, fixing without delay. On the laboratory form explain: 'left side of slide – first sweep of cervix; right side of slide – second sweep of cervix'. If the laboratory does not object, two slides could be sent marked '1st' and '2nd'.

If there is a mucus plug in the cervical os, this can be carefully lifted off without disturbing the cervical mucus with the tip of an Aylesbury spatula and discarded. If this plug of mucus were to get on to the slide it would be a very difficult specimen for the cyto-screener to look at.

If the cervix bleeds on the first sweep round with the spatula, do not make a second sweep. Spread the specimen immediately and fix and record the bleeding on the laboratory request form (all of the above will not be a problem with the new LBC method of collecting and sending the sample).

If the cervix looks sore and very red, take a high vaginal swab after the smear is taken and add a comment to the laboratory form. Your client should be told of the difference between cytology and bacteriology.

If there is a wide transformation zone on the ectocervix, take a first sweep with an Aylesbury spatula within the cervical os, and a second sweep with the blunt end of the spatula to sample the wide transformation zone. Spread the specimens side by side on the one slide and fix immediately.

A cervical polyp, which is an overgrowth of epithelial tissue (of varying sizes) often on a stalk and looking a little like a grape, may be seen (see Colour plate 4). Polyps are rarely associated with malignancy, but it is felt they are worth a referral to the gynaecological outpatients for removal. There is a chance that the polyp may originate from the endometrium on a long stalk, therefore profuse bleeding might occur on removal. Record on the laboratory form that you have seen 'polyp-type structure', explain to your client, and follow your policy for referral.

If the cervix looks unusual in any way it is appropriate to get a second opinion from another practitioner. It is quite acceptable for a client to be referred for further investigations/colposcopy on the look of the cervix alone.

Pelvic inflammatory disease (PID)

If PID is suspected then a chlamydia and endocervical swab needs to be taken. If there are no facilities for taking such swabs or you do not feel competent to undertake this kind of sampling then the procedure should not be attempted; your client should be referred to a clinic of genitourinary medicine (GUM) where the appropriate expertise is available.

A swab result returned as negative might still mean that *Chlamydia* is present if the correct sampling procedure has not been carried out. *Chlamydia* left undetected and untreated could lead to salpingitis and pelvic inflammatory disease with the high risk of future fertility problems.

Common faults when trying to locate the cervix

You can never judge by outward appearances (height, weight) exactly where and in what position your client's cervix will be. The 'one-finger' examination will be a good guide as to the position and angle of the cervix.

Incorrect position of the speculum

You have inserted the speculum into the vagina, open up the blades and all you see is a space surrounded by the vaginal walls. Often this is because you are in the posterior fornix.

Solution. Gently ease the speculum towards you while watching carefully to see if the cervix drops into view; it is useful to ask your client to cough. When having to manoeuvre your speculum while it is in the vagina, great care should be taken not to cause pain or discomfort. A useful tip is to hold the lower or posterior part of the speculum with your thumb and index finger and apply slight pressure which moves the speculum slightly.

Good idea. When inserting the speculum, open it up slightly when about half of it is inside the vagina; you may be surprised to see the cervix coming into view sooner than you would have thought. If it is seen, continue introducing the closed speculum towards the observed position of the cervix.

Acute position of the cervix (1)

The cervix is pointing into the anterior wall of the vagina, due to a retroverted uterus. You cannot encompass the cervix with your speculum.

Solution. Ask your client to half-sit-up resting on her elbows (if possible), keeping her informed of why you are asking her to do this, or ask her to put her hands underneath her buttocks to raise her pelvis.

Acute position of the cervix (2)

The cervix is pointing into the posterior wall of the vagina, due to a very anteverted uterus. You cannot encompass the cervix with your speculum.

Solution. Ask your client to press down with her hands over her lower abdomen (retro-pubic area) or ask her to bring her knees up against her abdomen holding them with her arms. Either of these solutions could help flip the cervix forward, allowing you to locate it with your speculum.

If these fail, ask her to get into the left-lateral position where, by inserting the speculum into the vagina from the back, the cervix should be able to be viewed. This may seem awkward initially, but when you have viewed a difficult cervix once this way, you will find it a useful alternative position. To undertake this you would need a moveable light source.

Prolapsed vaginal walls obscuring the view of the cervix

This is a common problem. You insert the speculum and can only see the lateral walls of the vagina fall into your field of view.

Solution. Instead of turning the speculum through 90° (just after you have inserted the tip into the introitus) keep the speculum in the position of having the blades remain in the lateral position, then continue introducing the speculum further into the vagina. The walls will be against the blades and unable to collapse. This method can only be used if the space or area around your client's inner thighs allow.

Alternatively, use a condom or the finger of a clinical glove with the closed end cut off and 'sheath' the speculum with this. Either method will hold back the vaginal walls.

A very deep (posterior) cervix

Solution. Use a Winterton speculum, or a large-size perspex disposable one, which has extra-long blades, or ask your client to press over her lower abdomen, or come up into the semi-sitting position, either of which may push the uterus down a little, allowing you to visualize and encompass the cervix.

It is important for you to remember the very delicate structures that your speculum may be pressed closely against:

◆ The clitoris

◆ The labia minora

◆ The labia majora – remember pubic hairs can easily be snagged in the tiny screws of the speculum hinges.

It is essential to keep checking that your speculum is not pressing on or pinching any of these structures.

It is also important to keep your client informed of what is happening during the examination and why you are asking her to do a certain thing. Reassure her that she is not abnormal and that each person has slight variations within their body which makes your job more 'interesting'.

A good standard to follow is to treat all your clients the way you would like to be treated yourself. As you progress and see more and more cervices, you will realize that there are indeed many different shapes and sizes, ranging from small flat, to long pointed ones.

The opportunistic smear

You should seize the chance of doing the 'opportunistic' smear when it presents itself, even if the woman has consulted you on an entirely different subject, as you may never see her again.

It is on such occasions when you have a woman with you and you have been trying to encourage her to have a smear, or she may have had a slightly abnormal result previously that, regardless of the fact that she may even be menstruating at the time, it is thought best to take the smear than not have one at all. A bloodstained slide is easier to read by the cyto-screener if it is spread thinly.

It will always be up to the individual to decide whether or not to take up the offer of a smear test and it is important not to become coercive or judgemental, but to offer all the known facts regarding screening and abnormalities of the cervix which will allow your client to make an informed choice.

You should discourage people from calling it the 'cancer smear' or 'cancer test' and try to dispel myths and misinformation surrounding the test. Elkind *et al.* (1989) explain how many women thought the test was inappropriate for them.

Any women who presents with the following symptoms will need further investigations which could include the taking of chlamydia and endocervical swabs and a gynaecological referral.

These are not reasons for taking a smear:

◆ Bloodstained vaginal discharge

◆ Intermenstrual bleeding

◆ Post-coital bleeding

◆ Post-menopausal bleeding.

Any woman who presents with abnormal vaginal bleeding should always be investigated and referred for a specialist opinion (NHS Executive, 1998).

Obstacles and dangers

Beware of the woman who always seems to have a 'period' so that she 'cannot have a smear today'. The 'period' that always gets in the way of a smear being taken could be due to some underlying pathology, or it might be that she is using her 'period' as an excuse for a smear not to be performed. You may well decide, with your client's permission, to take a smear at this time whether she is menstruating or not. Referral to a gynaecologist should be considered to investigate the bleeding.

Sometimes our clients are not as knowledgeable as we sometimes presume. The difference between a bacterial swab and a cervical smear can be confusing.

You may have a new client with you, whose records have not arrived from her previous doctor. On enquiring about her last smear test she says that she had one some time ago and that the result was negative. Hopefully her medical records will appear soon to verify this, but there is always the chance that she might only have had a swab taken and her last smear was abnormal and that she is overdue for the needed repeat.

Technological advances with the electronic transfer of patients' details between different primary care organizations make the scenario just discussed less of a problem. Good practice is to check if you are in any doubt at all regarding past smear history. This could be done simply by contacting your client's previous surgery (her records may still be there) or contact the Primary Care Agency concerned.

The postnatal smear

Before the setting up of the call/recall system in 1988, opportunistic smears were taken at the 6-week postnatal check. Many doctors and nurses are mistakenly continuing this practice. A smear should only be taken if it is due under the NHSCSP. If the smear is due, ideally it should be postponed until at least 12 weeks postnatally.

Often smears taken at 6 weeks have to be repeated due to 'postnatal, inflammatory or atrophic changes' and may cause needless anxiety.

Smear results and classifications

Waddell (1994) states that an 'adequate smear is one which is suitable for the purpose for which it was obtained', therefore it follows that an inadequate smear is unsuitable for the purpose for which it was obtained. The *Cervical Smear Results Explained* booklet (see Resources) describes the possible cervical screening outcomes and explains what they mean and the recommended action to be taken in each case.

Inadequate smears

There will always be a percentage of inadequate smears; over recent years the range nationally has been between 9.4% and 9.7% (NHSCSP, 2003).

Inadequate smears may be due to insufficient or unsuitable material being present; for example:

◆ Transformation zone not sampled sufficiently

◆ Excessive lubricant used

◆ Atrophic cervix, which can be due to low oestrogen levels not allowing exfoliation of cervical cells

◆ Cytolysis, which is the normal process of cell disintegration due to the high glycogen content in the cells during the second half of the menstrual cycle. Excessive cytolysis may render the smear unsuitable. If a repeat is requested the smear should be taken before ovulation, when the glycogen content is less

◆ Poor spreading of cervical mucus onto the slide

◆ Inadequate fixation; was the fixative shaken before use? Is the fixative out of date? Did you check to see that all the mucus was covered on the slide? Was the slide flooded too much, pushing off the cells? Was the slide laid horizontally and allowed to stand for at least 15 minutes to dry before putting it in the transport box?

◆ The smear consists mainly of blood/polymorphs/leucocytes or inflammatory exudate. Different laboratories use slightly different descriptions for these findings on a smear and, as the cervix should not be cleaned before sampling, this kind of result is out of the smear-taker's control. With the advent of LBC the laboratory will be able literally to wash away such debris.

If your laboratory reports a smear as 'inadequate' they will usually write details of why it is classified as such. If you have any concerns and need clarification about the result you should contact them for an explanation.

Incidental findings on smears

The cervical smear, although taken primarily to look for pre-cancer changes, may also identify or suggest the presence of infections. Care needs to be taken when discussing incidental findings on the smear as it is not commonly understood that possible infections (particularly sexually transmitted ones in this case) can be reported in this way on the asymptomatic woman.

Anaerobes or anaerobic bacteria

Organisms such as bacteria or fungi that can live without oxygen may be found in the moist airless genital tract.

Bacterial vaginosis or Gardnerella vaginalis

Laboratories no longer report on bacterial vaginosis or gardnerella, but may comment on 'organisms present, exclude infection' or 'cluecells present'. Clue cells are ordinary epithelial cells to which these bacteria become attached (see page 395).

Candida albicans/monilia/thrush

This is another quite innocent vaginal infection which often shows up on a smear and can give rise to 'many polymorphs' obscuring the cells on the slide. You should be guided by the laboratory's suggested action; if they are not happy with the sample, an early recall will be suggested.

Trichomonas vaginalis

This is a protozoan and is sexually transmitted, giving a frothy, fishy-smelling discharge with severe vaginal itching. The presence of *Trichomonas* makes cervical smears very difficult to read, often mimicking pre-cancer in the cervical cells. Your client and her partner should be treated with antibiotics. The laboratory will ask for a repeat smear after treatment. A *Trichomonas* infection can give the cervix the appearance of looking strawberry-like (see Colour plate 5).

Herpes Simplex Virus (HSV)

This can be identified on a cervical smear, and would be indicated by multinucleated giant cells.

Gonorrhoea and Chlamydia

These cannot be diagnosed from a cervical smear, but there can be intracellular detail that may suggest to the cyto-screener that one or the other is a possibility. The cytologist would suggest further bacterial investigations to be undertaken.

Actinomyces-type organisms

These are bacteria that live normally in the mouth and intestines. In women who have an intrauterine device (IUD) *in situ*, this bacterium can often colonize around the IUD and its threads, and show up on the cervical smear. Treatment of this will depend on whether the woman has any symptoms (see also page 285).

Human Papillomavirus (HPV) /koilocytosis

This is a very common result which has no treatment. Having HPV is not the same as having warts and this distinction is very important. HPV appearing alone on a smear result does not mean a referral for colposcopy is needed; it would be classified as 'borderline' and an early repeat requested.

Great care should be taken when discussing a result of HPV, as your client may wonder (particularly if she is in a stable, long-term relationship) how she came to have the virus. You should emphasize the fact that the natural history of HPV is fairly obscure, that it is very common and can lie dormant for many years before it is seen in cervical cells.

The main types (according to the DNA in the cell) of HPV associated with pre-cancer changes are HPV 16 and 18. These do not show up as genital warts in either women or men and there is no way of knowing if a man has it on his penis. To confuse things further, the genital warts that are visible are HPV 6 and HPV 11 and are not thought to be important as far as cervical cancer is concerned.

Your client may ask why men do not get penile cancer if they have HPV (albeit invisible). The answer lies in the difference between the soft vulnerable area of transformation zone on the cervix, compared to the tough squamous cells of the penis.

'Inflammatory smear' or 'inflammatory exudate'

These changes can be caused by a background infection. If there is a suspicion of an undiagnosed infection, full screening should be taken by yourself or GUM services. If all results from bacteriology are normal, but three consecutive smear results continue to be 'inflammatory', a colposcopy referral would be advised.

Borderline changes

This term is used to describe a cellular appearance that cannot definitely be described as normal. They are usually severe inflammatory changes on the borderline with mild dyskariosis.

The classification of inflammatory and borderline smears is very subjective, that is to say it depends on the particular cyto-screener who is looking at the cervical cells as to which classification is given. The presence of HPV infection is the main reason for recording borderline nuclear changes (Austoker *et al.*, 2003).

Cytology and histology

It is important to understand the difference between cytology and histology and to keep these distinctions in mind, as many people confuse cytological with histological terms.

Cytology

Cytology is the study of individual cells, focusing on the size and shape of the nucleus within the cytoplasm, giving due regard to the general shape of the cell itself. This screening is undertaken on cervical smears by cyto-screeners in the laboratory.

The outer layer of the cervix (ectocervix) is covered by thick, stratified squamous epithelium of up to 20 layers of cells in healthy women in their reproductive years. The cells arise at the basement membrane and mature in an orderly way, gaining increasing amounts of cytoplasm as they approach the surface of the epithelium.

They appear in the cervical smear as parabasal, intermediate and superficial squamous cells. If cell division at the basement membrane is defective, abnormal nuclei are formed: these are *dyskariotic* cells (dys means 'bad' or 'abnormal' and karyon means 'kernal' or 'nucleus', i.e. bad nucleus). The cyto-screener looking at the cervical cells can identify changes in the squamous cells which, in a high proportion of women, if left untreated might become cancer.

There are three grades of abnormality between a normal cell and a tumour cell which the cyto-screener can recognize (Figure 13.9):

◆ Mild dyskariosis

◆ Moderate dyskariosis

◆ Severe dyskariosis.

The British Society for Clinical Cytology is considering revising the terminology used in reporting

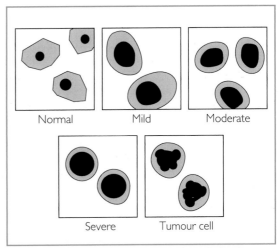

Figure 13.9 Dyskariotic changes in the cell. (Redrawn with permission from Barker, 1987.)

smears, but at present no final ratification has been given.

Histology

Histology is the study of a portion (or biopsy) of epithelium from the cervix, looked at under the microscope. This kind of sample could only be obtained at colposcopy.

Just as dyskariosis is a cytological term describing the abnormal nucleus, *dysplasia* is a histological term describing the abnormal architecture of the epithelium (dys means 'bad' and plasia means 'change', i.e. bad change).

Looking at a sample of cervical epithelium under the microscope, the histologist can see how far through the layers of squamous cells the dyskariotic cells have progressed.

Cervical intraepithelial neoplasia (CIN)

Cervical intraepithelial neoplasia (CIN) means 'new change in the outer layer of the cervix'. There are three levels of CIN (Figure 13.10):

◆ *CIN I* occurs if just the outer third of the epithelium is abnormal (mildly dyskariotic cells appear in the smear) and the epithelium is said to show *mild dysplasia*. CIN I may resolve without any intervention but more

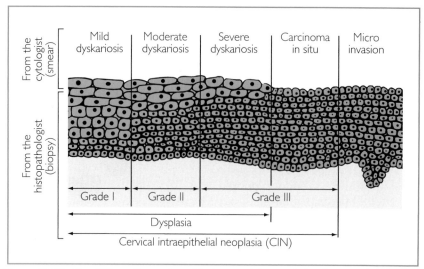

Figure 13.10 The CIN grading system. (Redrawn with permission from Barker, 1987.)

frequent smears may be necessary for a period of time following national guidelines

◆ *CIN II* occurs if one-half to two-thirds of the epithelium is involved (moderate dyskariotic cells appear in the smear) and the epithelium is said to show *moderate dysplasia*

◆ *CIN III* occurs if the full thickness of the epithelium is involved, with complete architectural chaos between the basement membrane and the surface of the epithelium (severely dyskariotic cells appear in the smear) and the epithelium is said to show *severe dysplasia*. This is also called *carcinoma in situ*. This CIN III is still 'skin deep', being confined by the basement membrane.

CIN I, II and III are histological findings, but many cytologists in a bid to give as much information as possible on the smear result will say 'moderate dyskariosis suggestive of CIN II', meaning that they are predicting that if a biopsy was taken the result would probably be CIN II.

Microinvasion

If the basement membrane has been breached by the abnormal cancer cells for a distance of 2 or 3 mm then microinvasion is said to have occurred. This is the first sign that the abnormal cells on the surface of the cervix are becoming malignant and starting to invade the cervix.

Invasive tumour

If the depth of invasion reaches 5 mm, involvement of the lymphatic channels and blood vessels becomes likely. At this stage the woman would no longer be asymptomatic but may present with a bloodstained vaginal discharge, intermenstrual bleeding, post-coital bleeding or post-menopausal bleeding.

On examination of the cervix the tumour may appear as a bleeding ulcer.

If left to invade further, the tumour may spread down the vagina, up into the uterus and out onto the ligaments on the side of the cervix and uterus (which holds the uterus in place). The tumour may invade forward into the bladder causing haematuria, or it may invade backwards into the rectum causing blood in the stools.

The woman may well have sought advice earlier with a low, dull, dragging backache.

Invasive cervical cancer is staged as described by (Barker, 1987):

◆ Ib   The cancer is confined to the cervix and uterus

- ◆ IIa The cancer has encroached onto the top of the vagina

- ◆ IIb The cancer has invaded the tissue around the cervix (parametrium)

- ◆ III There is extensive involvement of the vagina and invasion out to the bones of the side wall of the pelvis

- ◆ IV The cancer has invaded beyond the pelvis and adjacent organs such as the bladder or rectum.

The nurse's role in giving results

The cytology laboratory will report the result of the smear and recommend the timing for future recall or if treatment or referral is necessary. We all should comply with this and if we are in doubt or have a query should contact the laboratory. There are mechanisms that come into play when a smear result needs a referral to a colposcopy clinic. The NHSCSP document *Guidelines on Failsafe Actions* (NCN, 1992) explains this. If you are the nurse who took the cervical smear and your client has come to trust your approach, attitude and knowledge, then she may well come to you for clarification, reassurance or further information.

It is important for you to share with your client all the information written on the smear report, ideally reading the report together. This will only prove difficult if you are not sure of your facts. It is a recommendation that when a woman is sent a result that is not normal, the appropriate NHSCSP leaflet is enclosed (see Resources). We should be willing to act as advocates for our clients, and not fall into the trap of slightly altering the facts so that we feel more comfortable with the information we are giving.

Colposcopy

'Colpos' means bay, hollow or, in this case, vagina; 'oscopy' means to inspect. Therefore, colposcopy means inspection of the vagina (to enable viewing of the cervix). Colposcopy clinics are an important part of the NHSCSP, being the secondary screeners and the point of referral for GPs.

SCENARIO

The nurse had worked hard in encouraging Mary to have a long-overdue smear. They had got to know one another from Mary's visits to the surgery with each of her four children over a period of years. Now aged 46, Mary had a bit more time for herself and had come into the surgery for a 'check-up'. She had heard from a friend that she could come and have her blood pressure checked, and be given advice on diet. She said that she would love to try and stop smoking.

When the subject of having a cervical smear arose the nurse was aware of a feeling of apprehension in Mary and managed to give reassuring information and advice about the improved cervical screening service. Mary said she would make an appointment to see the nurse at one of the weekly well-woman sessions.

A few days later the nurse was pleased to see Mary at the surgery for her well-woman check. Mary was visibly relieved when everything was over. The nurse felt very pleased for having encouraged Mary to have the smear taken. One week later the nurse was shocked to see the smear result returned early as 'severe dyskariosis suggestive of CIN III. Invasion cannot be ruled out, requires urgent referral'. The nurse immediately felt as though she had just opened the proverbial 'can of worms'. She contacted Mary herself, as she had been the only person involved with the smear taking and consequent results.

The nurse explained exactly what all the terminology meant on the report which she saw was helpful to Mary. The most worrying thing for Mary was the next step – where, when and what would happen. The nurse told Mary all about the appointment for colposcopy that had been arranged, that it was an outpatient appointment, and what to expect there.

The colposcopy clinic sent Mary a leaflet of explanation before her visit which she discussed with the nurse. Mary came to see the nurse after she had been to the colposcopy clinic, where she had undergone investigations and treatment. Thankfully the cancer had not been invasive, but CIN III. Mary had been very aware that the nurse was actually feeling 'guilty' for being the one who had found the abnormality and reassured her that she was so thankful to have had the smear taken when she did. Mary admitted that she had been worried over the fact that she was very overdue in having a repeat smear and in a subconscious way was hoping that someone would talk her into having the test.

Mary thanked the nurse for all her help.

Colposcopy referrals are seen on an outpatient basis. There are parts of the country where laboratories are sending abnormal results direct to colposcopy clinics, which are then contacting women directly, thus removing the need for the referral to be made via the GP. Many colposcopy clinics also send out patient information leaflets giving details of what will happen at the consultation with clarification of some of the abnormalities that are being investigated (Box 13.7). This certainly helps to make the referral to a colposcopy clinic less of an ordeal due to fear of the unknown.

The colposcope

The colposcope is a binocular microscope which allows the whole cervix to be viewed in detail (Figure 13.11); it allows for magnification of up to 10 times life size (Barker, 1987). It can be used not only for inspection of the vagina and cervix but also of the vulva and anus. Hans Hinselman built his first colposcope in Germany in the 1920s, and this achieved widespread use in Britain from the 1960s onwards.

The woman can feel very frightened and alone, even though there will be a nurse present at colposcopy who will be able to give reassurance

> **Box 13.7** Useful information sent out by colposcopy clinics prior to a first consultation
>
> ◆ You should cancel your appointment if you are likely to be menstruating
>
> ◆ Bring a friend with you
>
> ◆ Arrange to have some time off work in case you have any treatment at your appointment; minor abnormalities may be dealt with the same day
>
> ◆ If you are pregnant you can still have colposcopy, but if you require treatment this may be deferred until after the birth of your baby
>
> ◆ Wear loose clothing, ideally in two halves, as you will be asked to remove your underwear
>
> ◆ It will be useful for you to know the first day of your last menstrual period
>
> ◆ Write down any questions that you would like to discuss.

and act as the 'vocal local' (Hopwood, 1990). Nowadays there may be the opportunity for the patient to see what is actually happening at the 'business end' of the couch on a television screen (via a video camera which is fixed to the colposcope). Some women may find this even more frightening, whilst others find it reassuring or even fascinating to watch the procedure. It is

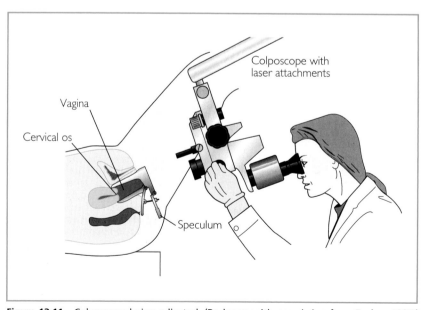

Figure 13.11 Colposcope being adjusted. (Redrawn with permission from Barker, 1987.)

important to be sensitive to the woman's feelings regarding this.

The procedure as far as the woman is concerned should be very similar to that of having a smear taken, apart from the fact she is on a special couch with her legs in a lithotomy position. A vaginal speculum is inserted and the colposcope is placed near to the vaginal opening. It is important for you to tell the woman that the rather complicated looking colposcope does not go into the vagina.

Nurse colposcopists

During the past decade many nurses have undergone further specialist training and have advanced their clinical role leading to a growing number of nurse colposcopists. Training requirements are laid down by the British Society of Colposcopy and Cervical Pathology (BSCCP) in conjunction with the Royal College of Obstetrics and Gynaecology (Shafi, 1999). There is an agreed curriculum for trainees with appropriate supervised clinical experience. Becoming a nurse colposcopist gives appropriately trained nurses the opportunity to use their experience and skills to their full potential, whilst also giving women increased choice (Flynn, 2000).

Three roles are recognized for nurses within the colposcopy service:

◆ A designated nurse with specialist skills to assist in the running of the clinic

◆ Nurses trained to perform colposcopy but not trained to perform treatment

◆ Nurses trained in diagnostic and therapeutic colposcopy.

The examination

Once the colposcope is in place, various procedures can be carried out:

◆ A repeat cervical smear may be taken

◆ The cervix may be swabbed with saline to remove any excessive discharge

◆ The colposcopist will note any polyps, retention cysts, ulcers or warts

◆ Dilute acetic acid is applied to the cervix to show up any protein-rich 'active' areas which will show up as extra white or 'acetowhite'. The degree of acetowhite change gives an indication of the likely severity of the underlying CIN, although the abnormality may not be the same throughout the affected area

◆ Lugol's iodine (1 part iodine, 2 parts potassium iodine, 97 parts distilled water) may be applied next. This is known as Schiller's test and is useful in delineating the extent of an abnormal area. The iodine reacts with glycogen (normally present in healthy, mature squamous cells), staining healthy areas dark brown. 'Active' areas produce less glycogen and so do not stain so darkly

◆ If the upper limit of the SCJ cannot be visualized then the extent of the lesion will not be known and it could extend much higher up in the endocervical canal. In such a case, local treatment at a colposcopy examination could not be carried out

◆ One or more colposcopically directed 'punch' biopsies may be taken from what appear to be the most severely affected areas. A local anaesthetic will be introduced into the cervix using a dental syringe with a very fine needle. Adrenaline may be added to the lignocaine to minimize bleeding.

Treatment of cervical intraepithelial neoplasia

Treatment of CIN can be achieved by local ablative therapy or by excision.

Local ablative therapy

Laser treatment

The laser beam is directed under colposcopic control and boils the water in the cells, vaporizing the tissue. The lesion is destroyed to a depth of approximately 1 cm. Sufficient depth is important as abnormalities often extend deep into the endocervical glands. The ablation should also extend beyond the margin of the lesion. This procedure has to a large extent been superseded by LLETZ. The advantages and disadvantages are listed in Box 13.8.

> **Box 13.8** Advantages and disadvantages of laser treatment
>
> **Advantages**
>
> ◆ Laser treatment is flexible; not only cervical but vaginal lesions can be treated
>
> ◆ The laser may also be used to take a cone biopsy for diagnostic purposes and as treatment
>
> ◆ The squamo-columnar junction remains accessible after treatment
>
> ◆ It does not affect childbearing.
>
> **Disadvantages**
>
> ◆ It may be uncomfortable and painful
>
> ◆ It uses an expensive piece of equipment
>
> ◆ The machine and extractor for smoke and vapour is noisy and can alarm people
>
> ◆ If an intrauterine device (IUD) is *in situ* it is difficult to avoid destroying the threads that protrude from the cervical os. Therefore the IUD is usually removed before the procedure, a new one being fitted straight away afterwards.

Cold coagulation

This is, in fact, not cold, but is not as hot as diathermy or laser. Probes are used depending on the contour of the area to be treated. They are heated electrically and are applied to the cervix for up to 30 seconds. This method has mainly been superseded by loop excision.

Cryocautery

This destroys the abnormal cells by freezing them via a cryoprobe which is applied to the cervix, through which a high-pressure gas such as nitrous oxide or carbon dioxide is released. This method has mainly been replaced by loop excision, but is still used for cervical ectopy (see page 358), an entirely physiological (normal) state which can sometimes cause excessive vaginal discharge or post-coital bleeding. Cryocautery is often used in this condition to 'seal' the affected area.

Excisional treatment

Diathermy – large loop excision

LLETZ (large loop excision of transformation zone) has become an increasingly popular method of treatment for CIN and could be used for routine management of CIN or reserved as a quick and acceptable outpatient alternative to other cone biopsy techniques.

There are different designs and sizes of loop which can be used to excise the abnormal tissue. The advantages and disadvantages are listed in Box 13.9.

After treatment a 'pack' of antibiotic or antiseptic cream is inserted into the vagina, which the woman will be advised to remove after a certain time. There will be a bloodstained vaginal discharge which may last for a few days. The patient should be advised to contact the clinic or her own doctor if she is concerned about this. She should also be advised to avoid sexual intercourse for about 4–6 weeks to allow the cervix to heal. Tampons should also be avoided for the first menstrual period after treatment.

Each colposcopy clinic may have a slightly different procedure for follow-up checks. There should be liaison between the clinic and the patient's own family doctor so that she does not slip through the net for follow-up. The first follow-up visit should ideally be at the centre in which treatment was offered, although the

> **Box 13.9** Advantages and disadvantages of LLETZ
>
> **Advantages**
>
> ◆ Cheaper than laser machine
>
> ◆ No noise or smell
>
> ◆ Can reduce the need for a biopsy and therefore a second visit for treatment
>
> ◆ Provides an interpretable specimen for histology with evidence that all the affected area has been removed.
>
> **Disadvantages**
>
> ◆ May be uncomfortable and painful
>
> ◆ Can cause excessive bleeding
>
> ◆ There is a possibility of over-treatment of minor abnormalities
>
> ◆ Can require a general anaesthetic for treating extensive areas
>
> ◆ If a deep cone is taken there could be implications for future childbearing.

patient's views should be considered when making arrangements for follow-up. Frequency of follow-up will vary according to grade of CIN and local protocols (Luesley, 1996).

Surgical cone biopsy

On the whole, the need for this operation has been superseded by LLETZ, but it should be noted that if a very deep cone is taken it is usually carried out under general anaesthetic.

The indications for conization are:

◆ The upper limit of the lesion cannot be visualized
◆ Microinvasion is suspected from colposcopy
◆ Previous unsuccessful local ablative treatment
◆ Where there is wide divergence between cytology and histology reports.

A cone biopsy that is very deep can lead to two problems:

◆ The external cervical os may become very tight after treatment, which can result in painful menstruation
◆ The internal cervical os may be damaged by treatment, weakening the muscle fibres. The internal os is responsible for keeping a pregnancy in the uterus, and after the 12th week of pregnancy an incompetent cervix might cause the pregnancy to miscarry.

If this problem is suspected, the treatment would be to have a stitch (like a purse string) inserted into the cervix: this is called a Shirodkar suture. It is removed once the patient has reached 38 weeks of her pregnancy and she then goes into labour normally.

With the advent of LLETZ problems of cervical incompetence are rarely seen.

Psychological and psychosexual problems

Following treatment for abnormalities of the cervix, psychological or psychosexual problems may occur for either the woman or her sexual partner. There may be time for discussion and counselling at the colposcopy clinic, but this is not always possible or ideal.

You may well be the person with whom your patient would like to discuss her anxieties following her treatment. You may feel as though you are not equipped to help, but you will soon find that one of the most important things about helping your patient is to be there to listen to her.

If you feel there is a need for more counselling than you can offer, be prepared to refer her to a local psychosexual counsellor.

Hysterectomy

A hysterectomy is indicated when there is:

◆ Recurrent abnormal smears or colposcopic abnormalities despite repeated local ablative therapy or conization
◆ A request for sterilization in the presence of severe or recurrent dysplasia
◆ Associated gynaecological problems such as menorrhagia or fibroids.

Invasive disease

If invasive disease has been diagnosed, the patient will be treated surgically and (depending on the stage of the disease) by radiotherapy or chemotherapy.

Wertheim's hysterectomy is the removal of the uterus and the upper third of the vagina with lymph node clearance. The ovaries may be removed if the woman is approaching the menopause or is post-menopausal (see page 561).

Innovative methods of screening for the future

Cervicography

Cervicography is the taking of a photograph of the cervix after 5% acetic acid is applied. The cervicograms obtained are projected on a screen, thus obtaining a magnification and resolution that compares to that at colposcopy. These can be interpreted by a colposcopist in much less time than it would take to perform a colposcopic examination. Szarewski *et al.* (1991) describe the use of cervicography in a primary screening service.

The Polarprobe

The Polarprobe prototype is a computerized diagnostic instrument specifically developed to detect pre-cancers and cancer of the uterine cervix. Studies in England are at present being carried out at the Whittington Hospital, London, by Professor Albert Singer and his team, and have been described by Coppleson *et al.* (1994). It is not envisaged that the Polarprobe will be used for primary screening (Polartechnics, personal communication, 1999).

Human papillomavirus (HPV) testing

The polymerase chain reaction (PCR) is a process by which the DNA of HPV is amplified to ascertain which type of HPV is present on the cervix. Research has demonstrated that the addition of HPV testing can substantially increase the detection rate of high-grade CIN. It may also be important in preventing the increasing proportion of invasive cancers among women with apparently adequate screening histories. More large randomized trials need to be done before it can be recommended for routine screening (Cuzick *et al.*, 1995).

Hybrid capture

Hybrid capture is a newer technique, which is considerably simpler than PCR technique with fewer pitfalls, easier to use and almost fully automated. Szarewski (1998) describes the procedure which leads to being able to 'capture molecules of DNA:RNA on the surface of an antibody-coated plate and detect with a chemiluminescent substrate'. So far in studies in London, this test appears to have only a 2% false-positive rate, and 100% of CIN 3 cases were detected. There is a low risk for development of high-grade CIN in women with borderline or mild smears who test negative for oncogenic HPV; this is the basis for further studies to look at expanding the use of such testing.

The Medical Research Council is at the moment evaluating the possibility of using HPV testing in the management of women with low-grade and borderline lesions, to follow up previously treated CIN and to screen whole populations either in addition to or as a replacement for Pap smears, results of which will be published in 2006 (Barton-Smith *et al.*, 2003). There are available 'self-testing kits' for HPV which women can purchase: advertisements for them are seen regularly in the popular press and some women who are anxious about abnormal smear results are using them. The general public are nowadays very well informed due to the availability of information on the internet, and some will decide to question or query matters relating to their health more than ever before. It is important for you to update regularly your own knowledge in order to give the correct advice to women.

Vaccination against HPV

Clinical trials are under way not only looking at the possibility of a vaccine for primary immunization, but also as a treatment for advanced stage cervical cancer (Crook *et al.*, 1996).

Video colpography

Video colpography, a new technique for secondary cervical screening, is currently being studied, and may be of great use in the future in the area of teaching, audit and cervical screening of low-grade smear abnormalities. Five per cent acetic acid is applied to the cervix, and a video recording is made of the cervix and vaginal fornices using a camera equipped with a macro lens (Etherington *et al.*, 1997). These images, along with vocal recordings of the patient's identity number, smoking habit and contraceptive practice, together with results of an index smear will assist the colposcopist reviewing the tape to form a diagnosis.

Conclusion – the way forward

This chapter started on an optimistic note with good news regarding the NHSCSP being 'up and running' and increasingly doing very well. It has been estimated that the incidence of cervical cancer in England and Wales fell by 42% between 1988 and 1997 (Sasieni and Adams, 1999). This message is backed up by statistics that show 'For the first time ever deaths from cervical cancer have fallen below 1000 in England. In 2002, 927 deaths were registered' (DoH, 2003).

New advances to improve the screening programme continue to be made. 'Modernizing the NHSCSP' includes the introduction of LBC and further use of HPV testing and changes to the screening interval. Our cervical screening programme is known to be one of the most organized in the world and the changes are based on the evidence and experience gained since the 1988 reforms. We should all be proud to be part of such a programme.

Sasieni in a review in 1998 (NHSCSP, 1998a) described clearly how we should view screening and its limitations:

> The cervical screening programme is not like a vaccine, it's not going to eradicate the cancer. The analogy must be more like wearing a seat belt; if you wear a seat belt there's no guarantee you won't be killed in a road accident, but it lessens the risks. Going for regular screening reduces the risk to 20 or 25% of what it would be if you didn't go. If every woman went for screening we could prevent 80% of all cervical cancers.

The chapter ends on a rather sombre note: discussing the treatment for invasive cervical carcinoma. As the smear-taker, you can do your very best to make sure that the cervical screening programme reaches all women who need (and want) to have a cervical smear.

In becoming a competent, sensitive smear-taker you will not only be helping to spread the positive news about the programme but also be helping to detect this disease in its early, very treatable stages.

Ideas for personal and professional development

- Practice holding, opening and closing a speculum to improve your dexterity before doing smears on a patient
- Discuss with colleagues the new guidelines for screening frequency (page 362) to enable full understanding of the changes and ensuring consistency of information to clients
  - Will there be exceptions allowed?
  - Do all staff know that smears taken outside the screening ages are not included in the targets for payment?
  - Would health professionals think it is a good idea to suggest having a smear taken in the private sector (for those whose level of anxiety is so high)?
- Consider making a patient information leaflet about how to prepare for a smear (see page 360)
- Audit the results of smears that you take. Are you obtaining satisfactory smears or do you have a high percentage of inadequate smears?
- Visit your local colposcopy unit and find out the treatment options available. Is there a nurse colposcopist at the unit? Do they have a video link so that the woman can see the procedure? What is the policy for follow-up checks?
- Get to know your local laboratory and in particular a named person whom you can contact to clarify any results of which you are not sure, or just to ask advice from. Your first contact with the laboratory may be as part of your cervical screening training course, which will be an ideal opportunity to 'build bridges'.

Patient education points

- A smear test is not the same as screening for infections, although both may be done at the same examination
- The cervical smear test is not a test for cancer, but is looking for very early changes that if left undiscovered and untreated could lead to pre-cancer and eventually cancer; this process could take many years to happen

- The cervical screening programme will not work like a vaccine, but it could be likened to wearing a seat belt, for which if you wear one, there is no guarantee you will not be killed in a car crash, but it lessens the risk

- If every woman went for cervical screening we could prevent 80% of all cervical cancers

- Condoms should be used in addition to other methods of contraception (pills, injections, implants) to reduce the risk of having HPV. This may be particularly relevant to young women under the new screening age of 25 who may be anxious about delaying a smear

- Advice should be sought from a health professional if there is any unexpected vaginal bleeding.

Resources

Video

British Society for Clinical Cytology (BSCC)
New video/CD with booklet/workbook 'Taking Cervical Smears'. Cost £75 including p&p (cheque payable to 'Cansearch Limited')
BSCC Office, PO Box 352, Uxbridge UB10 9TX
Tel: 01895 274020

Booklets
To order any of the following contact the NHS Response line on 08701 555 455 or e-mail doh@prolog.uk.com.
A Pocket Guide to Cervical Screening
NHSCSP (updated 2003)
Cervical Smear Results Explained (booklet). A Guide for Primary Care
NHSCSP (updated 2003)
Cervical Screening – The Facts (booklet)
Good Practice in Cervical Screening for Women with Learning Difficulties
NHSCSP, 2002
NHSCSP leaflets: 'What Your Abnormal Result Means'; 'The Colposcopy Examination'; 'Cervical Screening – The Facts'.

Useful addresses and web sites

Action on Smoking and Health (ASH)
Tel: 0207 739 5902
www.ash.org.uk

British Society for Colposcopy and Cervical Pathology (BSCCP)
Mrs E. Dollery, The Women's Hospital, Edgbaston, Birmingham B15 2TG
Tel: 0121 607 4716
E-mail: lizdollery@orbite.co.uk

CancerBACUP (British Association of Cancer United Patients)
3 Bath Place, Rivington Street, London EC2A 3JR
Tel: 0808 800 1234
www.cancerbacup.org.uk

Cancer Research UK
PO Box 123, London WC2A 3PX
Tel: 0207 242 0200
www.cancerresearchuk.org

Macmillan Cancer Relief
15–19 Britten Street, London SW3 3TZ
Tel: 0207 840 7840
www.macmillan.org.uk

Marie Curie Cancer Care
28 Belgrave Square, London SW1X 8QG
Tel: 0207 599 7777
www.mariecurie.org.uk

Medical Research Council
Tel: 0207 670 4855
www.mrc.ac.uk

NHS Cancer Screening Programmes
Director: Julietta Patnick
260 Ecclesall Road South, Sheffield S11 9PS
Tel: 0114 271 1060
www.cancerscreening.nhs.uk/ce

Nursing and Midwifery Council (NMC)
23 Portland Place, London W1B 1PZ
Tel: 0207 333 6541
E-mail: advice@nmc-uk.org

Further reading

HASLETT, S. (1994) *Having a Cervical Smear*. Beaconsfield, Bucks: Beaconsfield.
HASLETT, S. and JENNINGS, M. (1992) *Hysterectomy and Vaginal Repair*, 3rd edn. Beaconsfield, Bucks: Beaconsfield.
KUBBA, A., SANFILIPPO, J. and HAMPTON, N. (1999) *Contraception and Office Gynaecology: Choices in Reproductive Healthcare*. London: W.B. Saunders.

LUCAS and MARTIN (2004) *Practice Nurse Handbook.* Elsevier.

NHSCSP *'LINKS'* newsletter published quarterly for people working in the NHS Cervical Screening Programme.

PARKER, S. (1994) *Medico-Legal Aspects of Screening for Cancer in Women for the Practice Nurse.* London: Medical Defence Union.

QUILLIAM, S. (1992) *Positive Smear*, 2nd edn. London: Letts.

ROYAL COLLEGE OF NURSING (1994) *Female Genital Mutilation.* London: RCN.

SZAREWSKI, A. (1994) *A Woman's Guide to the Cervical Smear Test.* London: Optima.

References

ATKIN, K., LUNT, N., PARKER, G. and HIRST, M. (1993) *A National Census of Practice Nurses.* Report. York University.

AUSTOKER, J., BANKHEAD, C. and DAVEY, C. (2003) *Cervical Smear Results Explained: A Guide for Primary Care.* London: Cancer Research UK and NHSCSP.

AUSTOKER, J. and McPHERSON, A. (1992) *Cervical Screening*, 2nd edn. Oxford: Oxford University Press.

BARKER, G.H. (1987) *Your Smear Test.* London: Adamson.

BARTON, S.E., MADDOX, P.H., JENKINS, D., EDWARDS, R., CUZICK, J. and SINGER, A. (1988) Effects of cigarette smoking on cervical epithelial immunity. *Lancet* **11**:652.

BARTON-SMITH, P., THOMAS, V. and IND, T. (2003) Cervical screening in England and Wales: an update. *Reviews in Gynaecological Practice* **3**:5–10.

BROWN, J., HARDING, S. and BETHANE, A. (1997) Incidence of health of the nation cancers by social class. *Population Trends* **1997**:90.

CANCER RESEARCH UK (2003) Cancer Stats. January 2003. London.

CHOMET, J. and CHOMET, J. (1989) *Cervical Cancer.* London: Grapevine/Thorson Publishing.

COPPLESON, M., REID, B.L., SKLADNEV, V.N. and DALRYMPLE, J.C. (1994) An electronic approach to the detection of pre-cancer and cancer of the uterine cervix: a preliminary evaluation of the Polarprobe. *International Journal of Gynaecological Cancer* **4**:79.

CROOK, T. and VOUSDEN, K.H. (1996) Oncoprotein function. In Lacey, C. (ed.) *Papilloma Virus Reviews: Current Research on Papilloma Viruses.* Leeds: Leeds University Press, pp. 55–60.

CUZICK, J., SZAREWSKI, A., TERRY, G. *et al.* (1995) Human papillomavirus testing in primary cervical screening. *Lancet* **345**:1533–36.

CUZICK, J., TERRY, G., HO, L. *et al.* (2000). Association between high-risk HPV types HLA DRB1 and DQB1 alleles and cervical cancer in British women. *British Journal of Cancer* **82**(7):1348–52.

DoH (Department of Health) (1988) *Decontamination of Instruments and Appliances Used in the Vagina*, EL 88 MB 210. London: DoH.

DoH (1992) *The Health of the Nation.* London: DoH.

DoH (1994) *Instruments and Appliances Used in the Vagina and Cervix: Recommended Methods for Decontamination.* 'Safety Action Bulletin' SAB(94)22, June. London: DoH.

DoH (2002) Shifting the balance of power. Document 2002.

DoH (2003) Office of National Statistics Quarterly, summer 2003.

DYER, C. (1999) Three women win in cervical screening case. *British Medical Journal* **318**:484.

ELKIND, A.K., HARAN, D., EARDLEY, A. and SPENCER, B. (1989) 'Well you can come in but I'm not having it'. *Health Visitor* **62**:20.

ELUF-NETO, J., BOOTH, M., MUˆNOZ, N., BOSCH, F.X., MEIJER, C.J.L.M. and WALBOOMERS, J.M.M. (1994) Human papilloma virus and invasive cervical cancer in Brazil. *British Journal of Cancer* **69**:114.

ETHERINGTON, I.J., DUNN, J., SHAFI, M.I., SMITH, T. and LUESLEY, D.M. (1997) Video colpography: a new technique for secondary cervical screening. *British Journal of Obstetrics and Gynaecology* **104**:150–3.

FLYNN, C. (2000) The gentle touch. *Nursing Times* **96**(4):55.

GAGNON, F. (1950) Contributions to the study of the etiology and prevention of cervical cancer. *Journal of Obstetrics and Gynaecology* **60**:516–22.

GILLAM, S.J. (1991) Understanding the uptake of cervical cancer screening. *British Journal of General Practice* **41**:510.

HOPWOOD, J. (1990) *Background to Colposcopy and Treatment of the Cervix.* Burgess Hill: Schering Healthcare.

HOPWOOD, J. (1995) *Background to Cervical Cytology Reports*, 3rd edn. Burgess Hill: Schering Healthcare.

LUESLEY, D. (1996) *Standards and Quality in Colposcopy*, NHSCSP Publication No. 2. Sheffield: NHSCSP.

MARTIN-HIRSCH, P., LILFORD, R., JARVIS, G. and KITCHENER, H.C. (1999) Efficacy of cervical smear collection devices: a systematic review and meta-analysis. *Lancet* **354**:1763–70.

NCN (1991) National Co-ordinating Network of the NHS Cervical Screening Programme – The First Annual Report. London: NCN.

NCN (1992) *The NCN Guidelines on Failsafe Actions.* London: NCN.

NHSCSP (National Health Service Cervical Screening Programme) (1996) *Quality Assurance Guidelines for the Cervical Screening Programme.* Publication no. 3. Sheffield: NHSCSP.

NHSCSP (1998a) *A National Priority*, review. Sheffield: NHSCSP.

NHSCSP (1998b) *Resource Pack for Training Smear Takers.* Publication no. 9. Sheffield: NHSCSP.

NHSCSP (1999a) *A National Priority*, review. Sheffield: NHSCSP.

NHSCSP (1999b) *A Pocket Guide.* Sheffield: NHSCSP

NHSCSP (2000) *Achievable Standards, Benchmarks for Reporting, and Criteria for Evaluating Cervical Cytopathology*, 2nd edn. Sheffield: NHSCSP.

NHSCSP (2003) Review. Sheffield. NHSCSP. www.cancerscreening.nhs.uk/cervical.

NHSCSP (2004). Publication No. 1. www.cancerscreening.nhs.uk/cervical.

NHS EXECUTIVE (1998) *Cervical Screening Action Team – The Report.*

NMC (2002a) *Code of Professional Conduct.* London: NMC.

NMC (2002b) Guidelines for records and record keeping.

QUINN, M., BABB, P., BROCK, A., KIRBY, L. and JONES, J. (2001) *Cancer Trends in England and Wales. 1950–1999.* The Stationery Office.

RCN (Royal College of Nursing) (1994) *Female Genital Mutilation.* London: RCN.

RCN (1995) *Bimanual Pelvic Examination – Guidance for Nurses*. London: RCN.

RCOG, RCP, RCGP, FCM (Royal College of Obstetricians and Gynaecologists; Royal College of Pathologists; Royal College of General Practitioners; Faculty of Community Medicine) (1987) *Report of the Intercollegiate Working Party on Cervical Cytology Screening*.

SASIENI, P. and ADAMS, J. (1999) Effect of screening on cervical cancer mortality in England and Wales: analysis of trends with an age period cohort model. *British Medical Journal* 318:1244–5.

SASIENI, P., ADAMS, J. and CUZICK, J. (2003) Benefit of cervical screening at different ages: evidence from the UK audit of screening histories. *British Journal of Cancer* 89:88–93.

SCOTTO, J. and BAILAR, J.C. III (1969) Domenico Rigoni-Stern and medical statistics (a nineteenth century approach to cancer research). *Journal of the History of Medicine and Allied Sciences* 24:65–75.

SHAFI, M.I. (1999) *Nurse Colposcopists Point Towards the Future*. NHSCSP Review, pp. 8–9.

SIMONS, A.M., PHILLIPS, D.H. and COLEMAN, D.V. (1993) Damage to DNA in cervical epithelium related to smoking tobacco. *British Medical Journal* 306:1444–8.

SINGER, A. and SZAREWSKI, A. (1988) *Cervical Smear Test*. London: Optima.

SMITH, J.E., GREEN, J., BERRINGTON De GONZALES, A., APPLEBY, P., PETO, J., PLUMMER, M., FRANCESCHI, S. and BERRAL, V. (2003) Cervical cancer and use of oral contraceptives: a systematic review. *Lancet* 361(9364):1159–67.

SMITH, P.G. *et al.* (1979) Mortality of wives of men dying with cancer of the penis. *British Journal of Cancer* 41:422.

SOCIETY FOR GYNECOLOGIC (2000) Lost fragile histidine triad (FHIT) gene expression may link cigarette smoking and cervical cancer (abstract). Oncologists 31st Annual Meeting, 5–9 February 2000, San Diego, California.

SZAREWSKI, A. (1994) *A Woman's Guide to the Cervical Smear Test*. London: Optima.

SZAREWSKI, A. (1998) Advances in HPV testing to prevent cervical cancer. *Trends in Urology, Gynaecology and Sexual Health* 3(3):13–14.

SZAREWSKI, A. and CUZICK, J. (1998) Smoking and cervical neoplasia: a review of the evidence. *Journal of Epidemiology and Biostatistics* 3(3):229–56.

SZAREWSKI, A., CUZICK, J., EDWARDS, R., BUTLER, B. and SINGER, A. (1991) The use of cervicography in a primary screening environment. *British Journal of Obstetrics and Gynaecology* 98:313.

SZAREWSKI, A., JARVIS, M.J., SASIENI, P. *et al.* (1996) Effect of smoking cessation on cervical lesion size. *Lancet* 347:941–3.

TUNNADINE, P. (1970) *Contraception and Sexual Life*. London: Tavistock

VALINS, L. (1988) *Vaginismus*. Bath: Ashgrove Press.

VIZCAINO, A.P., MORENO, V. and BOSCH, F.X. (1998) International trends in the incidence of cervical cancer: adenocarcinoma and adenosquamous cell carcinomas. *International Journal of Cancer* 75:536–45.

WADDELL, C. (1994) Update in cytology with a focus on smear adequacy. *Journal of the National Association of Family Planning Nurses* 27:43–8.

WARDEN, J. (1998) Moves to end cervical screening failures in England. *British Medical Journal* 317:558.

WILSON, J.M.C. and JUNGER, O.G.H. (1968) *Principles and Practice of Screening for Disease*; World Health Organization. A report; Paper 34. Geneva: WHO.

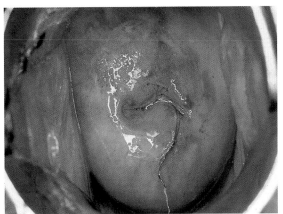

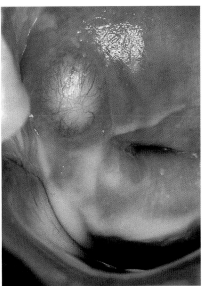

Plate 1 Multiparous os showing a typical transformation zone and IUD threads. (Reproduced with permission from Professor A. MacLean, The Royal Free Hospital, London.)

Plate 2 Nabothian follicle. (Reproduced with permission from Mr Peter Greenhouse, Bristol Royal Infirmary, Bristol.)

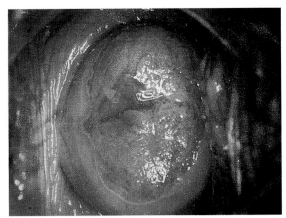

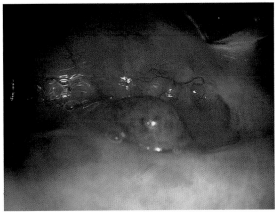

Plate 3 Cervical ectropion. (Reproduced with permission from Mr Peter Greenhouse, Bristol Royal Infirmary, Bristol.)

Plate 4 Cervical polyp. (Reproduced with permission from Professor A. MacLean, The Royal Free Hospital, London.)

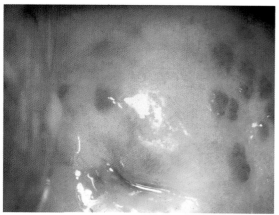

Plate 5 'Strawberry' cervix. Characteristic of infection with *Trichomonas vaginalis*. (Reproduced with permission from Professor A. MacLean, The Royal Free Hospital, London.)

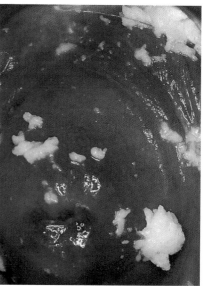

Plate 6 Candidiasis. Characterized by a thick, white lumpy discharge, adhering to the vaginal walls. (Reproduced with permission from Mr Peter Greenhouse, Bristol Royal Infirmary, Bristol.)

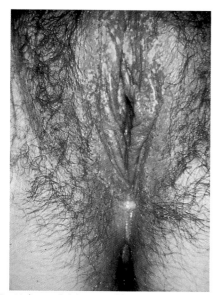

Plate 7 Vulvovaginitis caused by *candida*. (Bingham 1985, reproduced with permission.)

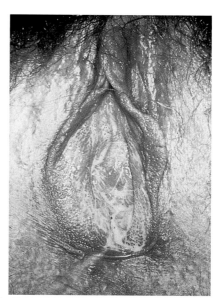

Plate 8 Bacterial vaginosis. Characterized by a grey malodorus discharge at the vulva. (Bingham 1985, reproduced with permission.)

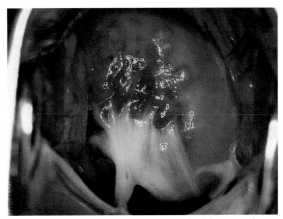

Plate 9 *Trichomonas vaginalis.* Characterized by a frothy greenish-yellow discharge exuding from the vaginal wall. (Bingham 1985, reproduced with permission.)

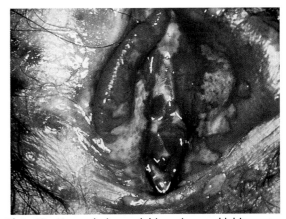

Plate 10 Purulent cervicitis associated with gonorrhoea and *Chlamydia.* (Reproduced with permission from Mr Peter Greenhouse, Bristol Royal Infirmary, Bristol.)

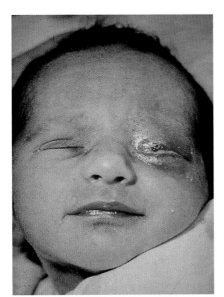

Plate 11 Ophthalmia neonatorum with gonorrhoea. Symptoms appear within 2–5 days of delivery. (Bingham 1985, reproduced with permission.)

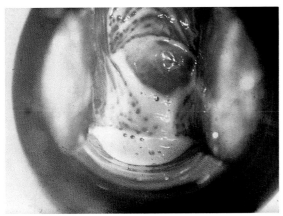

Plate 12 Herpes lesion on labia majora and labia minora associated with vulval oedema. (Bingham 1985, reproduced with permission.)

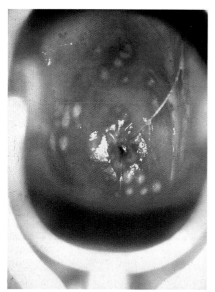

Plate 13 Herpetic lesions on the cervix. (Bingham 1985, reproduced with permission.)

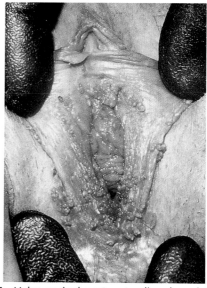

Plate 14 Vulvo-vaginal warts extending down into the perineum. (Bingham 1985, reproduced with permission.)

14: Sexual Health and Sexually Transmissible Infections

Alison Duffin ◆

OBJECTIVES

This chapter should help you understand:

◆ The importance of a good sexual/risk behaviour history ◆

◆ the importance of sexual health and sexual health promotion ◆

◆ some causes of vaginal discharge and genital ulceration ◆

◆ the basic features of sexually transmitted infections, with particular reference to women ◆

◆ issues for women with HIV and AIDS ◆

◆ the difficult emotional and practical problems that sexually transmitted infections can have on a woman's life and interpersonal relationships ◆

◆ nursing issues in sexual health. ◆

Introduction

In your professional role as a nurse, whether in primary care or in hospital departments and clinics, you will encounter women who are anxious about their sexuality, sexual health and particularly their vaginal discharge. It is within the context of the genito-urinary medicine (GUM) clinic that sexual health, vaginal discharge and sexually transmissible infections (STIs) in women are discussed in this chapter, but the philosophies of GUM can easily be adapted to your own clinical settings.

Vaginal discharge should never be trivialized or dismissed. When a pathological discharge is apparent it can be both psychologically and physically very distressing and can profoundly undermine a woman's sense of well-being. Consideration of this fact and sensitivity from nursing staff will make a visit to the sexual health clinic far less of an ordeal.

Sexual health in the new millennium

The World Health Organization (WHO, 1995) in a study estimated that at least 333 million new cases of *curable* STIs occurred in the world in 1995. These STIs, which are not only curable but also preventable, and their complications rank in the top 10 causes of healthy days lost by adults in the urban areas of the developing world and therefore have a large socio-economic impact on financial planning. According to the World Bank, 'provision of treatment for curable STDs represents one of the most cost effective interventions to improve health in the world' (WHO, 1995). This is of particular concern and relevance due to the links between STIs and the human immunodeficiency virus (HIV). Many of these curable STIs cause genital lesions and inflammation and there is strong evidence to suggest that these greatly increase the sexual transmission of HIV. Therefore every newly diagnosed STI could potentially be a new HIV infection, as it is an indicator that unprotected sex has taken place.

In the last two decades, the type of service provision provided for patients attending GUM clinics changed rapidly. The core service of GUM still diagnosed, treated, managed and maintained effective epidemiological control of sexually transmitted infections (STIs) but also increased the range of sexual health services available to clients. Such facilities now include family planning, counselling and psychosexual services, sexual health promotion and clinics for lesbian women. Other aspects of service provision include cervical cytology and colposcopy, and specialist clinics provided for patients who have HIV or who have developed acquired immune deficiency syndrome (AIDS).

The changes within GUM services cannot be divorced from the wider social changes that have occurred in the UK. These include greater freedom of sexual expression, improved standards of living, easier access to safe effective contraception, the use of recreational drugs, the rise of an articulate and informed women's movement and gay movement and the shift in the political and sexual arena. Sexual health is an idea that was forced on to the social agenda by the arrival of HIV, as individual needs, sexual and cultural diversity, and 'at risk' groups began to be recognized. The highest burden of sexual ill health is amongst women, men who have sex with men, teenagers, young adults and black minority and ethnic groups (Lacey et al., 1997; Low et al., 1997; Hughes et al., 2000). This shift within the social arena, and the rising incidence in STIs and HIV in the UK, has seen a rapid increase in demand for GUM services. The numbers of visits to clinics doubled during the last decade of the twentieth century and GUM clinics have been in crisis ever since, as increases in funding or resources do not match this demand. The Select Committee on Health (2003) suggests that as sexual health has not been seen as a public health priority, by either government or NHS organizations, this has contributed to the current crisis within GUM and sexual health services.

In response to the nation's failing sexual health, the first National Sexual Health and HIV Strategy (DoH, 2001) was produced. This document sets out three levels of service provision for sexual health services, and strongly recommends increasing the role of primary care in providing this service. All GPs will offer Level 1, which includes testing women for STIs and assessment and referral of men with symptoms of STIs. Primary care teams will offer Level 2 services with a special interest in sexual health including screening, treating and partner notification. Level 3 will be the specialist services such as GUM, abortion, and community family planning.

Although this is a welcome and long overdue strategic plan to improve the sexual health of the nation, it is disappointing that it has not been given the status of a National Service Framework (NSF), as one could argue that, again, it will still not be viewed as a priority within Primary Care Trusts (PCTs). Adler (2003) cites that this is clearly evident already.

Consent and confidentiality

The ethical perspectives of informed consent and confidentiality in GUM are of paramount importance. Every patient has the right to determine what is done to him or her. Patient consent is implied from their presentation at the clinic and request for help. The amount of information a patient receives should enable them to make a reasonable and informed decision about what is to happen to them. This respect for the patient's integrity and autonomy is crucial to the wider epidemiological management of STIs. A relationship of trust and confidence should be established by all levels of clinic staff, regardless of age, gender, ethnic, cultural or religious beliefs.

Young people under the age of sixteen may also seek advice and treatment for sexual health issues, but it is a legal requirement that their 'competence' be assessed first (see Chapter 7).

If a client is diagnosed as having an STI, the tracing of sexual contacts, also known as partner notification, needs to be undertaken, usually by a person employed within GUM, such as a health adviser.

The health adviser interviews the client in private and requires the client's full cooperation to motivate them to persuade their sexual contacts to attend the clinic to exclude infection. In most instances, the client is asked to contact all sexual contacts, from at least the previous three to six months, prior to diagnosis. The health adviser is able to acknowledge that telling a partner is not easy, particularly when the woman may be feeling hurt, angry, frightened or guilty. Some women may be in an abusive or violent relationship and therefore it is vital to ensure their personal safety is also considered. There is no right or wrong way to tell a partner, but the health adviser will be able to give advice and recommend different approaches to the discussion.

If the client is unable to do this or is too embarrassed, the health adviser, where appropriate, may need to undertake this responsibility personally, whilst maintaining the anonymity and preserving strict confidentiality for the client. Such a task requires tact, dedication and diplomacy. The wider role of the health adviser within GUM is now well accepted and includes counselling, health education, health promotion and discussion of safer sex. With the implementation of the national sexual health strategy, the health advisors role looks likely to extend into the community, to help co-ordinate partner notification (DoH, 2001).

The idea that clients attending GUM clinics are sexually irresponsible, reckless and indifferent to the welfare of others is a myth. The majority will make a considerable effort to contact sexual partners and encourage them to attend GUM clinics to seek treatment. For this to happen they need a clear idea of why it is necessary and also absolute confidence that respect will be given to the confidential nature of their disclosures. Some STIs are 'silent' infections, i.e. patients do not always have symptoms, and this may need to be explained to encourage disclosure to sexual contacts. Patients who attend GUM clinics are responsible, seeking appropriate advice and treatment. It is those who do not practise safer sex, or do not attend for check-ups, who are most at risk of long-term complications from untreated STIs.

Confidentiality is not an absolute concept and may be broken in a limited number of circumstances: with a patient's consent, by due legal process, or if on balance the doctor's duty to society outweighs their responsibility to the individual. However, this is rare in practice. Robertson *et al.* (1989) illustrate the issue of consent and confidentiality with examples of case law in STIs and conclude that 'compulsory measures are inappropriate' but persuasion, voluntary compliance and the knowledge that respect for patient confidentiality will prevail is more effective.

With regard to HIV antibody screening, informed consent must be obtained prior to testing individuals. The DoH has written guidelines for practitioners regarding this process (DoH, 1997a). Practitioners and individuals have often expressed concern regarding STI/HIV and other blood-borne viruses (BBVs) testing and life insurance policies. The British Medical Association (BMA) and the Association of British Insurers (ABI) have written joint guidelines (BMA and ABI, 2002), which state that in certain instances doctors should not reveal this information when writing reports and insurance companies will not expect this information to be provided. Insurance companies may ask, however, if a patient has tested HIV antibody positive or is receiving treatment for HIV/AIDS or hepatitis B or C. If insurance companies require a person to be tested, before issuing a policy for individuals, consent for testing must be given.

The ABI states that existing life policies will not be affected, even if someone tests positive, as long as the individual did not withhold any facts (e.g. activities that put them at an increased risk of HIV) when the policy was taken out.

Taking a sexual history and risk assessment for Blood-Borne Viruses (BBVs)

'A sexual history alerts the nurse to possible infections that will need to be screened during the physical assessment' (Andrist, 1988) and will also help to ascertain the woman's sexual health education requirements. Obtaining a sexual history and BBVs assessment takes practice, excellent communication and inter-personal skills, as well as expertise and time. It may create problems for the inexperienced health care professional, particularly if they are ill at ease not only with discussing sexual matters but also with their own sexuality. Box 14.1 briefly outlines the areas that need to be considered in order to gain the maximum knowledge about your client's sexual/risk history so that you can help her effectively. Before embarking on the process, it is important to explain to the patient that all the questions you will be asking her are questions you ask everybody in order to obtain the relevant information you need to assess her risk for STIs and BBVs. By doing this, you are less likely to cause her offence.

Bor and Watts (1993) state that 'patients are willing to answer questions about their intimate sexual behaviour and lifestyle provided that they do not feel judged or ridiculed'. A woman must be given time, space and a private place to discuss her sexual history.

Although the following list appears lengthy, you will find that with practice it should not take too long. Specific questions should include:

◆ What is the nature of the present problem and how long has she had this?

◆ Does she have any other symptoms: dysuria; vaginal discharge; lower abdominal pain; dyspareunia; post-coital bleeding; intermenstrual bleeding; any genital itches, lumps/bumps, rashes, sores or ulcers or anything else unusual?
(*Rationale: depending on clinic policy, this may affect which health professional she sees*)

◆ A brief medical history, prior to the sexual history is needed

◆ Has she any allergies to medications or any other allergies? These should be clearly documented, as it will affect her treatment options

◆ Has she any piercings or tattoos? If so, when and in what country were they performed? Was sterile equipment used?
(*Rationale: she may need to be screened for BBVs depending on the information she gives*)

◆ Has she ever been tested for HIV or hepatitis A, B or C? If so, when and what was the outcome?

◆ Has she ever been vaccinated for hepatitis A or B? If so, when, and did she complete the course?
(*Rationale: you may need to consider offering Hep A or B vaccination if she is at risk*)

◆ Has she ever been diagnosed with an STI before? If so, when, and what was the nature of the previous problem? Was she treated, if so, with what? If she has a partner, was he/she treated at the same time?
(*Rationale: she may not have been treated adequately, or she may have been re-infected*)

◆ Is she in a regular relationship at the moment? If so, how long, and what is her partner's gender?

◆ When was the last time she had sexual activity with anyone?

Box 14.1 Points to remember when taking a sexual history

◆ Ensure the woman understands why taking a sexual history is necessary and recognize that the issues involved are both personal and sensitive

◆ Recognize your own feelings in relation to discussing sex with a client. Try to acknowledge your own embarrassment, attitudes and your own belief and value systems, which may have an influence on the nature of the interaction between you and your client

◆ Do not be reluctant to use street language if appropriate to the context of the interview, particularly if that is more comfortable for your client

◆ Listen attentively to what the woman is saying and particularly note any non-verbal communication

◆ Be purposeful in your questions but do not make assumptions or apply sexual stereotypes. Adopt a non-judgemental attitude particularly in relation to lifestyle or sexual orientation and concentrate instead on sexual activity. Refer to all partners as partners and not by gender, until you clarify this point with the patient.

◆ Always work within your professional boundaries and within the framework of the law

◆ Protect the patient's right to confidentiality.

(Rationale: this will ensure when testing/ screening that incubation periods are taken into consideration)

◆ Who was this with? Regular, known or casual partner?

◆ Which country is their partner or contact from? *(Rationale: in some countries there are higher prevalences for some STIs/BBVs, plus antibiotic resistance which may affect treatment options)*

◆ What type of activity was it? Oral, vaginal or anal?
 Note: when asking about sexual activity, it is important to ascertain in each activity, whether she received it, gave it or both, and was a condom/dam used at any time, for any activity?

◆ Before this occasion, when was the last time, if any, that she had sex with anyone? (Then note all of the above, for this previous occasion only)
 (Rationale: this will enable you to assess her level of risk for STIs and BBVs. Also ask the level of condom use (i.e. 100% or less)

◆ Has she ever had sex with someone from overseas? If so, when and what country? *(Rationale: you may need to consider BBV screening)*

◆ Has she ever been paid for sex or paid someone to have sex with her? If so, when? Is she still working in the sex industry or paying to have sex?
 (Rationale: she may need additional information on safer sex, or if she is a sex worker, information on specific organizations who work with that particular group)

◆ Does she use a method of contraception? If so what? If not, is she trying to get pregnant?

◆ What was the date of her last menstrual period? Was it normal for her? How often does she have a period?

◆ When was her last cervical smear? Was it normal? Has she ever had an abnormal smear? If so, when and what was wrong? Has she ever had treatment following an abnormal smear? If so, when and what type of treatment?

◆ An obstetric history is also relevant. Has she ever been pregnant? When and what was the outcome?

◆ Does she use any recreational drugs? What is the type and frequency of the drug? Has she ever injected drugs? If so, what drugs, and has she ever shared needles or equipment? If so, when was the last time?
 (Rationale: you may need to consider BBV screening)

Additional questions to assess risk could include previous blood transfusions, alcohol intake (can lead to unprotected sex) and whether she has ever had sex with someone who she perceives to be at increased risk.

It is worth noting that women who have sex with women are also at risk of STIs/BBVs and cervical cancer, as many have had male partners in the past, or may have injected drugs (Conway and Humphries, 1994; Bevier *et al.*, 1995) or they may have sex with both sexes.

In order to take a satisfactory sexual history it is important to be aware of the barriers that can make effective communication between you and your client more difficult. These could include:

◆ *Gender*. A patient may have difficulty talking to someone of the opposite sex, or of the same sex

◆ *Culture*. Some women, for cultural or religious reasons, may have problems discussing sexual matters. If there are language problems, a professional interpreter should be used in preference to a member of the family or a friend

◆ *Age*. The young adult years are the time of highest sexual activity but you should remember that sexual activity continues well into later life. Preconceived notions that older people do not engage in active sex should be avoided and your recognition of the older individual's life experiences is important.

When taking a sexual history you must also discuss and offer advice on safer sex (see Chapter 11) and health education advice on lifestyle issues (see Chapter 3). This is an extremely important part of the health promotion work within GUM and by any health professional dealing with sexual health.

Vaginal discharge

A brief description of the anatomy and physiology of the vagina can be found on page 515.

Vaginal discharge is normal in all women, and does not necessarily indicate a pathological condition. Occasionally there will be a variation in the amount or colour of this normal discharge due to a number of different causes:

◆ The menstrual cycle – there will be an increase of clear mucus just prior to ovulation which is often described as looking like the white of an egg (spinnbarkeit mucus)

◆ Pregnancy

◆ Method of contraception – the contraceptive pill can cause a thicker discharge whilst spermicides, when recently used, make the vaginal discharge thinner

◆ Sexual arousal

◆ Stress.

A normal physiological discharge should not cause an offensive odour, irritation or soreness. A pathological discharge can be either infectious or non-infectious in origin. Whatever the cause of the discharge, the symptom is a very subjective one with the 'normal' discharge being a very arbitrary concept for some individuals. Often women may need reassurance that a vaginal discharge can be completely normal, and that the quantity differs for all women. When a woman complains of a vaginal discharge that is different from normal and causing her a problem, care needs to be taken that assumptions are not made that she is automatically suffering from an STI. However, assumptions should also not be made that the causative agent for the vaginal discharge is thrush as the woman may well have an underlying STI.

This case scenario demonstrates the importance of excluding all possible pathogens that may be causing a change in vaginal discharge. A full

SCENARIO

Alice, 22, presented at the GU clinic complaining of recent dysuria and lower abdominal pain, as well as infrequent thrush symptoms. She had previously seen her GP for the same symptoms and was treated for thrush.

Alice was not in a regular relationship and she had had unprotected vaginal intercourse with a casual partner 3 months previously. Alice had a full STI screen. The test for thrush was negative, although the test for chlamydia was positive.

screening of pathogens should be performed using: a high vaginal swab (HVS); an endo-cervical swab placed in a universal medium to be tested for gonorrhoea (one of the sites gonorrhoea affects can be the cervix); and an endo-cervical swab for chlamydia. Additionally, it is also important when screening for infections that should an STI be diagnosed, contact tracing of all sexual partners (usually, at least all within the last three months) is carried out in order to prevent re-infection.

The differences in the reproductive tract, and the respective anatomical structure between men and women, account for the greater risk of complications of STIs in women. In women the pattern of infection is more variable, often unapparent or asymptomatic, and several sites may be infected, including the cervix, urethra, rectum and pharynx. As Adler (1990) states 'Neither the patient's symptoms nor a subjective description of the colour and quantity of the discharge are of much value in reaching an accurate diagnosis'. The potential problems that also need to be considered are: (a) whether the cause of the vaginal discharge is due to more than one single cause; and (b) what the risk index is for sexual spread of an STI like syphilis or HIV infection.

Many of the organisms attributed to be responsible for producing vaginal discharge, e.g. *Candida albicans*, *Gardnerella vaginalis*, *Ureaplasma urealyticum* and *Mycobacterium hominis*, have been isolated from healthy women who are asymptomatic and not complaining of a particular problem. The development of signs and symptoms of vaginal discharge is discussed by Masfari *et al.* (1986), who suggest that a quantitative change occurs in the polymicrobial balance of the vaginal flora. A corresponding change to both the number and the yield of organisms may influence the vaginal environment which then allows some organisms to become pathogenic.

Common causes of vaginal discharge are listed in Box 14.2. Other possible causes of vaginal discharge include the cytomegalovirus which has been isolated from semen, the cervix and saliva. Enteric pathogens and B haemolytic streptococci have also been implicated as a cause of vaginitis and cervicitis.

An abnormal vaginal discharge is a common presenting complaint of women attending primary care or GUM clinic. Many women are embarrassed about their discharge and although they recognize the need for medical advice, will wash their genital areas excessively, or douche before going to seek medical attention. Unfortunately this may not only make diagnosis and treatment more difficult as the symptoms will be masked, but it also may exacerbate the condition due to the alteration of the vaginal pH. Frequently the discharge is accompanied by other symptoms, e.g. vaginal soreness or irritation, unpleasant odour, dyspareunia and bleeding. Sometimes women will also complain of 'cystitis', which may be an external dysuria due to vulval soreness or due to a urinary tract infection. Frequently women may complain of vaginal discharge when they actually need help with another problem, e.g. pregnancy, a psychosexual problem or domestic violence issues.

The standard management of a woman attending a GUM clinic complaining of vaginal discharge needs careful and considerate explanation at all stages. After a routine general and sexual history has been taken, the woman will undergo a general examination and a detailed genital examination. A bimanual examination should be performed on all symptomatic women and, depending on clinic policy, on all women attending.

◆ All lymph glands adjacent to the genital area will be checked for signs of inflammation or soreness

◆ The pubic area will be examined for anything abnormal including infestations or signs of genital warts or molluscum

◆ The genital/peri-anal area will be thoroughly examined for any of the above STIs, as well as ulcers, rashes, excoriation, pigment discolouration, fissuring in the skin, etc.

◆ A vaginal speculum will be inserted and specimens for both microscopy and cultures taken from the lateral vaginal wall, the posterior fornix and cervix. Depending on clinic policy a urethral swab may also be taken

◆ Depending on sexual practice, a rectal swab may also be taken

◆ A throat swab using a cotton-tipped applicator may be taken if appropriate

◆ A smear for cytology may be taken if appropriate. Women should be actively encouraged to have their cervical smears performed at the same place, e.g. GP surgery or family planning clinic. This is for continuity with reporting and follow-up

◆ A serological test for syphilis will be taken as part of the routine care and may be repeated

---

Box 14.2   Causes of vaginal discharge

Pathological discharge (infective)
◆ *Candida albicans*
◆ Bacterial vaginosis
◆ *Trichomonas vaginalis*
◆ *Chlamydia trachomatis*
◆ *Neisseria gonorrhoea*
◆ Genital ulceration, e.g. herpes.

Non-infective
◆ Cervical ectopy
◆ Cervical polyp
◆ Cervical neoplasm
◆ Retained products (e.g. tampon, broken condom or post-termination of pregnancy)
◆ Trauma
◆ Atrophic vaginitis
◆ Allergic reactions (e.g. douches)
◆ Genital washing with soaps or shower gels, particularly anti-bacterial products.

after 3 months as the incubation period for syphilis is variable

◆ A routine urinalysis is also performed

◆ Screening for hepatitis A, B or C or an HIV antibody test, following pre-test discussion, may be performed if required. An HIV test will be offered to all new GUM attendees as part of the sexual health strategy targets (DoH, 2001).

A good light source should be available for the routine examination. A hand lens is of particular value when trying to identify very small warts, infestations and in assisting to distinguish dermatological conditions of the vulva from STIs.

Physically, it takes longer to examine a woman and the examination is far more detailed. Specimen taking needs to be particularly accurate with sufficient material taken to inoculate cultures. Differential diagnosis can often be difficult to establish. The clinical picture may be made more complex if the woman is also experiencing a urinary tract infection.

Non-infective causes of vaginal discharge

It is worth noting that using soap or shower gel to wash the genital area (or douching the vagina) could potentially upset the acid balance thus causing more problems with discharge and potential odours. Women should be actively encouraged to stop using these products, and to use plenty of water instead.

Cervical ectopy
An explanation of cervical ectopy is given in Chapter 13, page 358.

Cervical polyp
An explanation of a cervical polyp is given on page 368 (see also colour plate 4).

Cervical neoplasm
Irregular bleeding (particularly post-coital) is the most common first symptom of a cervical neoplasm and there may be a watery discharge, which is often offensive.

Retained products
Postnatal or post-termination. Retained products of conception can cause symptoms of bleeding, lower abdominal pain and an offensive vaginal discharge, particularly if there is an accompanying infection. Treatment is with antibiotics and a surgical procedure called an evacuation of the retained products of conception (ERPC).

Retained tampon. A retained tampon, or part of tampon that has broken off, will very quickly give rise to a characteristically offensive discharge. This will settle on removal but occasionally antibiotics may be required if the tampon has been present for any length of time. There is obviously a risk of toxic shock syndrome associated with a retained tampon (see page 532).

Retained broken condom. A retained broken condom will very quickly give rise to a characteristically offensive discharge. This will settle on removal but occasionally antibiotics may be required if the condom has been present for any length of time.

Atrophic vaginitis
An explanation of atrophic vaginitis is given on page 456.

Pathological discharge

Vulvovaginal candidiasis
Vulvovaginal candidiasis or yeast infection (commonly known as thrush) is one of the most common causes of vaginal discharge throughout the world. It is a pathogen most associated with complaints of vulvovaginal irritation and itching (Hamill and Kaufman, 1990). Candidiasis thrives in a warm, moist and dark environment, which makes the vagina an ideal host for infection. *Candida* species may be present as blastospores in up to 20% of asymptomatic women (Sobel, 1990) or as germinated yeasts which have successfully adhered to vaginal epithelial cells in women with symptoms. Candidiasis is not considered to be sexually transmitted, although Sobel noted 'penile colonization with candida is present in approximately 20% of male partners of women with recurrent vaginal candidiasis'. Some specialists believe that *Candida* may be a normal

commensal in the vagina. For symptoms to develop the *Candida* must become activated and increase in number and this can occur when the vaginal environment becomes altered.

There are three yeasts that are commonly found in the vagina of asymptomatic women (Thin, 1982):

◆ *Candida albicans* 81%

◆ *Torulopsis glabrata* (now called *Candida glabrata*) 16%

◆ Other *Candida* species 3%.

The incubation period remains undetermined because it is difficult to establish at what precise moment the yeast begins to colonize the vagina.

Predisposing factors and clinical manifestations of candidiasis are listed in Boxes 14.3 and 14.4. Symptoms of candidiasis may be exacerbated

---

Box 14.4 Clinical manifestations of candidiasis (see Colour plates 6 and 7)

◆ Acute pruritus
◆ Vaginal discharge (which may range from watery to homogeneously thick and commonly described as looking like cottage cheese)
◆ Vulval erythema and burning
◆ Vaginal erythema and burning
◆ Dyspareunia
◆ External dysuria
◆ Odour (is often minimal and non-offensive)
◆ Fissuring and oedema (may occur).

---

a few days before the onset of menstruation and the soreness and excoriation may extend down to the peri-anal region.

Diagnosis

A high vaginal swab should be taken and microscopic examination by Gram stain or by wet mount preparation will usually demonstrate Gram-positive bacilli and yeast cells, mycelia and spores. A urine test should be performed to check for sugar and protein, as diabetic women are particularly prone to candidiasis. The vaginal pH is normal. No serological test is available to diagnose vulvovaginal candidiasis.

Treatment

A variety of preparations are now available to treat vulvovaginal candidiasis and the treatment regime will depend on whether the episode is a primary occurrence or recurrent and previously difficult to treat. No treatment is recommended for asymptomatic women.

A single episode. The following regimes are recommended to treat a single episode of candidiasis.

Topical intravaginal therapies:

Treating candidiasis intravaginally is necessary, as topical 1% cream on the vulva alone will not be effective. The following regimes may affect latex condoms and diaphragms so unless another method of contraception is used intercourse should be avoided.

Box 14.3 Predisposing factors for candidiasis

◆ Pregnancy
◆ The older generation contraceptive pill containing a higher dosage of oestrogen: the third generation pill is not considered a risk factor (Bowman, 1992)
◆ Diabetes mellitus
◆ Broad-spectrum antibiotics
◆ Steroid and immunosuppressive drugs
◆ HIV infection (when cell-mediated immunity is damaged)
◆ Tight restrictive clothing and nylon underwear, resulting in poor ventilation to the genital area
◆ Trauma to the vaginal mucosa due to vaginal dryness during sexual intercourse or the use of tampons
◆ The use of soaps or shower gels to wash the genital area; feminine hygiene products or douching. These chemical agents can alter vaginal pH. Women must be actively encouraged to wash with water only. A full explanation should be given to women so they understand this rationale
◆ Other factors that may cause a change in vaginal pH such as semen or menstrual blood
◆ Stress – this can trigger an increase in adrenaline, which in turn, can affect sex hormones which may lead to changes in the menstrual cycle, thus altering vaginal pH
◆ Anaemia.

- Clotrimazole 500 mg vaginal pessary at night once, or 200 mg vaginal pessary for three nights or 100 mg vaginal pessary for six nights
- Clotrimazole 5 mg 10% vaginal cream applied at night stat
- Econazole 150 mg pessary at night once or 150 mg vaginal pessary for three nights
- Fenticonazole 600 mg vaginal pessary at night once or 200 mg vaginal pessary for three nights
- Miconazole 1.2 g ovule at night stat
- Miconazole 100 mg vaginal pessary × 14 nights.

Oral therapies:

- Fluconazole 150 mg capsule stat
- Itraconazole 200 mg capsule b.d. × 1 day.

Oral regimes should not be used by pregnant or breastfeeding women (Clinical Effectiveness Group, 1999).

Recurrent and relapsing candidiasis. Women with recurrent candidiasis should be referred to GUM as this condition can cause considerable distress and is often difficult to treat, plus other pathogens could be involved. You should be able to reassure the woman that ultimately her condition is manageable. Treatment regimes may combine topical and oral therapy, involve the use of intermittent prophylaxis, and include the treatment of the partner.

The important aspect of the care of this group of women is the psychological support they need as recurrent problems can eventually put stress on a relationship as intercourse tends to be avoided due to discomfort and pain. Women will often self-medicate without medical advice and they should be advised against this. Recurrence of candidiasis may occur because a small number of organisms may persist and escape detection and re-emerge at another time. The need to ensure that clients comply with the full length of treatment is crucial in order to avoid recurrence.

Advice and follow-up

There are many useful patient information leaflets about candidiasis which you should have available to back up any verbal advice you offer. This advice should include the following:

- Avoid the use of douching as this may alter the acid/alkaline balance of the vagina therefore encouraging yeasts to multiply
- Use baths or salt baths to give relief from local discomfort but do not wash the genital area with bubble baths, disinfectants such as Dettol, strongly perfumed soaps and vaginal deodorants, as they can alter vaginal pH. Women should be actively encouraged to use water or aqueous cream to wash the genital area
- Change to a non-biological washing powder
- Avoid tights, nylon underwear, tight jeans, etc., and wear loose clothing with a high proportion of non-synthetic fibres. Women should be encouraged not to wear underwear in bed, in order to allow some airflow to the genital area
- Use pads and panty liners rather than tampons
- Take care with genital and anal hygiene (wiping from 'front to back') to avoid autoinoculation from the bowel of *Candida* species
- Apply live natural yoghurt to the vulva if an episode is not too severe. Although, this is thought to be soothing and relieve symptoms rather than actually treat symptoms
- If antibiotics usually give rise to candidiasis, then ask for prophylactic *Candida* treatment at the same time
- Avoid intercourse until all symptoms have disappeared, as this will naturally encourage local cellular repair
- Ensure that the genital area is thoroughly dried after washing. Some women use a hair dryer if too sore to dry with a towel
- In 1990 a study showed that potentially spores could be harboured in the gusset of damp underwear. It was suggested that after laundering, and whilst still damp, underwear is microwaved for a least 5 minutes or that a hot iron is run over the gusset area (Phillips and Friedrich, 1990)

◆ Tea tree oil has been recommended for treatment (see page 74).

If the episode of candidiasis is an isolated attack then follow-up is not necessary. For women who experience recurrent vulvovaginal candidiasis, a routine follow-up is recommended. Adler (1990) suggests male contacts should be seen 'firstly, if they have symptoms and secondly, if the woman is having repeated recurrences. The man should be thoroughly investigated, as was his female partner, to make sure that he has no concurrent sexually transmitted infection, since this is likely to predispose to candidal infection'.

Bacterial vaginosis

Bacterial vaginosis (BV) is a common cause of vaginal discharge affecting 12–20% of women of reproductive age (McDonald *et al.*, 1997).

There is constant debate as to whether BV is sexually transmitted, as the highest group of women experiencing the problem are seen at GUM clinics. However, the infection has been found in virgins (Bump and Buesching, 1988) and is also common in women who have sex with women (McCaffrey *et al.*, 1997).

Keane *et al.* (1997) indicated an association between BV and non-gonococcal urethritis (NGU). They argue that male partners may develop symptoms of NGU, when large numbers of the bacteria in BV are present in female partners. This suggests that BV is sexually transmissible but is not exclusively an STI. Despite all the conflicting opinions of researchers, women are informed that BV is not sexually transmitted and therefore their partners do not need screening and treatment.

BV is a complex condition which results in a shift in the ecological balance of the vaginal flora. The lactobacilli protecting the vagina are substantially reduced in number and replaced by a mixed anaerobic flora consisting of *Gardnerella vaginalis* and anaerobes such as *Mycoplasma hominis*, *Bacteroides* and *Mobiluncus* species.

The exact cause of BV is unknown. Keane *et al.* (1997) and Taylor-Robinson and Hay (1997) suggest that BV is associated with the following factors which alter the vaginal pH balance:

◆ Vaginal douching
◆ The use of soaps, shower gels and bath additives
◆ Hormonal changes during the menstrual cycle
◆ Genetic factors
◆ Residual semen after unprotected sexual intercourse.

BV is associated with pelvic inflammatory disease, infertility, spontaneous pre-term delivery in pregnancy and labour (McGregor *et al.*, 1994); late miscarriage as well as postoperative infection after hysterectomy (Easmon, 1993).

Consequently, there is a call amongst some GU physicians that antibiotic prophylaxis should be considered for women undergoing gynaecological procedures, or swabs taken for gonorrhoea and chlamydia PCR, prior to the procedure, to ensure there are no pathogens present. Some centres in the UK now routinely administer prophylaxis to women having a termination of pregnancy to reduce the incidence of pelvic inflammatory disease (PID) following this procedure.

BV has been found to be more common in African-Caribbean women, possibly due to ethnic differences in genital hygiene. It is common for African-Caribbean women to practise vaginal douching and to use Dettol/antiseptic products for genital washing (Rajamanoharan *et al.*, 1999), which could put them at a greater risk of developing symptomatic BV. The clinical manifestations are listed in Box 14.5.

Diagnosis

BV is primarily a diagnosis of exclusion. Other sexually transmitted pathogens need to be eliminated first as a possible cause of the pathology. The vaginal discharge is characteristic and may be viewed on the labia and fourchette prior to internal examination.

A Gram-stained slide is considered the definitive diagnostic test and shows the absence of lactobacilli and presence of mixed flora and 'clue cells'. Clue cells are epithelial cells which are readily identified under the microscope as their margins are crowded and they are often obscured

> **Box 14.5** Clinical manifestations of bacterial vaginosis (see Colour plate 8)
>
> ◆ Discharge – a malodorous vaginal discharge which is often described as milky-grey and watery with a fishy or cheesy odour and is frequently worse after sexual intercourse or at the time of a period. Occasionally there is an increase in the amount of discharge or a change of colour (grey or yellow)
> ◆ Abdominal discomfort (may be experienced)
> ◆ Pruritus
> ◆ Dysuria.
>
> There is little or no inflammation of the vaginal epithelium and no vulval erythema, oedema or fissuring present, unless a coexisting pathogen is also causing additional pathology which is why the infection is called vaginosis rather than vaginitis (Morse *et al.*, 1996).

by bacteria sticking to them. The vaginal pH is raised above 4.5. The amine test is often performed as part of the diagnostic criteria. This is when a drop of vaginal discharge is placed on a slide and mixed with a drop of 10% potassium hydroxide (KOH) which is then smelt immediately. KOH is an alkaline solution that allows the release of volatile amines, resulting in the characteristic fishy odour.

Another diagnostic method for BV that can be used is the Ison and Hay (2002) criteria. BV is diagnosed on Gram-stain, with little or no lactobacilli present, and the presence of *Gardnerella* and/or *Mobiluncus* species. A vaginal culture for BV is of limited value as mixed bacterial flora can be isolated in asymptomatic women.

Easmon (1993) believes that BV is underdiagnosed in the primary care setting for a variety of reasons:

◆ A shortage of consultation time
◆ A 'basic reluctance to undertake vaginal examination'
◆ The lack of a chaperone.

Easmon recommends that practice nurses should learn more about BV in order to improve the sexual health of their clients and to facilitate better management of the problem in primary care.

Treatment

Symptomatic patients require treatment, as do those undergoing some gynaecological surgical procedures. The current treatment is oral metronidazole 2 g given stat or metronidazole 400 mg twice daily for 5 days. Patients should be advised to avoid alcohol as this can produce a disulfiram-like reaction with nausea, flushing, headache and sweating. Extra care should be taken if women are also taking anticoagulants, as the prothrombin time may be prolonged. Metronidazole is relatively contraindicated in the first trimester of pregnancy because of its possible teratogenic risks. However, it can be used in the second trimester.

Alternatively clindamycin 2% cream used intravaginally with an applicator at night for 7 nights can be given and recent studies have shown cure rates of 90% after one week (Larsson, 1997). Clindamycin is the preferred treatment during the first trimester and early second trimester of pregnancy. It is also recommended for women with a high alcohol intake, who will not be able to refrain from alcohol consumption when taking metronidazole. It should be noted that clindamycin could affect the efficacy of condoms. Currently it is not a recommendation that all pregnant women should be screened and treated for BV. However, some health professionals may choose to discuss the evidence with women, particularly those with a history of preterm delivery, or late miscarriage. They in turn may choose to have treatment if indicated.

BV along with vaginal candidiasis are not sexually transmitted infections. However, women may experience similar anxieties and distress, because of the smell of the vaginal discharge and their discomfort, as women who present at a GUM clinic with an STI. It is important that you listen to your client's worries and discuss them thoroughly rather than dismiss them as trivial. Good communication is vital, because if the conditions are not clearly understood they can cause additional stress for the woman within her sexual relationship.

Trichomonas vaginalis

Trichomoniasis is an STI caused by a flagellated protozoan called *Trichomonas vaginalis* (TV).

It is the most common non-viral STI in the world (Petrin *et al.*, 1998). In women the organism is usually isolated from the posterior vaginal fornix where it attaches itself to areas of vaginal squamous epithelium. Columnar epithelium seems to demonstrate resistance to TV; however, the cervix can be involved in the inflammatory response, giving the cervix a characteristic strawberry appearance known as a 'strawberry cervix'. TV may also be present in the urethra, bladder, Skene's ducts and Bartholin's ducts (Gulmezoglu, 1996). Perinatal transmission is the main method of non-venereal spread. Up to 40% of women with trichomoniasis attending GUM clinics may also have gonorrhoea (Mohanty, 1990) and 10% may have candida (Adler, 1995).

TV is ovoid in shape and can be observed down the microscope making a jerky swaying motion. Four free anterior flagella and an undulating membrane provide movement. *Trichomonas* reproduce by binary fission and feed by phagocytosis. The incubation period is thought to be between 1 and 4 weeks. The reason for such a variable length of time for a woman to produce symptoms will depend on her susceptibility and reactivity.

The clinical manifestations are listed in Box 14.6 although the woman may well be asymptomatic and any clinical features present are variable. Many women notice the first symptoms during or immediately following a menstrual period (Catterel, 1972).

Box 14.6 Clinical manifestations of trichomoniasis (see Colour Plate 9)

◆ Vaginal discharge is most frequently described as profuse, yellow to green in colour, offensive in odour and frothy in appearance

◆ Vaginal pruritus and vulval soreness and erythema may be present although are not common

◆ Dyspareunia

◆ Dysuria (often with urinary frequency)

◆ Lower abdominal pain

◆ Colpitis macularis (small punctate haemorrhages of the cervix may be present, giving the cervix a characteristic 'strawberry' appearance, see Colour plate 5).

TV infection may assist in the transmission of the HIV virus (Sorvillo *et al.*, 2001). There is also increasing evidence suggesting an association between TV and premature delivery and low birth weight babies born to infected mothers (Cotch *et al*, 1997; Saurina and McCormack, 1997).

Diagnosis

Trichomoniasis can be diagnosed by using Amies transport medium or microscopy when a wet mount slide (with a coverslip) is viewed under the microscope. The flagella can be seen making a characteristic whiplash motion. The undulating membrane can also be seen pulsating. There are an increased number of polymorphonuclear neutrophils present as part of the acute inflammatory response. However, wet mount may fail to detect up to 50% of cases due to low sensitivity (Bickly *et al.*, 1989). The gold standard test for the infection is by culture (Sobel, 1997). No serological test is available. The vaginal pH is raised to 5.5. The amine test may also be positive.

Occasionally TV may be reported on a cervical smear result. However, it is difficult to identify it using this method, so it may lead to a large number of false positive results (Wiese *et al.*, 2000). It is important to confirm diagnosis by examination of vaginal secretions, and preferably culture medium. Evidence indicates that TV diagnosis by liquid-based cytology is accurate and merits treatment without any further investigation (Lara-Torre and Pinkerton, 2003).

Treatment

The treatment of choice is either metronidazole 2 g stat or 400 mg b.d. for 5 days given to the client and to all sexual partners within the last 3 months. The same advice outlined on page 396 should be given regarding the medication. Resistance to metronidazole is rising (Barat and Bloland, 1997; Petrin *et al.*, 1998), so alternative therapy needs to be considered and currently various treatment regimes are used, including intravaginal therapy. Coelho (1997) showed successful treatment for metronidazole-resistant TV using paromomycin, but how common this regimen could become is debatable.

All male partners need to be seen, examined and treated. Mohanty (1990) remarked that 'ninety per cent of male contacts of women with trichomonas are asymptomatic'. To isolate the organism in men is notoriously difficult and they should be treated epidemiologically in the absence of a definitive diagnosis if the female contact is positive. A follow-up test of cure is recommended for both partners.

For recurrent *Trichomonas* infections it is important to check that the partner has been correctly treated and to consider the possibility of re-infection. If the condition is more obstinate, then a further course of metronidazole 400 mg twice daily may be prescribed for 5 days. Abstinence from sexual intercourse at diagnosis is essential until a cure has been established.

Chlamydial infection

Chlamydia trachomatis is the most common curable STI in the developed world (Taylor-Robinson, 1996). With the exception of HIV, *Chlamydia trachomatis* has been associated with higher economic costs than any other disease in developed countries. The overall cost in the UK has been estimated at £200 million per annum. Chlamydial infection is a serious public health concern due to the long-term sequelae of untreated infection in women, as well as the infection enhancing HIV transmission (Wasserheit, 1992).

Chlamydia trachomatis is an obligate intracellular parasite and depends on the host cell to provide it with its energy source and other nutrients. The organism has a unique growth cycle that depends on attachment and penetration of the host cell using an enhanced phagocytic process. The incubation period is 7–21 days as confirmed from male urethral infection. Infection by *Chlamydia trachomatis* can be difficult to diagnose in women and may easily escape detection. It is usually acquired through unprotected vaginal, anal and, conceivably, oral sex (Winter *et al.*, 2000) or vertically at birth. The organism infects the columnar or transitional epithelium of the urethra, endocervix, and may spread to the endometrium, Fallopian tubes, peritoneal cavity and rectum, producing inflammation, ulceration and scarring. At least a third of women with *Chlamydia trachomatis* will have signs of local infection. However, up to 70% of women and 50% of men with *Chlamydia* will be asymptomatic (Cates and Wasserheit, 1991), and women may harbour the organism for a considerable length of time with few or no symptoms to suggest infection. Alternatively, women may present with PID (see also page 353), peri-hepatitis (Fitz-Hugh-Curtis syndrome), Bartholinitis or reactive arthritis. Some of the clinical manifestations are listed in Box 14.7.

Chlamydial infection is the commonest cause of PID in industrialized countries (Westrom, 1980; Stamm *et al.*, 1984). Of these, 10% will have an ectopic pregnancy and 20% may become infertile (Teare, 1986; Johnson *et al.*, 1996). The risk of infertility rises with each episode of PID – 10% after the first episode and 75% after the third (Adler, 1995). In babies born to untreated mothers, up to 50% will be infected with an eye disease and up to 20% will contract pneumonia (Adler, 1995).

Box 14.7 Clinical manifestations of chlamydial infection which may be present in women (see also Colour plate 10)

◆ Mucopurulent vaginal discharge
◆ Hypertrophic ectopy of the cervix, which becomes oedematous, congested and bleeds easily
◆ Urethritis
◆ Bartholinitis
◆ Endometritis
◆ Salpingitis (which may present as in the Fitz-Hugh-Curtis syndrome where the chlamydial infection has spread to the liver capsule causing right upper quadrant abdominal pain or shoulder pain)
◆ Dysuria or frequency
◆ Post-coital bleeding
◆ Lower abdominal pain
◆ A discharge from the anus
◆ Dyspareunia
◆ Dysmenorrhoea.

Some of the predisposing factors for *C. trachomatis* in asymptomatic women were discussed by Romanowski (1993) who noted that chlamydial infection was more common in the following groups of people:

◆ Sexually active women under 25 years of age

◆ Women who do not use contraception or those who use a non-barrier method

◆ Women who have had two or more sexual partners in the last year

◆ GUM clinic attenders having a partner with non-specific urethritis or gonorrhoea.

In 1996 the Chief Medical Officer set up an Expert Advisory Group to look at a national screening programme for *Chlamydia* in the UK (Central Audit Group in Genito-Urinary Medicine, 1997). This advisory group endorsed Romanowski's findings and recommended that the following groups should be routinely screened for *Chlamydia*:

◆ All GUM clinic attenders and their partners

◆ All women seeking termination of pregnancy and their partners

◆ Asymptomatic sexually active women aged under 25, especially teenagers

◆ Asymptomatic women aged over 25 who have had a new sexual partner or had two or more partners in a year.

Despite their recommendations, a national screening programme was not immediately implemented, and since 1997 there has been a massive 141% increase in diagnosed cases. In 2002 there were 82,206 new diagnosed cases of *Chlamydia* infection in England, Wales and Northern Ireland. In 2002 the highest rates were seen in young women between the ages of 16 and 19 (PHLS, 2003). Newly diagnosed complicated chlamydial infections (including PID) rose by 20% between 1997 and 1998 (PHLS, 1999).

Between 1999 and 2000 women between the ages of 16 and 24 were opportunistically screened in a variety of primary and secondary settings in a pilot chlamydial study, funded by the DoH, conducted in Portsmouth (chlamydial prevalence 9.8%) and in Wirral (chlamydial prevalence 11.2%)

(Pimenta *et al.*, 2003), using urine samples tested by ligase chain reaction (LCR).

Following this study, and the publication of the sexual health strategy (DoH, 2001), the DoH is finally introducing a phased rollout chlamydial screening programme. However, this is across a limited number of sites (and, at present, not amongst general medical services or general practice), and therefore will not capture all groups identified by the pilot study and the Chief Medical Officer's Expert Advisory Group's recommendations of nearly a decade ago. Also, as men are another known source of infection, it appears a little short-sighted to only screen women opportunistically. There are plenty of areas within health care where young men could be captured for opportunistic screening, e.g. accident and emergency departments. Until we have a national screening programme for both men and women, across primary and secondary care, the *Chlamydia* infection rates will undoubtedly continue to rise.

Diagnosis

Adequate specimen collection is essential in the diagnosis of *Chlamydia*. Swabs must be firmly rotated against tissue when sampling, as samples must contain cellular material. The most important site to sample in women is the endocervix. Any excess secretions should be removed prior to the sample being obtained. It is recommended that the swab is inserted 1–2 cm in the os and rotated for 15–30 seconds. Care should be taken not to touch the vaginal mucosa when removing the swab to prevent contamination.

Currently, in many clinical areas, the swab is used to detect chlamydial antigen, which is measured by enzyme-linked immunosorbent assay (ELISA). However, reliability of this test is dependent upon a good sample being obtained and is only about 70% accurate. This is a suboptimal test, and following the Select Committee's publication (2003) criticizing the use of ELISA for *Chlamydia* screening, the Government announced that it will be seeking bids for funding to ensure that all major laboratories in each region of England use nucleic acid amplification tests (NAATs) (DoH, 2003). NAATs available include polymerase chain reaction (PCR) and LCR.

Lee *et al.* (1995) reviewed DNA amplification techniques and although they are twice as expensive as the ELISA test, they can be 95% accurate, as even the smallest amount of bacteria present, in urine/vulval/vaginal/tampons and cervical swabs, can be amplified. As testing can be performed on urine and tampons, it has the advantage of being an acceptable alternative to invasive vaginal examination.

Serological tests for chlamydial antibodies are available but their use is of limited value, as they do not determine whether a patient has the infection at the time of collection. They only demonstrate that the patient has been in contact with the infection at some point (Goh and Forster, 1993).

A specific *Chlamydia* culture (a transport medium) is available. It is recommended that it should be used if a woman has been sexually assaulted, as it has high specificity, which is essential for medico-legal purposes. All female contacts of men with non-specific urethritis will routinely have an endocervical chlamydial test. Testing for *Chlamydia* prior to a termination of pregnancy or an IUD insertion is now routine in many units so that, if necessary, effective treatment can be commenced before the procedure is carried out.

Treatment

The first antibiotics of choice are either doxycycline 100 mg b.d. for 7 days or azithromycin 1 g stat oral dose. Azithromycin is as effective as doxycycline (Johnson *et al.*, 1996) but is twice as expensive. However, as compliance with azithromycin is greater, economic evaluations have shown it to be more cost-effective than doxycycline (Magid *et al.*, 1996). Studies of the use of azithromycin in pregnancy have shown substantially improved cure rates (Wehbeh *et al.*, 1998; Adair *et al.*, 1998), although its safety in this circumstance has not been fully established. Therefore, recommended treatment for pregnant or lactating women is erythromycin 500 mg q.d.s. for 7 days or b.d. for 14 days.

As it is conceivable that *Chlamydia* can be transmitted through oral sex, patients should be advised to abstain from all forms of sexual activity until a cure has been established and all partners treated. Transmission should be discussed and advice given about future safer sex.

Women should be followed up 1 week later to check treatment compliance and sexual abstinence, as well as contact tracing. Tests of cure are not indicated following treatment for uncomplicated infection, as long as the patient is asymptomatic, and there is not a risk that re-infection has occurred However, if required, evidence suggests that detection of *Chlamydia* during follow-up is greatest 3–5 weeks after completing treatment, and not earlier.

All patients found to be *Chlamydia* positive should see a health adviser for contact tracing of current and/or recent sexual partners. Women who are contacts of men diagnosed as having non-specific urethritis are treated epidemiologically for *Chlamydia* irrespective of whether the organism is isolated from them or not. Very often women who have *Chlamydia* at the time a cervical smear is taken may find the results show 'inflammatory changes'. A full bacterial and viral screen should then be performed, and if any infection is diagnosed it should be treated prior to repeating the smear. *Chlamydia* is often a co-infection when another STI (notably gonorrhoea) is present causing a vaginal discharge, or when a mucopurulent cervicitis is diagnosed with a non-specific cause.

Women need to be aware that *Chlamydia* can be transmitted through sex and vertically at birth. They should also know that the tests and treatment of *Chlamydia* are simple and effective. Raising awareness of *Chlamydia* infection and introducing a national screening programme is of utmost importance.

Gonorrhoea

Gonorrhoea (GC) is one of the oldest STIs and the historical epidemiology of gonorrhoea is linked to changes in sexual behaviour.

Recent statistics show that gonorrhoea is on the rise in the UK and indeed around the world. Almost half of all diagnosed UK cases are found in London (PHLS, 2002). Young women aged 16–19 have a higher incidence of GC than the national average (PHLS, 2002).

In approximately 70% of women gonorrhoea is asymptomatic or they may present with PID. Symptomatic women may present with any of the manifestations listed in Box 14.8.

Symptoms, if present, are often associated with a concurrent infection such as *Chlamydia trachomatis* in 20–40% of cases, or *Trichomonas vaginalis* in 20% of cases. The incubation period in men for urethral gonorrhoea is 3–7 days. For women the incubation period is more variable, but is approximately 10 days in women who are symptomatic.

The cause of gonorrhoea is an organism called *Neisseria gonorrhoea*. It was discovered by Albert Neisser, after whom it is named. *Neisseria gonorrhoea* is a Gram-negative diplococcus that is non-motile and non-spore-forming and characteristically grows in pairs. Serotyping of the gonococci has demonstrated at least 70 different strains.

Gonococci attach to cellular membranes of columnar and immature squamous epithelium causing substantial mucosal cell damage in a very short time. Submucosal invasion is accompanied by a heavy polymorphonuclear leucocyte response. In women the primary site is usually the endocervix, where the pH is neutral. However, other mucous membrane sites that can be infected are urethra, rectum, pharynx and conjunctiva. Transmission through sexual activity can be via oral, anal or vaginal sex and can occur by direct inoculation of secretions, via fingers or sex toys. Auto-inoculation may result in infection of the Skene's glands, Bartholin's ducts and colonization of the urethra and rectum, or conjunctiva. It can be acquired vertically at birth.

Diagnosis

A Gram-stain slide is taken to identify the Gram-negative intracellular diplococci. A wet-mount slide or HVS is also taken to exclude a co-infection with *Trichomonas vaginalis*. Primarily, swabs are taken from the cervix and/or urethra and cultured on blood agar plates or transported in Stuart's medium. If anal sex has been disclosed, then a rectal swab should be obtained as well. Women who are known contacts of partners with gonorrhoea, or complain of rectal discomfort will also have a rectal culture taken.

If the woman complains of a sore throat, or if her partner has GC, or she reports oral sex practices, an oropharyngeal swab test will also be performed (although >90% of pharyngeal infections are asymptomatic). Microscopy is not appropriate for pharyngeal specimens.

Taking cultures from women is essential as up to 50% of cases of gonorrhoea will be missed in women if the Gram-stain slide is relied on alone.

Blood tests are available to detect antibodies to *N. gonorrhoea*; however, they are not sufficiently sensitive or specific to be used in uncomplicated gonorrhoea.

In some clinical areas, first void urine gonorrhoea PCR tests may be taken if available. However, it should be noted that this particular test does not allow for antimicrobial sensitivity testing. If positive this would make treating resistant strains difficult, as no sensitivities would be available.

Treatment

Antibiotic-resistant strains of GC are increasing worldwide (PHLS, 1998), and there have been incidences of ciprofloxacin-resistant GC documented in the north of England (Corkill *et al.*, 2003; Tayal *et al.*, 1999). When treating GC, recent regional, national and global epidemiological GC treatment developments, as well as the patient's sexual contact history, must be married up, to ensure optimal success with first-line therapy chosen.

Box 14.8 Clinical manifestations of gonorrhoea (see also Colour plate 10)

◆ Mucopurulent vaginal discharge
◆ Cervicitis
◆ Intermenstrual uterine bleeding
◆ Menorrhagia (can be severe)
◆ Erythema and oedema of the cervix (may bleed on contact with a swab)
◆ Dysuria
◆ Dyspareunia
◆ Lower abdominal pain.

In uncomplicated cervical, urethral and rectal GC the usual treatment of choice is Ciprofloaxacin 500 mg stat oral dose or Ofloxacin 400 mg stat oral dose. In regional areas where there is minimal penicillin-resistant GC, treatment can be Amoxycillin 3 g stat and Probenicid 1 g stat orally. All pharyngeal GC should be treated with Ciprofloxacin 500 mg stat oral dose or Ofloxacin 400 mg stat oral dose or intramuscular Ceftriaxone 250 mg stat. Quinolones should not be used for pregnant women or in patients with a history of convulsions. These patients will require intramuscular antibiotic therapy listed below or Amoxycillin 3 g stat oral dose and Probenicid 1 g stat oral (bearing in mind epidemiological effects, mentioned earlier).

Quinolones are highly effective against penicillin-resistant strains of GC. If the GC is both penicillin- and quinolone-resistant, then intramuscular Cefotaxime 500 mg stat or Ceftriaxone 250 mg stat or Spectinomycin 2 g stat can be given. Mohanty (1989) explains that the reason for giving a single-dose treatment is based on the high default rate of follow-up examination for a test of cure'. It is possible that a rise in treatment failures could enhance transmission of GC.

French (1995) indicated that patients diagnosed with cervical and urethral gonorrhoea should also be treated with a course of doxycycline 100 mg twice daily for 7 days or Azithromycin 1 g stat oral dose in case of coexisting chlamydial infection. Routine screening for *Chlamydia* and other infections will be taken as part of the diagnostic procedure.

All patients with GC should be referred to the health adviser for contact tracing. They are advised to abstain from all forms of sexual activity until all partners are treated, and a follow-up set of swab tests have been performed a week following diagnosis and these results are proven to be negative (i.e. they will be abstaining for at least two weeks) to ensure the infection has been cured. Gonorrhoea can have serious sequelae if untreated. In the short term, complications like salpingitis, Bartholin's gland abscess and PID may ensue. Disseminated gonococcal infections can lead to septic arthritis and sexually acquired reactive arthritis, and longer term there is an increased risk of chronic pelvic pain, ectopic pregnancy and infertility. If a pregnant woman develops gonorrhoea, Godley (1993) reports a risk of intrauterine growth retardation, premature membrane rupture, chorioamnionitis and postpartum sepsis. There is the additional risk of ophthalmia neonatorum in the neonate (see Colour plate 11).

Genital ulceration

Most genital ulceration in young adults is likely to be infectious, whilst in the older woman the possibility of neoplastic disease has to be considered. The average age for developing vulval carcinoma is 60 years (Hall, 1993). When discussing genital ulceration the history-taking from the patient needs to be particularly detailed, particularly noting if the woman has recently had sexual intercourse abroad. This is for two reasons: first, because it may be necessary to consider a tropical STI; and second, genital ulceration is a co-factor throughout the world, implicated in the spread of HIV infection.

Other important questions to ask a patient about genital ulceration are:

◆ When was the last occurrence of sexual intercourse?

◆ Is the ulcer painful or painless?

◆ Is it a single ulcer or multiple?

◆ Is it the first occurrence or is it recurrent in nature?

◆ Has she taken any drugs recently? This could indicate Stevens-Johnson syndrome (a drug reaction causing genital ulceration usually associated with tetracyclines)

◆ Is there a history of any allergies?

◆ Is the area itchy and is there any excoriation present?

Common causes of genital ulceration are listed in Box 14.9.

Genital herpes

Anogenital herpes simplex virus (HSV) is the commonest ulcerative STI in the UK (PHLS *et al.*, 2001).

Box 14.9 Causes of genital ulceration

Infective

- ◆ Genital herpes
- ◆ Syphilis
- ◆ Tropical STIs
  - ◆ chancroid
  - ◆ lymphogranuloma venereum
  - ◆ granuloma inguinale

  (These tropical STIs are not detailed in this chapter. In the case of suspected tropical STIs, patients should be referred to a GUM clinic for management)
- ◆ Pyogenic infection
- ◆ Scabies and infestations
- ◆ Candidiasis (severe)
- ◆ Condylomata acuminata (genital warts – these do not usually ulcerate but if ulceration occurs it is often as a result of treatment, with the added risk of a secondary infection because of local tissue damage)

Non-infective

- ◆ Trauma
- ◆ Drug eruptions
- ◆ Carcinoma
- ◆ Behcet's disease
- ◆ Paget's disease
- ◆ Crohn's disease
- ◆ Dermatitis artefacta.

The notable feature of HSV is its ability to remain latent in the host, meaning it is not clinically apparent and the patient is asymptomatic. Although the process is not fully understood, the virus is somehow reactivated and moves to the nerve endings. Here it then replicates into the epidermis or cervical/vulval/oral mucosa and can cause a reoccurrence of the infection. At present there is no cure for herpes. The physical and psychological morbidity of the condition is of particular concern, as genital herpes tends to affect the woman's personal relationships due to its chronic nature. Breslin (1988) points out that 'emphasizing that the disease is not curable is non-productive'. When talking to women with herpes you should listen carefully to all their concerns and encourage them as far as possible to try to gain psychological control of the virus.

Several viruses are classified as herpes viruses. They are herpes simplex virus 1 and 2 (HSV-1 and HSV-2), varicella-zoster virus, Epstein-Barr virus, cytomegalovirus and human herpes virus 6. HSV-2 resides in the sacral ganglia causing anogenital lesions, whilst HSV-1 resides in the trigeminal ganglia and is principally associated with oral-facial lesions. However, both are sexually transmissible, to either site, depending on sexual practice, and auto-inoculation from one site to another is possible with a primary episode. Some population prevalence studies of HSV-2 have demonstrated an antibody level 25% higher than those who present with clinical disease. This may be because symptoms are mild, and therefore the infection is often not recognised as HSV, and therefore not reported.

Active HSV-2 infection has an incubation period of 2–20 days, or longer. HSV-2 has been demonstrated to be more virulent than HSV-1. Non-venereal spread of HSV-2 to the neonate can occur intrapartum and postpartum.

Transmission

The herpes virus is transmitted through direct skin contact, during genital-to-genital or genital-to-mouth contact, usually between mucosal surfaces. When the signs and symptoms of herpes are present, transmission can occur. However, studies have shown that transmission can occur when no signs or symptoms are present and this is known as asymptomatic viral shedding. This is more common in patients with HSV-2 and in the first year of infection, although this process is not fully understood (Mertz *et al.*, 1992).

This asymptomatic shedding obviously has clinical implications and patients need to be aware of current research findings, through a sensitive and supportive approach.

Clinical manifestations

Primary herpes. The first occurrence of primary herpes is usually the most severe, with a prolonged period of viral shedding, although some women may experience very mild localized symptoms only. The woman may have a systemic illness with fever, malaise, myalgias, headache, genital irritation, vaginal discharge, inguinal tenderness and lymphadenopathy. The lesions in a primary herpes episode of the genital area in women are frequently located on the vulva, vagina, perineum and may also occur on the thighs or buttocks (see Colour plates 12 and 13). Breslin (1988) noted that 'HSV cervicitis can be found in over 80% of women with initial genital disease'.

The lesions begin as erythematous papules which then develop into vesicles. The vesicles then rupture and leave ulcerative lesions; some of the ulcers coalesce, producing larger areas of ulceration. The ulcers then crust over and re-epithelialization takes place, usually without leaving a scar. The severity and duration of a first occurrence varies enormously and is dependent on many factors including: the amount of virus present at the time of exposure; previous exposure to either HSV types; and genetic factors. Some women find the lesions heal within a week, whilst in others the duration may be as long as 3–6 weeks. The median duration for viral shedding from the onset of the lesions is generally agreed to be approximately 12 days.

Complications of a primary herpes infection include: dysuria; retention of urine due to pain on urination; constipation due to pain on defecation; aseptic meningitis; and transverse myelitis. About 10% of patients are affected by neurological complications: headaches, photophobia and viral meningitis (Adler, 1993). Secondary infection, with either a fungus or bacteria can occur. The local symptoms can cause considerable psychological distress.

Recurrent herpes infection. Recurrent episodes of genital herpes are usually much milder and shorter in duration than the primary occurrence. This is partly due to the fact that women have established good levels of neutralizing antibodies to the virus. The recurrence rate for genital herpes will depend on a number of factors, including the amount of virus present at the initial time of exposure, immunological reactions in the host, past exposure to either HSV types and genetic factors. Lesions in recurrent episodes of herpes often occur at the initial infection site in small clusters and rupture within 48 hours. Viral shedding is for a much shorter period (about

5 days) and re-epithelialization takes place on average within 10 days. The constitutional symptoms associated with the primary occurrence are absent.

However, reoccurrence can appear at any site along the sacral dermatomes, the most common non-genital sites being the buttocks or natal cleft, perianal region, thighs or lower back.

Wilson (1995) notes that 50% of patients experience 'prodromal symptoms' or warning signs, which can occur up to 48 hours before an outbreak. These prodromal symptoms may consist of an itching or mild tingling sensation at the respective site and shooting pain to the buttock, leg or hip. There may also be mood alterations and the woman may become more irritable, tearful and easily upset. You can educate your client to recognize this prodrome, which will help her to manage the condition and encourage her to feel that she is more in control of the virus.

Diagnosis
The gold-standard method of diagnosing HSV is by taking a culture for viral isolation. The ideal specimen is obtained from a fluid-filled vesicle by rupturing the vesicle with a sterile needle or a cotton wool swab rubbed over the lesion. The fluid is collected on a sterile swab and transferred to a viral transport medium. In the laboratory the specimen is inoculated into a living cell maintained at body temperature to observe its growth and confirm diagnosis.

Obviously, the swab collection can cause pain and irritation to the woman but it is vital to obtain a good sample from the infected area. A speculum examination to observe and obtain HSV cultures from the cervix is good practice in the case of primary herpes. However, the woman often finds this too uncomfortable. The patient must be screened for other STIs, including syphilis, either at the initial visit or at follow-up.

Type-specific serological testing for HSV antibody is becoming more commercially available in the UK. However, there is a current debate amongst GU physicians regarding its value, as a positive result does not necessarily mean that current symptoms are HSV. Additionally, there may be heightened anxiety, relationship difficulties and psychological morbidity attached to a seropositive diagnosis when no actual symptoms have ever been apparent.

Treatment

As with all other STIs, treatment should aim at promoting comfort, promoting healing, preventing secondary infection and decreasing transmission of the infection. Oral treatments available are for a five-day period: Acyclovir 200 mg five times daily; Famciclovir 250 mg three times daily and Valaciclovir 500 mg twice daily. Treatment should begin within five days of an occurrence.

You should try to choose an appropriate moment to explain that treatment is not a cure for herpes, and the drugs act by suppressing viral replication. Saline bathing of the ulcerated area produces some relief of the discomfort. Mild analgesia is recommended for pain relief. The careful use of a hairdryer to dry the genital areas after bathing is recommended as the area may be too sore to towel dry. If the woman has difficulty passing urine, due to pain, it can be suggested that she either passes urine in a warm bath, or pours warm water over the front of her genitals, to reduce the burning sensation of the urine passing over the ulcers.

The use of suppressive therapy treatment as a prophylaxis against recurrent herpes appears to be limited, but women who experience more than 6 occurrences a year may qualify for oral suppressive therapy as a means of controlling the virus. A number of women are unhappy taking suppressive therapy as it is a constant reminder to them of their condition. However, suppressive therapy for some women has a beneficial effect on quality of life (Carney et al., 1993).

All women should see the health adviser for both contact tracing and education and counselling about the condition. Sexual intercourse should be avoided until lesions have completely re-epithelialized or prodromal symptoms have ceased.

Vaccine trials for genital herpes demonstrate that it is not effective in men, and is only effective in women who are negative for both HSV 1 and 2 (Stanberry et al., 2002). Potentially, this may be of benefit for women, in regards to prevention of infection, plus neonatal transmission. It may also assist in the future epidemiological control of HSV (Garnett et al., 2004).

Herpes in pregnancy

Acyclovir is not licensed for use during pregnancy, although it is often prescribed. Pregnant women who have previously suffered from herpes often express concern about the risk to their unborn baby. Corey (1990) points out that 'the vast majority of pregnant women with recurrent genital herpes deliver normal infants'. What is vital is that the woman informs her midwife and obstetrician of the fact that she has previously had the virus, as herpes in pregnancy and herpes of the neonate are complex and require an individual approach to care. The woman should be kept fully informed and encouraged to share in the decision-making process regarding delivery of her baby. If a woman has active lesions at the time of delivery then, to prevent neonatal herpes, it is recommended that a Caesarean section should be performed (Corey, 1990; Godley, 1993).

Godley (1993) points out that the results of routine viral cultures from the lower genital tract are of no predictive value in women who have asymptomatic viral shedding at the time of delivery and additionally a culture result takes an average of a week – frequently too late to be of value. Routine screening of pregnant women for genital herpes is not recommended. If a woman is suffering from a primary episode during pregnancy and has no HSV antibodies before pregnancy, there is a higher risk of transmission if lesions are present at the time of delivery. This risk is increased if she acquired the first episode during the third trimester. In this instance, Caesarean section should be considered, as the risk of viral shedding in labour is very high. There is a risk of pre-term delivery for all women who have acquired the infection during pregnancy. Neonates usually acquire the virus when they are in direct contact with the birth canal and secretions that carry the virus.

The psychological aspects of genital herpes

Breslin (1988) describes women as having a sense of shock, anger, isolation and loneliness on being made aware of the diagnosis of genital herpes. Initially the anger tends to be directed to the person thought to have given them the infection but is then frequently aimed at the medical profession for having diagnosed the condition and then not being able to provide a cure. Anxieties arise about relationships, childbirth and cancer. There is an increased incidence of psychiatric morbidity and depressive illness, and self-destructive feelings can be experienced. Breslin's comments have been validated and confirmed by Carney *et al.* (1994) who found the psychological impact of the first episode of genital herpes had a 'profound effect on patients'. If there were no recurrences of the condition then the woman's psychological state improved. However, if there was a recurrence the level of anxiety remained as high as for the primary occurrence.

Previously it was thought that there might be an association between herpes virus and cervical cancer. Evidence indicates that this is not the case.

The appropriate use of language is important when discussing genital herpes with patients. 'Occurrence/episode/re-occurrence', rather than 'attack' can be psychologically more acceptable – as 'attack' is a negative use of language and could make the patient feel somewhat 'invaded' by the virus.

Nurses therefore need to give positive assurances that the condition is manageable. Helping women to manage the disease means helping them to identify factors that may contribute to a recurrence. These may include:

◆ Hormonal changes, e.g. ovulation, menstruation

◆ Local heat from tight clothing or from prolonged exposure to sunlight

◆ Emotional distress and life-changing events

◆ Stress, lack of sleep, overwork and not taking sufficient time for emotional and physical repair and an opportunity to get things into perspective

◆ Friction/trauma during sexual intercourse

◆ Conditions that compromise the immune system.

In your clinical practice you should remember that listening to a woman's fears and anxieties about herpes can act as a major catharsis for her. This listening in itself may be enough to help, as many women feel isolated and unwilling to discuss the condition with others from whom they would normally draw support. Additionally, it will give you an idea whether the patient would benefit from psychological assistance or from joining a support group, such as the Herpes Association (see Resources).

Syphilis

Syphilis has been described as a social model for HIV and AIDS and called 'one of the most fascinating diseases of humans' (Sparling, 1990). It is impossible to do justice to the complexities of the condition of syphilis in an introductory chapter such as this on STIs.

Syphilis is divided into four stages: primary, secondary, latency and tertiary. It is rare amongst most women in the UK today (although there has been an increase amongst men who have sex with men within the UK and other areas of the world). Worldwide the disease still causes significant problems and you should be aware of this in patients who present with symptoms suggestive of syphilis. Any patient presenting with genital ulceration needs to be screened for syphilis as part of the diagnosis of exclusion.

The causative organism of syphilis is *Treponema pallidum*, which is classified as a spirochaete. It is one of a group of diseases referred to as the treponematoses, which includes yaws and pinta. These latter two conditions are described as 'variants of syphilis' and are acquired by non-venereal spread, usually in childhood (Arya *et al.*, 1980). Syphilis is acquired by sexual contact, except for congenital syphilis when the unborn infant acquires the condition by transplacental transmission from the infected mother.

The incubation period for primary syphilis is 9 days to 3 months. The median duration is 3 weeks. The reason for the varied incubation time is related to the amount of the *T. pallidum* inoculum. *Treponema pallidum* cannot enter the body through intact skin but will enter through small abrasions that occur in the mucous membrane during sexual intercourse. 'When a concentration of approximately 10 million organisms per gram of tissue is reached, clinical lesions appear' (Tillman, 1991).

Clinical manifestations

Primary syphilis. The primary stage is characterized by the appearance at the site of inoculation of a primary chancre (ulcer). The chancre is usually a painless ulcer that has a punched-in centre and indurated edge. There may be some oedema to adjacent tissue, and lymph glands local to the chancre site may be slightly enlarged. In women the common sites for the chancre are the vulva, labia, vagina and, in 25% of cases, the cervix. If untreated, the chancre heals spontaneously in a few weeks.

Secondary syphilis. The characteristic lesions of secondary syphilis usually occur 4–12 weeks after the appearance of the primary chancre. By this stage the disease has become systemic and the patient may present with malaise, headache, fever and a bilateral symmetrical rash. The rash occurs on the trunk, face, legs, arms and diagnostically on the soles of the feet and palms of the hands. Other lesions referred to by Adler (1990) include the appearance of condylomata lata (wart-like papules occurring on the labia and anus). These condylomata can be very infectious and are often a prime site for isolating the *T. pallidum*. The secondary stage of syphilis has a duration of approximately 2 years. It is important to realize that the stages of syphilis are very fluid and there is no clear demarcation line. Once the secondary stage subsides the patient enters the latent stage.

Late syphilis. This is usually characterized as a period absent of any clinical manifestations of disease although the serology would be positive. The patient may remain in the latent stage of syphilis for as little as 2 years or for as long as 40 years.

Tertiary syphilis. This is now a very rare condition and can be divided into three presenting categories: gummatous, cardiovascular and neurosyphilis. The two classic conditions of neurosyphilis are tabes dorsalis and general paralysis of the insane. It is not always appreciated by health care practitioners today that these conditions would have been extremely common in this country before the advent of penicillin and called for considerable nursing expertise. Today treatment for syphilis, at any stage of the disease, is successful.

Congenital syphilis. This is more accurately known as transplacental syphilis and can still be a problem in some parts of the developing world. A dramatic decline has taken place in the UK partly due to the serological screening of pregnant women.

Diagnosis

In the primary stage a dark ground microscopy is performed on the primary chancre to identify the *T. pallidum*. The serology may be negative at this stage but is positive within 10 days of the primary chancre appearing. Serological tests for syphilis vary, and you should consult with your pathology laboratory to ascertain what screening test they use for diagnostic procedure. Women should be screened for other STIs in the event of a positive syphilis diagnosis. Currently, the Health Protection Agency (HPA) is developing a mouth swab to detect antibodies from the gums (HPA, 2003), which would be more acceptable to patients, as well as be a useful tool for staff who perform outreach sexual health screening.

Treatment

The main treatment of choice for primary and secondary syphilis is procaine penicillin 750 mg intramuscularly daily for 10 days. Alternative oral therapies include: erythromycin 500 mg four times a day for 14 days; doxycycline 100 mg twice daily for 14 days; azithromycin 500 mg daily for 10 days. For late syphilis the treatment regime is increased both in dosage and length. Clients must be warned that it is essential to complete the medical treatment in order to stop asymptomatic disease progression.

Pregnant women are screened at antenatal visits, and if syphilis is confirmed, treatment should begin as soon as possible, as congenital syphilis is preventable. All clients with syphilis need to be seen by the health adviser for contact tracing and must abstain from sexual intercourse until two follow-up blood tests have been performed.

In dealing with women testing positive for syphilis, particularly those from other countries, it is important not to assume automatically that she has syphilis, as certain serological tests cannot distinguish between syphilis and non-venereal treponematoses like yaws, pinta and bejel.

Side effects of treatment

Jarisch-Herxheimer reaction (JHR). It is well documented that within a short time of receiving treatment for syphilis, particularly penicillin, the JHR occurs (Goldmeier and Hay, 1993). The reaction is more common with treatment of secondary syphilis, but can occur at any stage (Tramont, 1990). Before administering the first treatment, the nurse must advise the patient that they may develop a mild febrile reaction; mild pyrexia, myalgia and flushing. Patients should be advised to rest, drink plenty of fluids and to take aspirin or paracetamol. It is advisable after the administration of the first treatment that the patient rests for approximately 15 minutes. With follow-up treatment, it is advisable that the patient rests for approximately 5 minutes after each treatment. The reaction can be much more serious in the case of late syphilis.

It is possible for a JHR in the second or third trimester of pregnancy to induce uterine contractions resulting in premature labour (Zenker and Rolfs, 1990).

Procaine toxicity. Occasionally, patients may experience reactions to procaine penicillin and the nurse must be aware of this prior to administrating the injection. It can manifest itself as psychological disturbances such as severe anxiety and hallucinations, fever, hysteria, the patient feeling as though they are dying. The reaction passes off spontaneously and so the nurse will need to support and reassure the patient during this time.

The patient can further develop other symptoms of hypertension, tachycardia, hyperventilation and vomiting. Usually these symptoms are mild and settle within 30 minutes. However, cardiovascular collapse has been recorded and resuscitation may be required.

Genital warts

Genital warts are one of the most common STIs in the UK (PHLS, 1999). Between 1995 and 1998 diagnosis of genital warts increased significantly amongst females in the 16- to 19-year-old age group (PHLS, 1999).

Genital warts are a distressing problem for both male and female clients. Not only do they look aesthetically upsetting on the external genitalia but also women may have heard of a link with warts and cervical cancer. Genital warts are caused by HPV (human papilloma virus). There are over 100 genotypes of HPV, of which approximately one-third affect the genital tract. Papilloma viruses are classified according to their natural supporting host. HPVs are DNA viruses, meaning that they carry all their genetic information in a single strand of DNA. HPVs tend to be site-specific in infectivity, although auto-inoculation from one site to another can occur, but is very unusual (Adler, 1995).

Clinically, visible genital warts are usually associated with types HPV 6 and HPV 11. It has now been established that infection with specific sub-clinical HPV, DNA types, notably HPV types 16, 18, 31 and 33 is a causative link to cervical cancer (Etherington and Shafi, 1996; Wallin *et al.*, 1999). These types are less frequently associated with visible warts. The possible link between cervical cancer and genital warts was first discussed in oncology literature in the 1840s (see also Chapter 13).

The use of HPV DNA testing is debatable. Some clinicians believe it should be used in conjunction with the cervical screening programme. It may have a role in reducing the incidence and mortality of cervical cancer, making screening more cost effective and efficient. For example, clinicians will be able to refer women who have 'high-risk' types which are potentially destined to persist, and will be able to allow longer intervals between smears, as well as stop screening women at an earlier age if their tests are truly negative to HPV types associated with high-grade cervical lesions (Cuzick *et al.*, 1995). Clinical trials of HPV vaccine for types associated with high-grade cervical lesions show promising results (Harro *et al.*, 2001). It is currently being debated, if proven to be efficacious and safe, that young men and women should be vaccinated to protect them for their future sexual life (Lehtinen and Diller, 2002).

Transmission

The incubation period for HPV is very variable and can be anywhere between 3 weeks and 9 months, or in some cases even longer. Schneider (1993) states that 'sexual transmission is the main pathway for genital HPV; however, vertical, peripartal (during pregnancy and childbirth) and oral transmission are also possible'. Oral transmission through oral sex is rare, but the rate is increased if the woman is immunocompromised. HPV is transmitted by direct skin-to-skin contact. It enters through breaks in the skin and mucous membrane. Due to the method of transmission women who have sex with women are at risk of HPV (O'Hanlan and Crum, 1996; Bailey *et al.*, 2000).

Genital warts are described as hyperproliferative benign epithelial neoplasms, they are self-limiting tumours which may spontaneously regress. They are often exacerbated in pregnancy, old age and in immunocompromised patients.

Clinical manifestations

Clinical and sub-clinical warts can be present anywhere from the cervix to the anus. In women, the most common sites are the introitus, vulva, perineum and perianal area. Less often, they may be found on the cervix, vaginal walls, anal canal, pubic area, upper thighs and crural folds (see Colour plate 14). Tinkle (1990) describes clinical genital warts as 'flesh coloured verrucous lesions' that tend to occur on warm, moist areas of the genitalia.

Women with cervical or vaginal warts may experience bleeding, itching and a vaginal discharge following sexual intercourse.

Diagnosis

In clinical practice a diagnosis of clinical warts is made on their appearance. Any suspect or atypical growth will be biopsied to exclude a differential diagnosis such as carcinoma. The diagnosis of sub-clinical HPV might follow a cervical smear when the cytology report notes that koilocytes are identified, or during a colposcopy. The cervical transformation zone is particularly important, as this is the area where columnar epithelium undergoes a process of metaplasia, developing into squamous epithelium. This area of cellular change at the cervix is thought to make it more vulnerable to viral infection and to neoplastic change. Only 20% of women with genital warts will demonstrate clinical HPV of the cervix (Tinkle, 1990).

All women who present with a first episode of genital warts should be screened for other STIs. It is also good practice for a proctoscope to be passed, to allow the anal canal to be examined to exclude intra-anal warts if peri-anal warts are present.

Depending upon clinic protocol, a cervical smear may be performed if it is more than a year since her previous smear.

Treatment

The clinician should discuss the various treatment options available so that women can make an informed choice. Women should be advised that the warts might take a while to respond to treatment and that recurrence can occur. Keratanized (hard) warts respond better to cryotherapy, removal by surgical excision or electrocautery, whereas soft non-keratanized warts respond better to topical application of

SCENARIO

Lucy attended with lumps on her labia. She had sex with women only, and had never had sex with a man. A previous girlfriend of hers had had genital warts. She never considered it to be a problem, as health professionals in the past had told her she had nothing to worry about regarding STIs, as she only ever had sex with women. Lucy was diagnosed and treated for genital warts.

This demonstrates that although Lucy was exclusively a lesbian, she was at risk of genital wart infection due to sexual practices and would require screening for STIs and a cervical smear. She would also require information on safer sexual practices for the future.

Podophyllin, Podophyllotoxin or trichloroacetic acid (TCA).

A study by Lacey et al. (2003) demonstrated an increase in remission of all warts, associated with both Podophyllotoxin 0.15% cream and Podophyllotoxin 0.5% solution, compared to Podophyllin 25% solution. When comparing the cost effectiveness of all three treatments, Podophyllotoxin 0.5% solution was the most cost effective, then Podophyllotoxin 0.15% cream, followed by Podophyllin 25% solution.

The beauty of both Podophyllotoxin 0.15% cream and Podophyllotoxin 0.5% solution is that they are both home treatments and therefore can be a more convenient method for women. It is applied twice daily, for three consecutive days, then four days off without application. This cycle is repeated for three more occasions, or shorter if the warts are cleared. If warts remain after the fourth cycle, women should be reviewed, and further cycles prescribed if necessary. Home treatments will need clear written instructions and warnings about over-enthusiastic self-treatment, which can result in severe ulceration due to chemical burns.

Another home treatment, but more expensive, is Imiquimod 5% cream, which acts as an immune response modifier and produces a local cytokine response when applied to skin with HPV. It is applied three times a week at bedtime and washed off the next morning. Treatment continues until the warts have cleared or for a maximum of 16 weeks.

In clinical settings, the topical application of 25% Podophyllin to genital warts is applied once weekly and must be washed off within 4 hours. Surrounding skin can be protected with Vaseline beforehand. An accurate record should be kept of the number of treatments and the condition of the skin at each treatment. Some GU physicians believe that home treatments are now the way forward.

The treatments mentioned so far should not be used in pregnant women and should only be used in women of childbearing age if they are using adequate contraception. Treatments are for external use only and should be discontinued if adverse skin reactions occur.

Treatment regimes for genital warts are often very protracted and should be reviewed at least every 4 weeks. If treatment is not effective then alternative forms of treatment should be considered.

Cryotherapy, electrocautery, carbon dioxide laser, liquid nitrogen and treatment with trichloroacetic acid may be attempted. Some women with extensive genital warts, which have failed to respond to other forms of treatment, may eventually consider surgical excision.

Cervical warts can be treated by freezing techniques, laser and surgical procedures. Treatment to the cervix can often result in an increase in vaginal discharge about which women need to be informed. This discharge tends to be self-limiting as the treated area heals. Internal anal canal warts can take longer to clear, partly because the most caustic agents cannot be used in this area, so patients often have to be referred for surgical removal.

All of these treatments for clinical HPV are time-consuming, socially disruptive and often profoundly uncomfortable, and therefore can have a lasting psychological affect on the woman.

Information giving

Once diagnosed, women will need ongoing support and information regarding transmission, partner notification, reoccurrence of HPV, safer sex and condom use. They will also require information regarding cervical cytology. It is now firmly established that all women with genital warts must be encouraged to keep up to date with their cervical smears. The rationale for this is that if a woman has been in contact with genital wart viral types, then she may well have been in contact with the 'high-risk' HPV types associated with cervical dysplasia.

As HPV is a virus, women must be informed that once it has entered the body it is likely to be there for life. However, this does not mean that they will always have genital warts, because of treatment and immunity factors.

In order to maintain an adequate immune system, women are actively encouraged to lead a 'healthy' lifestyle. For example, smoking is known to lower the immune response and therefore women will require ongoing support either to cease smoking altogether or to reduce the amount they smoke (see Chapter 3). Genital hygiene is important, as warts are known to flourish in a wet warm environment. Therefore, adequate drying after bathing and the treatment of vaginal discharge, where appropriate, is vital.

Condom usage should be encouraged to prevent transmission to new partners. Within stable relationships, the use of condoms may not be needed, as the partner is likely to have already been in contact with the virus. However, the woman should discuss this with her partner, who may choose to use condoms, in case transmission has not occurred. Contact tracing should be encouraged for partners within the last 3–6 months.

Recurrences are common and can be distressing. Women should be encouraged to return as soon as they notice any new warts, so that treatment can be started quickly, before the warts become too extensive.

Molluscum contagiosum

Molluscum contagiosum (MC) is a pox virus and manifests itself as a benign papular condition of the skin and mucous membranes, with characteristic pearly, papular, smooth or umbilicated lesions/spots. Immunocompromised women, such as those with HIV/AIDS, may have larger, persistent lesions.

The incubation period is 3–12 weeks. The virus is probably passed on by direct skin-to-skin contact and may affect any part of the body, particularly the genitalia, in the case of sexual transmission. Diagnosis is usually based on the characteristic lesions themselves. The woman should be fully screened for other possible coexisting STIs.

The aim of the treatment is to eradicate the lesions themselves. Recommended treatment regimes are cryotherapy, chemical agents or electric current, although the simplest method is expression of the pearly core, either with a needle or sharpened orange stick, with or without the application of tincture of phenol to the expressed area. Follow-up treatments may

be necessary. Contact tracing is performed on an ad hoc basis.

Infestations

The main infestations seen in GUM clinics are the crab louse and scabies. Infestations of the genital area produce an intense itching which in turn may become secondarily infected. The woman may present with excoriation to the external genitalia resembling genital ulceration. Infestations are distressing and care needs to be taken in explaining treatment to the patient who also should be warned that purchasing additional proprietary products and over-treating the infestation can result in dermatitis.

All women should have a routine STI screen, as infestations are often the result of sexual contact.

Lice

Three species of lice infest humans. Transmission of *Phthirus pubis* is by 'intimate' sexual physical contact, usually sexual intercourse.

The nit of the crab louse is oval shaped and opaline in appearance. The incubation period is 5 days to several weeks. The grasp of the pubic louse's claw matches the diameter of the pubic and axillary hairs. It can therefore be found in other areas where there is axillary hair. The nits are secured to the base of the pubic hair by a cement-like substance and sometimes they can be seen by the naked eye. The louse is parasitic and feeds on human blood for its nourishment.

Diagnosis is usually made on the woman's symptoms, the primary symptom being itching. Treatment is preferably with topical lotions, rather than shampoos, which are applied to all body hair. Recommended regimes are:

- ◆ Malathion 0.5% applied to dry hair and washed off after 12 hours
- ◆ Permethrin 1% cream rinse applied to damp hair and washed off after 10 minutes
- ◆ Phenothrin 0.2% applied to dry hair and washed off after 2 hours
- ◆ Carbaryl 0.5% or 1% applied to dry hair and washed off after 12 hours.

Infestations in eyelashes can be treated with Permethrin 1% lotion and the woman should ensure her eyes remain closed during the 10-minute application. Permethrin is safe to use during pregnancy and breastfeeding. Clothing and bed linen should be washed on a hot cycle and close body contact avoided until treatment is completed.

Among the sexually active, pubic lice are more commonly found in females between the ages of 15 and 19 (Wistreich, 1992). Women should be screened for other STIs and contact tracing of sexual partners is required.

Scabies

Infestation with *Sarcoptes scabiei* results in severe itching in 2–6 weeks. The adult female burrows into the middle layer of skin and deposits 2–3 eggs a day. These eggs develop into adults in about 10 days. Transmission is by close social contact or it can be sexually acquired.

Diagnosis is made on the symptoms and the itching is worse at night when the body is warm. Burrows may be present and these can be opened using a sterile needle and the scabies mite observed under low-power light microscopy.

The mites are classically found on the flexor aspects of the wrists and between the finger webs, as well as the genitalia and abdomen. Other areas affected can be armpits, palms, buttocks, elbows, knees and nipples.

Treatment in adults is with Malathion 0.5% aqueous lotion or Permethrin 5% cream applied to all body surfaces except the face and washed off after 12 hours. Every time a woman washes her hands she must reapply the solution to prevent re-infection. Clothing and bed linen should be washed on a hot cycle and close body contact avoided until treatment is completed. For some women, itching may persist for several weeks post-treatment, so therefore reassurance must be given if re-infection has been eliminated.

Women should be screened for other STIs and contact tracing of sexual partners as well as members of the household or institution is necessary, as they may also require treatment.

Hepatitis A, B and C

Hepatitis means inflammation of the liver and can range from a sub-clinical chronic illness to a life-threatening disease. Viral hepatitis is caused by a group of viruses and this section will look very briefly at types A, B and C.

Hepatitis A virus (HAV) is spread via the oral-faecal route, so potentially can be sexually acquired through a sexual practice called 'rimming', i.e. there is oral–anal contact.

Hepatitis B virus (HBV) and hepatitis C virus (HCV) are blood-borne viruses. Routes of transmission include:

◆ Parenteral – via an activity that allows the transfer of infected blood, e.g. the sharing of needles by intravenous drug users, sharing of toothbrushes or razors, blood, blood products, unsterile skin piercing or tattooing techniques or occupational exposure

◆ Vertical transmission from mother to baby can occur with HBV infection and in some instances can occur with HCV. (The risk of HCV vertical transmission is higher if a woman is also HIV positive.)

HCV can also be found in other body fluids such as semen, vaginal secretions and saliva, but the amounts of virus present in these fluids are thought to be too low for transmission to occur.

Vaccinations are available for both hepatitis A and hepatitis B types but not hepatitis C. Safer sex can reduce the risk of transmission for all viral types, although sexual transmission of HCV remains relatively low (except in a few instances, mentioned later).

Regardless of the viral type, symptoms for hepatitis can be: jaundice, malaise, fever, anorexia, mild right upper abdominal pain and arthralgia.

HAV

The incubation period for HAV is 2–6 weeks. This viral type tends to cause an acute episode and treatment is conservative. This infection when sexually acquired in the developed world is more common amongst men who have sex with men.

HBV

Hepatitis B can be sexually, parenterally and vertically transmissible. The incubation period is 6 weeks to 6 months. Again, this infection when sexually acquired in the developed world is more common amongst men who have sex with men. However, in the last ten years, in the UK, there has been a rise in notifications amongst women. Most women make a full recovery from acute hepatitis and develop lifelong immunity, unless they were infected with hepatitis B at birth. In a small number of cases, the immune system does not completely clear the virus and these women can become chronic infected carriers with the possibility of chronic liver problems. Treatment is dependent upon liver function and there are various treatment options available.

All sexual and household contacts should be screened and vaccinated against HBV. Babies born to mothers with HBV are vaccinated from birth.

HCV

The incubation period is between 6 and 24 weeks. Approximately 75% of women who are acutely infected progress to chronic hepatitis and become carriers (Alberti, 1996). In a small number of cases women can develop hepatocarcinoma.

HCV is most prevalent within the intravenous drug user population, or in women who received blood or blood products prior to 1991. There is a *theoretical* risk of sexual transmission, *only* if there is blood-to-blood contact, through the use of sex toys or through sex that causes abrasions in the genital or anal area. Consequently in such circumstances, safer sex would be advocated if a woman or her partner were hepatitis C positive. The risk of sexual transmission would increase further if there was co-infection with HIV. Menstrual blood is thought to increase the *theoretical* risk of transmission, so if barrier methods are not being used intercourse/cunnilingus should be avoided during menstruation.

HIV infection and AIDS in women

It is now over 20 years since HIV and AIDS was first recognized in 1981 and the literature concerning the condition is extensive and, in some areas, controversial. Today, nurses and midwives face continuing challenges as prevention strategies and target groups change, as advances in anti-HIV treatments progress and as the very nature of the virus itself changes, mutates and develops resistance to certain drug therapies. This chapter can only briefly look at ongoing issues that concern women but further information can be obtained from the books, support groups, websites and helplines that are listed at the end of this chapter.

In the UK, although the large majority of women born in sub-Saharan Africa are HIV negative, this cohort of women currently remains the largest group of women infected with HIV in the UK (HPA *et al.*, 2003).

In order to gain an accurate picture of the impact of HIV and AIDS on women, it is important to bear in mind not only the national but also the global perspectives of the disease.

Globally, upwards of 14 million people have died from AIDS-related diseases, and UNAIDS and WHO (2003) estimated that up to 40 million people are living with HIV infection, of whom 17.6 million are women and 2.7 million are children under the age of 15 (WHO, 2003). Almost all of the new childhood infections are due to mother-to-child transmission, either before or during childbirth or through breastfeeding.

Over 13 million children under the age of 15 have lost both parents or their mothers to AIDS (WHO, 2003). This has a huge impact on traditional family structures, as extended families begin to break down under the strain of HIV. There is also a serious social economic impact as population growth and death rates change, with a marked reduction in life expectancy due to AIDS in most developing countries.

Thus, the two most effective methods of reducing HIV infection in children are:

◆ to protect their mothers from becoming infected in the first place, through health prevention strategies

◆ to prevent vertical transmission if maternal infection has already occurred. The risk of vertical transmission is 25%; however, this can be reduced to less than 5% if women accept the following interventions:

◆ the use of anti-HIV drugs during pregnancy
◆ careful obstetric management
◆ delivery by caesarean section
◆ bottle feeding.

Women have been targeted by HIV prevention messages since 1987. Since 1992 the focus has been to encourage women to test for HIV during pregnancy. In 1999 the NHS Executive published its report *Reducing Mother to Baby Transmission of HIV*. All expectant mothers are now offered and recommended an HIV test, routinely, along with other antenatal screening tests. The sexual health strategy has targets that anticipate that by the end of 2004 all attendees at GUM will be offered an HIV test as part of their first screening for STIs, and at follow-up visits, depending on risk factors (DoH, 2001). Although these HIV screening programmes are to be welcomed, testing is not yet encouraged at termination clinics. Hopefully, government initiatives in the future will target this population group as well.

A number of large studies have now shown that a woman is as much as 2-4 times at a greater risk of HIV infection from unprotected vaginal intercourse with an infected man than vice versa (WHO, 2000). It is also now widely recognized that the risk of being infected with HIV is even greater if a woman had an STI at the time intercourse took place. Studies of heterosexual HIV transmission have consistently found anal intercourse to be a highly predictive risk factor for seroconversion. Yet most AIDS prevention messages targeted at heterosexuals, presumably influenced by cultural taboos against acknowledging this sexual practice, continue to emphasize vaginal and, increasingly, oral sex transmission (Halperin, 1999). The health risks of anal sex appear to be severely underestimated by a substantial proportion of sexually active women and men, and need to be given greater emphasis in HIV and STI prevention programmes. Women-to-women transmission is rare, but has been documented (Kwakwa *et al.*, 2003) probably through the use of sharing sex toys, tinged with bloodstained body fluids. Health professionals need to be mindful of this and give women who have sex with women accurate information on safer sexual practices.

HIV has been isolated from blood, semen, cervical secretions, lymphocytes, cell-free plasma, cerebrospinal fluid, tears, saliva, urine and breast milk. However, the concentration of virus varies considerably, which means that not all of these fluids will transmit infection. Highly infectious are blood, semen, breast milk to the breastfeeding infant and possibly cervical secretions.

Other methods of transmission are through the receipt of infected blood or blood products, donated organs, semen and gametes in fertility procedures, sharing or re-using of contaminated needles.

Leading authorities in the field of HIV and AIDS are in accord that if the pandemic spread is to be controlled, then empowerment of women in relationships, and within society is vital. Blakey (1991) discusses how such strategies for reaching and empowering women may be achieved.

Empowerment is discussed in nursing in a very loose way and you should remember that it is a very sophisticated concept and takes considerable time for women to implement. A woman does not wake up one morning and say 'I think I will be empowered today'. Empowerment means fundamentally altering cognitive and behavioural patterns that have occurred and been instilled over years of socialization. This in turn has produced thinking and behavioural patterns in women that may never have been challenged. For many women, the concept of empowerment is an alien one.

Other issues that put women at a disadvantage include the socio-economic obstacles at both the microeconomic and macroeconomic level. Horton (1995) states a need for investigators and policy-makers to address the complexity of HIV disease in women and mentions that contributory factors like 'domestic violence, substance abuse, prison detention, mental illness, poverty and limited access to care all impinge on women at risk of HIV'. The sexual and economic subordination of women has certainly fuelled the HIV and AIDS pandemic. This does not mean that empowerment cannot happen, but you need to keep in mind that the change in attitude for some women may be difficult to understand and achieve. The whole concept of empowerment is complex and necessitates considerably more thought than merely teaching a woman to be responsible by carrying condoms in her handbag. A woman may be reluctant to request condom use from a partner, for fear of violence, withdrawal of financial support or fear of abandonment. Women may therefore need the support, whether it be emotional, financial or both, to be able to begin to make informed choices and changes to improve the quality of their lives.

The natural history of HIV and AIDS has altered since 1996 with the advent of effective anti-HIV drugs known as HAART (Highly Active Antiretroviral Therapy). There has also been an improved knowledge and understanding of HIV itself: improved diagnostic techniques, such as viral load testing which measures the amount of viral particles in the blood, and genotyping and phenotyping which is very important in treatment of HIV resistant virus to particular drug therapies.

Globally, as treatment costs are high, the advent of HAART has had a huge socio-economic impact. Currently, there are three classes of antiretroviral medications to make up 'combination therapy' or HAART. These are targeted at different stages of the virus's life cycle and are called protease inhibitors, non-nucleoside reverse transcriptase inhibitors and nucleoside reverse transcriptase inhibitors. In order for the drugs to prevent viral replication, increase CD4 counts and prevent resistance to treatment therapies, women need to adhere 90–95% to their treatment regimes. This of course, can be difficult if there are unwanted side effects to the medications and/or a high pill burden.

In most areas of the developed world, since the advent of combination therapy drug treatment regimes, the infection is becoming a more chronic illness. In practice, this means that prognosis is greatly improved and that women with an AIDS diagnosis, who are taking anti-HIV therapy, have a greater chance of continuing to lead healthy lives for longer periods. Clinically, as growing numbers of HIV-infected women live longer and feel better, pregnancy and contraceptive issues are becoming increasingly important.

Sexually active women will need advice and support when choosing a method of contraception. To date, there are no contraindications associated with any contraceptive method for women who have HIV infection (Boag, 1999). If a woman with HIV infection requests an intrauterine device, they, like non-infected women, must have a full STI screen prior to fitting. Clinicians may or may not prescribe prophylactic antibiotics to prevent pelvic infection during insertion. Many women with HIV infection prefer the IUS (intrauterine system) rather than the copper IUD (intrauterine device) because of its high efficacy, lower risk of pelvic infection and reduced menstrual flow. Condoms are actively encouraged to prevent either transmission of the virus to a non-infected partner, or, if both partners are positive, to prevent transmission of resistant virus. Women living with HIV will require annual cytological smears, as they are at a greater risk of cervical dysplasia.

Within nursing there has been the emergence of the nurse practitioner/specialist role. Many of these specialist practitioners are experts within the HIV/AIDS field and are therefore developing nurse-led clinics, and offering advice, support and treatment to HIV-infected women. Most GUM clinics have an HIV community nurse specialist who can provide an ongoing, invaluable holistic service for women infected with HIV. These nurses are an excellent resource for advice and information and can be contacted via your local GUM clinic.

It is now widely accepted that there are positive advantages for women who receive early diagnosis, advice and intervention. The whole perspective of HIV in women is markedly very different from men and you should be aware of these differences in your planning and implementation of nursing care. If your attitude is empathetic, understanding, caring and helpful then your client, her partner and her family will be able to benefit from your skills.

You also need to be aware and sensitive to your own feelings, beliefs and attitudes towards women who are HIV positive or who have AIDS. If you are uncomfortable about treating and talking to infected women, then you have a duty of care to refer them to other colleagues. However, as a registered nurse you also have a professional responsibility to educate yourself about HIV and AIDS, so that you can care for clients appropriately in the future.

Nursing issues in sexual health

Traditionally within GUM doctors examined patients and were responsible for taking a medical and sexual history, but this fixed role is changing. Increasingly, nurses and health advisers have gained responsibility for health promotion and counselling patients in relation to safer sex, harm minimization and sexual health. More nurse-led clinics have been established, which means that taking a history has become an integral part of the nurse's role. The general principles of sexual health care have remained the same, but the context in which that care is delivered has changed during the last decade. There has been the development of outreach work to cover schools, sex industry workers, drug users and the homeless. GUM clinics now have extended opening hours with longer appointments for consultation, examination and investigations. Patients who are HIV positive have regular check-ups and access to counselling, which is important for those who are living with this chronic infection or for those whose infection has progressed to an AIDS diagnosis. Additionally there has been the development of improved shared care with GPs for people living with HIV.

In light of the new sexual health strategy, GP and practice nurse roles will encompass sexual health issues and screening at some level. Evidence suggests that offering some sexual health services in primary care could enhance the control of STIs, since patients would be seen and treated at the first point of call (Catchpole, 2001). However, Cassell *et al.* (2003) suggest that barriers to access primary care, and the delay of treatment if patients are referred on to GUM services, need to be addressed when planning future services

and implementing the sexual health strategy within primary care services.

The need for 'one-stop shop' integrated sexual health services is becoming increasingly apparent and has been identified as a potential future service development by the sexual health strategy. The use of specific clinics with specific targets directed at a particular population group are by definition a better way of reaching the heterogeneous groups of women in society whose needs are very different in each group. However, Kane and Wellings (2003) comment that the move towards the integration of family planning and GUM has potentially progressed faster than the progress towards the staff training needed to underpin it.

Over the past two decades the National Health Service has undergone significant changes. Government initiatives have all been designed to ensure services are cost-effective and of a high quality, in order to improve patient care and meet local population needs. Changes have been instigated for the benefits of patients by setting national standards and by making health care providers more accountable for the services that are available (DOH, 1997b). Within this modernization agenda, nurses are set to become key players. The concept of nurse-led care has gathered momentum, following the Government's strategy to strengthen the nursing contribution to health and health care (DOH, 1999) by undertaking wider roles (DOH, 2000). The Chief Nursing Officer has stated 10 key roles for nurses, some of which include: ordering diagnostic tests; to make and receive referrals; to admit and discharge patients for specified conditions and within agreed protocols; to manage patient case loads; to run clinics; to prescribe medications and treatment; and to triage patients. This is an exciting time for nursing in the UK. We need to embrace these changes with vigour, in order ultimately to enhance our patients' care by expanding the range of services available to them. We now have the opportunity to expand our roles, to become expert practitioners in our own right, by offering comprehensive services alongside the medical profession.

The publication of the Government's modernization agenda, plus the national strategy for sexual health and HIV has added impetus to a growing body of evidence, both nationally and internationally, that clearly demonstrates the ability of sexual health and reproductive nurses to provide nurse-led clinics, within an existing sexual health service, that is an acceptable alternative to doctor-led clinics (Allen, 1998; Harinda *et al.*, 2001; Miles *et al.*, 2002a, 2002b, 2003a, 2003b). Given the current crisis within GUM, it is paramount that nurses within GUM challenge current working practices, based on the medical model of care, and drive nursing practice development forward within the specialty. In London, the Standing Conference for Nurses Working Group for Sexual Health was established in 2000 (see Resources) and is currently working in partnership with other groups to develop a competency framework for nurses working within the sexual health speciality.

Some GUM clinics have already developed a nurse specialist/practitioner or nurse consultant role, encompassing full assessment history and treatment by the nurse. This means that the role of the GUM nurse as a handmaiden to medical practitioners is well and truly over! GUM nurses are keen to expand and develop their roles, utilize their knowledge and skills, to become independent practitioners in their own right. However, across the country there remain inequalities in nursing roles within GUM that hopefully will be addressed following the advent of the sexual health strategy and the Government's modernization agenda.

In all clinical settings, information leaflets should be available about how to prevent STIs. These leaflets (some excellent ones are available from the Department of Health) should clearly explain safer sex, the use of barrier methods of contraception, the risks of multiple partners or a partner with multiple partners, how to tell a partner and where to go for appropriate help. Information that is given to women needs to be consistent with regard to universal precautions, safer sex practice and clinic policies and procedures. Lack of information, conflicting information and inconsistency between staff were some of the aspects of the service found to be most irksome to female patients (Whittaker, 1993).

The psychological response to STIs is another issue that nurses need to consider. A sexually acquired infection can affect an individual's self-concept and can lower self-esteem, resulting in anxiety, impaired social interactions, hopelessness, depression and a feeling of isolation. Most women will recover a sense of equilibrium in due course, and self-worth should be restored without recourse to psychological support. However, for a few, the consequences of a sexually acquired infection can be continued shock, pain and unresolved latent anger, hostility and aggression. This may disturb future relationships with feelings of mistrust and sexual dysfunction. When dealing with such women you should remember to let them express their anger and let them cry and validate their feelings. Assisting the woman to articulate her unhappiness can then lead to helping her develop effective coping skills. You should be caring, supportive, non-judgemental and sensitive to your client's anxieties and needs

In your dealings with clients from both sexes you should consider and reflect on the way men have little knowledge and have frequently been excluded from appreciating the woman's sexual health perspective. Educating both male and female clients about their sexual drive, sexual response time, sexual performance anxieties and sexual techniques, as well as sexual health promotion needs in the opposite sex will help to reduce the division and misunderstanding between them. A woman's sexual health will improve immeasurably if men are taught to value it. Recent research has shown men are equally ill-informed about their own health care needs and suggests much remedial work needs to be done in this area of health promotion as well.

Conclusion

Sexual health is a concept that means different things to different people. In your nursing role you should aim to have a holistic approach to sexual health which encompasses health promotion advice, recognizes varying sexual behaviour, understands that sexually acquired infection can interfere with sexual function, and most importantly accept that psychological factors impair and inhibit sexual functioning and relationships. In short, sexual health may be considered the physical and emotional state of well-being that enables women to enjoy and act on their sexual feelings (Boston Women's Health Book Collective, 1985).

Nurses, whether in primary care or in hospital departments and clinics, have an important role in maintaining the sexual health of women. You should be able to assess and identify sexual concerns and problems and be able to intervene effectively in order to help your clients. The key to successful and practical management of STIs lies in the accurate diagnosis and appropriate treatment for the condition.

STIs pose a serious threat not only to women's sexual and mental/psychological health but also to the general health and well-being of millions of women worldwide. Young women are a particularly vulnerable client group and need not only empowerment, in order to 'negotiate' safer sex, but they also need to be educated regarding their basic biological functions and sexual health needs. Until this is achieved they will potentially continue to have long-term complications and fertility issues.

Every newly diagnosed STI is a potential new HIV infection. Until the problem of STIs is tackled, both nationally and globally, the spread of STIs and HIV will continue. Do we not owe it to future generations to provide them with the knowledge and power to lead healthy sexually active lifestyles?

- Have you been on a study day recently for an update on HIV and AIDS? Do you understand why it is important that people adhere strictly to their treatment regimes? If not, you need to consider some professional development: contact your local health promotion unit for information on courses

- Do you want to expand your role within sexual health? Contact GUNA (see Resources) and your manager for advice as to how to drive nursing practice forward within your clinical area

- Do you know of local voluntary and government organizations to which to refer clients? Contact your local health promotion department for advice of contact names and addresses in your local area.

Patient education points

- Condoms, when used correctly, can protect against STIs, HIV and pregnancy. Oil-based products cause condoms to split

- Having swabs taken for an infection screen is not the same as a cervical smear test

- Screening for *Chlamydia* can be done when:
  - A cervical smear is done
  - Unprotected sex has taken place
  - There is a change of sexual partner

- Intermenstrual bleeding may be caused by an infection, rather than the method of contraception

- Lesbian women may require cervical screening and safer sex advice.

Ideas for personal and professional development

- Have you seen a sexual history being taken? Why not visit a local GUM clinic, to see how it is done? How comfortable would you be asking all these questions? What areas of professional development can you identify and how do you intend to develop these skills?

- How will you discuss genital washing with women in future? Can you identify areas of learning and development for yourself?

Resources

ACIA (African Community Involvement Association)
Eagle Court, 224 London Road, Mitcham, Surrey CR4 3HD
Tel: 020 8687 2400
www:acia-uk.org

AVERT (AIDS Education and Research Trust)
4 Brighton Road, Horsham, West Sussex
    RH13 5BA
Tel: 01403 210202
www.avert.org.uk

Body and Soul
9 Tavistock Place, London WC1H 9SN
Tel: 020 7833 4929
Tel: 020 7383 7678
www.bodyandsoul.demon.co.uk
Teenspirit for young people living with HIV.

Department of Health
PO Box 777, London SE1 6XH
Tel: 0870 155 5455
www.doh.gov.uk
Patient information leaflets on STIs.

Durex Information Service for Sexual Health
London International House, Broxbourne,
    Herts, EM0 6LN
Tel: 0800 338739
http://www.durex.com

George House Trust
77 Ardwick Green North, Manchester M12 6FX
Tel: 0161 274 4499
http://www.ght.org.uk
Support network for people affected by
    HIV/AIDS.

Health Protection Agency
http://www.hpa.org.uk
Produces statistics on STIs, HIV and
    other infections in the UK.

Herpes Association
41 North Road, London N7 9DP
Tel: 020 7609 9061
http://www.herpesalliance.org.uk

London Lighthouse
111–117 Lancaster Road, London W11 1QT
Tel: 020 7792 1200
Centre for people affected by HIV and AIDS
    including support groups and training. No
    in-patient services, although day-care available.

Mainliners
38-40 Kennington Park Road, London SE11 4RS
Tel: 0207 582 5434

Hep C advice line: 0207 735 7705
Provides information for drug users and
    those with Hep C, as well as info on
    HIV/AIDS.

NAM Publications
16a Clapham Common Southside,
    London SW4 7AB
Tel: 020 7627 3200
www.aidsmap.com
Information on HIV/AIDS, regularly
    updated.

National AIDS Helpline (all Freephone)
0800 567 123 (24 hours)
0800 555 777 for free copies of leaflets
0800 521 361 minicom for hearing impaired
    (10.00 am–10.00 pm)
0800 282 445 Bengali, Gujarati, Hindi,
    Punjabi, Urdu and English
    (Tues 6.00 pm–10.00 pm)
0800 282 447 Arabic and English
    (Wednesday 6.00 pm–10.00 pm)
www.playingsafely.co.uk

Positively Women
347–349 City Road, London EC1V 1LR
Tel: 020 7713 0444
www.positivelywomen.org.uk
Provides a range of free and confidential
    counselling and support services for
    women with HIV and AIDS.

**SASH (Society for the Advancement of
    Sexual Health)**
PO Box 17, Cheltenham GL54 2YU
Tel: 014541 822551
www.sheffhiv.demon.co.uk/sash

Terrence Higgins Trust
52–54 Grays Inn Road, London WC1X 8JU
Tel: 020 7831 0330
Helpline: 020 7242 1010
Legal Line: 020 7405 2381
(Mondays and Wednesdays 7.00 pm–9.00 pm)
www.tht.org.uk
Practical support, help, counselling and
    advice for people with or people
    concerned about AIDS, as well as advice
    regarding national support groups/
    networks.

Other websites

United Nations World AIDS Campaign
www.unaids.org

World Health Organization
www.who.org

Further training and professional development

Centre for HIV and Sexual Health Sheffield
22 Collegiate Crescent, Sheffield S10 2BA
Tel: 01442261900
www.sexualhealthsheffield.co.uk
This centre holds many training days for people working in sexual health, and those working with young people.

Family Planning Association
2–12 Pentonville Road, London N1 9FP
Tel: 0207 923 5235/5232
www.fpa.org.uk
Offers various training courses to health professionals about sexual health issues.

Genito-Urinary Nurses Association (GUNA)
www.guna.org.uk
See website for further information on clinical updates.

Health Promotion Units
These are within local PCTs and often offer various sexual health courses.

London Standing Conference for Nurses
Sexual Health Group, c/o South West Strategic Health Authority, 41–47 Hartfield House, Hartfield Road, London SW19 3RG
www.london.nhs.uk/lscn

Mainliners
Details as above. Offer courses mainly about HIV/hepatitis and drug use.

Royal College of Nursing
20 Cavendish Square, London W1G 0RN
Tel: 020 7409 3333

www.rcn.org.uk
Distance learning courses on sexual health now available.

Further reading

For nurses

ACHESON, D. (1998) *Independent Enquiry into Inequalities in Health: A Report.* London: The Stationery Office.
BENNETT, R. and ERIN, C.A. (1999) *HIV and AIDS: Testing, Screening, and Confidentiality.* Oxford: Oxford University Press.
COTTON, D. and WATTS, H.D. (1995) *Medical Management of AIDS in Women.* London: John Wiley.
CSONKA, G.W. and OATES, J.K. (eds) (1999) *A Textbook of Genito-Urinary Medicine.* London: Baillière Tindall.
CURTIS, H., HOOLAGHAN, T. and JEWITT, C. (eds) (1995) *Sexual Health Promotion in General Practice.* Oxford: Radcliffe Medical Press.
DOYAL, L. (1995) *What Makes Women Sick? Gender and the Political Economy of Health.* Basingstoke: Macmillan.
McMILLAN, A. and SCOTT, G.R. (2000) *Colour Guide: Sexually Transmitted Infections.* Elsevier.
MORSE, S.A., HOLMES, K.K. and BALLARD, R.C. (2002) *Atlas of Sexually Transmitted Diseases and AIDS,* 3rd edn. St Louis: Mosby.
PRATT, R. (2003) *HIV and AIDS: A Strategy for Nursing Care.* London: Arnold.
SOCIAL EXCLUSION UNIT (1999) *Teenage Pregnancy: Report: Cm 4342.* London: The Stationery Office.
SUTTON, A. and PAYNE, S. (1996) *Genito-Urinary Medicine for Nurses.* London: Whorr Publishers.
WAKLEY, G. and CHAMBERS, R. (2002) *Sexual Health Matters in Primary Care.* Oxford: Radcliffe Medical Press.
WAKLEY, G., CUNNION, M. and CHAMBERS, R. (2003) *Improving Sexual Health Advice.* Oxford: Radcliffe Medical Press.
WEISS, R.A, ADLER, M.W, and ROWLAND-JONES, S.L. (2001) *Changing Face of HIV and AIDS.* Oxford: Oxford University Press.
WESTON, A. (1999) *Sexually Transmitted Infections: A Guide to Care.* Guildford: Nursing Times Books.

For clients

KNOX, H. (1995) *SEXPlained: The Uncensored Guide to Sexual Health.* London: Knox Publishing.
MAIN, J., MOYLE, G., PETERS, B. and COKER, R. (eds) (1995) *What We Should All Know About HIV and AIDS.* London: Mediscript.
MOULTON, N. (2003) *New Body Book. The Modern Woman's Guide to Health, Beauty and Wellbeing.* Apple Press.
NORTHRUP, C. (1998) *Women's Bodies, Women's Wisdom.* London: Piatkus.
VILLAROSA, L. (2003) *Body and Soul: The Black Women's Guide to Physical Health and Wellbeing.* Vintage/Edbury.

References

ADAIR, C.D., GUNTER, M., STOVALL, T.G., McELROY, G., VEILLE, J.C. and ERNEST, J.M. (1998) *Chlamydia* in pregnancy: a randomized trial of azithromycin and erythromycin. *Obstetrics and Gynaecology* **91**(2):165–8.

ADLER, M.W. (1990) *ABC of Sexually Transmitted Diseases.* London: BMJ Publishing.

ADLER, M.W. (1993) *ABC of Sexually Transmitted Diseases,* 2nd edn. London: BMJ Publishing.

ADLER, M.W. (1995) *ABC of Sexually Transmitted Diseases,* 3rd edn. London: BMJ Publishing.

ADLER, M.W. (2003) Sexual health: report finds sexual health services to be a shambles. *British Medical Journal* **327**(12):62–3.

ALBERTI, A. (1996) *Clinical Gastroenterology.* London: Ballière Tindall.

ALLEN, D. (1998) Putting the experts in charge. *Nursing Standard* **12**(17):22–3.

ANDRIST, L.C. (1988) Taking a sexual history and educating clients about safer sex. *Nursing Clinics of North America* **23**(4):959–73.

ARYA, O.P., OSOBA, A.O. and BENNETT, F.J. (1980) *Tropical Venereology.* Edinburgh: Churchill Livingstone.

BAILEY, J.V., KAVANAGH, J., OWEN, C., McLEAN, K.A and SKINNER, C.J. (2000) Lesbians and cervical screening. *British Journal of General Practice* **50**:481–2.

BARAT, L.M. and BLOLAND, P.B. (1997) Drug resistance among malaria and other parasites. *Infectious Diseases Clinics of North America* **11**(4):969–87.

BEVIER, P.J., CHIASSON, M.A., HEFFERNAN, R.T. and CASTRO, K.G. (1995) Women at a sexually transmitted disease clinic who reported same sex contact: their HIV seroprevalence and risk behaviours. *American Journal of Public Health* **85**:1366.

BICKLY, L.S., KRISHER, K.K., PUNSALANG, A., TRUPEI, M.A., REICHMAN, R.C. and MENEGUS, M.A. (1989) Comparison of direct fluorescent antibody, acridine orange, wet mount and culture for detection of *Trichomonas vaginalis* in women attending a public sexually transmitted disease clinic. *Sexually Transmitted Diseases* **16**:127–31.

BLAKEY, V. (1991) Promoting sexual health: strategies for reaching and empowering women. In Curtis, H. (ed.) *Promoting Sexual Health.* London: Health Education Authority, pp. 87–95.

BOAG, F. (1999) Women and HIV. In Gazzard, B. (ed.) *Chelsea and Westminster Hospital AIDS Care Handbook.* London: Mediscript.

BOR, R. and WATTS, M. (1993) Talking to patients about sexual matters. *British Journal of Nursing* **2**(13):657–61.

BOSTON WOMEN'S HEALTH BOOK COLLECTIVE (1985) *The New, Our Bodies, Ourselves.* New York: Simon & Schuster.

BOWMAN, C.A. (1992) Recurrent vulvovaginal candidosis. *British Journal of Sexual Medicine* **19**(5):133–6.

BRESLIN, E. (1988) Genital herpes simplex. *Nursing Clinics of North America* **23**(4):907–15.

BRITISH MEDICAL ASSOCIATION (BMA) and ASSOCIATION OF BRITISH INSURERS (ABI) (2000) *Medical Information and Insurance: Joint Guidelines from the British Medical Association and the Association of British Insurers.* London: BMA.

BUMP, R.C. and BUESCHING, W.J. (1988) Bacterial vaginosis in virginal and sexually active adolescent females: evidence against exclusive sexual transmission. *American Journal of Obstetrics and Gynecology* **158**(4):935–7.

CARNEY, O., ROSS, E., BUNKER, C., IKKOS, G. and MINDEL, A. (1994) A prospective study of the psychological impact on patients with a first episode of genital herpes. *Genito-Urinary Medicine* **70**:40–5.

CARNEY, O., ROSS, E., IKKOS, A. and MINDEL, A. (1993) The effect of suppressive oral acyclovir on the psychological morbidity associated with recurrent genital herpes. *Genito-Urinary Medicine* **69**(6):457–9.

CASSELL, J.A., BROOK, M.G., MURPHY, S. and JOHNSON, A.M. (2003) Treating sexually transmitted infections in primary care: a missed opportunity. *Sexually Transmitted Infections* **79**:134–6.

CATCHPOLE, M. (2001) Sexually transmitted infections: control strategies. *British Medical Journal* **322**:1135–6.

CATES, W. and WASSERHEIT, J.N. (1991) Genital chlamydial infections: epidemiology and reproductive sequelae. *American Journal of Obstetrics and Gynecology* **164**(6):1771–81.

CATTEREL, R.C. (1972) Trichomonal infection of the genital tract. *Medical Clinics of North America* **56**:1203.

CENTRAL AUDIT GROUP IN GENITOURINARY MEDICINE (1997) *Clinical Guidelines and Standards for Genital* Chlamydia *Infection.* London: Health Education Authority.

CLINICAL EFFECTIVENESS GROUP (Association for Genitourinary Medicine and the Medical Society for the Study of Venereal Diseases) (1999) National guideline on the management of vulvovaginal candidiasis. *Sexually Transmitted Infections* **75**(Suppl 11):S19–20.

COELHO, D.D. (1997) Metranidazole-resistant trichomoniasis successfully treated with paromomycin. *Genito-Urinary Medicine* **73**(5):397–8.

CONWAY, M. and HUMPHRIES, E. (1994) Bernhard Clinic: meeting need in lesbian sexual healthcare. *Nursing Times* **90**(32):40–1.

COREY, L. (1990) Genital herpes. In Holmes, K.K., Mardh, P.A., Sparling, P.F. *et al.* (eds) *Sexually Transmitted Diseases.* New York: McGraw-Hill.

CORKILL, J.E., KOMOLAFE, A.J., NEAL, T.J., MORTIMORE, A., ALAWATTEGAMA, A.B. and HART, C.A. (2003) Molecular epidemiology of endemic ciprofloxacin-resistant Neisseria gonorrhoea in Liverpool. *International Journal of STD and AIDS* **14**:379–85.

COTCH, M.F., PASTOREK, P.G., NUGENT, R.P., HILLIER, S.L., GIBBS, R.S., MARTIN, D.H., ESCHENBACH, D.A., EDELMAN, R., CAREY, J.C., REGAN, J.A., KROHN, M.A., KLEBANOFF, M.A. and RHOADS, G.G. (1997) Trichomonas vaginalis associated with low birthweight and preterm delivery. *Sexually Transmitted Diseases* **24**:353–60.

CUZICK, J., SZAREWSKI, A., TERRY, G. HO, L., HANBY, A., MADDOX, P., ANDERSON, M., KOCJAN, G., STEELE, S.T. and GUILLIBAUD, J. (1995) Human papilloma virus testing in primary cervical screening. *Lancet* **345**(17): 1533–6.

DoH (DEPARTMENT OF HEALTH) (1997a) *HIV testing; Guidelines for Pre-test Discussion.* London: DOH, The Stationery Office.

DoH (1997b) *The New NHS: Modern, Dependable*. London: DOH, The Stationery Office.

DoH (1999) *Making a Difference. Strengthening the Nursing, Midwifery and Health Visiting Contributions to Health and Healthcare*. London: DOH, The Stationery Office.

DoH (2000) *The NHS Plan – A Plan for Investment. A Plan for Reform* (Cm 4817-I). London: HMSO.

DoH (2001) *The National Strategy for Sexual Health and HIV*. London: DOH, The Stationery Office.

DoH (2003) Government response to the Health Select Committeee's third report of session 2002–2003 on sexual health. London: Crown Copyright. Online. Available: http://www.doh.gov.uk/sexualhealthandhiv/pdfs/response_to_health_select_comm_three.pdf (accessed 15th January 2004).

EASMON, C.S.F. (1993) *The Diagnosis and Management of Bacterial Vaginosis*. London: Royal Society of Medicine.

ETHERINGTON, I. and SHAFI, M. (1996) Human papilloma viruses and cervical screening. *Genito-Urinary Medicine* **72**(3):153–4.

FRENCH, P. (1995) *The Clinic Guide* (unpublished). Mortimer Market Centre, Mortimer Market (off Capper Street), London WC1E 6AU.

GARNETT, G.P., DUBIN, G., SLAOUI, M. and DARCIS, T. (2004) The potential epidemiological impact of a genital herpes vaccine for women. *Sexually Transmitted Infections* **80**:24–9.

GODLEY, M.J. (1993) The management of sexually transmitted diseases in pregnancy. *Medicine International* **21**(3):74–81.

GOH, B.T. and FORSTER, G.E. (1993) Sexually transmitted diseases in children: chlamydial oculo-genital infection. *Genito-Urinary Medicine* **69**:213–21.

GOLDMEIER, D. and HAY, P. (1993) A review and update on adult syphilis, with particular reference to its treatment. *International Journal of STD and AIDS* **4**:70–82.

GULMEZOGLU, A.M. (1996) Trichomoniasis treatment during pregnancy. In Neilson, J.P., Hofmeyr, G.J., Renfrew, M.J. and Keirse, M.J.N.C. (eds) *Pregnancy and Childbirth Module of the Cochrane Database of Systematic Review*. The Cochrane Library. The Cochrane Collaboration; Issue 1. Oxford: Update Software.

HALL, J. (1993) Management of genital ulceration in general practice. *British Journal of Sexual Medicine* May/June.

HALPERIN, D.T. (1999) Heterosexual anal intercourse: prevalence, cultural factors, and HIV infection and other health risks, Part 1. *AIDS Patient Care STDs* **13**(12):717–30.

HAMILL, H. and KAUFMAN, R. (1990) Vaginal candidiasis: tailoring the treatment. *Physician Assistant* **14**(7):41–4.

HARINDA, V., TOBIN, J.M, and TUCKER, L.J. (2001) Triage clinics: a way forward in genito-urinary medicine. *International Journal of STD and AIDS* **10**:539–42.

HARRO, C.D., PANG, S.Y-Y., RODEN, R.B.S, HILDESHEIM, A., WANG, Z., REYNOLDS, M.J., MAST, T.C., ROBINSON, R., MURPHY, B.R., KARRON, R.A., DILLNER, J., SCHILLER, J.T and LAWY, D.R. (2001) Safety and immunogenicity trail in adult volunteers of a human papilloma virus 16 L1 virus-like particle vaccine. *Journal of the National Cancer Institute* **93**:284–94.

HORTON, R. (1995) Women as women with HIV. *Lancet* **345**:531–2.

HPA (HEALTH PROTECTION AGENCY) (HIV/STI DEPARTMENT, CDSC) and SCOTTISH CENTRE FOR INFECTION AND ENVIRONMENTAL HEALTH (2003) AIDS/HIV Quarterly surveillance tables: cumulative UK data to end September 2003, No.6: 03/3.

HPA (2003) The Health Protection Agency Five-Year Corporate Plan. Press release, 5 August 2003. Online. Available: http://www.hpa.org.uk/hpa/news/articles/press_release/2003/030805_corplan.htm (accessed 10 January 2004).

HUGHES, G., CATCHPOLE, M., ROGERS, P.A., BRADY, A.R., KINGHORN, G., MERCEY, D. and THIN, N. (2000) Comparison of risk factors for four sexually transmitted infections: results from a study of attenders at three genito-urinary medicine clinics. *Sexually Transmitted Infections* **76**:262–7.

ISON, C.A. and HAY, P. (2002) Validation of a simplified grading of Gram stained vaginal smears for use in genito-urinary medicine clinics. *Sexually Transmitted Infections* **78**:413–15.

JOHNSON, A.M., GRUN, L. and HAINES, A. (1996) Controlling genital chlamydial infection. *British Medical Journal* **313**(7066)1160–1.

KANE, R. and WELLINGS, K. (2003) Staff training in integrated sexual health services. *Sexually Transmitted Infections* **79**:354–6.

KEANE, F.E., THOMAS, B., RENTON, A. *et al.* (1997) Investigation into a possible causal role of bacterial vaginosis in non-gonococcal urethritis. *Genito-Urinary Medicine* **73**(5):373–7.

KWAKWA, H.A. and GHOBRIAL, M.W. (2003) Female-to-female transmission of human immunodeficiency virus. *Clinical Infectious Diseases* **36**:40–1.

LACEY, C.J.N., MERRICK, D,W,. BENSLEY, D.C. and FAIRLEY, I. (1997) Analysis of the socio-demography of gonnorhoea in Leeds. *British Medical Journal* **314**:1718–19.

LACEY, C.J.N., GOODALL, R.L., RAGNARSON TENNVALL, G., MAW, R., KINGHORN, G.R., FISK, P.G., BARTON, S. and BYREN, I. (2003) Randomised controlled trial and economic evaluation of podophyllotoxin solution, podophyllotoxin cream, and podophyllin in the treatment of genital warts. *Sexually Transmitted Infections* **79**:270–5.

LARA-TORRE, E. and PINKERTON, J.S. (2003) Accuracy of detection of trichomonas vaginalis on a liquid-based papanicolaou smear. *American Journal of Obstetrics and Gyneacology* **188**(2):354–6.

LARSEN, S.A., HUNTER, E.F. and CREIGHTON, E.T. (1990) Syphilis. In Holmes, K.K., Mardh, P.A., Sparling, P.F. *et al.* (eds) *Sexually Transmitted Diseases*. New York: McGraw-Hill.

LARSSON, P.G. (1997) Treatments for bacterial vaginosis: an update on the expected cure. *International Journal of STD and AIDS* **8**(Suppl 1):35–6.

LEE, H.H., CHERNESKY, M.A., SCHACTER, J. *et al.* (1995) Diagnosis of chlamydia trachomatis genito-urinary infection in women by ligase chain reaction assay of urine. *Lancet* **345**(8944):213–16.

LEHTINEN, M. and DILLER, J. (2002) Preventative human papilloma virus vaccination. *Sexually Transmitted Infections* **78**:4–6.

LOW, N., DAKER-WHITE, G., BARLOW, D. and POZNIAK, A. (1997) Gonorrhoea in London: results of a cross sectional study. *British Medical Journal* **314**(7096):1719–23.

MAGID, D., DOUGLAS, J.M. and SCHWARTZ, J.S. (1996) Doxycycline compared with azithromycin for treating women with genital chlamydia trachomatis infections: an incremental cost-effectiveness analysis. *Annals of Internal Medicine* **124**:(4)359–99.

MASFARI, A.N., DUERDEN, B.I. and KINGHORN, G.R. (1986) Quantitative studies of vaginal bacteria. *Genito-Urinary Medicine* **62**:256–63.

McCAFFREY, M., VARNEY, P.A., EVANS, B. and TAYLOR-ROBINSON, D. (1997) A study of bacterial vaginosis in lesbians. *International Journal of HIV and AIDS* **8**(Suppl 1):11.

McDONALD, H.M., O'LOUGHLIN, J.A., VIGENE SWARAN, R. *et al.* (1997) Metronidazole treatment of bacterial vaginosis flora and its effect on pre-term birth. *International Journal of STD and AIDS* **8**(1):37–8.

McGREGOR, J.A., FRENCH, J.I., JONES, W. *et al.* (1994) Bacterial vaginosis is associated with prematurity and vaginal fluid mucinase and sialiclase: results of a controlled trial of topical clindamycin cream. *American Journal of Obstetrics and Gynecology* **170**:1048–59.

MERCEY, D. (1992) Clinical audit in genito-urinary medicine: 'why, who, what, how and when?' *Genito-Urinary Medicine* **68**:205–6.

MERTZ, G.J., BENEDITTI, J., ASHLEY, R., SELKE, S.A. and COREY, L. (1992) Risk factors for the transmission of genital herpes. *Annals of Internal Medicine* **116**(3): 197–202.

MILES, K., PENNY, N., MERCEY, D.E. and POWER, R. (2002a) A postal survey to identify and describe nurse-led clinics in genito-urinary medicine services across England. *Sexually Transmitted Infections* **78**:100.

MILES, K., PENNY, N., MERCEY, D.E. and POWER, R. (2002b) Sexual health clinics for women led by specialist nurses or senior house officers in a central London GUM service: a randomized controlled trial. *Sexually Transmitted Infections* **78**:93–7.

MILES, K., PENNY, N., MERCEY, D.E. and POWER, R. (2003a) Comparing doctor- and nurse-led care in a sexual health clinic: patient satisfaction questionnaire. *Sexually Transmitted Infections* **42**:64–72.

MILES, K., KNIGHT, V., CAIRO, I. and KING, I. (2003b) Nurse-led sexual health care: international perspectives. *International Journal of STD and AIDS* **14**:243–7.

MOHANTY, K.C. (1989) Gonorrhoea. *British Journal of Sexual Medicine* May:206–7.

MOHANTY, K.C. (1990) Trichomoniasis. *British Journal of Sexual Medicine* July:210–12.

MORSE, S.A., MORELAND, A.A., HOLMES, K.K. and TAYLOR, P.K. (1996) *CD – Atlas of Sexually Transmitted Diseases and AIDS*. London: Mosby International.

NHS EXECUTIVE (1999) *Reducing Mother to Baby Transmission of HIV*. London: NHS Executive (HSC 1999/183).

O'HANLAN, K. and CRUM, C. (1996) Human papilloma virus associated cervical intraepithelial neoplasia following lesbian sex. *Obstetrics and Gynecology* **88**:702–3.

ORIEL, J.D. (1978) Genito-urinary medicine. *British Journal of Venereal Diseases* **54**:291–4.

PETRIN, D., DELGATY, K., BHATT, R. and GARBER, A. (1998) Clinical and microbiological aspects of trichomonas vaginalis. *Clinical Microbiology Review* **11**(2):300–17.

PHILLIPS, L.E. and FRIEDRICH, E. (1990) Microwaving underwear. *American Journal of Nursing* **90**:9–17.

PHLS (PUBLIC HEALTH LABORATORY SERVICE): CDSC (COMMUNICABLE DISEASES SURVEILLANCE CENTER) (1998) *Communicable Disease Report CDR Weekly* **8**(22):194–6.

PHLS: CDSC (1999) New cases seen at genito-urinary medicine clinics: England 1998. *Communicable Disease Report Supplement* **9**(6) December.

PHLS, DHSS and PS and SCOTTISH ISD (D) 5 COLLABORATIVE GROUP (2001) *Sexually Transmitted Infections in the UK: New Episodes Seen at Genitourinary Medicine Clinics, 1995 to 2000*. London: PHLS.

PHLS: CDSC (2002) Sexually transmitted diseases quarterly report: gonorrhoea in England, Wales and Northern Ireland. *Communicable Disease Report CDR Weekly* **12**:4.

PHLS: CDSC (2003) *Communicable Disease Report CDR Weekly* **13**(05).

PIMENTA, J.M., CATCHPOLE, M., ROGERS, P.A., PERKINS, E., JACKSON, N., CARLISLE, C., RANDALL, S., HOPWOOD, J., HEWITT, G., UNDERHILL, G., MALLINSON, H., McLEAN, L., GLEAVE, T., TOBIN, J., HARINDA, V. and GHOSH, A. (2003) Opportunistic screening for genital chlamydial infection: I. Acceptability of urine testing in primary and secondary healthcare settings. *Sexually Transmitted Infections* **79**:16–21.

RAJAMANOHARAN, S., LOW, N., JONES, S.B. and POZNIAK, A.L. (1999) Bacterial vaginosis, ethnicity and the use of genital cleaning agents: a case control study. *Sexually Transmitted Diseases* **26**(7):404–9.

ROBERTSON, D.H.H., McMILLAN, A. and YOUNG, H. (1989) *Clinical Practice in Sexually Transmitted Diseases*. Edinburgh: Churchill Livingstone.

ROMANOWSKI, B. (1993) Sexually transmitted diseases in women: symptoms and examination. *Medicine International* **21**(3):82–6.

SAURINA, G.R. and McCORMACK, W.M. (1997) Trichomoniasis in pregnancy. *Sexually Transmitted Diseases* **24**:361–2.

SCHNEIDER, A. (1993) Pathogenesis of genital HPV infection. *Genito-Urinary Medicine* **69**:165–73.

SELECT COMMITTEEE ON HEALTH (2003) Sexual health, third report of session 2002–2003: conclusion and recom-mendations. Online. Available: http://www.publications.parliament.uk/pa/cm200203/cmselect/cmhealth/69/6917.htm (accessed 14 November 2003).

SOBEL, J.D. (1990) Vulvovaginal candidiasis. In Holmes, K.K., Mardh, P.A., Sparling, P.F., *et al.* (eds). *Sexually Transmitted Diseases*. New York: McGraw-Hill.

SOBEL, J.D. (1997) Vaginitis. *New England Journal of Medicine* **337**(26):1896–903.

SORVILLO, F., SMITH, L., KERNOTT, P. and ASH, L. (2001) Trichomonas vaginalis, HIV and African Americans. *Emerging Infectious Diseases* **7**(6):927–32.

SPARLING, P.F. (1990) Biology of neisseria gonorrhoea. In Holmes, K.K., Mardh, P.A., Sparling, P.F. *et al.* (eds) *Sexually Transmitted Diseases*. New York: McGraw-Hill.

STAMM, W.E., GUINAN, M.E., STARCHER, T., HOLMES, K.K. and McCORMACK, W.M. (1984) Effect of treatment regimens for neisseria gonorrhoea on simultaneous infection with chlamydia trachomatis. *New England Journal of Medicine* **310**(9):545–9.

STANBERRY L.R., SPRUANCE, L.S., CUNNINGHAM, A.L., BERNSTEIN D.I., MINDEL, A., SACKS, S., TYRING, S., AOKI, F.Y., SLAOUI, M.DENIS, M., VANDEPAPELIERE, P. and DUBIN, G. (2002) Glycoprotein-D-adjuvant vaccine to prevent genital herpes. *New England Journal of Medicine* **347**:1652–61.

TAYAL, S.C., SANKAR, K.N., PATTMAN, R.S., WATSON, P.G. and GALLOWAY, A. (1999) Neisseraia gonorrhoea in Newcastle upon Tyne 1995–1997: increase in ciprofloxacin resistance. *International Journal of STD and AIDS* **10**:290–3.

TAYLOR-ROBINSON, D. (1996) Tests for infection with chlamydia trachomatis. *International Journal of STD and AIDS* **7**(1):19–26.

TAYLOR-ROBINSON, D. and HAY, P.E. (1997) The pathogenesis of the clinical signs of bacterial vaginosis and possible reasons for its occurrence. *International Journal of STD and AIDS* **8**(Suppl 1):13–16.

TEARE, E.L. (1986) How to … diagnose and treat chlamydial infections. *British Journal of Sexual Medicine* January:20–2.

THIN, R.N. (1982) *Lecture Notes on Sexually Transmitted Diseases.* Oxford: Blackwell Scientific.

TILLMAN, J. (1991) Syphilis an old disease, a contemporary perinatal problem. *Journal of Obstetric and Gynaecological Neonate Nursing* **21**(3):209–13.

TINKLE, M.B. (1990) Genital human papilloma virus infection: a growing health risk. *Journal of Obstetric and Gynaecological Neonate Nursing* **19**(6):501–7.

TRAMONT, E.C. (1990) Treponema pallidum (syphilis). In Mondell, G.L., Douglas, R.G. and Bennett, J.E. (eds). *Sexually Transmitted Diseases,* 2nd edn. New York: McGraw-Hill.

UNAIDS and WHO (2003) *AIDS Epidemic Update: December 2003.* Geneva: Joint United Nations Programme on AIDS and World Health Organization.

WALLIN, K.L., WIKLUND, F., ANGSTROM, T. *et al.* (1999) Type specific persistence of human papilloma virus dva before the development of invasive cervical cancer. *New England Journal of Medicine* **341**(22):1633–8.

WASSERHEIT, J.N. (1992) Epidemiological synergy: inter-relationships between human immunodeficiency virus infection and other sexually transmitted diseases. *Sexually Transmitted Diseases* **19**(2):61–77.

WEHBEH, H.A., RUGGEIRRIO, R.M., SLAHEM, S., LOPEZ, G. and ALI, Y. (1998) Single dose azithromycin for chlamydia in pregnant women. *Journal of Reproductive Medicine* **43**(6):509–14.

WESTROM, L. (1980) Incidence, prevalence and trends of acute pelvic inflammatory disease and its consequences in industrialised countries. *American Journal of Obstetrics and Gynecology* **138**(7, Pt 2):880–92.

WHITTAKER, D. (1993) *'In The Room' – Invisible Work and Hidden Experiences of Women Nurses and Women Patients in a Genito-Urinary Medicine Clinic: An Exploratory Study* (unpublished). Mortimer Market Centre, Mortimer Market, London WC1E 6AU.

WHO (1995) *Sexually Transmitted Diseases: Three Hundred and Thirty-Three Million New Curable Cases in 1995.* Press Release WHO/64. Geneva: World Health Organization.

WHO (2000) Fact sheets on HIV/AIDS for nurses and midwives. Geneva: World Health Organization.

WHO (2003) HIV-infected women and their families: psychological support and related issues. A literature review. Occasional Paper 7. Geneva: World Health Organization.

WIESE, W., PATEL, S.R., PATEL S.C., OHL, C.A. and ESTRADA, C.A. (2000) A meta-analysis of the Papanicolaou smear and wet mount for the diagnosis of vaginal trichomoniasis. *American Journal of Medicine* **108**(4):301–8.

WILSON, J.D. (1995) *Female Genital Infections: Infections of the Vulva.* London: Martin Dunitz.

WINTER, A.J., GILLERAN, G., EASTWICK, K. and ROSS, J.D.C. (2000) Comparison of a ligase chain reaction-based assay and cell culture for detection of pharyngeal carriage of Chlamydia trachomatis. *Journal of Clinical Microbiology* **38**(9):3502–4.

WISTREICH, C.A. (1992) *Sexually Transmitted Diseases: A Current Approach.* East Los Angeles College: WCB Group.

ZENKER, P.N. and ROLFS, R.T. (1990) Treatment of syphilis, 1989. *Reviews of Infectious Diseases* **12**(Suppl 6):S590–S609.

15: Premenstrual Syndrome

Gilly Andrews

OBJECTIVES

This chapter should help you understand:

◆ Some of the theories about the possible causes of PMS ◆

◆ The variety of symptoms and the devastating effect that severe PMS can have on a woman's life ◆

◆ How to recognize and help to diagnose when a woman is suffering from PMS rather than a psychiatric problem ◆

◆ How to advise a PMS sufferer about self-help options ◆

◆ The different treatment options available for severe PMS. ◆

Introduction

Premenstrual syndrome (PMS) is a topical and controversial issue, with increasing interest in the subject both in medical journals and in women's magazines. Many doctors, however, still refuse to believe that PMS exists, making it extremely difficult for a sufferer to find understanding and supportive advice for a problem that she feels is ruining her life – not only her personal and social relationships but also in her work environment.

Too often sufferers will hear dismissive comments such as: 'It is all part of being a woman', 'It's that time of the month again – ignore it and you will feel better in a few days' time' or 'Pull yourself together'. Such remarks and lack of understanding only serve to isolate women even further in their misery and despair – many feel that they have a psychiatric illness and are terrified that they are 'going mad'. Even worse, some women will have been given the wrong treatment which can be more harmful than no treatment at all.

Attitudes towards PMS are slowly changing as women take an active and positive role in trying to understand health issues that affect their life. This chapter will give you an insight into this bewildering and occasionally frightening disorder to enable you to counsel clients who ask for your advice. You might find it helpful to remind yourself of the fluctuating hormonal influences in the normal menstrual cycle (see page 516).

Historical perspective

Premenstrual syndrome is frequently thought of as a twentieth-century disorder that the modern woman may use to provide a convenient excuse for occasions when she does not live up to her own lifestyle expectations. However, Hippocrates in 460 BC observed that 'women are subjected to intermittent "agitations" and as a result the "agitated" blood finds its way from the head to the uterus whence it is expelled'. He also noticed that 'shivering, lassitude and heaviness of the head denote the onset of menstruation' (Chadwick and Mann, 1950). The fact that this correlation of psychological symptoms with menstruation was observed and written about two and a half thousand years ago clearly contradicts the idea that PMS is a new phenomenon.

425

In spite of Hippocrates' mention of these typical premenstrual symptoms it was not until 1931 that the term 'premenstrual tension' was used. Frank (1931) published a description of a small group of women who had symptoms of tension, depression, headaches and weight gain for 7–10 days before menstruation. Greene and Dalton in 1953 first used the term 'premenstrual syndrome' when they recognized and wrote about the wide range of symptoms which may occur with the menstrual cycle. PMS is the term that is now more generally accepted. Five decades later, despite considerable scientific and medical research, we are little further forward in understanding the disorder. There is confusion and disagreement in the medical profession over the definition of PMS, its causes, the diagnostic criteria and the best methods of treatment. It is hardly surprising that women who suffer from premenstrual syndrome often find it extremely difficult to obtain information, advice and help for their symptoms when doctors cannot agree amongst themselves.

Definition

The World Health Organization (WHO) does not acknowledge PMS as an illness, so consequently there is no officially recognized definition. Reading through medical and nursing journals you will come across numerous definitions which can only add to your confusion in trying to understand the disorder. The diverse nature of PMS symptoms necessitates a definition that is broad enough to cover the variability of symptoms, which will also vary from cycle to cycle in individual women in their severity, timing and duration.

A definition of PMS by Magos and Studd (1984) is 'distressing physical, psychological and behavioural symptoms not caused by organic disease which regularly recur during the same phase of the ovarian (or menstrual) cycle, and which significantly regress or disappear during the remainder of the cycle'. It is the repetitive cyclical nature, not the type of symptoms, which is important to the definition and diagnosis of PMS. Additionally Reid (1991) stressed that the severity of symptoms was important. Many women suffer premenstrual symptoms but in most cases they are mild. It is only a minority of women whose symptoms are of such extreme severity as to interfere with function, and it is only this latter group who should be said to suffer from PMS. Premenstrual dysphoric disorder (PMDD) is a severe form of PMS and affects 3–5% of menstruating women.

Menstruation itself is not necessarily a prerequisite of the diagnosis, as cyclical symptoms may continue to occur following hysterectomy if the ovaries have been conserved (Backstrom et al., 1981). This condition would be better termed 'ovarian cycle syndrome' and women who suffer from it may not realize what their problem is, as they have no outwardly visible signs (i.e. menstruation) which would signal a relief of their distressing symptoms. Consequently they often suffer many months and even years of cyclical symptoms following a hysterectomy without realizing that their problem is identical with premenstrual syndrome. Once diagnosed, the treatment of these women is very straightforward.

Some researchers have tried to classify PMS into different subgroups (Abraham, 1980) but these 'subtypes' are often arbitrary and women report their own unique combinations of symptoms.

Incidence

Although PMS has been described as 'one of the world's commonest diseases' the true prevalence is difficult to assess. This is mainly due to the wide differences in the definition and diagnostic criteria.

Up to 90% of women are aware of some body changes or symptoms during the fourth week of their menstrual cycle, which forewarn them of the imminent start of their period. These changes are mild and may only consist of a slight increase in breast tenderness. True PMS is said to affect approximately 40% of women, with about 5–10% so severely incapacitated that it dominates their life during this phase of the cycle (Reid and Yen, 1981). This means that a GP with an average number of 2500 patients might expect between 25 and 50 women to have severe PMS (Figure 15.1).

PMS is no respecter of class. Snowden and Christian (1984) in a WHO global study of patterns and perception of menstruation suggest that PMS is a phenomenon of Western 'civilized' society. Other studies have found PMS to be just as prevalent in Third World countries when questions are specifically asked (Shershah *et al.*, 1991). Age, parity, race, socioeconomic groups and familial predisposition are thought likely to have distinct effects on the incidence of PMS, but studies show conflicting results.

A young woman's attitude to her periods develops from those who first introduced her to menstruation, e.g. her mother, her teacher or friends. If they viewed menstruation in a negative way and if a young woman has been told since childhood that PMS exists and has experienced these problems at first hand with her mother, then the daughter will expect that time of the month to be problematic. It is a self-fulfilling prophesy.

Nowadays the average age for puberty is 12 years, and for the menopause 51 years. An average woman may thus expect to have over 450 menstrual cycles in her life, with only short breaks for pregnancy and breastfeeding. If she is adversely affected during the premenstrual phase of her cycle, even for only 2 or 3 days

a month, it can be seen that PMS can create a significant problem throughout her life.

Changes in social structure during the twentieth century and contemporary lifestyle expectations mean that the modern woman, who is frequently trying to juggle the varied demands of a job, alongside those of being a wife, lover, mother and carer, is no longer prepared to tolerate symptoms which result in her feeling less than at her best. Attitudes differ though and an ardent feminist has said 'you can't have equality and PMS!'

A leading women's magazine recently quoted a female psychologist as saying that 'PMS becomes a very convenient way to explain why we burnt the toast, shouted at our partner or were bitchy to a colleague. It allows us to be forgiven and means we can hang on to our perfection a bit longer' (Einon, 1997).

Symptoms and effects

The symptoms of PMS are less frequent during the early reproductive years, tend to become progressively worse with age and then merge with similar climacteric symptoms as the menopause approaches. Symptoms are frequently said to start after stopping the oral contraceptive pill or following a pregnancy. The severity of the symptoms may fluctuate from cycle to cycle but the type of symptoms will usually remain constant.

The symptoms of PMS are numerous – over 150 different symptoms have been recorded in research literature (Moos, 1969). Unfortunately as PMS symptoms are so diverse and are also symptoms of other disorders (which can be experienced by both men and postmenopausal women), it can often lead to difficulties when trying to make a diagnosis.

Magos and Studd in 1985 wrote about the effects of the menstrual cycle on medical disorders and noted that the severity of symptoms of over 160 medical conditions fluctuated with the menstrual cycle. You might find it helpful to enquire whether any of your female patients with pre-existing medical conditions such as asthma, epilepsy, migraine, rheumatoid arthritis and herpes find that these conditions worsen

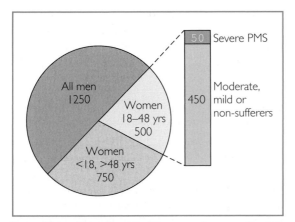

Figure 15.1 Approximately 50 women in a practice list of 2500 may have severe PMS.

during the premenstrual phase of their cycle. You will then be able to give advice and reassure them of the cyclical nature of their symptoms.

PMS symptoms are numerous and diverse and almost any system of the body can be affected. Symptoms are often broadly classified into three categories and women may often have a mixture of symptoms from each group:

◆ Physical
◆ Psychological
◆ Behavioural.

Physical symptoms

Typical physical symptoms are listed in Box 15.1. The common symptoms of bloating, fluid retention and mastalgia cause the uncomfortable *sensation* of weight gain, but the majority of women show no demonstrable premenstrual weight increase. Interestingly some PMS sufferers clearly experience an altered perception of body image premenstrually, which may at least partially explain this (Faratian *et al.*, 1984). There is possibly a redistribution of body fluids rather than fluid retention which could account for these differences. Such symptoms cause considerable distress to many PMS sufferers who often have to wear looser, more comfortable clothes and a larger and more supportive bra. One woman

describes her wardrobe as her 'normal clothes' and her 'fat clothes'. Wald *et al.* (1981) showed that gastrointestinal transit time is significantly increased during the luteal phase of the cycle when there is an increase in progesterone levels which inhibit the smooth muscle of the gut. This will then give rise to constipation, gaseous distension and the sensation of being bloated.

The impression of putting on weight premenstrually is in itself depressing and the effect can be devastating for those who are on a diet. Many women experience cravings for certain types of food in the few days before their period. These cravings may be for unusual, highly savoury meals, but more frequently are for sweet, high-carbohydrate snacks such as bread, cakes, chocolate and fizzy drinks. Women who are normally vigilant about their diet and weight often find their will-power will suddenly desert them and they can munch through one or two bars of chocolate. Whether these are genuine cravings, or whether women eat because they are feeling miserable and food is a comforter, is a point that is difficult to determine. As a result of their extra eating and cravings they consequently feel more bloated and fat and this makes them even more miserable – a vicious circle!

Some PMS sufferers complain of headaches during the premenstrual phase of their cycle. These headaches can vary from mild diffuse pain to a classic migraine associated with nausea, vomiting, visual disturbances and a blinding unilateral headache. Headaches and migraine

---

Box 15.1 Typical physical symptoms of PMS
◆ Breast tenderness and swelling
◆ Abdominal bloating
◆ Peripheral oedema
◆ Headaches and migraine
◆ Hot flushes
◆ Dizziness
◆ Palpitations
◆ Visual disturbances
◆ Pelvic discomfort
◆ Altered bowel habits
◆ Appetite changes or cravings
◆ Nausea
◆ Acne or skin blemishes
◆ Reduced coordination.

SCENARIO

Jenny, a fitness instructor, who is normally conscientious to the point of being obsessive about her diet, found her will-power deserted her in her premenstrual week and she craved highly flavoured crisps and salted nuts. These salty foods then made her want to drink plenty of fluids and she then felt bloated, obese and miserable. She would then push herself even harder during her exercise classes to try and offset the effects of her cravings – making her feel even more guilty and miserable.

are unpredictable in whether they respond to treatment and how long they last. You should advise all women who present with headaches as part of their PMS problems to take appropriate analgesia at the first symptoms so that an ordinary headache does not develop into a full-blown migraine.

Clumsiness and lack of coordination can increase premenstrually and some women drop and break crockery, cut themselves on knives, burn themselves whilst cooking and continually bump into furniture. It is tempting to assume that these women are normally clumsy, uncoordinated and accident-prone throughout the month but this is not the case. Perhaps this clumsiness is caused by a lack of concentration when women feel edgy and tense premenstrually. Women who play a lot of sports find their coordination and concentration is lacking, and they frequently get angry and aggressive both towards themselves and their opponents.

Psychological symptoms

Many women find the psychological manifestations of premenstrual syndrome the hardest group of symptoms to tolerate, as they often feel totally out of control and are completely bewildered by their own behaviour. Colleagues, friends and relatives offer kindness and understanding for physical problems such as headaches and breast tenderness but rarely give sympathy and support for symptoms of depression, mood swings, irritability and tension.

The most common psychological symptoms are listed in Box 15.2.

Women or their partners will frequently complain of a 'Jekyll and Hyde' personality. A woman who is normally even-tempered and calm may find that some small and trivial incident can completely upset her equilibrium and she can rapidly lose her temper and become aggressive. This is frequently followed by feelings of guilt and tearfulness at her own unreasonable behaviour and occasionally she might even develop suicidal ideas.

Leather *et al.* (1993) in a study of 100 women found that PMS influenced most daily activities

---

Box 15.2 Common psychological symptoms of PMS

- ◆ Tension
- ◆ Irritability
- ◆ Depression
- ◆ Mood swings
- ◆ Anxiety
- ◆ Restlessness
- ◆ Lethargy
- ◆ Lack of libido
- ◆ Lack of concentration.

---

but the greatest effect was felt in the home. Relationships with their partner were severely affected in 82% of PMS sufferers, and 61% said their relationships with their children were also severely affected. Fortunately, women seem more able to control their mood swings and anger at work with only 22% saying that their work relationships were severely affected (Table 15.1).

Clare (1983) found that women presenting with PMS are more likely to complain of interpersonal conflicts and marital disharmony, and that they also have high anxiety levels. Laws (1985) suggests that women focus on the complaints of premenstrual syndrome instead of acknowledging and dealing with existing problems such as stressful relationships or adverse circumstances. Therefore in dealing with women who claim to have PMS it is important for you to distinguish between those who have genuine PMS and those who are just 'complaining' and unhappy about their stressful situations.

Table 15.1 Effect of PMS on lifestyle in 100 women with PMS (Leather *et al.*, 1993)

	Not applicable	Number affected	Severely affected (%)
Work performance	14	80	27.5
Work relationships	23	70	22.1
Household chores	1	97	45.5
Relationship with partner	6	93	82.8
Relationship with children	22	77	61.0
Social relationships	2	94	41.5

Alice and John came to a specialist PMS clinic together for the first time. This was the third appointment that Alice had been sent as she had failed to attend on two previous occasions. Alice explained that she missed these appointments as they had coincided with times when she was not premenstrual and she was feeling very positive about herself and felt in control of her PMS. This third clinic appointment was also at such a time but John insisted that both he and Alice should attend as he was finding it very difficult to cope. Alice suffered violent mood swings and John occasionally feared for the safety of their 6-year-old twins. Twice in the past week he had come home from work and found the children on their own. On one occasion the children were left alone in the kitchen with broken glass all over the floor, which Alice had dropped when they had been naughty. The second time he had arrived home to find that Alice felt that she could not cope any longer with the boys and had just walked out, leaving them to cope on their own for over two hours.

John was very keen to relate how dreadful the situation was becoming and how important it was for Alice to get some expert help. He was anxious that as this third clinic appointment coincided yet again with a postmenstrual phase, that Alice would not explain how desperate the situation was at home. Alice was treated with oestrogen therapy and within 3 months was back to a more even-tempered disposition. John later said that if she had not received treatment when she did, that he could see that their marriage was in imminent danger of breaking up. John, needless to say, was delighted with the result.

Eighteen months later John again attended the clinic with Alice – she had forgotten how bad she had been with her premenstrual mood swings and was intending to see how she could manage without treatment. John was very keen for her to continue as he really feared for the safety of the twins and for the future of their marriage if she reverted back to her aggressive mood swings.

It is also important to distinguish women who have premenstrual syndrome from those with a psychiatric disorder whose symptoms are not related to the ovarian cycle. Failure to make these two distinctions can lead to inappropriate and ineffective treatment. However, women with depression or underlying psychiatric disorders will often experience a premenstrual exacerbation of their symptoms (Halbreich *et al.*, 1983)

which can be severe enough to warrant admission to a psychiatric hospital.

Behavioural symptoms

A wide range of behavioural changes are reported to increase during the premenstrual phase. These include agoraphobia, absenteeism from work, loss of concentration, decreased work performance and avoidance of social activities (Moos, 1969). Accidents, alcoholic binges, criminal behaviour (Dalton, 1961), suicide attempts and psychiatric admissions (Glass *et al.* 1971) all seem to occur more frequently during the premenstrual phase.

PMS and its behavioural symptoms have occasionally been used as a defence in criminal proceedings. This obviously has important legal implications since, although many of these prosecutions may be for minor offences, the issue has occasionally been raised during trials for murder or manslaughter. In the absence of agreement within the medical profession about a definition of PMS, it is difficult for the legal profession to know how to proceed.

It should be your professional duty to try and ensure that a genuine sufferer from PMS receives the help and treatment she needs rather than a criminal record. You also have to ensure that the

Lesley, a 44-year-old housewife, had been seeing her doctor for the past 2 years complaining of increasing premenstrual symptoms. Her doctor had tried Lesley on a variety of tranquillizers and antidepressants but basically told her 'it was a woman's lot'. Lesley felt her premenstrual behaviour was becoming increasingly out of control and after a particularly tearful session with her GP she was eventually referred to a specialist PMS clinic. Unfortunately the week before her first appointment she stole a pair of woollen gloves from a department store, an item she clearly did not need as it was the middle of summer and she had plenty of money in her purse. The store had a policy of prosecuting shoplifters and Lesley wondered if the clinic would write a letter to the court confirming that she suffered from PMS and was premenstrual when the crime was committed.

plea of PMS is not abused by those who do not suffer from the problem.

Positive symptoms

PMS is not necessarily all about distressing symptoms and bad news. Logue and Moos (1988) found that between 5 and 15% of women actually feel better during the premenstrual phase of the cycle. They reported an increase in well-being, energy and confidence. Libido is also said to improve during this phase as testosterone levels rise premenstrually.

SCENARIO

Jane, a 28-year-old advertising executive, found that she was at her most dynamic and resourceful in the week leading up to her period. She would find a tremendous surge of energy and enthusiasm, often clearing her desk of all the paperwork that had been accumulating over the past 3 weeks. She got her best creative ideas for work during this phase and due to an increased libido and sex drive her relationship with her partner was also at its best.

Causes of PMS

Numerous theories have been put forward to explain why PMS occurs (Box 15.3), but as yet the precise cause remains unknown despite extensive research. Psychological, endocrine, social, environmental and dietary theories have been widely investigated and extensively reviewed in the medical literature (O'Brien, 1987; Sampson, 1989) but none of these hypotheses has been proved to be solely relevant.

Progesterone deficiency has been the most fashionable theory for many years, but there is no evidence of such a deficiency, or that it causes PMS. Studies demonstrate contradictory and varying levels of progesterone between patients and controls (Backstrom and Carstensen, 1974; O'Brien *et al.*, 1980). This is hardly surprising since the secretion of progesterone is pulsatile and occasional blood sampling will fail to detect the subtle differences that were thought to exist.

> **Box 15.3**   Possible causes of PMS
>
> ◆ Psychological
> ◆ Progesterone deficiency
> ◆ Oestrogen/progesterone imbalance
> ◆ Sodium and water retention
> ◆ Prostaglandin deficiency/excess
> ◆ Prolactin excess
> ◆ Vitamin B_6 deficiency
> ◆ Trace element deficiency
> ◆ Hypoglycaemia
> ◆ Thyroid abnormality
> ◆ Serotonin deficiency.

Some research indicated there might be a central neurotransmitter abnormality as there was reduced platelet uptake of serotonin and reduced peripheral blood serotonin levels in PMS sufferers during the luteal phase of the cycle (Menkes *et al.*, 1992; Sundblad *et al.*, 1992).

The symptomatology of PMS in many women bears a close resemblance to that of depression. This has led to the theory that PMS is a form of cyclical depression which has become 'entrained' to the menstrual cycle. That is, the hormonal changes themselves do not cause PMS, but merely act as a cue for an independently cycling primary depressive disorder (Schmidt *et al.*, 1991).

The best information that we have at present is that there is an obvious link between PMS and cyclical ovarian activity (Studd, 1979) as symptoms only occur between puberty and the menopause. They disappear during anovulatory cycles and pregnancy, yet persist after hysterectomy if the ovaries have been conserved (Backstrom *et al.*, 1981). Studd (1992) described that there are three well-recognized peaks of depression in women that correspond to times of profound hormonal change:

◆ Postnatal depression
◆ Premenstrual syndrome
◆ Climacteric depression.

Cronje (2003) concludes that fluctuating levels of ovarian hormones, particularly progesterone, would seem to be a fundamental factor.

If ovarian function is completely suppressed by gonadotrophin-releasing hormone analogues or by bilateral oophorectomy then PMS symptoms will disappear. This does not mean that the primary abnormality is in the ovaries – it could lie anywhere in the hypothalamus–pituitary–ovarian (HPO) axis or in the higher centres that influence this HPO axis. This association with ovarian function is not in conflict with a central neurotransmitter theory of the cause of PMS, as there is increasing evidence that ovarian hormones can influence neurotransmitter function (Guicheney et al., 1988).

Considerable research has been conducted and numerous papers written on all the above hypotheses but there is no real evidence that any of them explains the true cause of PMS. Although researchers have been keen to find one particular reason for PMS it is more probable that there are several factors and PMS is probably a combination of physiological, psychological and social factors that interact with life events.

Assessment and diagnosis

Correct diagnosis is essential for the successful treatment of PMS. Unfortunately, there are no universally agreed objective diagnostic criteria for PMS and no biological markers, such as blood tests, which can be used to confirm a diagnosis. Many 'informed' women have read that PMS is caused by a hormone imbalance and so will often request a 'hormone measurement test'. Such tests are useless in diagnosing PMS but can be more appropriately used in excluding other disorders which might be causing similar symptoms, e.g. anaemia, hypothyroidism, polycystic ovarian disease and the peri-menopause.

A full menstrual, contraceptive, gynaecological and obstetric history should be obtained. Women should be asked when they first noticed symptoms of PMS and whether these symptoms were absent during pregnancy. The onset of PMS has often been linked to starting or stopping the contraceptive pill, the birth of a child or sterilization.

As mentioned earlier, symptoms can vary from cycle to cycle. It is important to find out what type of symptoms the woman is complaining of (both positive and negative), when these start in relation to the onset of menstruation and how quickly they resolve after bleeding has commenced. Some women might have minor symptoms for a day or two with which they can easily cope, whilst others have symptoms which start at ovulation and become progressively more severe during the next 14 days until menstruation starts. If they then also suffer from menorrhagia and dysmenorrhoea these women, unfortunately, do not have many 'good' days in a month.

The contribution of any underlying psychological disease and previous psychiatric history should also be taken into account – although in practice this can be difficult. The major pitfall is to confuse PMS with psychological and psychiatric disorders that are unrelated to the ovarian cycle.

Many self-assessment questionnaires, visual analogue scales and menstrual diaries have been introduced in an attempt to make it easy for the woman and her doctor to assess whether she suffers from premenstrual syndrome (Boxes 15.4 and 15.5).

Box 15.4   Menstrual Distress Questionnaire

The 'Menstrual Distress Questionnaire', developed by Moos in 1968, is widely used to assess symptoms on a daily basis. It consists of 47 symptoms divided into 8 symptom clusters.

◆ Pain
◆ Concentration
◆ Behavioural change
◆ Autonomic reactions
◆ Water retention
◆ Negative effect
◆ Arousal
◆ Control.

The eighth 'control' group consists of 6 symptoms not normally associated with the menstrual cycle and is included to help to identify 'complainers'. Women are asked to complete the chart every evening for two or three cycles scoring their symptoms on a scale of 0–3 (0 = none, 1 = slightly, 2 = moderately, 3 = a lot). They are also asked to chart when they start and stop bleeding. An adaptation of this menstrual questionnaire is shown in Box 15.5.

Box 15.5 Symptom assessment chart for use in the menstrual distress questionnaire

Name: ....

Please complete every evening.

Describe how you felt during the day, scoring each symptom from 0–3: 0 = none; 1 = slight; 2 = moderate; 3 = a lot. If applicable, indicate days of period with a 'p'.

		Mon	Tue	Wed	Thu	Fri	Sat	Sun
Pain	Muscle stiffness							
	Stomach pains/cramps							
	Backache							
	Tiredness							
	General aches/pains							
Concentration	Difficulty sleeping							
	Forgetfulness							
	Confusion							
	Difficulty concentrating							
	Clumsiness							
	Accidents, e.g. cutting finger							
	Difficulty making decisions							
Behavioural Changes	Lowered work performance							
	Taking naps, staying in bed							
	Staying at home from work							
	Avoid social activities							
	Loss of efficiency							
Autonomic Reactions	Dizziness or faintness							
	Cold sweats							
	Feeling sick/vomiting							
	Hot flushes							
Water Retention	Weight gain							
	Skin disorders (spots, rash)							
	Painful or swollen breasts							
	Feeling swollen/bloated							
Negative Effect	Crying spells							
	Loneliness							
	Anxiety							
	Restlessness							
	Irritability							
	Mood swings							
	Depression							
	Tension							
Arousal	Feeling affectionate							
	Orderliness							
	Excitement							
	Feelings of well-being							
	Bursts of energy/activity							
Control	Feelings of suffocation							
	Chest pains							
	Ringing in the ears							
	Heart pounding							
	Numbness, tingling							

When symptom assessment charts are analysed after two or three cycles, it is readily apparent whether a woman is suffering from the cyclical symptoms of PMS, or perhaps has some other underlying physical or psychiatric disorder which is present throughout the month.

Management of PMS

Numerous approaches and treatments for PMS have been advocated since Frank first described premenstrual tension over seven decades ago. The fact that so many treatments are available suggests that the majority of them are ineffective, and confirms that researchers are no further forward in understanding the aetiology of PMS or the treatment of the condition. Harrison (1982) says it is the *woman* with PMS who should be treated rather than the PMS itself.

Hallman (1986) estimated that only 7.5% of women with PMS seek the advice of a doctor. This means that the vast majority of women will try many different approaches and self-help remedies in order to obtain relief from their cyclical symptoms.

All women can be helped by simple, straightforward discussion and counselling with advice regarding diet, stress avoidance and their general lifestyle. It is difficult to find an effective drug therapy for mild to moderate symptoms and thus the treatment for this grade of PMS is often unsatisfactory. Paradoxically, women who have severe PMS are easier to treat than those who suffer from mild to moderate PMS. This is because severe symptoms can have such a disruptive effect on women's lives that they are willing to try more active intervention by suppressing the ovarian cycle.

However PMS is managed, it is important to realize that the syndrome demonstrates a *high placebo response rate*. This rate has been reported to be as high as 94% (Magos *et al.*, 1986) although the generally agreed figure is nearer 50%. Some studies have shown that the placebo response has been more marked with psychological rather than physical symptoms but other studies disprove this. Why a placebo response is so high is uncertain – it may be due to the effect of counselling and having the problems validated and taken seriously that symptoms become better tolerated, together with a real desire to improve. Such placebo responses, however, usually disappear within 3 months.

Reports of successful, but uncontrolled, treatments are consequently impossible to interpret and virtually meaningless. Drug trials that make no attempt to compare the effects of placebo should be ignored.

Self-help measures

General advice
The advice listed in Box 15.6 may seem basic but can make a considerable difference when trying to cope with PMS.

Discussion
Discussion about the different symptoms that the woman is experiencing will help you to establish the severity of her problem. You should find out how long her symptoms last, how severe they are and whether they are relieved immediately by menstruation. In an ideal world we should also try to establish the woman's threshold of complaining and tolerance, and the degree of disruption that PMS has on her normal life. In practice, however, it can be very difficult to ascertain these facts.

As a nurse, you are often perceived by your patients as being more approachable than other

---

Box 15.6   General advice for women with PMS

◆ If your main symptom is abdominal bloating then do not try to squeeze into a garment that you usually wear, but try some looser, more comfortable clothes with elasticated waistbands

◆ If breast tenderness is a problem then wear a well-fitting supportive bra

◆ Do not arrange to go out and socialize when you do not feel like it, but stay in and read a book or watch a video

◆ Get a good night's sleep

◆ Some women find that sex is helpful as an orgasm is a powerful way of relieving tension (Masters and Johnson, 1966).

health care professionals. Nurses are also seen as having more time to chat about a problem that might seem 'too trivial to bother the doctor with'. Discussion with an empathetic nurse can be very therapeutic, especially for those women who have found other health professionals not so understanding. If you can give the woman a greater understanding and knowledge about menstruation and PMS it will reduce her anxiety and hopefully lessen her symptoms. Once pre-menstrual problems have been voiced, you should encourage the woman to talk to others who may not have appreciated that there was a problem. These can include colleagues at work, friends, her partner and her family.

A sympathetic ear can be very comforting. Simple reassurance that she is not 'going mad' and that there is 'light at the end of the tunnel' can have an enormous psycho-therapeutic effect. Women frequently report that their worst fear is that they are 'going crazy' and that this fear is not being taken seriously. You should listen carefully to what they have to say, support them as women and confirm that their experiences are real and that other women also experience similar problems.

It can be helpful to find out why the woman is coming forward at this particular moment in time for help and advice. Has she experienced any major changes in her life during the past few months that have tipped the balance, and made symptoms she was normally able to tolerate become unbearable? Such problems can range from relationship difficulties, job changes, stresses with children or ageing parents to financial crises. Being able to talk to someone about them can be very therapeutic and you might well be able to refer the woman to local organizations for help. Some helpful suggestions you could make include:

◆ Belonging to a mother and baby group
◆ Relationship counselling
◆ Joining a local carers' group
◆ Referral to social services to see if extra financial support is available.

These suggestions, although they seem simple, might be all that is needed to tip the balance back again from seemingly unmanageable and distressing problems into tolerable but manageable difficulties.

Dietary changes

There is an abundance of conflicting advice that women are given about how to modify their diet to improve the symptoms of PMS. The best advice that you as a nurse can give to any woman, whether or not she suffers from PMS, is to eat a diet that is low in fat and refined carbohydrates and high in unrefined starchy food. High protein diets are not recommended for women with PMS. (See Chapter 3 for general advice about healthy eating.)

Recommendations that some women have found helpful include those listed in Box 15.7.

Box 15.7   Dietary recommendations to alleviate PMS

◆ *Reduce the intake of salt* Excess salt – whether added during cooking or at the table – can cause fluid retention leading to feelings of bloatedness and mastalgia. Foods with a high salt content should also be restricted, e.g. cheese, preserved meats or fish, salted nuts, etc.
◆ *Reduce fluid intake* This advice is particularly suitable for women whose main symptoms include bloating and mastalgia
◆ *Limit intake of caffeine* Restrict the amount of coffee, tea or cola. Caffeine can increase levels of anxiety and irritability. Many women find decaffeinated coffee or herbal teas are acceptable alternatives. Camomile tea is a great relaxant, peppermint tea helps with nausea and lime blossom tea settles mood swings
◆ *Reduce dietary fat intake*
◆ *Reduce intake of 'junk foods'* Eat as much fresh, unrefined food as possible. Have a varied diet containing a broad spectrum of nutrients
◆ *Eat regularly* It is amazing how many women skip meals or pick at their food at exactly the time of the month when they should be eating regularly and having a well-balanced diet

Continued

Box 15.7 Dietary recommendations to alleviate PMS – Cont'd

◆ *Eat more starch, fibre, vegetables and fruit* Slow-release carbohydrates are the best to eat when you have PMS, and include muesli, oats, granary bread, brown and basmati rice. Some experts consider that starchy foods assist serotonin production

◆ *Do not overeat* Some women have been advised to keep their blood sugar levels up (therefore avoiding the risk of hypoglycaemic-like symptoms of tiredness, irritability and headaches). Consequently they nibble at frequent intervals on sugary snacks and chocolate. This should be avoided as they will only end up fat and premenstrual rather than just premenstrual! If they feel the desire to nibble frequently then fresh fruits and vegetables should be substituted

◆ *Limit intake of alcohol and tobacco* Women often use alcohol or tobacco for short-term relief of mood symptoms but both can lead to long-term problems.

Your patients may find it helpful if you remind them not to expect an instant result from altering their diet. It can often take a few months for the beneficial effects to be felt both on their general health and on their PMS symptoms.

Self-help groups

Unfortunately there are few PMS self-help groups in the UK but advice about starting a local group can be obtained from the organizations and societies listed at the end of this chapter. These societies also supply further advice about suitable books, leaflets and videos. It is important to read these books yourself before recommending them to PMS sufferers as the information might be very biased towards a particular method of treatment and not give a well-balanced overview of PMS.

In general practice it is sometimes more practicable for PMS support groups to be set up and run alongside other clinics and activities that involve women, e.g. family planning clinics and mother and baby clinics, rather than being a separate entity of their own.

Many PMS sufferers have their own small, unofficial self-help groups. Neighbours, friends and colleagues at work can all get together and swap experiences and remedies that they have tried and found to be beneficial (or useless). It is hardly surprising that women get a lot of support and encouragement from others who can empathize with their problems, and it can also reveal a wealth of successful strategies for dealing with PMS.

SCENARIO

Sue, a normally calm mother, found that her main premenstrual problem was that she was becoming increasingly bad tempered and aggressive. She would shout at her children for trivial reasons, stamp around the house and slam doors in her fury. She eventually found an outlet for all this pent-up anger by realizing that if she made bread when she was premenstrual she could knead and pummel the dough very heavily, thereby calming her anger and filling her freezer with bread for the next few weeks!

Exercise and relaxation techniques

Any form of exercise is beneficial for women who have PMS and should be encouraged. It is thought that exercise triggers the production of endorphins, natural opiates, that promote a sense of well-being and self-esteem and may increase a woman's tolerance to premenstrual change, thus reducing the impact that PMS has on her life (Goodale *et al.*, 1990).

Walking, jogging, aerobics, swimming and yoga are all therapeutic and are recommended. Some women find relief from their symptoms by using meditation, breathing exercises and relaxation techniques similar to those used in antenatal classes.

You should advise women who suffer from PMS that they should try to find some time every day in which they can be on their own and free from outside interruptions. In practice, unfortunately, this is often difficult when women are trying to juggle the varied demands of having a busy career with those of being a wife and mother. Reading, watching television, listening to music or even masturbating are all effective ways of relaxing.

Stress management

In general, advice about stress management can seem very simple and basic but it is surprising how few women have actually thought logically about how they can effectively manage their lives in order to help themselves. Many women, if they are able to plan when they are likely to suffer from PMS, can benefit by making minor adjustments to their normal work schedule or family life. Suggestions that you could make might include:

◆ Arrange appropriate childcare to give a 'break'

◆ Avoid having in-laws or guests to stay

◆ Avoid having friends to supper

◆ Postpone driving tests

◆ Do not start a strict new diet

◆ Postpone a starting date for a new job.

Some women (and their families) have found it helpful if days that are likely to be stressful are marked on the family calendar. This means that both partners and children might be able to avoid discussing potentially difficult issues during these few days and hopefully avoid head-on clashes. This form of stress management, whilst being very successful, does unfortunately mean that PMS can effectively dominate the rest of the month as women constantly have to refer to the calendar to check where they are in their menstrual cycle.

Women who have demanding and stressful jobs often find that PMS can have a very debilitating effect on their working relationships and how they are perceived by their colleagues. They may be extremely competent for most of the month, but need only lose their temper once, or walk out of a meeting in tears, and their credibility is immediately diminished. Potentially awkward meetings should be arranged, if possible, for times when a woman is not at her most vulnerable. If this cannot be managed, then advice in relaxation techniques should help the woman cope with the strains and responsibilities of her employment.

Complementary and alternative therapies

Many women have found relief from various alternative or complementary therapies. These can include aromatherapy, reflexology, herbal medicine, hypnotism, homeopathy and acupuncture (see Chapter 4). Although there have been few controlled trials to show the beneficial effects of alternative therapies on PMS, many women have found them extremely useful in reducing stress levels and helping them adapt to the strains of PMS and a busy lifestyle. Most are generally only available privately but some do have sliding scales of fees for those who are unable to afford the full rate. It is useful to compile a list of locally recommended therapists that you could give to any women who might be interested. It might also be helpful to have a price list and a note of who has recommended them.

Domoney *et al.* (2003) in a study of women attending a specialist PMS clinic found that over 90% had used at least one form of complementary therapy to manage their symptoms, but few continue with long-term usage. They concluded by saying that as use is so prevalent, but with few randomized controlled trials to show benefits and risks, it is important to improve awareness, both in qualitative and quantitative terms.

Whilst no specific studies have been carried out, aromatherapy can be helpful in alleviating PMS symptoms by reducing stress. A couple of drops of oil can be used in the bath, in massage oil or for inhalation. The aroma plays a part in affecting mood, whilst the chemicals within the various oils act pharmacologically. You should be aware that essential oils are as powerful as drugs and must be used carefully.

Although there have only been a few scientific studies into acupuncture and how it helps PMS, practitioners report good success rates (Habek *et al.*, 2002).

Herbal therapies

Evening primrose oil (EPO) is a fashionable therapy. It is rich in an oil containing the essential fatty acid gamolenic acid, and has been strongly promoted in recent years as a treatment for PMS. Gamolenic acid is thought to correct a disorder of E_1 prostaglandins which have many complicated functions within the body. Supplements of gamma-linolenic acid are believed to correct the theoretical disorder that exists between E_1 prostaglandins and essential fatty acids.

There are a bewildering number of formulations of EPO available which either combine EPO with marine oils, or with other sources of gamolenic acid such as borage seed oil and star flower oil. All these preparations are expensive and their value is doubtful. There are wide variations between the doses recommended by different manufacturers, ranging from 295 mg to 3000 mg daily.

Mansel et al. (1990) showed that EPO was effective in the treatment of cyclical mastalgia and benign breast disease. Controlled studies using EPO for the general treatment of PMS are lacking and their results are contradictory (Khoo et al., 1990). Little benefit seems to be gained from using EPO and the therapeutic efficacy of it has most likely been overstated. However, EPO certainly does not have any adverse side effects, and women may find it worth trying to see if they have any symptom relief.

St John's wort (Hypericum perforatum), a herbal preparation, has gained popularity over the past few years as an antidepressant. The levels of active ingredients vary from one preparation to another. Following a report regarding the safety of St John's wort (Ernst, 1999), the Committee on Safety of Medicines highlighted there could be interactions of St John's wort with certain prescribed medicines. This is particularly important for women taking the contraceptive pill as its efficacy could be reduced (Committee on Safety of Medicines, 2000).

Vitex agnus castus (derived from the chasteberry tree and rich in plant oestrogens) has been used for many years for the treatment of menstrual problems, and Schellenberg (2001) found it more effective than placebo in treating PMS.

Red clover contains a high proportion of isoflavones which have mild oestrogenic activity. Preliminary studies have shown improvement in some premenstrual symptoms but larger studies are needed to confirm these effects.

Black cohosh has been shown to relieve menopausal and premenstrual symptoms, particularly psychological symptoms, but more studies are needed.

Light therapy

Research has shown promising results in a small study using a form of light therapy known as photic stimulation (Anderson et al., 1997). The treatment involves wearing a mask that covers the eyes for about 15 minutes a day in the second half of the cycle. The mask contains miniature lights which gently flicker in pre-programmed rhythms, and it is suggested that it has an action on circadian rhythms.

Magnetic therapy

A recent small trial with static magnets attached to underwear has shown considerable relief from pelvic pain and dysmenorrhoea (Brown et al., 2002). Some women also experienced an improvement in their PMS symptoms with magnetic therapy. It is thought that this improvement is due to the effect of the magnet improving circulation in the pelvic area, which re-oxygenates the blood, enabling the uterine muscles to work more effectively. Larger clinical trials are underway, including one studying magnet therapy and endometriosis.

Nutritional supplements and non-hormonal drugs

In addition to the above measures, many women will try preparations that are readily available at chemists and health food shops. As a nurse, you might often find that you are consulted first for advice on any 'over-the-counter' remedies that might help. The woman may not be visiting you ostensibly to discuss her PMS but will often ask for advice following a cervical smear or a contraceptive check.

You should remember that, as mentioned previously, any medication has a high placebo response and that if you can 'add in' some counselling as well, then your patient may feel much better. Any improvement in symptoms, even if it is only a placebo response from non-prescription therapies, should be valued. The woman should be encouraged to continue with her treatment no matter how illogical the therapy seems, as it certainly will not be causing her any harm, unlike the side effects that may occur from wrongly prescribed drugs for PMS.

Our knowledge about the effectiveness of many of these supplements is limited and larger placebo-controlled trials are needed.

Pyridoxine (vitamin B₆)

Pyridoxine is an important co-factor in the synthesis of neurotransmitters serotonin and dopamine and is easily available from chemists and health food shops. It appears to be the most widely used self-prescribed medication with up to 92% of women with PMS having tried it (Leather et al., 1993).

Trials of pyridoxine therapy have shown conflicting results. A systematic review of published and unpublished randomized placebo-controlled trials of vitamin B₆ in the management of PMS suggested that doses up to 100 mg a day are likely to be of benefit (Wyatt et al., 1999).

Women with PMS often self-medicate with vitamin B₆ in high doses. Concern was raised (Dalton and Dalton, 1987) that in high doses B₆ produced symptoms of neurotoxic syndrome. On reviewing their evidence the government's Committee on Toxicity restricted health food shops to selling tablets of 10 mg per day. Doses between that and 50 mg daily are restricted to sale at pharmacies, and 50 mg and above are available only on prescription. These restrictions were met with astonishment by many groups, who have been actively lobbying for them to be withdrawn.

Multivitamin and mineral supplements

The best advice is for women to have a healthy, well-balanced diet with plenty of fresh food as discussed earlier (see also Chapter 3). However, many women will supplement their dietary intake by taking extra nutritional treatments which are widely advertised and marketed as helpful in the treatment of PMS.

Many types and varieties of multivitamin and mineral supplements are available at chemists and health food shops. They differ enormously both in content and in price. The cheapest are of little use as they contain only small amounts of nutrients, whilst the most costly contain ingredients of doubtful relevance and can be prohibitively expensive at the recommended dosage. Walker et al. (1998) investigated the daily supplement of magnesium and concluded that a dose of 200 mg daily reduced mild premenstrual symptoms of fluid retention.

General advice that can be given is that extra vitamins and mineral preparations taken in moderation will not cause any harm. As they might have a placebo effect it may well be worth trying them for a three-month period to see if PMS symptoms improve.

Medical treatments

All the means of managing PMS symptoms that have so far been described are methods that the PMS sufferer can use and try on her own, or buy at a chemist or health food shop without a prescription. Women have usually investigated and tried many of these different treatment approaches and remedies to see if they can help their symptoms. If symptoms show no significant improvement then they may well consult a health care professional for advice and help.

Nurses are well placed in the medical setting to talk to the woman before she sees the doctor and can often offer valuable advice and support. Confirmation of the validity of her experiences and an understanding attitude will often be a great relief in itself.

Unfortunately, some doctors only have a passing interest in PMS and are not able to give the support and help that is needed. They may be unsympathetic towards PMS sufferers and show little sensitivity in dealing with their problems. 'It is something women have to live with' and 'pull yourself together' are comments that sufferers hear all too frequently. The message should be conveyed to the woman that PMS has a physical basis related to her hormones, that she is not going mad and that effective treatments are available. Treatments have to take account of the needs and requirements of the individual woman, which differ according to her age, wishes for future pregnancy, the severity of her symptoms and her menstrual pattern.

Diuretics

Many women experience bloating and a feeling of weight gain, although, as mentioned earlier, very few have a demonstrable weight increase. The use of diuretics should be reserved for those who have an appreciable weight increase during the luteal phase of their cycle. If diuretics are prescribed then they should be taken on alternate days, although women then tend to increase the dosage and frequency if they get no immediate relief from their symptoms.

Care is needed in the prescribing of diuretics as electrolyte imbalances can occur if the course is extended, and continuous use can exacerbate fluid retention, consequently worsening the condition that it was meant to improve. This can be prevented to some extent by the use of an aldosterone agonist such as spironolactone. Wang *et al.* (1995) used 100 mg spironolactone in a double-blind, placebo-controlled, crossover study which showed beneficial effects over placebo on negative mood changes and somatic symptoms.

Prostaglandin inhibitors

Prostaglandin levels fluctuate throughout the cycle in response to the changing levels of oestradiol and progesterone. Prostaglandin inhibitors have many effects on the central nervous system, including sedative and analgesic properties, and they also reduce menorrhagia. In PMS where generalized aches and pains, headaches and fatigue are reported then mefenamic acid (250–500 mg three times a day) has been found to be more beneficial than placebo in a double-blind crossover study (Mira *et al.*, 1986).

If a woman suffers from premenstrual migraine, pelvic pain, dysmenorrhoea and menorrhagia then prostaglandin inhibitors may well be worth considering. Treatment should start from about day 16 of the cycle, and you should advise the woman that gastrointestinal side effects can be reduced if the drug is taken with food.

Antidepressants

Rapkin *et al.* (1987) demonstrated that women suffering from PMS have lower levels of serotonin than the control group in the luteal phase of the menstrual cycle. The use of SSRIs would therefore make a rational approach to the management of the many women who have coexisting PMS and an underlying depressive illness. A meta-analysis by Dimmock *et al.* (2000) of all published clinical trials of SSRIs in the treatment of PMS showed that fluoxetine was effective in treating physical and behavioural symptoms. Fluoxetine is usually prescribed for daily use, although some studies have shown benefit when an SSRI is used only during the luteal phase of the cycle (Freeman *et al.*, 1999).

Some women are reluctant to be treated with an antidepressant for what they consider to be a gynaecological problem, but intermittent dosing of fluoxetine during the luteal phase may overcome this reluctance.

Fluoxetine was the only product in the UK licensed to treat PMDD, a severe form of PMS, but this licence was withdrawn at the end of 2003 when the pharmaceutical company developed a Summary of Product Characteristics (SPC) that was adopted by all European member states. Their reasoning was that PMDD is not a well-established disease in Europe and that it is purely a research diagnosis by the American Psychiatric Association with a number of complicated diagnostic criteria. This does not mean that doctors cannot continue to prescribe SSRIs for PMS, particularly as there is a large body of evidence of the clinical benefits, but they will need to explain to the woman why it is an appropriate treatment for her condition.

Bromocriptine

Bromocriptine inhibits the release of prolactin and is useful in treating mastalgia, but it has no effect on general PMS. It is a powerful drug and many women experience unpleasant side effects and it is therefore no longer widely used.

Progestogens and progesterone

Despite no scientific evidence that progesterone deficiency is a cause of PMS, progestogens and progesterone continue to be among the most commonly used first-line treatments prescribed by doctors. This method of treatment has been strongly advocated and enthusiastically promoted by Dalton (1984). However, her views on the treatment of PMS with progesterone must be considered controversial and are unsubstantiated by controlled trials.

As this method of treatment has been widely written about in women's magazines, many PMS sufferers will request progesterone treatment. This is usually given as Cyclogest® suppositories or dydrogesterone, which is structurally similar to natural progesterone. There is no evidence of a lack of progesterone during the luteal phase, and Wyatt et al. (2001) in a meta-analysis of 14 trials of progestogen or progesterone therapy concluded that there was no convincing evidence for their use in the management of PMS.

Research into hormone replacement therapy (HRT) at the menopause has shown that cyclical progestogen (norethisterone 5 mg), given to prevent endometrial hyperplasia, causes symptoms that are very similar to those of PMS (Magos et al., 1986), so it seems even more bizarre that women with PMS are given treatment that can worsen an existing condition which they were trying to avoid!

If progesterone has any place in PMS it is one of causation rather than therapy.

Suppression of the ovarian cycle

The most successful treatments for severe premenstrual symptoms are those that suppress ovulation and ablate the cyclical biochemical changes that cause PMS.

All methods that suppress the ovarian cycle need to be used in conjunction with sympathetic counselling and a supportive medical team. Discussion needs to be centred around future pregnancy plans as all these treatments will affect fertility in the short term.

Pregnancy itself will effectively treat PMS but this may not be a convenient or appropriate solution. Women should be advised that pregnancy is an option and will certainly 'cure' their PMS in the short term, but that symptoms will most likely return after delivery. Many women may then decide to 'speed up' their pregnancies and then seek effective treatment once their family is complete.

The following medical treatments all act by suppressing ovulation and are reversible.

Combined oral contraceptive pill

The combined oral contraceptive pill would seem to be the ideal treatment for PMS as it effectively suppresses ovulation and also gives contraceptive cover. Endocrine cyclicity remains, however, as hormones are only given for three weeks out of four, or in fluctuating doses with the biphasic and triphasic pills.

Surprisingly there have been few conclusive placebo-controlled studies to assess the effect of the combined oral contraceptive pill on premenstrual symptoms, and those studies that have been done show conflicting results. Moos in 1969 showed that the pill reduced the incidence and severity of premenstrual complaints, especially psychological symptoms, whilst Walker and Bancroft (1990) showed that the response is generally unpredictable.

The pill though is a suitable first-line option for a large percentage of women, particularly those who also require effective contraception. Women will experience the additional benefits of reduced dysmenorrhoea and menorrhagia. A multicentred study into a new contraceptive pill, Yasmin, containing the progestogen drospirenone (a derivative of spironolactone), showed benefits to general well-being and to fluid-related symptoms associated with the menstrual cycle (Parsey and Pong, 2000; Apter et al., 2003). Borenstein et al. (2003) using the same pill and charting symptoms with the Moos Menstrual Distress Questionnaire showed a significant reduction in premenstrual symptomatology.

Symptoms may reappear during the pill-free week and, if this is the case, it may be more logical to take the combined pill continuously for 3 months without any break between packets, followed by a 7-day break (tricycle regime). This will reduce the number of pill-free intervals and withdrawal bleeds with their associated symptoms per annum, but there is a small incidence of breakthrough bleeding, particularly in the first cycle.

Anna, a 19-year-old student, needed contraception. Whilst taking a full history Anna mentioned to the nurse that she always felt moody and irritable for 4 or 5 days before her period, but had learned to cope with this so long as it did not occur just before exams. She started on the combined oral contraceptive pill but returned 3 months later complaining of general moodiness and depression throughout the cycle which worsened during the pill-free week. Anna was given a pill with a different progestogen which certainly improved her generalized depression, but symptoms definitely returned when she did not take the pill for a week. It was decided to see if Anna would be symptom free if she avoided the pill-free week by taking three packets without a break.

Anna returned at her next follow-up visit feeling pleased as she was having no cyclical symptoms and also had the added benefit of fewer episodes of bleeding.

The symptoms of a significant number of women appear to get worse whilst they are on the pill. This is thought to be due to the side effects of the progestogen element of the contraceptive pill (Cullberg, 1972). It is well worth changing to a different pill with a different progestogen content to see if this might help. Any change of pill should be tried for a minimum of 3 months before any conclusion can be made about the benefits or otherwise.

The exact role and the effect of the combined oral contraceptive pill in the treatment of PMS are unresolved. There is a great need for proper prospective randomized placebo-controlled studies to look at this area and, in particular, the use of tricyclic regimes needs to be fully evaluated.

The progestogen-only pill and depot progestogens for contraception have not been carefully evaluated regarding PMS. Again, some women have reported a relief of symptoms, but others say their problems get much worse.

Danazol

Danazol is a synthetic steroid which has multiple effects on the pituitary–ovarian axis. Given continuously and in high doses (400 mg daily) danazol will suppress ovulation and menstruation. It has been shown to be beneficial for those women with severe mastalgia and other PMS symptoms (Halbreich *et al.*, 1991). However, many women discontinue treatment at these doses as they experience androgenic side-effects which they find unacceptable, e.g. acne, hirsutism, bloating and weight gain (Watts *et al.*, 1987).

Danazol has been shown to be effective at reducing symptoms in some women at lower doses (Deeny *et al.*, 1991), thus avoiding the masculinizing side effects. O'Brien and Abukhalil (1999) showed that danazol 200 mg daily given in the luteal phase of the menstrual cycle was effective in relieving premenstrual mastalgia but had no effect on the general symptoms of PMS.

Given over a long term, danazol has a detrimental effect on lipids and regular monitoring needs to take place. It should not be given for more than 6 months.

Gonadotrophin-releasing hormone analogues

At high continuous doses, gonadotrophin-releasing hormone (GnRH) analogues suppress ovarian function completely, thereby causing a 'medical oophorectomy' and complete absence of cyclical and premenstrual symptoms. These drugs, widely used in the treatment of endometriosis, are usually given as subcutaneous or intramuscular injections. They are also available as nasal sprays but these give less precise suppression of the ovarian cycle and symptoms may recur intermittently.

GnRH analogues have been shown to be more effective than placebo (Muse *et al.*, 1984) but the consequences of causing a medical oophorectomy limit their use to only 6 months. Long-term treatment cannot be justified because of the risks of osteoporosis associated with low oestradiol levels. Women tolerate the menopausal symptoms of hot flushes and night sweats if adequately counselled before therapy starts and in fact will often prefer these new symptoms to the cyclical tyranny of PMS.

Studies have been made to see if the skeleton can be protected by supplementing the treatment of GnRH analogues with conventional low-dose

HRT ('add-back' therapy). The progestogens in such therapy may cause symptoms to recur to a degree in some women but others experience relief (Leather *et al.*, 1999). Bone loss and menopausal symptoms may also be prevented with the use of 'add-back' tibolone (Livial) (Rymer *et al.*, 1998).

The use of GnRH analogues, even in the short term, is beneficial in a number of cases as it can convince the woman, her family and her colleagues at work that her symptoms are in fact caused by her ovarian cycle and not by an underlying personality or psychiatric disorder. They are also useful in testing the potential value of performing a bilateral oophorectomy in women undergoing a hysterectomy (O'Brien and Chenoy, 1995).

SCENARIO

Margaret, a solicitor in her early thirties, had been in a stable relationship with Tony for over 4 years. The relationship had come under increasing strain when the responsibilities of Margaret's job took her overseas for short periods. Margaret had always complained of PMS and had some insight into the problem, but normally kept her symptoms at a manageable level using stress avoidance, exercise and relaxation techniques. She also took vitamin B_6, although she admitted that this most likely gave little benefit. The problems between Margaret and Tony increased over 6 months with Margaret becoming increasingly depressed, irritable and aggressive in the 10 days before her period. Tony thought that Margaret was 'going mad' and threatened that unless she received psychiatric help urgently he would leave her as he felt completely unable to cope with her moods.

Fortunately Margaret's doctor referred her to a specialist clinic where she was initially treated with GnRH analogues. Margaret and Tony began to notice a distinct improvement in her depression and mood swings, in spite of experiencing menopausal symptoms of hot flushes and night sweats. Their relationship began to return to an even keel, despite the increasing pressures of Margaret's work. This 6-month trial of treatment with GnRH analogues was enough to convince both Tony and Margaret that her problems were related to her menstrual cycle and that she certainly did not have an underlying psychiatric problem.

Oestrogen therapy

Cronje *et al.* (2003) suggest that the oestrogens that are widely used in HRT are the most important hormone for the treatment of severe PMS (see also Chapter 16). This oestrogen therapy needs to be in the form of subcutaneous implants or transdermal patches as oral HRT will not sufficiently suppress the ovarian cycle and thus symptoms may remain.

Oestradiol implants and patches contain natural rather than synthetic oestrogens and their route of administration avoids the liver. They can safely be given to women regardless of blood pressure, weight or smoking habits as they do not have the same restrictions that apply to the contraceptive pill.

The use of these highly effective percutaneous oestrogen treatments for PMS is made more complicated in women with a uterus by the need to take a cyclical progestogen. This is important in order to prevent endometrial hyperplasia (Sturdee *et al.*, 1978) but it does mean that some women develop mild PMS-like symptoms during this phase of treatment. These symptoms are usually less severe and less prolonged than their previous symptoms but if persistently troublesome the dose and duration of the progestogen may be reduced, or a different progestogen can be tried. The levonorgestrel intrauterine system (IUS) is another way of minimizing progestogenic side effects, thereby maximizing the treatment benefits of oestrogen (Panay and Studd, 1998). Women should be advised that if they do experience side effects, they are due to the progestogen element of the treatment and are not symptoms of untreated PMS.

Oestradiol implants

The ovarian cycle can be suppressed by subcutaneous implants of oestradiol (Greenblatt *et al.*, 1977) and the benefit of this in treating PMS sufferers was demonstrated in a placebo-controlled study (Magos *et al.*, 1986). This study showed a superior response of active treatment against placebo for all of the Moos symptom clusters in the Menstrual Distress Questionnaire despite an initial placebo response of 94%.

Implants (100 mg decreasing to 75 mg and then to 50 mg as symptoms are controlled) are given at 6-monthly intervals and many women find this method of administration convenient and cosmetically more pleasing than wearing oestradiol patches. Testosterone 100 mg can be added if there are problems of loss of libido, loss of energy and profound depression. As this is often the case with PMS sufferers, combined oestradiol and testosterone implants are often the best initial treatment.

This therapy is usually well liked and tolerated by women, but it does require a degree of

SCENARIO

Claire, a 38-year-old divorced mother, had suffered from PMS for most of her life. Her symptoms got progressively worse after the birth of her two daughters. Initially she put this deterioration down to the stresses of coping with two boisterous and demanding children, and the added financial anxieties of her husband's business. Claire's main problem was of aggression and violent mood swings – she even once threw the television out of the window during an argument over which programme to watch.

The marriage eventually ended and Claire hoped that her PMS might improve as one stressful area in her life had gone. However, the duration of her PMS symptoms gradually increased despite the fact that she had modified her diet, did regular exercise and had tried most 'over-the-counter' remedies. She eventually sought the advice of her doctor after she became violent towards her youngest daughter. The strength of her anger and aggression had really frightened Claire and had persuaded her that she urgently needed help.

Her doctor referred her to a gynaecologist with a particular interest in PMS who decided after discussion with Claire that she would benefit from an oestradiol implant. The improvement was dramatic – her family and friends could not believe the transformation that took place over the next few months – no more mood swings and anger. Claire returned for a repeat implant every 6 months for 2 years but then did not attend for a further 10 months. On enquiry it transpired that Claire had felt so well and 'in control' of herself that she thought she no longer needed oestrogen therapy and could discontinue treatment. Unfortunately her symptoms were beginning to reappear as her ovarian cycle was not sufficiently suppressed and her new partner persuaded Claire to return for treatment.

commitment because of the prolonged duration of action of the implants and the consequent need to continue with cyclical progestogens to prevent endometrial hyperplasia. This prolonged action may last for approximately 2 years after the last implant and makes implant treatment unsuitable for women who may be planning a pregnancy in the foreseeable future. It is ideal for women who have completed their families and for those who have worsening PMS symptoms as they approach the menopause.

Oestradiol patches

Oestradiol patches provide an attractive alternative to implants. High doses are needed initially (100–200 µg) – which is a much higher dose than that used for the menopause.

Studies have shown that patches are more effective than placebo in relieving psychological, behavioural and physical symptoms of PMS by more than 50% (Watson *et al.*, 1989). Treatment should be started on the first day of a period and a progestogen such as norethisterone or medroxy-progesterone acetate should be taken from days 17 to 26 of the cycle for endometrial protection.

Some women experience transient breast tenderness and nausea when starting treatment but you should encourage them to continue with the patches as these symptoms will normally resolve by the second or third month. Oestrogen patches can have adhesion problems and may cause skin reactions in some women – you can give simple advice regarding rotation of the patch site. If problems are encountered with the progestogen phase of the treatment then it is always possible to alter the type of progestogen, the dosage or the duration or to try the intra-uterine system (Panay and Studd 1998).

It is clear that oestrogen therapy either as an implant or as patches is the only convincingly effective pharmacological treatment for severe PMS that is well tolerated by women and should be the first-line therapy for severe PMS.

Surgery

The ultimate, if drastic, solution – as for so many gynaecological problems – may be hysterectomy and bilateral salpingo-oophorectomy followed by straightforward HRT. This HRT can be with oestrogen alone, as progestogen need not be added as endometrial protection would not be required. The ovaries must be removed at surgery in order to alleviate PMS symptoms, otherwise the ovarian cycle remains and will continue to give rise to cyclical problems.

Although total abdominal hysterectomy with bilateral oophorectomy is curative (Casson *et al.*, 1990), it should be reserved for those women who have severe PMS, or whose PMS is compounded by menstrual and gynaecological problems.

Leather *et al.* (1993) showed that nearly 40% of women whose families were complete were prepared to consider such major surgery in order to be relieved of their cyclical symptoms. That such a substantial number of women are prepared to consider major surgery in an attempt to be free of the stresses of PMS confirms the inadequacies of current treatment options and the extent to which severe PMS can destroy women's professional and domestic lives.

A summary of different treatment approaches is shown in Figure 15.2.

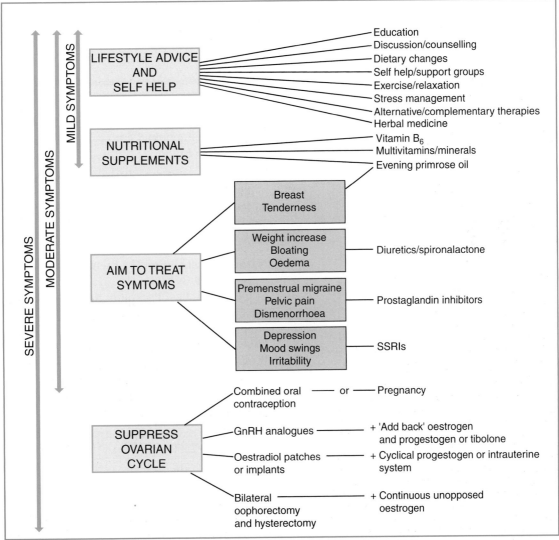

Figure 15.2 Summary of treatment approaches to PMS.

Conclusion

PMS can affect up to 90% of women and includes a wide range of physical and emotional changes. The broad range of symptoms can vary from cycle to cycle in their severity, duration and their effect on women's lives. PMS unfortunately is not a straightforward problem as there is no recognized cause, and there is a wide range of management approaches and conflicting treatment options. It is important when women first seek help and advice that they are able to discuss their problems with a sympathetic nurse who will be able to listen, counsel and support them through a variety of self-help approaches.

In severely affected women who have not been helped with these therapies then cycle suppression may be considered a suitable option. Women can also be referred to a small number of specialist PMS clinics which may be run by gynaecologists who have an interest in PMS and menopausal problems.

Ideas for personal and professional development

- Contact the support agencies listed below and review the information and advice they offer

- Compile a list of local support networks, complementary therapists, etc., so that you can pass the details to sufferers

- Contact your local menopause clinic and enquire whether they see women with severe PMS. If they do, try and arrange a visit

- Think of a woman who has consulted you recently with PMS. Reflect on this consultation. Did you listen to all that she was trying to tell you and were you able to offer any helpful advice? Remember listening can be very therapeutic

- Consider writing a leaflet for PMS sufferers giving general advice about diet, stress relief, etc. Mention local support agencies and helplines.

Patient education points

- Encourage your patients who think they might have PMS to keep a diary and chart their symptoms in relation to their periods

- Reassure women that they are not 'going mad', and their symptoms are real and should resolve as soon as their period starts

- Try and eat a healthy well-balanced diet

- Exercise is an excellent form of stress relief and promotes general well-being

- Any new therapy should be tried for at least three months before being dismissed as of no benefit.

Resources

Light Therapy Centre
A member of the Dezac Group, 54–56 Bath Road, Cheltenham, Glos GL53 7HG
Tel: 0870 516 8143

Magno-Pulse Ltd (suppliers of LadyCare magnets)
24 Emery Road, Brislington, Bristol BS4 5PF
Tel: 0117 972 8883
www.ladycarehealth.com

National Association for Premenstrual Syndrome (NAPS)
41 Old Road, East Peckham, Kent TN12 5AP
Tel: 0870 7772178
Helpline: 0870 7772177
www.pms.org.uk
Provides information and support to PMS sufferers and provides literature and study days for professionals.

PREMSOC (Premenstrual Society)
PO Box 429, Addlestone, Surrey KT15 1DZ
Tel. 01932 872560

Women's Health
52 Featherstone Street, London EC1Y 8RT
Tel: 020 7251 6333
www.womenshealthlondon.org.uk

Women's Nutritional Advisory Service

PO Box 268, Lewes, East Sussex BN7 2QN
Tel: 01273 487366
www.wnas.org.uk

Further reading

GLENVILLE, M. (2002) *Natural Solutions to PMS*. London: Piatkus.
HAYMAN, S. (1996) *PMS: The Complete Guide to Treatment Options*. London, Piatkus.
O'BRIEN, P.M.S. (1987) *Premenstrual Syndrome*. Oxford: Blackwell Scientific.
STEWART, M. (1997) *No more PMS*. London: Vermilion.
WESTCOTT, P. (2004) *Food Solutions: Premenstrual Syndrome: Recipes and Advice to Control Symptoms*. London: Hamlyn.

References

ABRAHAM, G.E. (1980) Premenstrual tension. *Current Problems in Obstetrics and Gynecology* **3**:1–48.
ANDERSON, D.J., LEGG, N.J. and RIDOUT, D.A. (1997) Preliminary trial of photic stimulation for premenstrual syndrome. *Journal of Obstetrics and Gynaecology* **17**(1):76–9.
APTER, D., BORSOS, O., BAUMGARTNER, W., MELIS, G.-B., VEXIAU-ROBERT, D., COLLIGS-HAKERT, A., PALMER, M. and KELLY, S. (2003). Effect of an oral contraceptive containing drospirenone and ethinylestradiol on general well-being and fluid-related symptoms. *European Journal of Contraception and Reproductive Health* **8**:37–51.
BACKSTROM, T. and CARSTENSEN, H. (1974) Estrogen and progesterone in plasma in relation to premenstrual tension. *Journal of Steroid Biochemistry* **5**:257–60.
BACKSTROM, T., BOYLE, H. and BAIRD, D.T. (1981) Persistence of symptoms of premenstrual tension in hysterectomised women. *British Journal of Obstetrics and Gynaecology* **88**:530–6.
BORENSTEIN, J., YU, H.T., WADE, S., CHIOU, C.F., and RAPKIN, A. (2003). Effect of an oral contraceptive containing ethinyl estradiol and drospirenone on premenstrual symptomatology and health-related quality of life. *Journal of Reproductive Medicine* **48**(2):79–85.
BROWN, C.S., LING, F.W., WAN, J.Y., and PILLA, A.A. (2002). Efficacy of static magnetic field therapy in chronic pelvic pain: a double-blind pilot study. *American Journal of Obstetrics and Gynaecology* **187**(6):1581–7.
CASSON, P., HAHN, P., VAN VUGT, D.A. and REID, R.L. (1990) Lasting response to ovariectomy in severe intractable premenstrual syndrome. *American Journal of Obstetrics and Gynaecology* **162**:99–105.
CHADWICK, J. and MANN, W.N. (1950) *The Medical Works of Hippocrates*. Oxford: Blackwell.
CLARE, A.W. (1983) Psychiatric and social aspects of premenstrual complaint. *Psychological Medicine Monograph Supplement* **4**:1–58.

COMMITTEE ON SAFETY OF MEDICINES (2000) *Important Interactions Between St John's Wort (Hypericum perforatum) Preparations and Prescribed Medicines*. London: Medicines Control Agency.
CRONJE, W., HAWKINS, A. and STUDD, J.W.W. (2003) Premenstrual syndrome. In Studd, J.W.W. (ed) *Progress in Obstetrics and Gynaecology*, vol. 15. Edinburgh: Churchill Livingstone.
CULLBERG, J. (1972) Mood changes and menstrual symptoms with different gestagen/estrogen combinations: a double-blind comparison with placebo. *Acta Psychiatrica Scandinavica (Suppl.)* **236**:1–86.
DALTON, K. (1961) Menstruation and crime. *British Medical Journal* **2**:1752.
DALTON, K. (1984) *Premenstrual Syndrome and Progesterone Therapy*, 2nd edn. London: William Heinemann Medical Books.
DALTON, K. and DALTON, M.J.T. (1987) Characteristics of pyridoxine overdose neuropathy syndrome. *Acta Neurologica Scandinavica* **76**:8–11.
DEENY, M., HAWTHORN, R. and McKAY HART, D. (1991) Low dose danazol treatment of the premenstrual syndrome. *Postgraduate Medical Journal* **67**:450–4.
DIMMOCK, P. W., WAYTT, K.M., JONES, P.W. and O'BRIEN, P.M.S. (2000) Efficacy of selective serotonin-reuptake inhibitors in premenstrual syndrome: a systematic review. *Lancet*. **356**:1131–6.
DOMONEY, C., VASHIST, A. and STUDD, J.W. (2003) Use of complementary therapies by women attending a specialist premenstrual syndrome clinic. *Gynaecological Endocrinology*. **17**(1):13–18.
EINON, D. (1997) Is PMS a reason to behave badly or just an excuse? *Options* December:79–81.
ERNST, E. (1999) Second thoughts about safety of St John's wort. *Lancet* **354**:2014–16.
FARATIAN, B., GASPAR, A., O'BRIEN, P.M.S., JOHNSON, I.R., FILSHIE, G.M. and PRESCOT, P. (1984) Premenstrual syndrome: weight, abdominal swelling, and perceived body image. *American Journal of Obstetric Gynaecology* **150**:200–4.
FRANK, R.T. (1931) The hormonal causes of premenstrual tension. *Archives of Neurology and Psychiatry* **26**:1053–7.
FREEMAN, E.W., RICKELS, K., ARREDONDO, F., KAO, L.C., POLLACK, S.E. and SONDHEIMER, S.J. (1999) Full-or half-cycle treatment of severe premenstrual syndrome with a serotonergic antidepressant. *Journal of Clinical Psychopharmacology* **19**(1):3–8.
GLASS, G.S., HENINGER, G.R., LANSKY, M. and TALAN, K. (1971) Psychiatric emergency related to the menstrual cycle. *American Journal of Psychiatry* **128**:705.
GOODALE, I.L., DOMAR, A.D. and BENSON, H. (1990) Alleviation of premenstrual syndrome symptoms with the relaxation response. *Obstetrics and Gynaecology* **75**:649–55.
GREENBLATT, R.B., ASCH, R.H., MAHESH, V.B. and BRIGNER, J.R. (1977) Implantation of pure crystalline pellets of estradiol for conception control. *American Journal of Obstetrics and Gynecology* **127**:520–4.
GREENE, R. and DALTON, K. (1953) The premenstrual syndrome. *British Medical Journal* **1**:1007–14.
GUICHENEY, P., LEGER, D., BARRAT, J. *et al.* (1988) Platelet serotonin content and plasma tryptophan in peri- and

postmenopausal women: variations with plasma oestrogen levels and depressive symptoms. *European Journal of Clinical Investigation* **18**:297–304.

HABEK, D., HABEK, J.C. and BARBIR, A. (2002). Using acupuncture to treat premenstrual syndrome. *Archives of Gynecology and Obstetrics* **267**(1):23–6.

HALBREICH, U., ENDICOTT, J. and NEE, J. (1983) Premenstrual depressive changes. Value of differentiation. *Archives of General Psychiatry* **40**:535–42.

HALBREICH, U., ROJANSKY, N. and PALTER, S. (1991) Elimination of ovulation and menstrual cyclicity (with danazol) improves dysphoric premenstrual syndrome. *Fertility and Sterility* **56**:1066.

HALLMAN, J. (1986) The premenstrual syndrome – an equivalent of depression? *Acta Psychiatrica Scandinavica* **73**:403–11.

HARRISON, M. (1982) *Self-help for Premenstrual Syndrome*, revised edn. New York: Random House.

KHOO, S.K., MUNRO, C. and BATTISTUTTA, D. (1990) Evening primrose oil and treatment of premenstrual syndrome. *Medical Journal of Australia* **153**:189–92.

LAWS, S. (1985) Who needs PMT? A feminist approach to the politics of premenstrual tension. In Law, S., Hey, V. and Eagan, A. (eds) *Seeing Red. The Politics of Premenstrual Tension*. London: Hutchinson, pp. 16–64.

LEATHER, A.T., HOLLAND, E.F.N., ANDREWS, G.D. and STUDD, J.W.W. (1993) A study of the referral patterns and therapeutic experiences of 100 women attending a specialist premenstrual syndrome clinic. *Journal of the Royal Society of Medicine* **86**(4):199–201.

LEATHER, A.T., STUDD, J.W.W., WATSON, N.R. and HOLLAND, E.F.N. (1999) The treatment of severe premenstrual syndrome with goserilin with and without 'add-back' estrogen therapy: a placebo-controlled study. *Gynaecological Endocrinology* **13**:48–55.

LOGUE, C.M. and MOOS, R.H. (1988) Positive perimenstrual changes: towards a new perspective on the menstrual cycle. *Journal of Psychosomatic Research* **32**:31–40.

MAGOS, A.L. and STUDD, J.W.W. (1984) The premenstrual syndrome. In Studd, J.W.W. (ed.) *Progress in Obstetrics and Gynaecology*, vol. 4. Edinburgh: Churchill Livingstone.

MAGOS, A.L. and STUDD, J.W.W. (1985) Effects of the menstrual cycle on medical disorders. *British Journal of Hospital Medicine* **33**:68–77.

MAGOS, A., BRINCAT, M. and STUDD, J.W.W. (1986) Treatment of the premenstrual syndrome by subcutaneous oestradiol implants and cyclical norethisterone; placebo-controlled study. *British Medical Journal* **292**:1629–33.

MANSEL, R.E., PYE, J.K. and HUGHES, L.E. (1990) Effects of essential fatty acids on cyclical mastalgia and non-cyclical breast disorders. In Horobin, D.F. (ed.) *Omega-6 Essential Fatty Acids. Pathophysiology and Roles in Clinical Medicine*. New York: Wiley-Liss, pp. 557–66.

MASTERS, W.H. and JOHNSON, V.E. (1966) *Human Sexual Response*. Boston, MA: Little, Brown.

MENKES, D.B. TAGHAVI, E., MASON, P.A., SPEARS, G.F.S. and HOWARD, R.C. (1992) Fluoxetine treatment of severe premenstrual syndrome. *British Medical Journal* **305**:346–7.

MIRA, M., McNEIL, D., FRASER, I.S., VIZZARD, J. and ABRAHAM, S. (1986) Mefenamic acid in the treatment of premenstrual syndrome. *Obstetrics and Gynaecology* **68**:395–8.

MOOS, R.H. (1968) The development of a menstrual distress questionnaire. *Psychosomatic Medicine* **30**:853–67.

MOOS, R.H. (1969) Typology of menstrual cycle symptoms. *American Journal of Obstetrics and Gynecology* **103**:390–402.

MUSE, K.N., CETEL, N.S., FUTTERMAN, L.A. and YEN, S.C. (1984) The premenstrual syndrome effects of medical ovariectomy. *New England Journal of Medicine* **311**:1345–9.

O'BRIEN, P.M.S. (1987) *Premenstrual Syndrome*. Oxford: Blackwell Scientific.

O'BRIEN, P.M.S. and ABUKHALIL, I.E. (1999) Randomized controlled trial of the management of premenstrual syndrome and premenstrual mastalgia using luteal phase-only danazol. *American Journal of Obstetrics and Gynecology* **180**(1):18–23.

O'BRIEN, P.M.S. and CHENOY, R. (1995) Premenstrual syndrome. *The Diplomate* **2**(2):87–94.

O'BRIEN, P.M.S., SELBY, C. and SYMONDS, E.M. (1980) Progesterone, fluid and electrolytes in premenstrual syndrome. *British Medical Journal* **ii**:1161–3.

PANAY, N. and STUDD, J.W.W. (1998) Non-contraceptive uses of the hormone releasing intrauterine systems. In Studd, J.W.W. (ed.) *Progress in Obstetrics and Gynaecology*, vol. 13. Edinburgh: Churchill Livingstone, Chapter 25, p. 387.

PARSEY, K.S. and PONG, A. (2000). An open-label, multi-center study to evaluate Yasmin, a low-dose combination oral contraceptive containing drospirenone, a new progestogen. *Contraception* **61**(2):105–11.

RAPKIN, A.J., EDELMUTH, E., CHANG, L.C. *et al.* (1987) Whole-blood serotonin in premenstrual syndrome. *Obstetrics and Gynaecology* **70**:533–7.

REID, R.L. (1991) Premenstrual syndrome. *Current Problems in Obstetrics and Gynecology and Fertility* **8**:1–57.

REID, R.L. and YEN, S.S.C. (1981) Premenstrual syndrome. *American Journal of Obstetrics and Gynecology* **139**:85–104.

RYMER, J.M., MORRIS, E.P. and FOGELAMN, I. (1998) Gonadotrophin-releasing hormone analogues and addback therapy in current gynaecological practice. In Studd, J.W.W. (ed.) *Progress in Obstetrics and Gynaecology*, vol. 13. Edinburgh: Churchill Livingstone, Chapter 23, p. 353.

SAMPSON, G.A. (1989) Premenstrual syndrome. *Baillière's Clinical Obstetrics and Gynaecology* **3**:687–704.

SCHELLENBERG, R. (2001) Treatment for the premenstrual syndrome with agnus castus fruit extract: prospective, randomized, placebo controlled study. *British Medical Journal* **322**(7278):134–7.

SCHMIDT, P.J., NIEMAN, L.K., GROVER, G.N., MULLER, K.L., MERRIAM, G.R. and RUBINOW, D.R. (1991) Lack of effect of induced menses on symptoms in women with premenstrual syndrome. *New England Journal of Medicine* **324**:1174–9.

SHERSHAH, P.J., MORRISON, J.J. and JAFAROY, S. (1991) Prevalence of premenstrual syndrome in Pakistani women. *Journal of the Pakistan Medical Association* **41**:101–3.

SNOWDEN, R. and CHRISTIAN, B. (1984) *Patterns and Perceptions of Menstruation*. New York: St Martins Press.

STUDD, J.W.W. (1979) Premenstrual tension syndrome. *British Medical Journal* **277**:410.

STUDD, J.W.W. (1992) Oestrogens and depression in women. *British Journal of Hospital Medicine* **48**:211–13.

STURDEE, D.W., WADE EVANS, T., PATTERSON, M.E.L., THOM, M.H. and STUDD, J.W.W. (1978) Relations between bleeding pattern, endometrial histology and oestrogen treatment in post menopausal women. *British Medical Journal* **i**:1571–7.

SUNDBLAD, C., MODIGH, K., ANDERSCH, B. and ERIKSSON, E. (1992) Clomipramine effectively reduces premenstrual irritability and dysphoria: a placebo controlled trial. *Acta Psychiatrica Scandinavica* **85**(1):39–47.

WALD, A., VAN THIEL, D.H., HOECHSTETTER, I. *et al.* (1981) Gastrointestinal transit: the effect on the menstrual cycle. *Gastroenterology* **80**:1497–500.

WALKER, A. and BANCROFT, J. (1990) Relationship between premenstrual symptoms and oral contraceptive use. *Psychosomatic Medicine* **52**:86–96.

WALKER, A.F., De SOUZA, M.C., VICKERS, M.F., ABAYASEKERA, S., COLLINS, M.L. and TRINCA, L.A. (1998) Magnesium supplementation alleviates premenstrual symptoms of fluid retention. *Journal of Women's Health* **7**(9):1157–65.

WANG, M., HAMMARBACK, S., LINDHE, B.A., *et al.* (1995) Treatment of premenstrual syndrome by spironalactone: a double-blind, placebo-controlled study. *Acta Obstetrica Gynaecologica Scandinavica* **74**:803–8.

WATSON, N.R., STUDD, J.W.W., SAVVAS, M., GARNET, T. and BABER, R.J. (1989) Treatment of severe premenstrual syndrome with oestradiol patches and cyclical norethisterone. *Lancet* **ii**:730–2.

WATTS, J.F., BUTT, W.R. and LOGAN-EDWARDS, R. (1987) A clinical trial using danazol for the treatment of premenstrual tension. *British Journal of Obstetrics and Gynaecology* **94**:30–4.

WYATT, K.M., DIMMOCK, P.W., JONES, P.W. and O'BRIEN, P.M.S. (1999) Efficacy of vitamin B-6 in the treatment of premenstrual syndrome: systematic review. *British Medical Journal* **318**:1375–81.

WYATT, K., DIMMOCK, P., JONES, P., OBHRAI, M. and O'BRIEN, P.M.S. (2001) Efficacy of progesterone and progestogens in the management of premenstrual syndrome: systematic review. *British Medical Journal* **323**:776–80.

16: The Menopause

Kathy Abernethy

◆

OBJECTIVES

This chapter should help you understand:

◆ How the menopause occurs and the hormonal changes that occur ◆

◆ The short-, intermediate- and long-term effects of the menopause ◆

◆ Hormone replacement therapy (HRT) and its uses, indications, contraindications and possible long-term risks ◆

◆ How to counsel a woman before she starts HRT and how to monitor effectively HRT once treatment is established ◆

◆ Non-hormonal treatments for menopausal symptoms ◆

◆ Factors, other than hormones, which influence a woman approaching the menopause. ◆

A woman in the autumn of her life, deserves an Indian summer, rather than a winter of discontent.

(The late Robert B. Greenblatt MD, formerly Professor of Endocrinology, Georgia, USA)

Introduction

All women who live long enough will experience the menopause. The menopause marks the end of fertility and the end of periods. Alongside this often comes acute menopausal symptoms and anxiety about long-term effects such as cardio-vascular disease and osteoporosis. Emotionally, the menopause can signify a time of great change as women take the opportunity to make an assessment of life, perhaps having to adapt to a changing role in the family and in society, and also to come to terms with a changing body and changing expectations in life. Physical changes in her body, social and emotional changes in life and psychological changes make the time of menopause one of great turbulence and self-analysis for some women. The menopause is such an individual event, with its differing associated 'mid-life' problems, that how each woman perceives and experiences this time of physical change will vary enormously. Medicine will help some, counselling may be necessary for others and for some the time of menopause will slip by barely recognized.

This chapter aims to highlight the physical aspects of the menopause along with recognizing some of the non-physical effects and suggesting ways in which you can help women through this phase of their life in a positive way, using both medical and non-medical means.

Definitions

The 'menopause' is a term used to describe the final menstrual bleed in a woman's life. The term 'climacteric' covers the phase of time either side of the last bleed. It is during this climacteric phase that menopausal symptoms commonly occur. Both women and health professionals alike tend to use the term 'menopause' to describe the phase in a woman's life when fertility

451

disappears and periods stop. The following terms are also used:

◆ *Pre-menopause* The time prior to periods stopping, usually before symptoms start

◆ *Peri-menopause* The time around the menopause when bleeding can be irregular and symptoms may occur. Conception is still theoretically possible although cycles may be anovulatory

◆ *Post-menopause* The time in a woman's life after periods have stopped for at least a year.

Age of menopause

In the UK the average age at which periods stop is 51 years. This has remained constant for many years although general improvements in health care provision have resulted in a much greater life expectancy than was known by previous generations. Women now expect to live much longer after the menopause and it is partly for this reason that women themselves are thinking more about the long-term effects of oestrogen deficiency. Although 51 years is the average age of the menopause, it commonly occurs between the ages of 45 and 58 years and can occur much earlier in some women. A menopause that occurs earlier than age 40 years is described as a premature menopause and these women deserve special attention.

The age of menopause is affected by smoking which can bring this forward by 1–2 years (Cooper *et al.*, 1999).

The following factors do not seem to affect whether a woman has an early or late menopause:

◆ Race
◆ Use of oral contraception
◆ Number of pregnancies
◆ Age of menarche
◆ Socio-economic factors.

Some women experience a gradual stopping of periods over a couple of years whilst others will find that their periods stop suddenly. Others may see more frequent periods initially, gradually becoming less frequent. All of these patterns are normal.

In relation to types of menopause the following terms are used:

◆ *Natural/spontaneous* – periods stop of their own accord

◆ *Surgical* – the ovaries are removed by surgery thus producing an instantaneous menopause

◆ *Premature* – menopause occurs under the age of 40 years, for whatever reason

◆ *Induced* – menopause is brought on by external factors such as chemotherapy or radiotherapy.

Hormonal changes at the menopause

During the peri-menopausal phase, oestradiol levels fall and levels of follicle stimulating hormone (FSH) and luteinizing hormone (LH) rise. However, there is wide fluctuation in levels around the time of menopause. The rise in FSH is gradual and reaches a peak after the final bleed has occurred. The levels drop again about 10–20 years after the menopause (Berger *et al.*, 1995).

Prior to the menopause, oestradiol and oestrone are the principal oestrogens circulating in the body. They are produced mainly by the ovaries, with oestradiol the predominant hormone. Oestrone is also available through conversion of a hormone, androstenedione, which is secreted by the adrenal glands. After the menopause, levels of both oestradiol and oestrone drop markedly and oestrone becomes the dominant oestrogen.

Women themselves often believe that they need to have a blood test to measure hormone levels at the time of menopause. In practice, this is hardly ever useful or even necessary. Symptoms of the menopause do not correlate to actual oestrogen levels, with some women seemingly able to tolerate very low oestrogen levels with few symptoms, whilst others will experience profuse symptoms despite only a small change in oestrogen levels. FSH levels fluctuate widely around the time of the menopause and can be unreliable. A series of two or three measurements would be required for a diagnosis of the menopause and again would be of little value in predicting the need for hormone replacement therapy. FSH levels may be useful in a hysterectomized woman who is experiencing early symptoms of the climacteric. FSH levels are also used to diagnose a premature menopause when the medical implications are going to be greater than for the average age woman.

Premature menopause

Whilst it is common for the natural menopause to occur in the late forties or early fifties, some women experience the menopause much earlier. A menopause prior to age 40 years is described as premature. Long-term consequences for such women are greater than with a so-called 'normal menopause', and many specialists would now agree that this group of women deserves special attention because of their additional physical needs. They also deserve special attention with regard to the psychological and emotional upsets that some women experience when undergoing an early menopause.

Causes of premature menopause

Surgery
If both ovaries are removed, the menopause occurs immediately. Symptoms can be quite severe after even a very short time. Hormone replacement therapy should be given not only to prevent symptoms but also to help protect against osteoporosis and cardiovascular disease. Hysterectomy alone (i.e. with conservation of one or both ovaries) has been shown to bring forward the age of menopause in some women (Siddle *et al.*, 1987). Women should no longer be assured therefore that their remaining ovaries will necessarily carry on working until the normal age of menopause. Professionals should now listen more carefully to those women who may complain of menopausal symptoms soon after hysterectomy: FSH levels may be indicated. It remains controversial as to whether it is necessary

SCENARIO

Deborah is 42 years old. She had a hysterectomy with conservation of ovaries 2 years ago. Apart from her initial postoperative check she has not seen her doctor since. She now feels extraordinarily tired and often wakes at night feeling very hot. Eventually she sought medical advice. After checking her thyroid function was normal, the GP decided to do a series of FSH levels. He was surprised to discover they were in the post-menopausal range. Deborah started HRT and within a few weeks her symptoms were improved. Deborah was reassured to have the risks of HRT explained to her, especially with regard to younger women.

to do regular annual FSH measurements in premenopausal women who have had their ovaries conserved at the time of a hysterectomy.

Natural
Occasionally the menopause occurs spontaneously at an unusually early age. This may be associated with chromosomal abnormalities or autoimmune diseases affecting the ovaries. Sometimes no cause is found for the early menopause. Typical menopausal symptoms may or may not be present, so careful investigations are needed. For women who want children it is particularly important that a prompt diagnosis is made, as implications with regard to their fertility are immense.

Iatrogenic
Iatrogenic early menopause, i.e. caused by outside influences, such as chemotherapy or radiotherapy, can be quite traumatic, especially when the woman has successfully faced malignant disease but has to come to terms with an early menopause as a result of her treatment.

Consequences of an early menopause

Menopausal symptoms
These are likely to be worse in a woman who experiences a sudden menopause, as a result of surgery, for example, than in those

women who experience a gradual ovarian failure (Anasti, 1998).

Cardiovascular disease

Early studies in the 1950s showed a higher incidence of heart disease in women with early menopause (Oliver and Boyd, 1959). The US Nurses Study demonstrated that the risk of myocardial infarction increased as the age of the menopause decreased and that bilateral oophorectomy under the age of 35 years incurred a sevenfold risk compared to pre-menopausal women (Rosenberg *et al.*, 1981). A later study showed that women who took oral hormone replacement therapy after oophorectomy had no increased risk in cardiovascular disease (Colditz *et al.*, 1987). It is now accepted that premature menopause incurs a more significant risk of heart disease than a menopause at the normal age (Hu *et al.*, 1999). Recent studies showing a possible increased risk of coronary heart disease and stroke with oestrogen therapy have not included women with a premature menopause (WHI, 2002).

Osteoporosis

Premature menopause is associated with an earlier onset of osteoporosis (Anasti *et al.*, 1998). This is preventable by the use of long-term hormone replacement therapy or other bone sparing therapies (Eastell, 1999).

Premature menopause and hormone replacement therapy

A woman with an early menopause needs special care with regard to HRT. She is likely to be taking it for many years so care must be taken to find a regime which suits her and gives acceptable hormonal replacement. The woman herself should be involved in a decision as to how she wants to take her HRT and every effort should be made to minimize side effects. Younger women may need higher doses of oestrogen not only in order to feel well but also to maintain an adequate protection of the skeleton (Gangar and Key, 1993). The consequences of stopping

treatment are potentially more damaging in women with premature menopause, so it is particularly important that they understand why the HRT is necessary and are given ample opportunity to express anxieties and ask questions about treatment.

Women with a premature menopause (natural or surgical) have traditionally been encouraged to continue HRT until the age of 50 years. Although evidence is lacking, most specialists continue to advise this as it is thought that the potential risk of breast cancer with HRT use is simply equivalent to those women who do not have a premature menopause (British Menopause Society, Consensus Statement, 2003).

Psychological effects of premature menopause

Experiencing an early menopause, whether natural or surgical, can cause emotional difficulty. Issues relating to sexuality in particular can become very important and for some women these issues can be difficult to handle. These may include:

◆ Loss of fertility
◆ Change in body image
◆ Feelings of loss of femininity
◆ Fear of ageing prematurely
◆ Feeling 'out of control' of their body
◆ Feeling that their body has 'let them down'.

It is helpful if women are given the opportunity to discuss such issues openly. Some women value being able to talk within a group of other women who have also undergone early menopause. Young women often feel very isolated at the time of premature menopause and this is not helped by the fact that almost all literature on the subject of menopause is aimed at women in their fifties. Women undergoing planned surgery may have time for discussion within the gynaecology unit but those who undergo a natural early menopause are often left feeling angry, frightened and alone with nobody to turn to.

SCENARIO

Isobella is 34 years old. She has two children and had considered her family to be complete until she was diagnosed as experiencing an early menopause. Once confronted with the inevitability of having no more children, she had a constant desire for one more child, even though she knew it was not possible. She felt very bitter that this decision was taken from her. She did not tolerate HRT very well and was reluctant to take it. She was eventually seen by an experienced menopause counsellor who, over time, helped her to adjust to her new situation. As she came to terms with her infertility, she became more willing to try other HRT regimes and eventually found one that suited her.

Short- and intermediate-term effects of oestrogen deficiency

For many people, the most obvious symptom associated with the menopause is the hot flush. Almost all women and probably many men would be able to associate hot flushes with 'the change'. However, there are many other symptoms that can arise around the time of the menopause, some of which can be quite distressing, particularly if the woman herself does not realize that they may be related to her menopause. Symptoms are summarized in Box 16.1.

Box 16.1   Summary of typical menopausal symptoms

Short term
- Flushes/sweats
- Psychological complaints
- Insomnia.

Intermediate
- Sexual difficulties
- Dyspareunia
- Vaginal atrophy
- Bladder symptoms.

Long term
- Osteoporosis
- Cardiovascular disease.

Vasomotor symptoms

Approximately 75% of post-menopausal women in the UK do experience acute menopausal symptoms. Symptoms sometimes start before periods even become irregular and can continue for many years after the last bleed (Studd *et al.*, 1990). The average length of time that symptoms last is 2 years with 25% of women continuing to experience them for 5 years and 5% of women still experiencing them many years after the menopause (McKinlay *et al.*, 1992).

The hot flush

Women describe a flush as a feeling of intense heat, sometimes accompanied by sweating, starting in the chest area and rising through the neck and face. The frequency and length of flushes varies from woman to woman. Flushes that occur at night often result in profuse sweating, the so-called 'night sweat'. These can occur night after night for months or even years. The actual cause of the hot flush is not known although various theories have been suggested. Hormone levels cannot predict the onset of flushes and sweats and it seems that the fluctuation in oestrogen levels which occurs around the time of the menopause is more important than the actual physiological levels. Vasomotor symptoms respond extremely well to oestrogen therapy, which remains the treatment that has been most widely researched for this problem (Maclellan *et al.*, 2001). There is a strong placebo response with treatment for hot flushes so any study has to be carefully controlled if a true therapeutic effect is to be demonstrated.

If left untreated, vasomotor symptoms will eventually subside, leaving no long-term effects. The decision as to whether to treat them or not can only be taken by the woman herself according to her individual circumstances, a decision that will be based on how severe and unbearable her symptoms are.

Other treatments apart from oestrogen therapy which have been suggested to relieve hot flushes include:

- Black cohosh (see page 72)
- Clonidine

◆ Natural progesterone

◆ Phytoestrogens (see also page 475)

◆ Complementary therapies (see Chapter 4).

Psychological symptoms

Many women complain of psychological problems at the time of the menopause but it is difficult to establish whether they are a true result of oestrogen deficiency or whether they are secondary factors related to other symptoms, such as flushes and sweats. Prolonged episodes of night sweats may lead to a very poor sleep pattern, which in turn results in poor concentration, poor memory, mood changes and even physical symptoms such as headaches and fatigue. This is described as the 'domino effect'. Studies are difficult to perform objectively because of the strong placebo effect and because of the difficulty of allowing for all the external influences on psychological well-being.

Nevertheless, many studies have shown that minor psychological disturbances often precede the actual last bleed and seem to correlate with fluctuating oestrogen levels (Ballinger, 1975; Montgomery and Studd, 1991). These symptoms can include:

◆ Loss of confidence

◆ Depressed mood

◆ Fatigue

◆ Feelings of unworthiness

◆ Forgetfulness

◆ Difficulty in making decisions.

It should be remembered that many external factors will influence how a woman is feeling emotionally and psychologically around the time of the menopause and these should be taken into account when considering the effects of the menopause. These factors are discussed later in the chapter.

Sexual function

Sexual function is another area where many influences other than simply that of the menopause have an important role. Satisfaction within a relationship, emotional stability and psychological well-being will all help to contribute to a satisfactory sex life. Sexual activity involves both partners and we should not assume that a problem at mid-life is always due to the woman and her hormones. The male partner also may be changing and male sexual dysfunction, such as impotence or loss of desire, may also contribute to a less than satisfactory sexual relationship. In the same way that we must not always blame the menopause for sexual disorders at the time of the menopause, we should not assume that HRT is always the answer.

Psychosexual counselling may be necessary even if oestrogen deficiency is playing an important role. Sexual difficulties that are likely to respond to HRT are:

◆ Lack of lubrication

◆ Loss of libido

◆ Dyspareunia.

The vaginal epithelium changes markedly after the menopause, resulting in the vaginal walls becoming thinner and less elastic. Vaginal secretions diminish and the vagina becomes more susceptible to infection because of the changing pH. This is known as atrophic vaginitis.

It is likely that simply relieving vaginal dryness and discomfort can break the cycle which is often seen, where a woman makes love but it is painful, so next time the desire is absent, leading to even less lubrication and therefore even more discomfort. If intercourse is expected to be painful, it occurs less and less frequently, resulting in further atrophy and consequently more discomfort. Oestrogen can help to break this cycle.

Some studies have shown that testosterone increases sexual desire and for some women this can be combined with their oestrogen therapy (Sherwin and Gelfland, 1985). Testosterone is given by implant and may be particularly useful for the hysterectomized woman. A trial of therapy may be necessary to see if the effects will be beneficial.

There is evidence that Tibolone, a gonadomimetic, is more effective than oestrogen–norethisterone combination, but no more effective than oestrogen alone, for improving libido and sexual enjoyment (Moore, 1999).

Bladder symptoms

Bladder symptoms worsen with age and are often assumed to be directly associated with the hormonal effects of the menopause (see also Chapter 17). However, no studies have been able to relate directly menopausal status with specific urinary symptoms, although beneficial effects of oestrogen therapy have been shown (Hilton and Stanton, 1983). This beneficial effect may be due to collagen factors in the tissue around the urethra. It has been estimated that 50% of women attending a menopause clinic have urinary symptoms, such as stress incontinence, frequency of micturition, urgency, and nocturia (Cardozo, 1990). Whether these are a genuine response to oestrogen deficiency or are caused by other factors, they none the less need a sympathetic ear and helpful advice. A trial of oestrogen therapy may well be of benefit.

Long-term effects of oestrogen deficiency

Osteoporosis

More and more women are now becoming aware of the condition called osteoporosis, and the fact that it particularly affects women after the menopause. The National Osteoporosis Society, a national charity, has ensured that osteoporosis is much more fully understood now than in the past. The media has also covered the subject extensively, and many women are now presenting to their GPs expressing concern about the condition of their bones.

Osteoporosis is a condition in which bone mass per unit volume reduces to such an extent that fractures may occur, even following minimal trauma. This definition does not require a fracture to have occurred, but simply for the risk of fracture to be increased because of reduced bone mass. Some women, therefore, are said to have osteoporosis even though they have not yet experienced a fracture.

Normal bone structure

Bone is a living part of the body, being constantly removed and renewed, with new bone being deposited on a continuous basis. Four main cells are found in bone, but the two most relevant to osteoporosis are the *osteoclasts*, which remove old bone, and *osteoblasts*, which replace it. In children and young adults, there is a net increase in bone density, resulting in skeletal growth. However, at around the age of 30–35 years, peak bone mass is achieved and less bone formation takes place. The bone becomes less dense as a result of greater bone destruction and less formation, resulting in a demineralization, leaving a less dense and consequently weaker bone structure (Figure 16.1).

This gradual thinning of the bone particularly affects trabecular bone, of which the long bones and vertebrae are mainly comprised. This trabecular bone is surrounded by a hard cortical shell. Osteoporotic bones lose strength as they become less dense as a result of less bone formation. Therapies aimed at preventing osteoporosis aim either to increase bone formation (building) or to reduce bone resorption (destruction). Hormone replacement therapy is thought to work partly by preventing bone resorption, thus helping to restore the balance between bone resorption and formation.

Causes

Osteoporosis can be caused by various factors. Peak bone mass is achieved by early adult life and appears to be largely genetically predetermined, although lifestyle factors such as diet and

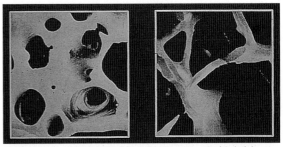

Figure 16.1 Normal (left) and osteoporotic (right) bone. (Reproduced with permission from Dempster, D. *et al.*, 1986.)

exercise may be influential in promoting a healthy bone mass during skeletal development. Race is also an important factor, with Afro-Caribbean people having a greater bone mass than white people, who in turn have a greater bone mass than Asians (Ellerington and Stevenson, 1993).

Once peak bone mass is achieved, bone loss then occurs at varying rates throughout the rest of a person's life. Men lose bone density more slowly and also often achieve a greater peak bone mass in the first place, so are less at risk of osteoporosis. By far the greatest influence on the bone density of a woman is the menopause, after which bone density may be lost very rapidly. How much at risk of developing osteoporosis a woman is will depend on how great a peak bone mass she achieves as a young adult, combined with how fast she subsequently loses bone density after the menopause. A woman who achieves a good peak bone mass may subsequently lose bone rapidly, putting her at as much risk as the woman who has a lower peak bone mass, but after the menopause loses bone density more slowly. The initial 5–10 years after the menopause is the time when the greatest bone loss occurs, with a general slowing down of the rate some 10 years or so after the menopause. Measures for preventing osteoporosis are therefore most effective in the first ten years after the menopause although benefit will still be achieved many years later (Nilas and Christiansen, 1988).

Although osteoporosis occurs most commonly in women after the menopause, it can also occur in both men and women as a result of the following contributory factors:

◆ Corticosteroid therapy (above 7.5 mg prednisolone daily or equivalent on a regular basis)

◆ Hyperparathyroidism

◆ Cushing's syndrome

◆ Some malignant diseases

◆ Long-term immobilization

◆ Excessive exercise, such as with athletes or ballet dancers

◆ Chronic diseases, such as hepatic or renal failure

◆ Rheumatoid arthritis.

Box 16.2   Risk factors for osteoporosis

◆ Race
◆ Heredity
◆ Early menopause
◆ High alcohol intake
◆ Cigarette smoking
◆ Low body weight
◆ Nulliparity
◆ Episodes of amenorrhoea
◆ Sedentary lifestyle
◆ Secondary contributory factors.

Risk factors

Various risk factors (Box 16.2) have been identified to try and predict women at risk of osteoporosis, but it has proved difficult to correlate these with actual incidence of osteoporosis in individual women. Some women seem to have all the risk factors and not develop osteoporosis, whilst others are not apparently at high risk yet develop the disease. At best such risk factors will only identify 30% of those people who will subsequently develop osteoporosis (Slamender et al., 1990).

Incidence

Osteoporotic fractures are extremely common. It is estimated that 40–50% of all women will experience a fracture related to osteoporosis during their lives (Cummings et al., 1989). The three most common sites for fracture as a result of osteoporosis are the wrist, the spine and the hip.

The wrist. There are approximately 50,000 cases of Colles' fracture in the UK each year, with a dramatic rise in numbers among women over the age of 50. Men do not experience a rise in incidence such as occurs among women.

The spine. Vertebral fractures occur when osteoporosis causes the vertebral bodies to collapse because of weakened bone mass. These fractures may occur without causing pain and only subsequently be shown by X-ray, or they may result in sudden, acute back pain requiring medical attention. Repeated vertebral fractures cause the so-called 'dowager's hump' (Figure 16.2)

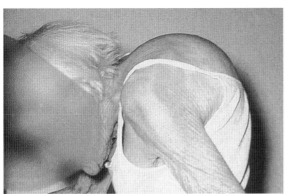

Figure 16.2 A woman with severe osteoporosis. (Reproduced with permission from slide set *A Woman's Guide to the Menopause*, produced by Wyeth Laboratories.)

which typifies the image of an elderly lady and frightens so many younger ones.

The hip. Hip fractures are potentially very serious and there are approximately 70,000 per year in the UK. Treatment of hip fractures is generally by surgery which carries the risks associated with general anaesthetic as well as risks from immobility in a generally frail and elderly person. Many elderly women who experience a hip fracture never regain their independence and have to rely on their family or society for help and support. About 20% of those who sustain a hip fracture will die within a year (Kanis, 1994).

The incidence of hip fractures in the UK is high, with figures likely to rise as we experience an increasing elderly population. The cost to the NHS is enormous and the cost in terms of personal suffering, immeasurable (Hillard *et al.*, 1991).

Measuring bone density

Conventional X-rays are of little value in assessing osteoporosis because bone loss will only be evident when very severe. Obvious fractures will show up and past vertebral fractures which may have occurred without pain will also be evident. However, as a means of predicting those at risk of osteoporosis and subsequent fracture, X-rays are seldom used.

The most usual way of currently assessing bone density is dual energy X-ray absorptiometry (DXA). This measures bone density at various sites and is said to give an accurate result of bone density at the spine and hip. Fracture risk is directly related to bone density and even a single measurement at around the time of the menopause will give a good indication of future risk of fracture (Hui *et al.*, 1988). A further scan 18 months to 2 years later will also help to assess the actual rate of bone loss over this period of time.

Measurements such as these are particularly helpful to the woman who would prefer not to intervene medically but who would do so if there was evidence that she was likely to benefit. They also help to determine how long a woman may wish to stay on therapy, as a woman with more severe bone loss is more likely to remain on a treatment than one with only slight bone loss. Bone density measurements also help in assessing the effectiveness of a particular therapy, as repeat scans over a period of time will demonstrate the benefit of the therapy for an individual.

There is no evidence to support screening women with DXA at the time of the menopause. We try to identify those women who we perceive to be most at risk, which particularly includes those women experiencing an early menopause, those who have had long episodes of amenorrhoea earlier in life and those on long-term steroid therapy (Miller *et al.*, 2003).

Other methods of measuring bone density include photon absorptiometry (single and dual) and quantitative computerized tomography (CAT) scans. The use of quantitative ultrasound (QUS) to measure bone strength is under investigation. A number of systems are available and further research is needed to assess their reliability and sensitivity. It would appear that a low bone density in the heel correlates with a low bone density in the hip or spine (Stewart *et al.*, 1996). Research is being conducted to establish whether it is possible to measure bone density at sites other than the hip and spine with equal validity.

High bone turnover is associated with a fast rate of post-menopausal bone loss. Bone markers, measured in blood or urine assay, may be useful in identifying women at risk of fracture. They could also be used to monitor response and compliance with therapy, as levels fall with effective therapy.

Calcium

Women sometimes believe that if they simply take extra calcium, they will prevent osteoporosis. Unfortunately this is too simplistic. Calcium, like all vitamins and minerals, is an essential part of a normal diet. If it is lacking during the years that the skeleton is forming, then the bones will suffer as a consequence. However, most people do get sufficient calcium in a modern Western diet. After the menopause, taking extra calcium alone will not stop osteoporosis. Women at the time of the menopause sometimes cut back on the calcium in their diet inadvertently whilst trying to diet, by reducing the amount of dairy products they eat. These women should be encouraged to maintain an adequate intake of calcium, either through dairy products or through other foods. Women on special diets for moral or religious reasons may not be getting sufficient calcium and supplements may be useful for these women.

Calcium may be useful as a treatment for established osteoporosis, particularly in an elderly person. Some regimes for established osteoporosis incorporate extra calcium, e.g. bisphosphonates.

Hormone replacement therapy and osteoporosis

HRT has been shown to protect against fracture of the hip and spine (WHI, 2002). For the greatest benefit to the skeleton, HRT should be started soon after the menopause and continued long term (Kanis, 1996). This is the phase when women lose bone density very rapidly and therefore conserving bone at this stage is valuable in the long term. If HRT is started some years after the menopause the bone density will not be substantially reversed although further loss will be prevented (Kanis, 1996). Short courses of HRT (less than 5 years) at a young age may not significantly reduce fracture risk in old age, many years after HRT has been stopped (Barrett-Connor *et al.*, 2003). HRT will reduce bone loss in women of all ages, regardless of menopausal age or type of HRT (Kanis, 1996). However, the dose required for individual women will vary, with standard doses needed for peri-menopausal women and women in the early post-menopausal years

(Lindsay *et al.*, 1984). Older women or women who are some years past the menopause may gain benefit to bone from lower doses of oestrogen (Eastell, 1999).

The use of HRT solely for osteoporosis prevention has been a matter of discussion, and in 2003 the Committee on Safety of Medicines stated that it should not be used as a first-line treatment for most women, because of the associated risks (Committee on Safety of Medicines, 2003). Some professional groups have disputed this and issued counter statements demonstrating the evidence supporting the use of HRT (British Menopause Society Statement, 2003). However, for those of us advising women, it is important to be fully aware of these recommendations and the implications for clinical practice. At the time of writing, the prevention and treatment of osteoporosis is a subject being discussed by NICE (National Institute for Clinical Excellence) and guidelines are expected in 2005.

Exercise

It is known that long periods of immobilization lead to a decrease in bone density; however, research has been unable positively to demonstrate whether taking extra exercise around the time of the menopause can increase bone mass on its own accord. Such studies would be difficult to conduct because of other influencing factors such as diet, drugs and lifestyle. It does seem evident, however, that weight-bearing exercises such as walking, running and dancing are of more benefit to the skeleton than swimming which is still of course an excellent exercise, particularly for the cardiovascular system (Stevenson *et al.*, 1990). Exercise also increases muscle tone, general fitness and agility, perhaps reducing the likelihood of a fall and consequent risk of fracture.

Excessive exercise such as that undertaken by athletes or ballet dancers reduces body weight to such an extent that periods may stop. This results in a loss of bone density pre-menopausally which will increase the risk of fracture later in life, particularly when combined with a later loss associated with the menopause (Drinkwater *et al.*, 1984).

Cardiovascular disease

Heart disease is the major cause of death in women aged over 50 years in the UK (OPCS, 2002). Heart disease has always been considered to be predominantly a male problem, and it is true that until the age of 50 years it is men who are far more likely to suffer a heart attack or stroke. After this age, the incidence in women comes closer to that of men. This is considered to be partly due to a fall in oestradiol levels after the menopause, which appears to have a strong influence on various factors relating to heart disease (Barrett-Connor, 1997). It is not clear which factors are most important, whether it is to do with changing lipids alone or whether other changes occur in blood vessels themselves as a result of oestrogen deficiency. The role of HRT and its effect on heart disease is controversial and is discussed later in this chapter.

Other factors

Of course the menopause is not the only factor that will influence whether a woman gets cardiovascular disease. Lifestyle, medical and genetic factors all play an important role (Box 16.3). When assessing health in relation to women at the time of menopause, a combination of factors should be taken into account and appropriate advice offered and information given.

The role of HRT in preventing cardiovascular disease

The role of oestrogen therapy as primary or secondary prevention of coronary heart disease is controversial. Longstanding epidemiological evidence seems to conflict with recent randomized trials. The publication of the Women's Health Initiative (WHI) study in 2002 and other papers has led to more uncertainty (WHI, 2002; British Menopause Society Consensus Statement, 2003) among clinicians.

The combined arm of this large US study demonstrated a small increased risk of heart disease, stroke and breast cancer after long-term use. A reduction in incidence of colorectal cancer and osteoporotic fracture were also seen. Limitations of this study (WHI, 2002) are that only one drug

> **Box 16.3** Risk factors for cardiovascular disease
>
> Lifestyle
> ◆ Smoking
> ◆ Obesity
> ◆ Sedentary lifestyle
> ◆ High-fat diet.
>
> Medical
> ◆ Menopausal status
> ◆ Hypercholesterolaemia
> ◆ Family history of heart disease
> ◆ Hypertension
> ◆ Diabetes.

regimen was used (conjugated equine oestrogen 0.625 mg and medroxyprogesterone acetate 2.5 mg), which is not available in the UK; the average age of women was 63 years and the average body mass index was high. Consequently many women might already have pre-existing medical conditions related to heart disease, and were not the healthy post-menopausal younger woman that is more typical with UK HRT usage.

Interestingly, results of the oestrogen-only arm of the study indicated a similar risk of stroke as that demonstrated with the combined regimen, but failed to demonstrate an increased risk of heart disease or breast cancer after 7 years of follow-up (WHI, 2004). This is encouraging news for the many women who need oestrogen replacement following hysterectomy.

The risks and benefits of HRT in this study are summarized in Table 16.1.

In the light of this and other studies the following recommendations have been made (Royal College of Physicians of Edinburgh, 2003; British Menopause Society Statement, 2003):

◆ There is no evidence to justify using oestrogen therapy solely for prevention of coronary heart disease or stroke

◆ The effects of different oestrogens and progestogens may be different from that reported in the WHI (2002) study

◆ In women with existing heart disease, the risks and benefits of HRT should be considered on an individual basis.

Table 16.1 Increase/decrease in health events per 10,000 women annually for those taking combined HRT and for those taking placebo (WHI, 2002)

	10,000 women/year taking placebo	10,000 women/year taking oestrogen/progestogen HRT	Differences per year per 10,000 women
Breast cancer	30	38	8 more women with breast cancer
Heart attacks	30	37	7 more women with heart attacks
Strokes	21	29	8 more women with strokes
Venous thrombolic events	16	34	18 more women with blood clots
Colorectal cancer	16	10	6 fewer women with colorectal cancer
Hip fractures	15	10	5 fewer women with hip fractures

Alzheimer's disease

Whilst oestrogen therapy may delay or reduce the risk of Alzheimer's disease, it does not appear to improve established disease (Kesslak, 2002). It may be that there is a critical age for exposure to oestrogen that makes it more effective (British Menopause Society Consensus Statement, 2003). Further studies are under way.

Colon cancer

Recent studies suggest that oestrogen may offer a protective effect against colon cancer, dependent on dose and duration of treatment. Preliminary studies have shown a reduction in incidence and mortality of the disease (Troisi et al., 1997). The WIH study was the first randomized trial to confirm the benefit of oestrogen therapy on colorectal cancer risk, showing a one-third reduction in risk (WHI, 2002).

Hormone Replacement Therapy

HRT has become a hot issue for discussion among women in their late forties and fifties. 'Should I or shouldn't I take it?'; 'Do I need it?'; 'Will it harm rather than help?'. These and other questions are very important to women as they go through their menopause. The decision to take HRT is a personal one for most women, with conflicting advice often being offered by doctors,

nurses, friends and the media. As a health professional you must give accurate and up-to-date information to women so that they can make an informed choice for themselves.

Principles of HRT

HRT consists of the two female hormones oestrogen and progestogen. In hysterectomized women, oestrogen is used on its own, but women with a uterus are generally prescribed both oestrogen and progestogen in order to prevent the endometrial stimulation which has been associated with oestrogen-only therapy (Grady et al., 1995).

Oestrogens used in HRT are natural rather than synthetic. Natural oestrogens, which include oestradiol, oestrone and oestriol, cause the level of oestrogen circulating in the bloodstream to be similar to normal pre-menopausal levels. Synthetic oestrogens such as those found in the oral contraceptive pill have a much more potent effect and are not used in modern forms of HRT. Conjugated equine oestrogens (e.g. Premarin, a common form of HRT) act in a similar way to human oestrogens and are considered to be 'natural' rather than synthetic.

In most current forms of HRT in the UK, oestrogen is given on a continuous basis, i.e. without a break. Progestogens may be added on a monthly or 3-monthly basis, resulting in a withdrawal bleed, or continuously – the so-called 'period-free' treatment (Figure 16.3). This 'period-free' HRT is

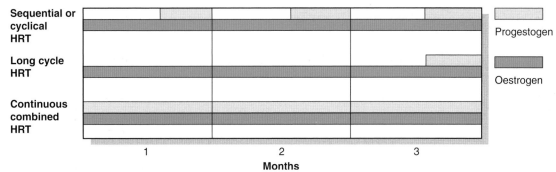

Figure 16.3 HRT preparations for women with a uterus.

an attractive option for *post*-menopausal women wanting to start HRT. Studies have shown irregular bleeding and spotting are common in the first few months but these usually settle. Tricyclical or quarterly regimens minimize the likelihood of progestogenic side effects and produce a withdrawal bleed only once every 3 months. The choice of regimen should be tailored to the individual woman, depending on her menopausal status. During the perimenopause, cyclical or tricyclical regimens should be used, changing to a continuous regimen when she is thought to be postmenopausal. Women who start HRT more than 1 year after their periods stop, should be offered 'period-free' HRT from the start.

Routes of administration

HRT can be given in various forms, and for the majority of women the final decision should be influenced by a personal choice. A woman who has chosen her favoured route of receiving HRT is more likely to continue the therapy than the woman who has been persuaded to use a regime with which she does not feel comfortable. HRT can be given in the following ways:

◆ Oral
◆ Transdermal
◆ Implants
◆ Vaginal creams/pessaries/rings
◆ Intranasal.

The main difference between the oral and non-oral routes of HRT is the avoidance of the gastrointestinal tract in non-oral routes and the subsequent 'first-pass effect' on the liver. Tablets also result in a greater change of oestradiol to oestrone, changing the ratio from that which is normally found in a pre-menopausal woman. Variation in circulating oestrogen levels between women is common as rates of absorption vary from individual to individual.

First-pass effect
The so-called 'first-pass effect' means that the liver receives a bolus of oestrogen after each dose, rather than a steady release. It results in metabolism of much of the oestrogen into a less active form. This means that a higher dose is necessary in order to achieve similar therapeutic effects to non-oral routes. This first pass will have an effect on various factors, including clotting and lipids. It is generally recommended that oral therapy should be avoided in women who are considered to be particularly susceptible to effects in the liver, such as those with hypertension, hypertriglyceridaemia or a previous history of venous thrombosis (Stevenson, 1996). Women who have previously experienced severe gastrointestinal upset, such as Crohn's disease, may also benefit from a non-oral route, because of possible absorption problems.

Tablets
Tablets are the commonest way of receiving HRT. They have been available longer than any other

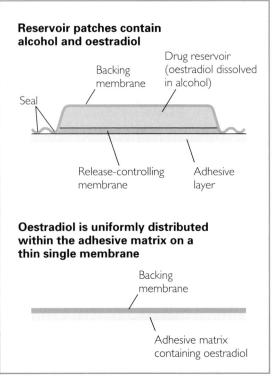

Figure 16.4   Reservoir patches (top) contain alcohol and oestradiol. In matrix patches (below) the oestradiol is uniformly distributed within the adhesive matrix on a thin single membrane. (Reproduced courtesy of Janssen Cilag Ltd.)

form of HRT and much of the research into the long-term effects of HRT has been carried out using oral forms of therapy. They are available in different doses containing various natural oestrogens and in combination with a choice of progestogens. The advantages and disadvantages are listed in Box 16.4.

Transdermal

HRT can be given transdermally by:

◆ Patches
◆ Gel preparation.

Oestradiol patches deliver a constant dose of oestrogen over a 24-hour period. The patch is stuck to the abdomen or buttocks and changed once or twice weekly and is generally kept on during bathing and swimming. The first patch to be developed was the 'reservoir' patch, which consists of oestradiol dissolved in alcohol in a drug reservoir. An adhesive layer holds the patch in position on the skin whilst the alcohol carries the drug through the skin. The newer 'matrix' patches contain no alcohol and the oestradiol is contained in the matrix of the adhesive itself (Figure 16.4). These patches seem to stick better and for some women cause less skin irritation. Patches are available in different doses and can be used in combination with progestogen, either

orally or in a combined oestrogen/progestogen patch.

The advantages and disadvantages of transdermal HRT patches are listed in Box 16.5.

HRT in the form of a gel is now available in the UK, after many years of use in France. It is recommended to be rubbed into the skin (upper arm and shoulders or alternatively the inner thighs) daily and it works in a similar way to patches. Women with a uterus must also take progestogen in order to prevent endometrial stimulation.

Implants

Oestradiol implants are small pellets containing oestrogen which are inserted under the skin of the abdomen or buttock through a small incision (Figure 16.5). The oestrogen is released slowly over a period of months. They are available in

> **Box 16.5** Transdermal HRT patches: advantages and disadvantages
>
> **Advantages**
> ◆ No need for tablets. A combined oestrogen/progestogen patch is available
> ◆ Physiologically normal ratio of oestradiol to oestrone
> ◆ Avoids first-pass effect on the liver
> ◆ Perceived as more natural by some women.
>
> **Disadvantages**
> ◆ Some women develop a skin irritation
> ◆ Degree of adhesion may vary between women
> ◆ Visual reminder to the woman of her HRT
> ◆ Must remember to change the patch regularly.

varying doses: the higher the dose, usually the longer they last. Levels of oestrogen in the blood-stream tend to be higher than with other forms of HRT, but there is no evidence that this is damaging. Indeed some women seem to benefit from these higher levels. Implants can last a long time with great variation between individuals. The physiological effect of an implant can continue for up to 2 years and progestogen therapy may be necessary for that time if the woman has a uterus. Rarely, a condition described as 'tachyphylaxis' has been observed, where women return for an implant at increasingly shorter intervals (Gangar *et al.*, 1989). Symptom control becomes poor even though oestrogen levels

are high. So far there has been no evidence that this is harmful but some specialists consider it wise to try and offer lower doses less frequently until levels return to a more normal level. This may be difficult for a woman who has become used to high oestrogen levels.

The advantages and disadvantages of HRT implants are listed in Box 16.6.

Intranasal

Intranasal administration of medicines has been successfully used in other therapeutic areas and is now available as an oestrogen-only HRT. Intranasal absorption is facilitated by the highly vascularised nature of the nasal mucosa. The pharmokinetics of intranasally administered oestradiol differ from that of oestradiol taken orally (Devassaguet *et al.*, 1999). With intranasal administration there is a rapid uptake of oestradiol, with maximum plasma levels being achieved within 10–30 minutes. Within 12 hours the level has dropped back to untreated levels, but sustained relief of symptoms appears to occur with repeated doses (Studd *et al.*, 1999). The advantages and disadvantages of intranasal HRT are listed in Box 16.7.

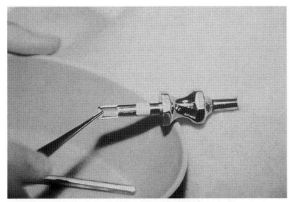

Figure 16.5 Insertion of an oestradiol implant. (Reproduced courtesy of Organon Laboratories.)

> **Box 16.6** HRT implants: advantages and disadvantages
>
> **Advantages**
> ◆ Inserted twice a year and then nothing more to remember
> ◆ Compliance is ensured
> ◆ No first-pass effect
> ◆ Physiologically normal oestradiol to oestrone ratio
> ◆ Can be given alongside testosterone therapy
> ◆ Very convenient for women who do not need progestogen
> ◆ Cheap.
>
> **Disadvantages**
> ◆ Has to be inserted by a medical practitioner
> ◆ Minor surgical procedure
> ◆ Prolonged action in some women
> ◆ 'Tachyphylaxis' in some women.

Box 16.7 Advantages and disadvantages of intranasal oestrogen

Advantages

◆ Flexible doses
◆ Avoids first-pass effect on liver
◆ No need for tablets
◆ Different pharmokinetics suits some women.

Disadvantages

◆ Method does not appeal to some women
◆ Added progestogen needed for hysterectomized women
◆ An unfamiliar route for most women.

Box 16.8 Advantages and disadvantages of local vaginal oestrogen

Advantages

◆ No need for bleed
◆ Can be used alongside other HRT if necessary for women with severe urogenital symptoms
◆ Vaginal tablets very convenient to use
◆ Offers good relief of urogenital symptoms
◆ Vaginal ring offers more long-term relief with less intervention.

Disadvantages

◆ Some creams seem messy to use
◆ Older women may find an applicator or ring difficult to use
◆ Regulation of dose can be difficult.

Vaginal treatments

Oestrogens administered directly to the vagina are useful for some women.

Local vaginal oestrogens have a direct beneficial effect on atrophic vaginitis without the systemic effects of other routes. They are particularly useful for the older woman whose main complaint is of vaginal discomfort.

The oestrogens used in modern forms of local vaginal preparations are oestriol and oestradiol. These are not absorbed systemically when administered at the recommended doses, and therefore will not have an effect on vasomotor symptoms or confer benefit to the skeleton. Preparations that comprise creams, pessaries or vaginal tablets are recommended to be used 4–5 times a week for 2–3 weeks and then reduced to twice a week as a maintenance dose for 2–3 months. Many women then repeat the course a few months later. A soft flexible ring containing oestradiol is also available and should be changed after 3 months. This has the advantage of being less intrusive on a woman's lifestyle and yet offers good relief of vaginal symptoms. It can be inserted either by a medical practitioner or, after instruction, by the woman herself.

Systemic vaginal treatments are also available: a soft vaginal ring containing oestrogen of a sufficient dose to be systemically absorbed is available. Changed every three months by the woman herself it offers relief of vaginal symptoms and general symptoms. If used by a non-hysterectomized woman, added progestogen is necessary.

The advantages and disadvantages of vaginal HRT treatments are listed in Boxes 16. 8. and 16.9.

Progestogens

Progestogen is added to oestrogen in order to offer protection to the endometrium. Studies have reported an increased risk of endometrial hyperplasia in users of oestrogen-only regimes and that these regimes have a prolonged effect on the endometrium even after treatment has stopped. The implication of this is that if women receive even a relatively short course of oestrogen-only therapy they would theoretically need medical follow-up for several years after stopping treatment (Rees, 1996).

Box 16.9 Advantages and disadvantages of systemic vaginal oestrogen

Advantages

◆ Daily dosing not required
◆ Offers urogenital and general symptoms relief.

Disadvantages

◆ Oestrogen-only treatment, so will need progestogen if non-hysterectomized
◆ Not all women are comfortable with self-insertion.

> **Box 16.10** Recommended daily doses of various progestogens in combination with oestrogen used in cyclical HRT
>
> | | |
> |---|---|
> | Norethisterone | 0.7–2.5 mg (1 mg is most common) |
> | Levonorgestrel | 150 μg |
> | Dydrogesterone | 10/20 mg |
> | Medroxyprogesterone acetate | 5/10 mg |
> | Progesterone vaginal gel | 4% |

This incidence of hyperplasia can be prevented by giving a cyclical progestogen alongside the oestrogen therapy (Box 16.10). It is currently recommended that 10–13 days offers maximum protection and most cyclical HRT preparations work on this principle.

Progestogen-only therapy. If a woman has severe vasomotor symptoms and is concerned about osteoporosis, but cannot or will not take oestrogen therapy, progestogen on its own may be useful. Doses necessary would be medroxyprogesterone acetate 10–20 mg or norethisterone 5–10 mg daily.

Bleeding. Approximately 80–90% of women who take a cyclical HRT regime will experience a monthly withdrawal bleed. You should counsel a woman that this bleed should be regular, lasting up to about 6 or 7 days, but could be much shorter. It should not be painful or too heavy and should settle into a predictable pattern.

Breakthrough bleeding (i.e. unrelated to the progestogen) should not occur and repeated episodes need investigation. Occasional episodes may be due to:

◆ Poor compliance – progestogen is missed
◆ Interaction with other drugs – such as antibiotics
◆ Gastrointestinal upset – progestogen is not absorbed
◆ Stress.

Heavy prolonged bleeding may be caused by:

◆ Poor compliance
◆ Fibroids

◆ Endometrial polyps
◆ Inadequate dose of progestogen
◆ Endometrial hyperplasia.

Progestogen-releasing intrauterine system (IUS)

A T-shaped IUD containing levonorgestrel in a sleeve around the stem is available and marketed in the UK under the name 'Mirena'. The insertion of this IUS means there is a progestogenic effect directly on the endometrium with minimal systemic absorption. Potentially this has several advantages for the woman: cyclical progestogen is unnecessary as the endometrium is protected from hyperplasia by the steady release of levonorgestrel, progestogenic side effects are minimized, reduced bleeding or amenorrhoea occurs in a substantial number of women and contraception would be provided for the peri-menopausal woman.

This product is licensed in the UK for contraception and also for the treatment of idiopathic menorrhagia for 5 years. It has also recently been licensed for HRT use for 4 years.

Women appreciate the simplicity of the method (no regular pill taking or patch changing combined with minimal bleeding) and that this increased the acceptability and convenience of HRT (Suhonen *et al.*, 1995).

Tibolone

Tibolone (termed a gonadomimetic) is a therapy for relief of acute menopausal symptoms which is given continuously and theoretically does not produce a bleed. It has oestrogenic, progestogenic and androgenic properties and has been shown to be effective at reducing flushes, sweats, sleeplessness and in improving mood and libido in women (Moore, 1999). Irregular bleeding may occur in peri-menopausal women so it is only recommended for use in women who have had one year without periods. The majority of post-menopausal women on Tibolone will have amenorrhoea, but any irregular bleeding on this therapy should be investigated (Sturdee, 1993). Tibolone appears to be well tolerated and prevents bone loss in early post-menopausal women and women with established osteoporosis

(Rymer *et al.*, 2001). Tibolone is included in the advice about HRT in statements from the Committee on Safety of Medicines.

Contraindications to hormone replacement therapy

In the past both health professionals and the lay public alike have been concerned about which women should not take HRT because of pre-existing medical conditions. Data based on research into the oral contraceptive pill have been wrongly applied to HRT and confusion has consequently arisen.

Absolute contraindications

Absolute contraindications are considered to be those medical conditions that will be worsened by the use of HRT. In these circumstances HRT use should be avoided, although occasionally women with such conditions seek the advice of a menopause specialist and may be prescribed HRT under close medical supervision. This would be on an individual basis, however, and should not be taken as general guidelines.

Absolute contraindications to HRT are:

◆ Endometrial cancer
◆ Breast cancer
◆ Pregnancy
◆ Undiagnosed abnormal vaginal bleeding
◆ Severe, active liver disease.

Relative contraindications

In the past, some other conditions have been taken as contraindications but are no longer always considered to be so. Some specialists would, however, recommend the use of the non-oral route as a preference for women with these conditions, because of the avoidance of the first-pass effect on the liver and subsequent lipid and clotting changes (Stevenson, 1996). The conditions listed in Box 16.11 could be considered relative contraindications and referral to a specialist may be preferred. However, it is important that women with these conditions are not led to believe that HRT would be out of the question.

Box 16.11   Medical conditions and HRT

◆ *Hypertension* Untreated hypertension should be treated prior to starting HRT but is not a contraindication

◆ *Myocardial infarction or angina* Specialist advice is suggested

◆ *Previous thrombosis* Thrombophilia screens are recommended in women who have had a previous thrombosis, or in women who are thought to be at greater risk of venous thrombosis (Royal College of Obstetricians and Gynaecologists, 1999)

◆ *Varicose veins* Not a contraindication

◆ *Heavy smoker* Not a contraindication unless accompanied by other risk factors for heart disease

◆ *Diabetes* Glucose levels should be monitored in case insulin requirements change initially

◆ *Gallstones* If a woman actually has gallstones HRT is usually avoided. Treated gallstones are not a problem

◆ *Migraine* It is impossible to predict how migraine will respond to HRT. The only answer is for a woman to try it and monitor the migraines

◆ *Otosclerosis* A condition of progressive deafness which has been shown to worsen in pregnancy. It has been suggested that HRT should be used with caution in case the changing oestrogen status worsens the condition, although referral to an ENT specialist may be helpful.

Venous thrombosis and oestrogen use

Prior to 1996 it was generally thought that there was no increased risk of thromboembolic disease with use of oestrogen in HRT. In 1996 two papers were published which documented an increased risk. The increased risk appears small and may be limited to the first year of oestrogen use, although the WHI study demonstrated a slightly higher risk (WHI, 2002). It does not seem to be related to type or dose of HRT (Jick *et al.*, 1996; Daly *et al.*, 1996).

Breast cancer and HRT

One of the greatest anxieties which is shared by both women and health professionals is the possibility of increasing the risk of breast cancer whilst taking HRT. Unfortunately, breast cancer is a common disease with hormonal factors being known to play an important role. The following are known risk factors for breast cancer:

◆ Early menarche
◆ Obesity (which is associated with higher levels of circulating oestrogen)
◆ Late first pregnancy
◆ Late menopause.

Breast cancer is naturally a very emotive issue and one that frightens many women. The idea of increasing the risk of developing cancer is unthinkable for many women even though the risk of developing other diseases, e.g. heart disease, may be greater without HRT. Women therefore look for reassurance that they will not get cancer and although the data about HRT is reassuring, especially in short- to medium-term use, it is impossible to give women the absolute reassurance they want. As more and more women are prescribed HRT it is inevitable that some will develop breast cancer, and it will be very difficult to persuade these women that the HRT was unrelated.

The Collaborative Group on Hormonal Factors in Breast Cancer (1997) reanalysed about 90% of the worldwide epidemiological evidence on the relation between risk of breast cancer and HRT. They found that the cumulative incidence of breast cancer between the ages of 50 and 70 in never-users of HRT is about 45 per 1000 women. For every 1000 women who began HRT at age 50 and used it for 5 years it is estimated that 2 additional women will be diagnosed with breast cancer. After 10 years on HRT this additional number increases to 6, and after 15 years to 12 women.

The WHI study showed a similar level of risk in the combined treatment arm (WHI, 2002) but not in the oestrogen-only arm (WHI, 2004). A large, non-randomized, questionnaire study appeared to show a stronger link between HRT and breast cancer and, in particular, demonstrated a higher risk for women using combined oestrogen and progestogen HRT (Million Women Study Collaborators, 2003). This effect is reduced after cessation of use of HRT and has largely, if not wholly, disappeared after about 5 years. These findings should be considered in the context of the benefits and other risks associated with the use of HRT (Collaborative Group on Hormonal Factors in Breast Cancer, 1997).

Preparing a woman for hormone replacement therapy

You should encourage women to make an informed choice about HRT, to decide for themselves whether or not to take it and how long they may take it for. Many doctors wait for a woman to ask for HRT rather than offering it to her and indeed some doctors appear only to prescribe for those women with unmanageable symptoms. Yet some women find accurate information about HRT difficult to find and making an informed choice can be very difficult for them. It is hardly surprising then to discover that many start HRT only to stop it at a very early stage because of anxiety about side effects.

Information

Women read about issues relating to menopause and HRT in the media. These articles are not always well researched or accurate, yet women often believe them because they are in print. Some articles over-sensationalize HRT, making it out to be a modern wonder drug, whilst other articles emphasize only the negative aspects of HRT and encourage women to 'think natural' rather than trying HRT.

Women also receive information about HRT from sketchy medical consultations where time is short and the opportunity for discussion limited. It is therefore essential that you carefully consider how you can provide the necessary information for women so that they are better placed to make decisions for themselves. Some would suggest that all women attending for a medical consultation in their forties should be provided with information about the menopause so that they are prepared when the time comes. You could also consider the menopause to be a time in a woman's life, like pregnancy, where help and advice is essential but that ultimately the woman makes decisions for herself regarding the options open to her.

Ways of providing this information include:

◆ Leaflets/books/videos

One general practice decided to offer monthly information evenings on the subject of the menopause. Women were targeted with invitations through the age/sex register and offered a suitable date. The evenings were run jointly by the practice nurse and the health visitor. A video was shown which prompted discussion and questions of a general nature, and the opportunity was taken to discuss the menopause and health issues surrounding it. Women were then encouraged to return for a personal consultation in order to discuss their own individual situation. They came to these consultations better informed and able to ask relevant questions because they had been to the information evening.

◆ Group discussions
◆ Menopause information evenings
◆ Support groups
◆ Talks to local women's groups.

Unrealistic expectations

If you are able to, it is well worth evaluating with a woman about to start HRT what she is hoping it will do for her. Some women start HRT with hopelessly unrealistic ideas and, not surprisingly, are disappointed a few months later. You can assess which symptoms are most likely to be helped by HRT and warn her that some may take longer to improve than others. If she has the idea that HRT will make her look and feel 20 years younger, it is helpful to try and dispel this myth. Some women also expect HRT to repair broken relationships, restore sexual desires and generally perform miracles!

Side effects

Women do worry about risks of HRT and unwanted side effects (Box 16.12). It is therefore important that *you* raise these issues even before a woman starts HRT. You should have honest discussion about issues such as breast cancer, bleeding and other side effects so that a woman starts treatment confident that she has received all the necessary advice. She will then start it with an open mind, prepared for early side effects

---

Box 16.12 Understanding the side effects of HRT

Often oestrogen-related and temporary:
◆ Breast tenderness
◆ Nausea
◆ Leg cramps
◆ Headaches.
Usually progestogen-related:
◆ PMS-type symptoms
◆ Fluid retention
◆ Bleeding problems.

---

but willing to persevere. You should advise her as to when to expect her bleed and warn her that the first one is not necessarily an indication of how future bleeds will be. You should also warn her of early side effects that are caused by the sudden rise in oestrogen levels when HRT is started. If you do not prepare women for these side effects they may cause greater anxiety as women become concerned about underlying problems. For example, the woman with breast tenderness thinks the HRT is causing breast cancer, or the woman with leg cramps thinks she is getting a thrombosis. It is often these early side effects that cause women to give up HRT after only a very short time.

Understanding her HRT

Many women are prescribed HRT without understanding of what the treatment comprises.

Jill started HRT for relief of flushes. These disappeared rapidly but her breasts felt very sore and she experienced headaches for 10 days out of the month. After a few weeks Jill decided the treatment was not worth the benefits and discontinued the HRT. She failed to keep her follow-up appointment. Her symptoms returned but she did not realize that the breast problem would probably have subsided and that the progestogen may have been the cause of the headaches and that this could be altered. The resulting flushes caused her to go without a good night's sleep for nearly 2 years.

Most HRT regimes are 'user-friendly' but women can still misunderstand the therapy and take it incorrectly. As with the contraceptive pill it is worth taking the time to explain the regimen and reinforce how to take it. In the case of patches, it may be helpful to actually demonstrate them to some women. Women who are taking a combined oestrogen and progestogen therapy need to understand why the progestogen is important and necessary or they may be tempted to miss this part out, particularly if it is causing side effects.

SCENARIO

Karen commenced on HRT for acute menopausal symptoms. She felt much better on it and her symptoms subsided. However, she noticed that the extra tablets at the end of the packet caused her to feel bloated and generally less well. She decided to experiment and initially missed every other tablet and eventually missed them all. The bloated feeling disappeared yet her menopausal symptoms were still well controlled. It was a further 5 months before she told her doctor, and she was alarmed to realize that she had been potentially damaging the womb by taking unopposed oestrogen. She had thought all the tablets in the treatment were simply to control her symptoms.

Tailoring the dose

Women are often unaware that HRT is a whole spectrum of medications, doses and types of hormones. They may simply stop a treatment which is unsuitable thinking that they have 'given it a go' when in fact a different regimen may be much more suitable. You need to encourage women to return with their complaints so that a different regimen can at least be tried. This will sometimes mean moving away from the convenient packs of combined oestrogen and progestogen and prescribing the two hormones separately. It is particularly important that a woman on a 'tailored' dose understands when to take each component. Women on such regimens may find it easier to take the progestogen on a calendar month basis rather than on her own cyclical one, e.g. commencing the progestogen on the first day of every month.

Perseverance

You should prepare women for the fact that the first HRT regimen they try may not be the one that is most suited to them. An open mind is necessary when starting HRT and a willingness to try different treatment variations. As a practitioner you also need to be open to the woman who wants to try different regimes until she finds the one that most suits her needs.

Pre-treatment counselling

The secret to a woman's confidence in her HRT often lies in the information you offer her before she even starts it and in the way you deal with her anxieties once she is on therapy. Women want and deserve open and frank discussion before starting HRT with ample opportunity to ask questions.

Anxieties women have about HRT

Fear of cancer

The word 'hormone' can be off-putting for some women and cause them to have anxieties about how they will be affected if they take HRT. Education and information is the answer to ensure that women fully understand both the risks and benefits of HRT. The issue of breast cancer must be discussed and not avoided and the need for progestogen in the non-hysterectomized woman must be stressed.

Weight gain

Some women are anxious about taking HRT because of the fear of gaining weight. Although there may be a small fluctuation in weight initially, and certainly women may feel fuller around the breasts on HRT, there is no evidence to suggest that substantial weight increases are common with any type of HRT (Rees and Purdie, 2002).

Fertility

Some women worry that if they resume a monthly bleed, then fertility will also return.

An explanation about the mechanics of conception and of how HRT works will be helpful. Women should also be reminded that HRT is not contraceptive in its actions.

Side effects

A careful explanation of common side effects, e.g. nausea, leg aches and breast tenderness, is appreciated by most women, who would prefer to be forewarned and therefore prepared for any possible problems.

HRT is unnatural

Many people have the idea that if something is natural it must be good for you, and if it is unnatural it must be harmful. Women look to those of previous generations for whom HRT was not available, and ask 'Why do I need it and they did not?' forgetting that life expectancy and the expected quality of life in old age has improved dramatically. You could argue that the menopause is a state of hormone deficiency and that by giving HRT you are simply replacing the hormones, but to discuss whether this is natural or not is rarely helpful. Each woman should be encouraged to look at the facts for herself and then make her choice.

Bleeding

For many women, stopping the monthly periods is the only real advantage of the menopause. If a woman is to start HRT she should be prepared for the possibility of bleeding and be told when to expect it and how long it may last.

Media scares

HRT is a hot topic both for the media and for health professionals. Women are sometimes alarmed by what they read in the papers or women's magazines and simply stop their HRT, without seeking advice. It is frightening for women to read the statistics of a recent study published in a stark, sensationalized manner and unless they come for consultation, they may overestimate the risks involved. As health professionals we can try to put into perspective the data and apply them on an individual basis.

SCENARIO

Jean is 56 years old. She has recently stopped HRT after 5 years because of recent media scares, although she was generally well on HRT. She stopped gradually as she had been advised, but 5 months later was still experiencing dreadful flushes and sweats. On returning to her doctor, she was given information about alternative therapies, which she tried for 6 months. Finally, keen to return to feeling well again, she asked her doctor if she could go back on her HRT. Her doctor assessed her as being at a relatively low risk of heart disease and explained the risks to her as best he could, given current knowledge. He offered Jean a lower dose than before and within a month, Jean was feeling greatly improved. She intends to review the situation in another year, but at present is confident with her treatment and felling well again.

Sometimes this will result in a woman stopping her HRT, but in a controlled, supervised manner. On other occasions, women may be reassured enough to continue their treatment.

Monitoring and evaluation of HRT

When a woman starts any form of HRT, she wants to be sure that it is safe for her to do so and be confident that she will be adequately monitored whilst on therapy. The following baseline investigations are usually performed prior to a woman starting HRT:

◆ Height
◆ Weight
◆ Blood pressure
◆ Medical history/health assessment

These represent basic well-woman checks and ensure that there are no true contraindications to the use of HRT. Regular cervical smears and mammography should be recommended according to local policy for all women. These are not required more frequently because of HRT use.

Other investigations

Some women will require extra investigations because of a particular medical or family history.

These should be assessed on an individual basis but may include the following:

◆ Thyroid function test
◆ Clotting screens
◆ Lipid profiles
◆ Mammography
◆ FSH levels
◆ Bone densitometry.

These tests may be clinically indicated prior to starting HRT but an abnormal result will not necessarily preclude the woman from taking HRT. Treatment for the relevant condition may be initiated, followed by HRT. Some of the results, e.g. low bone density, may give a stronger indication for using HRT than for not using it.

Ongoing evaluation

Initial evaluation is generally done after 3 months on HRT or after starting a new regime. Once established on a satisfactory treatment regime, follow-up visits can be every 6–8 months. Assessments at follow-up visits will include:

◆ Weight
◆ Blood pressure
◆ Symptom assessment
◆ Assessment of side effects
◆ Monitoring of bleeding
◆ Encouraging breast awareness.

Pelvic examination

A pelvic examination may be performed prior to a woman starting HRT, but is no longer routinely performed either before starting or once on HRT unless clinically indicated (Committee of Safety of Medicines, 2001). Such indications may include:

◆ Abnormal bleeding pattern on HRT
◆ Presence of fibroids which require monitoring
◆ Presence of endometriosis
◆ Post-coital bleeding
◆ Pelvic pain.

Breast examination

The prescribing doctor may perform a breast examination if clinically indicated, but it is not routinely recommended (Committee on Safety of Medicines, 2001). All women are advised to attend the National Breast Screening Programme every three years from the age of 50 to 70 years, whether or not they are on HRT.

Who should monitor?

As with many areas of medicine, preparing a woman for HRT and monitoring her whilst she takes it, has in the past been the responsibility of doctors, either general practitioners or consultants. As nurses widen their roles, particularly in the community, it is becoming more common for women to turn to them for help and advice about well-woman and menopause-related issues. Nurses are already running health promotion clinics, and advice and care at the time of the menopause could be incorporated into these. For some nurses, the role of nurse practitioner will encompass health at the menopause. However, you must ensure the following:

◆ Education provision for the nurse
◆ Supervision and support from the GP
◆ Willingness to work as a team by both GP and nurse
◆ Consistency of information among team members.

Areas in which nurses are most likely to be involved are:

◆ Health assessment
◆ Information and explanations about HRT
◆ Information about non-hormonal therapies
◆ Answering specific enquiries, especially by telephone
◆ Organizing a specific clinic
◆ Providing literature and recommending books/videos
◆ Liaising with self-help groups
◆ Monitoring of women who are established on any therapy

◆ Discussing menopausal health issues unrelated to HRT.

It is important that you make it as easy as possible for women to ask questions once on HRT. Appointments may be busy but a helpline will ensure that those women with anxieties are dealt with speedily and in time to prevent them simply stopping their HRT. This helpline may only need to be available for a couple of hours a week, but it is very useful for women to know that if they phone at a certain time on a certain day they will receive adequate advice. In the long term this will probably reduce the number of appointments needed as many minor issues can be easily dealt with over the telephone.

Non-hormonal treatments for oestrogen-deficiency symptoms

One of the commonest questions asked by women considering the use of hormone replacement therapy is, 'Is there an alternative?' Those women who are advised against HRT for medical reasons seek other ways of relieving acute menopausal symptoms. Other women see HRT only as a 'last resort' and would prefer to use anything but HRT to help symptoms. Some view taking HRT as failure to cope with life, believing that if they live a healthy, positive lifestyle, then they should not need it. However, women soon find that menopausal symptoms are non-discriminatory and even the woman with the healthiest lifestyle and strongest positive attitude may get unpleasant menopausal symptoms. The ability to cope with the symptoms may vary and some women will turn to HRT much sooner than others, whilst a few women will persevere with all sorts of other therapies before eventually turning to HRT. Many women will never need HRT, successfully coping with symptoms in other ways.

There have been few large studies to evaluate the success or otherwise of non-hormonal treatments, particularly alternative therapies which are becoming so widely talked about and tried by women. Reports are therefore often anecdotal rather than scientific and we can only suggest to women that they try them with an open mind. Menopausal symptoms have been demonstrated to have a strong placebo response to any treatment so a woman needs to try a therapy for quite a while to be sure of its long-term effectiveness. Some would argue that even a placebo effect is worthwhile if it improves quality of life for a while without being harmful. Some non-hormonal treatments are aimed more at assisting the woman to cope with her symptoms, rather than actually curing them. For many women this is sufficient to substantially improve quality of life.

Short-term symptom relief

Each symptom needs assessment individually and treatment offered accordingly. Clonidine may be offered for relief of hot flushes but results are conflicting (Eden, 2000); vaginal lubricants are for vaginal discomfort and sedatives for sleep problems. Obviously these do not treat the underlying cause but may achieve good symptom control at least in the short term. Oil of evening primrose is widely quoted as being useful for menopausal symptoms although scientific evidence is not conclusive. Other therapies that have been suggested for relief of menopausal symptoms are (see also Chapter 4):

◆ Herbal remedies, e.g. black cohosh
◆ Acupuncture
◆ Aromatherapy
◆ Reflexology
◆ Shiatsu
◆ T'ai Chi
◆ Yoga
◆ Phytoestrogens
◆ Natural progesterone cream
◆ Homeopathy.

Coping strategies
Some women discover ways of coping with their symptoms, particularly vasomotor symptoms, which enable them to continue a normal life. These include:

◆ Wearing several layers of light clothing which can be easily removed

- Reducing caffeine/alcohol intake
- Showering frequently and avoiding hot baths
- Avoiding 'trigger' foods such as spices and curries
- Cutting down on smoking
- Opening plenty of windows
- Avoiding stressful situations where possible
- Wearing a lightweight towelling dressing gown in bed to help absorb perspiration and reduce the need to change sheets so frequently.

Some women also find that relaxation techniques, stress management and counselling may help in coping with symptoms and also in coming to terms with this transitional life phase.

At the time of the menopause, many women take the opportunity to re-evaluate their lifestyle, perhaps making adjustments to their habits related to smoking, diet and exercise.

Whatever a woman decides about whether to take HRT or not, it is important that she realizes that these 'natural' therapies may not be totally free from drawbacks themselves and that although her symptoms may improve, she should not assume that she is also benefiting her skeletal, cardiovascular and urogenital systems.

Phytoestrogens

Phytoestrogens are naturally occurring oestrogen-like substances, contained in foods such as soya products and linseed. A high dietary intake of phytoestrogens has been associated with a lower incidence of menopausal symptoms and a decreased incidence of diseases such as breast and colon cancer as well as atherosclerotic disease (Mackey and Eden, 1998). The link has been made partly because the incidence of these so-called 'Western diseases' is higher in countries where a Western diet has been adopted. In parts of the world where phytoestrogens are an integral part of the diet, the incidence of such diseases is lower (Parkin, 1989; Oldenhave and Netelenbos, 1994). Research into phytoestrogens in relation to menopause has been promising, with evidence that they may help reduce or relieve menopausal hot flushes (Mackey and Eden, 1998).

Women can increase their dietary intake of phytoestrogens (the best known are isoflavones and lignans) through foods such as linseed, sunflower seeds, sesame seeds, nuts, tofu and through soya products. Alternatively, dietary supplements are available in health food shops, e.g. Red Clover, Estroven and others.

Osteoporosis and cardiovascular disease

Other factors that influence the rate of osteoporosis and heart disease should be considered. These include:

- *Exercise* This is beneficial to the whole body, leading to a general feeling of well-being and improved physical strength and suppleness. Beneficial to both the cardiovascular system and to the skeleton
- *Diet* A good, varied diet is necessary to maintain a healthy body. Recommendations include low total fat intake, low sugar intake, low salt intake, increased fibre intake, good calcium intake. Calcium is an essential part of a balanced diet and women are particularly encouraged to think about this at the time of the menopause. Most women who take a healthy diet probably achieve a good calcium intake, but those women who have a restricted dairy intake may need supplements
- *Lifestyle* Reducing alcohol intake and cutting back on smoking will help to promote good health. Cigarette smoking in particular is known to be harmful to the cardiovascular system and women who are serious about improving their health should stop smoking.

Other medications

Alternative drug therapies are available for the treatment or prevention of osteoporosis:

- *Calcitonin* This is given as an injection and as a nasal spray. It has some analgesic properties and is generally used for treatment, not prevention, of osteoporosis

◆ *Bisphosphonates* This is a group of medications which works on bone in a similar way to HRT. Most commonly available as tablets, either daily or once weekly, they are occasionally administered intravenously

◆ *Progestogen alone* This cannot be described as 'non-hormonal' but is useful for those women who cannot take HRT for medical reasons (see page 468)

◆ *Selective estrogen receptor modulators (SERMs)*, e.g. Raloxifene, are compounds that act on oestrogen receptors in the body to display oestrogen-like effects on the bone and on lipids without stimulating the endometrium or the breast. They are therefore said to have a 'selective' action (Delmas *et al.*, 1997). Raloxifene is licensed for the prevention and treatment of vertebral osteoporosis. Side effects are minimal, with some women experiencing mild hot flushes. The risk of venous thromboembolism is similar to that associated with HRT use. Initial studies of Raloxifene have shown a favourable effect on breast tissue (Cummings *et al.*, 1999)

◆ *Teriparatide* This acts to generate new bone by anabolic action (i.e. bone building). It is administered once daily by injection, increasing bone strength and reducing risk of fracture (Neer, 2001).

It is helpful to point out to women that whilst lifestyle changes are important they may not be of sufficient value to fully replace the benefits of therapeutic interventions. A healthy lifestyle is always to be encouraged but we must ensure that we do not lead women to think that this alone is an effective alternative to medical treatment.

Other factors that influence a woman at the climacteric

The menopause is a time in a woman's life when her body undergoes immense physical change. The consequences can be long lasting and can affect how she copes with other stresses which may arise at around the same time. It is all too easy to blame the menopause for every physical and emotional upset which occurs at around the age of 50. This would be wrong, but it is true that areas of a woman's life with which she has always coped successfully can suddenly become difficult to manage. Some women find life at the time of the menopause to be one of great change, whilst others find life continues as normal. Whether the physical effects of a changing body lead to the woman feeling less able to cope, or whether the emotional upsets appear to make physical symptoms worse, is unclear. Nevertheless, the woman, her problems and her hormones must be viewed together rather than in isolation from each other. Some women will need treatments and therapies other than HRT in order to help them cope with some aspects of their lives. Some problems that arise around mid-life will be better treated by these other therapies than by simple HRT.

Changing body image

It is an unfair fact of life that society accepts the concept of a youthful figure as one for which to be constantly strived. In the UK women spend large sums of money trying to keep slim, with no wrinkles and youthful-looking hair. The cosmetics industry would have us believe that this is not only desirable but also essential for the modern lifestyle. Both men and women need to accept that our bodies do change as we get older. Fat distribution changes, metabolic rate slows down and skin and hair may lose their youthful texture.

A change in how women view their body image is therefore required from women around mid-life if they are to come to terms with their changing bodies. This does not mean that women should resign themselves to being overweight and unattractive but they may need to make more effort to keep to the same weight. Extra exercise will be necessary to firm up sagging muscles and lifestyle changes become more pertinent at this time. The menopause occurs at a similar time to these other body changes and women tend to blame their hormones alone for all these changes.

Relationships

Mid-life can be a time when women re-evaluate the things that are important to them. Marriages that have become stale, relationships that are faltering may be re-assessed and decisions made about the future. Women sometimes take the opportunity to discuss issues that have remained unspoken for many years. Relationships with children can become confrontational as teenagers become more rebellious and independent.

Failed dreams

Some women look upon the time of the menopause as a landmark in their lives and a time to evaluate their life. They may be disappointed that they have not achieved all that they had hoped for. Perhaps they did not succeed at work as they had expected. Maybe they did not have the longed-for children and the menopause has finally closed that door. Sometimes the disappointment may lie with their partner, the promotions that were never realized and the expectations that were not met.

Ageing parents

Some women expect the menopause to signify a time when they will be free of some of their previous responsibilities, particularly if children are getting older and more independent. It can therefore come as a shock to realize that their own parents or those of their partner are becoming more dependent on them. Women may find themselves the unpaid carer, leading to feelings of frustration and sometimes resentment that their own freedom has been restricted.

'Empty nest'

The so-called 'empty nest syndrome' can occur in women who have dedicated their lives to the upbringing of their children to the exclusion of their own independence. When the children leave home it leaves a gap which is hard to fill. With more and more women having responsibilities both inside and outside the home, this phenomenon seems to be lessening. Indeed many women cannot wait for the last child to fly the nest!

Sexuality

Some women view the menopause as being the culmination of fertile years. The ability to bear children was a driving force behind sexual satisfaction and once fertility declines, new desires and expectations must be met. Women may feel less attractive and therefore consider themselves less desirable to their partner. For others, the freedom from the need for contraception can be a release and sexual relationships improve. For some, the stability of a longstanding relationship represents freedom for sexual expression, whilst for others it can lead to feelings of boredom and frustration. Physical symptoms of the menopause such as vaginal dryness may lead to sexual frustrations as women try to avoid painful and uncomfortable intercourse, as well as emotional upsets.

Fear of death

For some, the menopause may mark the beginning of old age. Fear of getting older and of death in particular may influence how they feel. Attitudes to ageing vary from individual to individual and it is important that we consider this when discussing mid-life problems and the menopause. For some, the menopause prompts a sad realization that life is getting shorter and that old age, and ultimately death, are inevitable.

Work

In a society that values youth, it is easy for a woman to feel undervalued in the workplace despite her greater experience. Finding a job in her fifties is much more difficult than in younger years, even though she may be better qualified for the job than some younger applicants. Some women find that symptoms of the menopause cause them to give up a job because they feel less able to cope with difficult situations, a decision they may then regret when their symptoms subside, only to discover that it is not easy to find work again.

Contraception at the peri-menopause

For many women, a real advantage of the menopause is that the fertile years are over and concerns about contraception can be forgotten. A freedom from these anxieties can lead to a renewed sexual enthusiasm and greater satisfaction within a relationship. Whilst one must appreciate that for some women, particularly the childless, this end of fertility marks a sad disappointment that children will not now be born, for others the relief that contraception can stop can be just as great.

Yet some women do not realize the point at which fertility stops is very difficult to pinpoint and, in theory, can only be done retrospectively. Fertility begins to decline during the late thirties continuing into the forties. Women may consider themselves infertile during the peri-menopausal phase when in fact they could still conceive. With the well-known physical risks attached to pregnancy in older women and the psychological trauma this can bring, it is particularly important that you counsel women appropriately about the ongoing need for contraception at this time.

The current Family Planning Association (FPA) recommendations are that contraception should continue in women over 50 years until they have not had a period for 1 year. Women under the age of 50 should continue using contraception for 2 years after their last period. The FPA recommendations are easily understood for those women who do not start HRT, but because HRT often causes bleeding to continue or to resume, the actual last period can be masked. This means that advising a woman when to stop contraception can at best only be a guide. HRT cannot be considered to be contraceptive, so some women will need to consider a change of contraception at this time.

The pill or contraceptive patch and the menopause

If a woman is using the combined oral contraceptive pill then she is unlikely to notice menopausal symptoms as the levels of oestrogen in the pill will be controlling them. They may, however, be noticed in the pill-free week. Regular bleeds are likely to continue and the last physiological period will be masked. Healthy, non-smoking women, who are of normal weight and normotensive, may continue using the combined pill until the age of 50 years, providing that they are considered to be at a low risk of thrombosis and heart disease (Gebbie, 2003). In the light of recommendations from the Committee on Safety of Medicines (1995), it is particularly important that women are carefully assessed before continuing to use the combined pill. Women themselves must be informed of the small risk of thrombosis when considering the risks and benefits (Mills *et al.*, 1996).

Those women who decide to come off the pill may find either that their periods return, in which case they can follow the usual FPA guidelines and use contraception for a further 1 or 2 years after they stop, or that their periods have stopped. Measurement of FSH levels on two or three occasions over a 6-month period can confirm that the menopause has occurred. Alternative contraception should be used whilst awaiting confirmation of FSH levels.

The progestogen-only pill

Use of the progestogen-only pill will not usually mask menopausal symptoms, although bleeding patterns may be unpredictable. Amenorrhoea should not be assumed to indicate that the menopause has occurred. Measurement of FSH levels on several occasions can help to give an indication of menopausal status. Occasionally the progestogen-only pill is prescribed alongside conventional HRT. Theoretically this should be contraceptive, but no studies have been carried out to confirm that the mini-pill continues its effect alongside exogenous oestrogen. Women who stop the progestogen-only pill and go straight on to HRT will not know when their last period occurs.

Depot progestogens

The main drawback of this method is its irreversibility and long-lasting effect. Menopausal symptoms can occur and if oestrogen therapy is required irregular bleeding can result. In practice this method is rarely used by peri-menopausal women, particularly those wanting HRT.

Intrauterine devices and HRT

Women can continue using modern IUDs until the time of the menopause. An IUD inserted from the age of 40 years onwards need not be replaced unless it causes problems, and can simply be removed after the menopause (Gebbie, 2003). One disadvantage is that if the IUD is left *in situ* for the recommended 1 or 2 years after the last bleed, it may be more difficult to remove than if a woman were still menstruating because of stenosis of the cervical os. The levonorgestrel releasing system (Mirena) is often ideal for the peri-menopausal woman.

Sterilization

Sterilization of one or other partner is a very secure way of preventing a pregnancy. It is unlikely, however, that a couple would choose this method at a time close to the menopause, because of the need for surgery. Sterilization at an earlier age will have no effect on the woman's subsequent menopause.

Natural methods of family planning

It is not recommended that women rely on natural methods of family planning around the time of the menopause. Irregular periods and changing vaginal and cervical mucus will make these methods unreliable.

Barrier methods

Barrier methods, such as the condom, cap and spermicides provide an effective method of contraception at the peri-menopause. They will not alter menstrual pattern and will not influence symptoms of the menopause. If a couple are already familiar with the use of cap or condoms it is relatively easy to continue using them. It may be more difficult for those women who have not been used to barrier methods to start at this time. The decline in fertility leading up to the menopause means that those methods that might be considered unreliable in younger women, such as spermicides used alone, will probably offer sufficient protection for this group of women. Barrier methods are easily stopped when contraception is no longer required.

The issue of contraception is one that must be discussed alongside advice about HRT. Some women think that HRT will act as a contraceptive and the consequences of such a belief could be disastrous for that individual. The question of when to stop using contraception is much more difficult to answer and will vary from woman to woman. If the actual date of the menopause is not known, only an arbitrary guess can be made as to when to stop contraception. To be on the safe side, some would say this should be continued to the age of 55 years (Gebbie, 2003).

Future developments

Newer compounds

It is likely that newer drugs which mimic oestrogen and progestogen will be investigated in an attempt to reduce risk, minimize side effects and enhance overall health benefits.

More low-dose treatments

With the trend towards using shorter regimens of HRT at a lower dose, we may see doses of oestrogen therapy becoming even lower than are currently used.

Testosterone patches and gels

These are available for use in men. We may see them being developed as an adjunct to HRT for some women.

Intrauterine progestogens

With the development of the intrauterine system, Mirena, for contraceptive use, we may see smaller devices being developed specifically for use with HRT.

'Natural' alternatives

As more studies are completed, we may have a clearer idea of the risks and benefits of natural or complementary therapies. More products are becoming available for women to purchase and evaluation of them is required on the basis of evidence accumulated.

Conclusion

HRT is a rapidly changing field and one in which there is great deal of scientific controversy. Whilst a greater variety of regimens and products are available, there is still a need for more research. Women are becoming more informed about alternative ways of alleviating symptoms and our emphasis should be on ensuring a healthy life around the time of the menopause and into the years beyond. At the lowest effective dose, HRT may be part of the picture for some women and it falls to us as health professionals to ensure that these women receive safe and appropriate treatments.

Ideas for personal and professional development

● Think about symptoms that women commonly experience at the time of the menopause. With a colleague, choose three and consider how each of the symptoms might affect your life at home or at work, if you experienced them

● Find out where your local menopause clinic is and how women access their services. What support do they offer to women and how would women access it?

● Visit a local health food shop and list some of the products available for women to buy at the time of the menopause. Choose one or two and consider how much they cost and what evidence they claim to have for their use

● Consider how you would prepare a woman for HRT. Plan an information sheet for women covering the points you consider to be important.

Patient education points

● The menopause is a natural event; women sometimes need help and information to understand therapy options and make appropriate choices

● HRT encompasses a wide variety of products and women may need to try more than one to find one that suits

● The decision to take HRT is individual and the risks and benefits of HRT will not be identical for all women. A personal health assessment is essential before starting HRT

● The menopause commonly occurs around the time of mid-life and it is common for factors other than just your hormones to influence how you feel

● A premature menopause (under 40 years) is considered differently to one occurring at the so-called normal age and you may be offered treatment for longer than a woman in her fifties.

Resources

Amarant Trust Helpline
Helpline: 01293 413000 (11 am–6 pm Mon–Fri)
www.amarantmenopausetrust.org.uk

British Menopause Society
4–6 Eton Place, Marlow, Bucks SL7 2QA
Tel: 01628 890199
www.the-bms.org

Daisy Network
PO Box 183, Rossendale BB4 6WZ
www.daisynetwork.org.uk
Premature menopause information and support.

Hysterectomy Association
Aynsley House, Chester Gardens, Church Gresley, Swadlincote DE11 9PU
www.hysterectomy-association.org.uk

Institute of Psychosexual Medicine
11 Chandos Street, London W1G 9DR

Tel: 020 580 0631
www.ipm.org.uk

National Osteoporosis Society
Camerton, Bath
Tel: 01761 471771
www.nos.org.uk
Please enclose SAE.

**Natural Progesterone Information
Service**
PO Box 24, Buxton SK17 9FB

Relate
Herbert Gray College, Little Church Street,
Rugby, Warwickshire CV21 3AP
Tel: 01788 573241
www.relate.org.uk

Women's Health Concern
PO Box 2126, Marlow, Bucks SL7 2NB
Tel: 01628 483612
Please enclose SAE.
www.womens-health-concern.org

Women's Nutritional Advisory Service
PO Box 268, Lewes, East Sussex BN7 2QN
www.wnas.org.uk

Other useful websites

www.menopause-online.com
www.menopause.org
www.hormone.org
www.menopausematters.co.uk

Further reading

ABERNETHY, K. (2001) *The Menopause and HRT*, 2nd edn. London: Baillière Tindall.
HOPE, S., REES, M. and BROCKIE, J. (eds) (1999) *Hormone Replacement Therapy: A Guide for Primary Care*. Oxford: Oxford University Press.
REES, M. and PURDIE, D. (eds) (2002). *Management of the Menopause, Handbook of the British Menopause Society*. Marlow: BMS Publications.
REES, M., PURDIE, D. and HOPE, S. (2003) *The Menopause – What You Need To Know*. Marlow: BMS Publications.
SHEEHY, G. (1993) *The Silent Passage*. London: Harper Collins.
SINGER, D. and HUNTER, M. (eds) (2000) *Premature Menopause – A Multidisciplinary Approach*. London: Whurr Publishers.
STEWART, M. (1998) *The Phyto Factor*. London: Vermillion.

References

ANASTI, N. (1998) Premature ovarian failure: an update. *Fertility and Sterility* **70**:1–15.
ANASTI, J.N., KALANTARIDOU, S.N., KIMZEY, L.M. *et al.* (1998) Bone loss in young women with karyotypically normal spontaneous premature ovarian failure. *Obstetrics and Gynaecology* **91**:12–15.
BALLINGER, C.B. (1975) Psychiatric morbidity and the menopause: screening of general population sample. *British Medical Journal* **3**:344.
BARRETT-CONNOR, E. (1997) Sex differences in coronary heart disease. Why are women so superior? The 1995 Acel Keys Lecture. *Circulation* **95**:252–64.
BARRETT-CONNOR, E., WEHREN, L.E., SIRIS, E.S. *et al.* (2003) Recency and duration of postmenopausal hormone therapy: effects on bone mineral density and fracture risk in the National Osteoporosis Risk Assessment (NORA) Study. *Menopause* **10**(5):412–19.
BERGER, H.G., DUDLEY, E.C., HOPPER, J.L. *et al.* (1995) The endocrinology of the menopause transition: a cross-sectional study of a population based sample. *Journal of Clinical Endocrinology and Metabolism* **80**:3537–45.
BRITISH MENOPAUSE SOCIETY CONSENSUS STATE-MENT ON HRT (2003) Managing the menopause: Writing Group for the British Menopause Society Council. *Journal of the British Menopause Society* **9**(3):129–32.
BRITISH MENOPAUSE SOCIETY STATEMENT (2003). December. www.the-bms.org.uk.
CARDOZO, L. (1990) Oestrogen deficiency and the bladder. In Drife, J.O. and Studd, J.W.W. (eds) *HRT and Osteoporosis*. London: Springer-Verlag, p. 57.
COLDITZ, G.A., WILLETT, W.C., STAMPFER, M.J. *et al.* (1987) Menopause and the risk of coronary heart disease in women. *New England Journal of Medicine* **316**:1105.
COLLABORATIVE GROUP ON HORMONAL FACTORS IN BREAST CANCER (1997) Breast cancer and hormone replacement therapy: collaborative reanalysis of data from 51 epidemiological studies of 52,705 women with breast cancer and 108,411 women without breast cancer. *Lancet* **350**:1047–59.
COMMITTEE ON SAFETY OF MEDICINES (1995) Combined oral contraception and thromboembolus (letter). London: CSM.
COMMITTEE ON SAFETY OF MEDICINES (2001) Working Group Report: Breast and pelvic examination in women taking hormone replacement therapy. London: CSM.
COMMITTEE ON SAFETY OF MEDICINES (2003) Further advice on safety of HRT: risk/benefit unfavourable for first line use in prevention of osteoporosis. London: CSM.
COOPER, G.S., SANDLER, D.P. and BOHLIE, M. (1999) Active and passive smoking and the occurrence of natural menopause. *Epidemiology* **10**: 771–3.
CUMMINGS, S.R., BLACK, D.M. and RUBIN, S.M. (1989). Lifetime risk of hip, colles or vertebral fracture and coronary heart disease among white postmenopausal women. *Archives of Internal Medicine* **149**:2445–8.
CUMMINGS, S.R., ECKERT, S., KRUEGER, K.A. *et al.* (1999) The effect of Raloxifene on risk of breast cancer in postmenopausal women. Results from the MORE randomised trial. *Journal of the American Medical Association* **281**(23):2189–97.

DALY, E., VESSEY, M.P., HAWKINS, M.M. *et al.* (1996) Risk of venous thromboembolism in users of hormone replacement therapy. *Lancet* **348**:977–80.

DELMAS, P.D., BJARNASON, N.H., MITLAK, B.H. *et al.* (1997) Effects of Raloxifene on bone mineral density, serum cholesterol and uterine endometrium in postmenopausal women. *New England Journal of Medicine* **337**:1641–7.

DEMPSTER, D.W., SHANE, E., HORBERT, W. and LINDSAY, R. (1986) A simple method for correlative scanning electron microscopy of human ileac crest biopsies. *American Journal of Bone Mineral Research* **1**(1):15–21.

DEVISSAGUET, J.-Ph., BRION, N., LHOTE, O. *et al.* (1999) Pulsed estrogen therapy: pharmokinetics of intranasal 17B estradiol in postmenopausal women and comparison with oral and transdermal formulations. *European Journal of Drug Metabolism and Pharmokinetics* **24**(3):265–71.

DRINKWATER, B.L., NILSON, K., CHESHUNT, C.H. *et al.* (1984) Bone mineral content of amenorrheic and eumenorrheic atheletes. *New England Journal of Medicine* **311**:277.

EASTELL, R. (1999) Treatment of postmenopausal osteoporosis. *New England Journal of Medicine* **338**:736–46.

EDEN, J. (2000) Managing menopausal symptoms after breast cancer. In Studd, J.W.W. (ed.) *The Management of the Menopause: The Millennium Review*. London: Parthenon, pp. 221–4.

ELLERINGTON, M.C. and STEVENSON, J.C. (1993) *Osteoporosis, Questions and Answers*. Kingston, UK: Merit Communications.

GANGAR, K. and KEY, E. (1993) Individualising HRT. *Practitioner* **237**(1525):358.

GANGAR, K., CUST, M. and WHITEHEAD, M. (1989) Symptoms of oestrogen deficiency associated with supraphysiological levels of plasma oestradiol concentrations in women with oestradiol implants. *British Medical Journal* **299**:601.

GEBBIE, A. (2003). Contraception in the peri-menopause. *Journal of the British Menopause Society* **9**(3):123–8.

GRADY, D., GREBETSADIK, T., KARLIKOWSKE, K., EMOKE, V. and PETITTI, D. (1995) HRT and endometrial cancer risk: a meta analysis. *Obstetrics and Gynecology* **85**:304–13.

HILLARD, T.C., WHITCROFT, S., ELLERINGTON, M.C. *et al.* (1991) The long term risks and benefits of HRT. *Journal of Clinical Pharmacology and Therapeutics* **16**:231.

HILTON, P. and STANTON, S.L. (1983) The use of intravaginal oestrogen creams in genuine stress incontinence. *British Journal of Obstetrics and Gynaecology* **90**:940.

HU, F.B., GRODSTEIN, F., HENNEKENS, C.H. *et al.* (1999) Age at natural menopause and risk of cardiovascular disease. *Archives of Internal Medicine* **159**:1061–6.

HUI, S.L., SLAMENDA, C.W. and JOHNSTONE, C.C. (1988) Age and bone mass as predictors of fracture in a prospective study. *Journal of Clinical Investigation* **81**:1804.

JICK, H., DERBY, L., MYERS, M.W. *et al.* (1996) Risk of hospital admission for idiopathic venous thromboembolism among users of postmenopausal oestrogens. *Lancet* **348**:981–3.

KANIS, J.A. (1994) *Osteoporosis*. London: Blackwell Science.

KANIS, J.A. (1996) Estrogens, the menopause and osteoporosis. *Bone* **19**(Suppl):185–90.

KESSLAK, J.P. (2002) Can estrogen play a significant role in the prevention of Alzheimer's disease? *Journal of Neural Transmission* **62**(Suppl):227–39.

LINDSAY, R., HART, D.M. and CLARK, D.M. (1984) The minimum effective dose of estrogen for prevention of postmenopausal bone loss. *Obstetrics Gynaecology* **63**:759–63.

MACKEY, R. and EDEN, J. (1998) Phytoestrogens. *Journal of the British Menopause Society* **4**:18–23.

MACLENNAN, A., LESTER, S. and MOORE, V. (2001) Oral estrogen replacement therapy versus placebo for hot flushes: a systematic review. *Climacteric* **4**(1):58–74.

McKINLAY, S.M., BRAMBILLA, D.J. and POSNER, J.G. (1992) The normal menopause transition. *Maturitas* **14**:103–15.

MILLER, P.D. (2003) Bone mineral density – clinical use and application. *Endocrinology and Metabolism Clinics of North America* **32**(1):159–79, vii.

MILLION WOMEN STUDY COLLABORATORS (2003) Breast cancer and hormone replacement therapy in the Million Women Study. *Lancet* **362**:419–27.

MILLS, A.M., WILKINSON, C.L., BROMHAM, D.R. *et al.* (1996) Guidelines for prescribing combined oral contraceptives (letter). *British Medical Journal* **312**:121.

MONTGOMERY, J.C. and STUDD, J.W.W. (1991) Psychological and sexual aspects of the menopause. *British Journal of Hospital Medicine* **45**:300.

MOORE, R.A. (1999) Livial: a review of clinical studies. *British Journal of Obstetrics and Gynaecology* **106**(Suppl 19):1–21.

NEER, R.M. (2001) Effect of parathyroid hormone on fractures and bone mineral density in postmenopausal women with osteoporosis. *New England Journal of Medicine* **344**:1434–41.

NILAS, L. and CHRISTIANSEN, C. (1988) Rates of bone loss in normal women: evidence of accelerated trabecular bone loss after the menopause. *European Journal of Clinical Investigation* **18**:529.

OLDENHAVE, A. and NETELENBOS, C. (1994) Pathogenesis of climacteric complaints: ready for the change? *Lancet* **342**:649–53.

OLIVER, M.F. and BOYD, G.S. (1959) Effect of bilateral ovariectomy on coronary artery disease and serum lipid levels. *Lancet* **ii**:690.

OPCS (Office of Population Censuses and Surveys) (2002) *Mortality Statistics: Cause of Death England and Wales*. London: HMSO.

PARKIN, D.M. (1989) Cancers of the breast, endometrium and ovary: geographical correlations. *European Journal of Cancer and Clinical Oncology* **25**:1917–25.

REES, M. (1996) HRT and the endometrium. *Journal of the British Menopause Society* **2**(2):23–5.

REES, M. and PURDIE, D. (eds) (2002) *Management of the Menopause, Handbook of the British Menopause Society*. Marlow: BMS Publications.

ROSENBERG, L., HENNEKENS, C.H., ROSNER, B. *et al.* (1981) Early menopause and the risk of myocardial infarction. *American Journal of Obstetrics and Gynecology* **139**:47.

ROYAL COLLEGE OF OBSTETRICIANS AND GYNAE-COLOGISTS (1999). HRT and venous thromboembolism guidelines, No 19. London: RCOG.

ROYAL COLLEGE OF PHYSICIANS OF EDINBURGH (2003) Consensus Conference Summary. Edinburgh: RCP.

RYMER, J., ROBINSON, J. and FOGELMAN, I. (2001) Effect of 8 years of treatment with Tibolone 2.5 mg daily on postmenopausal bone loss. *Osteoporosis International* **12**:478–83.

SHERWIN, B.B. and GELFLAND, M.M. (1985) Differential symptom response to parenteral oestrogen and/or androgen administration in the surgical menopause. *American Journal of Obstetrics and Gynecology* **151**:153.

SIDDLE, N., SARRELL, P. and WHITEHEAD, M.L. (1987) The effect of hysterectomy on the age of ovarian failure: identification of a subgroup of women with premature loss of ovarian function. *Fertility and Sterility* **47**:94.

SLAMENDER, C.W., HUI, S.L., LONGSCOPE, C., WELLMAN, H. and JOHNSTONE, C.C. (1990) Predictors of bone mass in perimenopausal women. A prospective study of clinical data using photon absorptiometry. *Annals of Internal Medicine* **112**:96–101.

STEVENSON, J.C. (1996) Handling hormone replacement therapy: key issues for the prescriber. *European Journal of Obstetrics, Gynecology, and Reproductive Biology* **64**(Suppl):S25–7.

STEVENSON, J.C., LEES, B., FIELDING, C. *et al.* (1990) Exercise and the skeleton. In Smith, R. (ed.) *Osteoporosis.* London: RCP.

STEWART, A., TORGERSON, D.J. and REID, D.M. (1996) Prediction of fracture in perimenopausal women: a comparison of dual energy x-ray absorptiometry and ultrasound attenuation. *Annals of Rheumatological Diseases* **55**:140–2.

STUDD, J.W.W. *et al.* (1999) Efficacy and acceptability of intranasal 17B oestradiol for menopausal symptoms: randomised dose response study. *Lancet* **353**:1574–8.

STUDD, J.W.W., WATSON, N.R. and HENDERSON, A. (1990) Symptoms and metabolic sequelae of the menopause. In Drife, J.O. and Studd, J.W.W. (eds) *Hormone Replacement Therapy and Osteoporosis.* London: Springer-Verlag, pp. 23–4.

STURDEE, D. (ed.) (1993) *Managing The Menopause II.* London: Fusion Communications.

SUHONEN, S.P., ALLONEN, H.O. and LAHTEEMAKI, P. (1995) Sustained-release estradiol implants and a levonorgestrel-releasing intrauterine device in hormone replacement therapy. *American Journal of Obstetric Gynecology* **2**:562–7.

TROISI, R., SCHAIRER, C., CHOW, W.-H. *et al.* (1997) A prospective study of menopausal hormones and risk of colorectal cancer (United States). *Cancer Causes Control* **8**:130–8.

WHI (WRITING GROUP FOR THE WOMEN'S HEALTH INITIATIVE INVESTIGATORS) (2002) Risks and benefits of estrogen plus progestin in healthy postmenopausal women: principal results from the Women's Health Initiative randomised controlled trial. *Journal of the American Medical Association* **288**:321–33.

WHI (WOMEN'S HEALTH INITIATIVE STEERING COMMITTEE) (2004) Effects of conjugated equine oestrogen in post-menopausal women with hysterectomy. The WHI randomised controlled trial. *Journal of the American Medical Association* **291**:1701-12.

17: Continence Issues

Mary Dolman

OBJECTIVES

This chapter should help you understand:

◆ Urinary incontinence and its relationship to female sexuality ◆

◆ How incontinence can affect the quality of life of healthy women ◆

◆ Whether hormones affect urinary incontinence ◆

◆ How to inform women about how self-help can ameliorate the symptoms of incontinence ◆

◆ How to encourage women to seek early treatment by informing them of conservative treatments and discuss the surgical options. ◆

Introduction

Being incontinent makes me feel I am no longer a woman. I feel as though I have lost my femininity.

These words were said by a young woman during an assessment at the continence clinic. This is not an isolated case and similar expressions are heard all too frequently.

During the last decade more has been acknowledged and researched on the subject of incontinence and its effect on sexuality, but nurses often fail to recognize that this symptom can be a real problem to women at any age. Dorey (2003) points out 'some women fake an orgasm to keep their partner happy'. Incontinence during sexual activity most usually occurs during penetration or at orgasm. It is not known how common this is so it is not surprising that it is difficult to investigate. However, in a survey by Dolman (1995), 13.5% of the sample ($n = 155$) indicated leakage during sexual intercourse.

While assessing women at a continence clinic, nurses have an opportunity to ask if they experience dyspareunia. This is an excellent way to introduce the subject of incontinence during intercourse without asking a direct question. It may be difficult for a woman to talk about this problem and you should provide the opportunity and give appropriate prompts to make such a discussion possible. One woman attending my clinic admitted that she leaked during orgasm, but related that she had solved the problem by never allowing herself to have an orgasm.

What causes urinary incontinence during sexual activity is unknown, but it is thought that mechanical pressure as in penetration of the penis (Hilton, 1988) or a detrusor contraction underlie the problem. Sometimes treatment for a diagnosed overactive bladder will cure the problem, but reassurance that the symptom has no pathological significance is needed along with advice on how to possibly avoid the problem in future, e.g. by emptying the bladder before sexual intercourse and thinking positive rather negative thoughts.

When women are too embarrassed to talk to their partner about urinary incontinence during intercourse they make endless excuses for avoiding sex. It can sometimes lead to a breakdown of the relationship. Wet bedclothes and the fear of odour lead to such anxieties that intimate moments are avoided.

Incidence of urinary incontinence in women

Prevalence studies have been well documented (RCP, 1995; Thomas *et al.*, 1980; Norton, 1990) but the results vary according to the type of incontinence and age of the sample. However, it has been estimated that 1 in 4 women experience urinary incontinence varying from mild to severe leakage sometime in their life. One of the difficulties for accurate reporting of the symptom is the fact that many women are too embarrassed or ashamed to mention it. Recently the subject has gained more publicity in women's magazines and other media, and incontinence has even been mentioned in the 'soaps'! This has helped women realize that they are not alone with such a symptom, that treatment should be sought early and that surgery is not the only answer to the problem. For the last decade there has been a much greater awareness of how bladder/bowel problems can be assessed and treated. Campaigns organized by the Continence Foundation and pharmaceutical companies have helped in this, and the internet has a plethora of information.

The so-called 'taboo' subject of urinary incontinence is now out in the open in many Western countries and you must feel confident to give advice to women in your care. This chapter provides you with the information and knowledge required to help women who may have urinary problems. It must be stressed that sexual counselling is a speciality in itself (see Chapter 5) and you must recognize your own limitations on counselling women with urinary incontinence and sexual dysfunction. After all, the incontinence may be the best excuse the woman has thought to use!

Before the 1970s the aetiology of urinary incontinence was poorly understood and women tended to put up with it as an inevitable event following childbirth. In the last 25 years bladder and bowel dysfunction has been better understood, and together with urodynamic investigations, ultrasound and other scientific studies for diagnosing bladder problems, the outlook for women with urinary incontinence has greatly improved.

Development and anatomy of the lower urinary tract

The lower urinary tract is composed of the bladder and the urethra (Figure 17.1) and has a complex nerve supply from both the sympathetic and para-sympathetic branches of the central nervous system (Figure 17.2). Urine is conveyed from the kidneys via the ureters which enter the bladder obliquely. The triangular area of the bladder bounded by the two ureteric orifices and the proximal part of the urethra (bladder neck) is known as the trigone. The bladder consists of the detrusor and trigone muscles which are composed of smooth muscle fibres. The capacity for urine storage is assured by elasticity of the detrusor

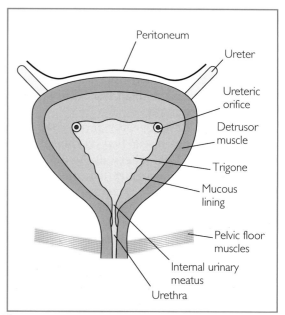

Figure 17.1 Cross-section of the female bladder.

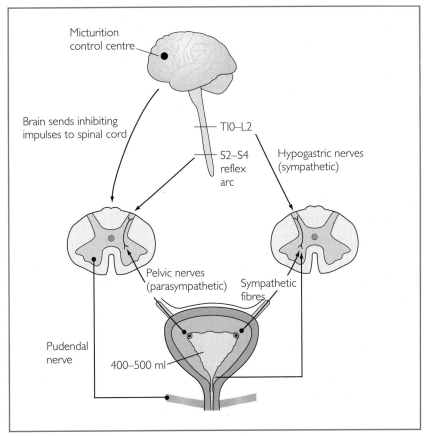

Figure 17.2 Diagram of nerve pathways to the bladder.

muscle which allows the bladder to stretch to accommodate urine with minimal increase in pressure (Mundy, 1984).

The female urethra is about 4–5 cm long and conveys urine from the bladder to the external surface of the body at the meatus. The urethra is lined by transitional cell epithelium but distally the lining becomes stratified squamous epithelium. The submucosal folds along the urethra help to provide a watertight seal for maintaining continence. The mucosal folds are sensitive to oestrogen and, when fully oestrogenized, provide the watertight seal. When there is an oestrogen deficiency at the menopause, the mucosal folds become less effective and this may contribute towards stress incontinence.

The main support for the bladder is the pelvic floor striated muscle which forms a hammock-like sling from the public bone to the coccyx known as the levator ani. This subdivides into the pubococcygeus and iliococcygeus and the ischiococcygeus muscles through which the urethra, vagina and the rectum pass (Figure 17.3).

During the embryological development of the lower urinary tract, it is important to know that by the 12th week of intrauterine life the upper bladder and lower part of the urethra have a common embryological origin with the vagina (Cardozo *et al.*, 1993). This will help you to understand the effects of oestrogen and progesterone which are discussed later in the chapter.

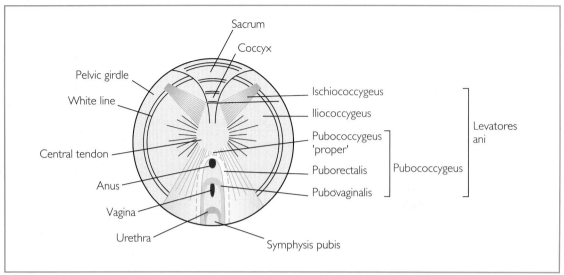

Figure 17.3 The female pelvic floor muscles viewed from above.

Physiology of micturition and continence control

According to Mundy (1984), the bladder should fill to a capacity of about 500 ml and empty at a rate of 20–25 ml/second to completion. Emptying should be under voluntary control which commences with the relaxation of the pelvic floor muscle. This allows the bladder neck to open and then the detrusor bladder muscle contracts, thus voiding begins.

The bladder can fill to 400–500 ml because the detrusor muscle does not contract until voluntary voiding begins. As a result, the pressure within the bladder stays low (less than 15 cm H_2O). This is partly due to the inherent physical properties of the bladder wall, which allow it to be stretched without causing a rise in intravesical pressure, and partly due to a neurological mechanism which prevents nervous impulses being transmitted to the bladder, thereby preventing detrusor contraction until a capacity of approximately 400–500 ml is reached.

Continence is maintained as long as (a) the bladder neck stays closed and (b) the pressure within the urethra (the intraurethral pressure) is greater than the pressure within the bladder (the

intravesical pressure). These two functions are achieved by two sphincter mechanisms:

◆ The *internal sphincter* ensures that the bladder neck only opens when the detrusor muscle contracts, regardless of any rise in pressure around the bladder, e.g. coughing, sneezing or physical activity

◆ The high urethral closure pressure below the bladder neck is maintained by the *external sphincter*. This comprises the striated muscle of the levator ani and the rhabdosphincter.

The bladder fills with urine at the rate of about 1 ml/minute by a series of ureteric, peristaltic contractions. As the bladder fills, sensory fibres send impulses from the stretch receptors in the detrusor to the sacral roots of S2, S3 and S4 (Figure 17.2). These are suppressed by unconscious inhibitions mediated from the level of the basal ganglia. As the urine volume increases, impulses are relayed up the lateral spinothalamic tracts to the cerebral cortex, bringing the desire to micturate to a conscious level. This is suppressed by the cortex until a suitable time and place has been selected for micturition.

When the correct time and place has been selected, an appropriate position is adopted and, through the organization of the frontal lobes and hypothalamus, the bladder becomes converted to an active, dynamic, well-coordinated expulsive unit. At the same time, active relaxation of the striated and smooth muscle components of the urethra causes a marked fall in intraurethral pressure. The inhibitory activity of the higher centres on the sacral reflex arc is lifted, allowing a rapid flow of efferent, parasympathetic impulses to cause the detrusor to contract and pull open the bladder neck. As a result, the intravesical pressure rises smoothly, sometimes augmented by the voluntary contraction of the abdominal muscles. As soon as the intravesical pressure exceeds the intraurethral pressure, urine flow commences.

At the end of micturition, the intravesical pressure falls and the urine flow diminishes. Eventually, the pelvic floor and external urethral sphincter are voluntarily contracted, causing the terminal flow to stop in the region of the midurethra, with 'milking back' of urine in the proximal urethra into the bladder. At the same time the abdominal muscles relax and inhibition of the higher centres on the sacral reflex is reapplied, so that the bladder becomes passive once again to allow the recommencement of the next micturition cycle.

Continence control

Under normal conditions, urine is retained in the bladder because the intravesical pressure is very much less than the intraurethral pressure. This is achieved by suppression of the sacral reflex arc by the higher centres which prevents detrusor contractions occurring during the filling phase.

The urethra is kept closed at a higher pressure than the bladder by a combination of the smooth and striated muscle components around the bladder neck. The urethra is also held forward and upwards by the pubourethral ligaments so that increases in intra-abdominal pressure are equally transmitted to the bladder and upper third of the urethra which lie above the pelvic floor, thus maintaining the pressure gradient between the two. In addition, a reflex contraction of the levator ani compresses the mid-urethra; this is innervated by the pudendal nerve.

Urinary tract infection, cystitis and sexuality

Although a urinary tract infection alone does not cause incontinence, it can certainly affect sexual function and can cause considerable discomfort. At least 20% of women will have a urinary tract infection (UTI) during their lifetime and 3% experience recurrent infection (Nicolle and Ronald, 1987). It is probable that the majority of infections in adult women are asymptomatic and clear spontaneously; however, many women will be troubled by recurrent symptomatic infections. For women who do experience recurrent UTIs, the frequency of episodes is highly variable.

Factors that precipitate infection are poorly identified, but sexual intercourse and method of contraception, particularly diaphragm use, are two well-documented associations (Nicolle *et al.*, 1982). According to Cardozo *et al.* (1993), there is a double peak in the prevalence of UTI in women: one occurs in the 30–40 age group and the other between 55 and 65 years. In the younger of these two age groups, with a higher level of sexual activity, it is thought that intercourse predisposes women to UTI by microorganisms readily entering the bladder from the vagina and perineum. Newly sexually active women on honeymoon frequently experience cystitis and this is often called 'honeymoon cystitis'.

In the post-menopausal age group, the incidence of recurrent UTIs may be related to the reduced oestrogen status.

Urinary pathogens

The indigenous intestinal bacterial flora is the primary source for urinary pathogens. These organisms contaminate the vagina and perineum and ascend into the bladder. The most common organism is *Escherichia coli*, which accounts for up to 85% of acute infections. Less common pathogens are *Proteus mirabilis, Klebsiella pneumoniae, Aerobacter aerogenes* and, rarely, Gram-positive cocci.

A UTI can affect any part of the urinary tract, but it is the 'adherence' of the bacteria that is an important factor in the pathogenesis of infections. The urinary tract has a natural ability to resist bacterial colonization and the intruding bacteria are efficiently eliminated by the interaction of multiple mechanisms. Urine acidity, osmolality, organic acids and urea have a role in inhibiting bacterial adherence and growth. Bladder mucosa has intrinsic antibacterial properties and destroys those bacteria remaining on its surface after micturition. However, if a woman does not empty her bladder completely and leaves a residual urine, it reduces the host defence and makes her susceptible to UTI (Iravani, 1988).

Symptomology

A patient with a UTI will present with frequency of micturition, but may or may not complain of pain or difficulty in passing urine. With cystitis, however, frequency of micturition, urgency, dysuria and suprapubic discomfort are characteristic symptoms. Twenty to thirty per cent of women presenting with classic symptoms of cystitis will not have a urinary tract infection.

Many women with frequent episodes of cystitis live in dread of the next episode, and sexual dysfunction may occur due to the apprehension of acute cystitis following intercourse.

Investigation

In the investigation of UTI or cystitis, a midstream urine specimen is essential and antibiotic treatment should only be commenced according to the results of the culture and sensitivity. It is unsound practice to treat a patient with a presumptive diagnosis as many cultures are negative and antibiotics will not be required.

Upper-tract pathology may be adequately investigated by renal ultrasound along with a plain X-ray of kidneys, ureters and bladder. Cystourethroscopy may be performed and a bladder biopsy may show evidence of chronic inflammation. Cystourethroscopy is more relevant in the elderly, as recurrent UTIs may be the presenting symptoms of a transitional cell carcinoma.

Women under 40 years old should have a urodynamic investigation to rule out an overactive bladder, as this symptom is one of urgency.

Urodynamic studies will also reveal mechanical outflow obstruction which may have resulted from previous bladder neck surgery. These women may not be emptying the bladder completely and this predisposes to the likelihood of a UTI.

Treatment

Most UTIs can be treated with an appropriate antibiotic, depending on the urine culture. However, before going ahead with treatment, you should check for underlying conditions or practices that may predispose to recurrent UTI (Box 17.1).

Various non-prescription treatments and hints can be recommended to your clients:

◆ Increase fluid intake by at least 2 litres per day. The diuresis will help to 'wash out' low-grade infections

◆ Take a mixture of potassium citrate, 3 g in water, three times daily. This will relieve mild UTIs by restoring the urine pH

◆ Take sodium bicarbonate, 3 g in water, every 2 hours. This also helps by reducing the acidity of the urine

◆ Drink three glasses of cranberry juice daily (Box 17.2). Women taking warfarin should be advised to limit or avoid drinking cranberry juice as there have been a few reports of changes in INR values (Committee on Safety of Medicines, 2003).

Box 17.1 UTI: predisposing factors

◆ *An incorrectly fitted diaphragm* This may be causing pressure during intercourse, followed by dysuria and sometimes the onset of infection

◆ *Spermicidal preparations* These may cause dysuria secondary to a vaginitis due to an allergy

◆ *Sexual partners* Establish whether there has been any recent change in sexual partner or sexual practice. This may be a contributory factor

◆ *Incomplete bladder emptying*

◆ *Bladder overactivity* (see page 503)

◆ *Atrophic vaginitis* This can be treated with oestrogen supplements (see page 466).

Box 17.2 Effects of cranberry juice

As early as the last century, American Indians used crushed cranberries as a herbal remedy for the treatment of urinary infections (Bodel *et al.*, 1959). Many studies have focused on the anti-adherence activity of cranberry juice and its alteration of the urinary pH (Blatherwick and Long, 1923; Schmidt and Sobata, 1988).

Although there is no conclusive evidence that cranberry juice is a cure for urinary infection and cystitis, it can be effective for some people. It has been found with some women who complain of recurrent cystitis that drinking three glasses of cranberry juice a day during the acute phase can often help to alleviate the symptoms. As cranberry juice is quite harmless, it may be worth trying! Cranberry juice is available in most supermarkets, some chemists and independent health food stores.

You can also recommend that she consults her pharmacist. Many preparations can be bought over the counter without a prescription that can relieve symptoms.

Women should be advised that if their symptoms are not considerably improved after 48 hours then they should consult their doctor.

Interstitial cystitis

Frequent episodes of cystitis do not inevitably lead to interstitial cystitis (IC), a chronic and painful inflammation of the bladder wall. A woman suffering from suprapubic pain, frequency of micturition and continuous bladder pain must be referred to a urological consultant, as specialized treatment is required. Additionally there may also be pain associated with sexual intercourse, which in the long-term can lead to avoidance of sex and relationship problems.

According to Allan (1998) the symptoms of interstitial cystitis are:

◆ Severe suprapubic pain
◆ Unremitting bladder, urethral and lower back pain as the bladder fills
◆ Chronic day/night frequency and urgency (up to 60 times in 24 hours)
◆ Dyspareunia
◆ Pelvic pressure
◆ Spasms.

There are many combination therapies to try to help alleviate IC symptoms and these range from anti-inflammatory medication, avoidance of some foods and drinks, complementary therapies and surgical intervention. When vulval pain is involved it may be due to the inability to relax the pelvic floor muscles (Dolman, 1998) and biofeedback can be used to teach relaxation of this group of muscles.

Sometimes patients with IC feel isolated and joining a support group can be helpful (see Resources). There is also a very informative web site, www.ic-network.com, which has support chat, a newsletter, sections for patients, research, and covers sexual relations and infidelity, etc. In fact there is so much to see on this site, it is worth a visit. To quote: 'Thanks for all the time you spend helping interstitial cystitis patients. I was 16 when I was diagnosed four years ago and found, and continue to find, the Interstitial Network an invaluable resource.'

Types of incontinence

Urinary incontinence can be divided into different categories according to the symptoms. It is not unusual to experience more than one type simultaneously and this is referred to as 'mixed incontinence'. However, there is more emphasis nowadays on treating pelvic floor dysfunction (Davis and Kumar, 2003). Bladder problems do not always result in incontinence and most treatments start with pelvic floor rehabilitation to control the bladder (and also the bowel).

Stress incontinence. The most common type, especially in women. This occurs when the pelvic floor muscles are weakened or the urethral sphincters are damaged. Typical symptoms are leakage of small amounts of urine on coughing, sneezing, lifting, running or exercise

Urge incontinence. There is loss of urine with a very strong desire to void due to an overactive bladder contraction. The symptoms are frequency and urgency of micturition and nocturia more than twice during the night

Mixed incontinence. A mixture of symptoms as described above. This will be due to both an overactive bladder contraction and weak pelvic floor muscles

Overflow incontinence. A feeling of not emptying the bladder completely, frequency, passive dribbling and recurrent urinary infections. This type of incontinence is due to outflow obstruction, underactive bladder contraction or detrusor-sphincter dyssinergia (as in multiple sclerosis)

Functional incontinence. Unable to reach the toilet in time due to mobility problems or lack of cognitive awareness; unable to remove clothing, or poor environmental conditions

Nocturnal enuresis. Wetting the bed while asleep. The cause is often unknown but an overactive bladder and bladder capacity should be investigated

Transient incontinence. Temporary episodes of incontinence which might be due to some medication, infection or severe constipation

Surgical-induced incontinence. A result of some surgery such as hysterectomies, caesarean sections, prostatectomies, lower intestinal surgery or prolapse repairs.

Another good web site dealing with urinary incontinence and patient information on bladder control is at www.types-of-incontinence.com.

Quality of life and incontinence

The challenge in measuring quality of life (QoL) lies in its uniqueness to the individual. Many existing measures of QoL fail to take this into account and impose standardized models of QoL and preselected domains. Carr and Higgins (2001) debated whether QoL measures were patient-centred and felt a general health status rather than QoL is being measured. They explored newer individualized approaches which allow patients to define their QoL in relation to their own goals and expectations. Studies are continuing in this field of research.

In clinical practice, the appropriate questions need to be asked relating to the impact urinary (or faecal) incontinence has on that individual's everyday life. The perceived frequency or quantity of incontinence will vary from person to person. To assess the symptoms and their effect, patients record their own voiding diaries, which includes fluid intake, frequency, volume, episodes of incontinence and pad usage. Additionally they answer questions from their perspective of the problem, and about how it disrupts their well-being and social life (Kelleher *et al.*, 1997).

Measurement of QoL is not simple but typical key points include:

◆ Activities of daily living, e.g. self-care, cooking, shopping, walking

◆ Psychological well-being, e.g. memory, anxiety, levels of depression

◆ Social functioning, e.g. relationships, participation in activities, interaction with people

◆ Life satisfaction, e.g. a perception of how good/bad life is

◆ Health status, e.g. how an individual perceives their well-being

◆ Pain, e.g. severity or impact on daily activities.

The most used questionnaire in the UK, which has been validated and tested for reliability for symptom assessment specific to incontinence and the impact on QoL in women is the King's Health Questionnaire (Kelleher *et al.*, 1997).

To improve QoL there are a number of treatment options which aim to reduce the frequency of incontinent episodes, or to limit the impact of incontinence on everyday life (see following sections in this chapter).

Incontinence and sexual function

A number of studies, without validated questionnaires, have attempted to assess the impact of incontinence on sexual function. However, a woman should be given the opportunity to answer a simple question: 'Do you leak urine during intercourse?' This gives her an opening to discuss her problem and she often feels grateful the subject has been raised and she has been able to voice her concerns.

A study (Sutherst and Brown, 1980) indicated that urinary symptoms interfered with sex lives either by reducing frequency (of intercourse) or ceasing intercourse altogether. Patients with an overactive bladder experienced more sexual difficulties than those with stress incontinence.

Stress incontinence

Stress incontinence is the most common type of incontinence found in females of all ages, and will be discussed in detail. It is defined as 'the involuntary loss of urine when the intravesical pressure exceeds the maximum urethral closure pressure in the absence of detrusor activity' (Abrams *et al.*, 1990).

Stress incontinence occurs due to the deficiency in the urethral closure mechanisms when there is an increase intra-abdominal pressure such as coughing, sneezing, running, etc. (Figure 17.4).

Weak pelvic floor muscles are rarely due to a single event (although there may be congenital weakness of the muscles which may go undetected) and usually it is a combination of factors that contribute to the weakening of the pelvic floor muscles. It is associated with pregnancy, vaginal delivery, previous incontinence surgery, the menopause, constipation and obesity (Box 17.3).

'Don't make me laugh or I will wet myself.'

Women frequently complain of small amounts of urine loss during activities such as playing with the children, running, jumping, laughing, dancing, etc. The degree of urine loss will be variable: for some it is only mild (damp pants) and for others it is quite severe (wet underclothes and wet outerclothes which require changing). One woman said 'I can no longer wear trousers as the wetness cannot be hidden'.

Careful history taking and a physical examination will give a nursing diagnosis of stress incontinence. However, assessment with urodynamic studies will be necessary to make a clinical diagnosis, and is essential prior to most surgical procedures. Typically women try to keep the bladder empty prior to engaging in physical

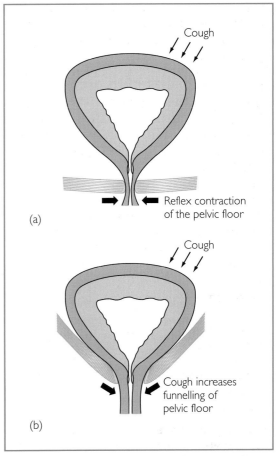

Figure 17.4 (a) Normal contraction of the pelvic floor with raised abdominal pressure. (b) Contraction of the pelvic floor with stress incontinence. (Reproduced with permission from Norton, 1986.)

Box 17.3 Causes of stress incontinence
◆ Pregnancy and childbirth
◆ Obstetric trauma to pelvic floor muscles (episiotomy, tears, forceps)
◆ Laxity of pelvic floor muscles
◆ Prolapse of uterus
◆ Atrophy of pelvic supports
◆ Oestrogen depletion
◆ Collagen disorder in some women
◆ Obesity
◆ Chronic constipation.

activity, and as such, may then develop voluntary frequency and perhaps urgency, thus presenting with 'mixed' symptoms.

Incontinence related to pregnancy and childbirth

Pregnancy

About 46% of women complain of incontinence during pregnancy (Chiarelli, 1991), but Cardozo and Cutner (1993) state that up to 55% of pregnant women have stress incontinence, depending on the gestation. When it occurs antenatally it is normally transient and will resolve postpartum. When it occurs for the first time postnatally it is likely to be more severe and permanent due to a weakened urethral sphincter closure.

There may be an additional problem due to the hormone relaxin, which begins to circulate even before the ovum is fertilized in the Fallopian tube. Relaxin is responsible for softening all the ligaments and muscles of the pelvic outlet so that the baby's head can be pushed out during childbirth. When the ovum is fertilized, the levels of relaxin continue to rise and reach a peak at about the 12th week of pregnancy. Relaxin needs to start softening tissues early in the pregnancy so that the baby's increasing weight acts as a stretching force.

Allen and Warrell (1987) found stress incontinence in pregnancy to be significantly increased due to partial denervation of the striated muscle of the pelvic floor, which is supplied by the pudendal nerve and pelvic branches of the sacral plexus. This partial denervation caused by the expanding uterus results in reduced postural tone of the sphincter mechanism. It is usually resolved postpartum.

Labour and delivery

Intrapartum events, which may have a profound effect on postpartum lower urinary tract function, include the method of delivery, the length of labour and the weight of the baby (Cardozo *et al.*, 1993). A long first stage and a long active second stage (pushing) have both been shown to result in urethral sphincter damage. Changes in the position of the bladder neck during labour may result in the stretching of supporting muscles and ligaments which can also cause damage to the urethral sphincter closure.

Poor bladder management during labour can result in voiding difficulties such as overflow incontinence, particularly if a spinal epidural has been administered (Dolman, 1992). Labour causes a decrease in bladder sensation and this, combined with epidural analgesia, may result in an overdistension of the bladder. Urine output must be monitored carefully during the first 24 hours postpartum as it has been shown that a single episode of overdistension of the detrusor can result in long-term voiding difficulties (Weil *et al.*, 1983).

Women who have a caesarean section will not have urethral sphincter damage, which is the main cause of postpartum stress incontinence, but the effects of hormones and the pregnancy itself will still apply.

As most women return home only hours after delivering a baby, midwives could use the factors listed in Box 17.4 to make a risk assessment of pelvic floor damage and advise the woman to seek advice as soon as any bladder or bowel symptoms occur. Most continence advisory centres take direct referrals from the patient, but physiotherapist referrals must be made through the general practitioner.

Box 17.4 Summary of risk factors for women developing postnatal incontinence

- Baby over 4.25 kg
- Forceps delivery
- Parity
- Long active second-stage labour
- Perineal suturing
- Epidural
- Obesity
- Chronic constipation
- Pudendal nerve damage (trauma/denervation).

Perineal damage: episiotomy and forceps-assisted delivery

Trauma to the perineal body, perineum and layers of the pelvic floor muscles which results from overstretching, forceps, tearing or episiotomy will cause damage to the pudendal nerve. Denervation causes loss of sensation and the ability to exercise the muscles. If suturing has to take place, this will leave scar tissue, which will not be innervated. The muscle around the scar tissue needs to be kept healthy and strong by pelvic floor exercises.

Other factors precipitating stress incontinence

Other factors that put pressure on the pelvic floor muscles causing weakness are obesity, chronic chest problems with coughing, constipation and occupations that require heavy lifting (see Figure 17.5). An eminent male urogynaecologist advises that women should never lift anything heavy as the strain damages the pelvic floor, so they should always ask a man to do the lifting for them!

Treatment for stress incontinence

The various options for treatment of stress incontinence are discussed in the following section and are summarized in Box 17.5.

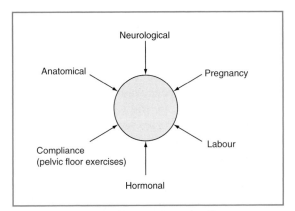

Figure 17.5 Factors affecting the pelvic floor.

> **Box 17.5** Summary of treatment for stress incontinence
>
> ◆ Pelvic floor exercises
> ◆ Electromuscular stimulation
> ◆ EMG/biofeedback
> ◆ Vaginal cones
> ◆ Surgery
> ◆ Macroplastique injections
> ◆ Oestrogen replacement.

Pelvic floor exercises

The American gynaecologist Arnold Kegel (1948) was the first to describe pelvic floor exercises in the treatment of urinary incontinence in women and the exercises are often referred to as 'Kegel exercises'. He reported a 'cure' rate of 84%, although 'cure' was not defined. Little activity in this field initially followed Kegel's presentation, although there has been extensive research in the last three decades.

Early published data on these exercises showing a 'cure' or improvement were based on the patients' own reports. The variation in success rates may be partly explained by the different duration of exercise periods, which varied from 4 weeks to 4 months. It may also be explained by the lack of reliable and valid measurements of the degree of urinary leakage and pelvic floor muscle strength. On an uncontrolled study of 500 women, Kegel recommended 300 contractions a day with the added use of a perineometer for resisted exercises twice a day. He reported that 84% became continent, including obese and elderly women. He described the weak muscles as a 'syndrome of lack of awareness of function and co-ordination of the pubococcygeus muscle'. He also noted that 30% of women could not elicit a contraction on command.

In 1963 Gomer-Jones adopted Kegel's methods of exercises and he emphasized the importance of teaching awareness of the pubococcygeus muscle and its ability to draw in, draw up and retract the perineum. He also emphasized the need to hold the muscles in this contracted state and then relax the muscles completely during half-hourly exercise sessions. Gomer-Jones maintained that more than 10 contractions at each session would cause fatigue and would therefore be counterproductive. Studies by Laycock *et al.* (1992), however, suggest that individual exercise programmes are needed to ensure maximum effort without fatigue and such exercise programmes will depend on the initial pelvic floor assessment.

Research on compliance with pelvic floor exercises was investigated by Dolman and Chase (1996) and the dominant factor found was that women had trouble remembering to do the exercises. It was suggested that they be incorporated into a daily activity so that they became a natural part of life. There is ongoing research into why women do not continue with pelvic floor exercises as a life-long activity.

Purpose of pelvic floor exercises

Simply explained, the purpose of pelvic floor exercises is to increase the muscle volume. A strong, healthy pelvic floor muscle will result in an increase of maximum urethral closure pressure and stronger reflex contractions following a quick rise in intra-abdominal pressure (Bo *et al.*, 1991). The striated muscle comprises fast and slow twitch fibres which are innervated by the pudendal nerve. When re-educating the pelvic floor muscle, attention must be paid to the needs of these fast and slow twitch muscle fibres (Gosling, 1979). These two fibre types have differing roles to play in maintaining continence and will respond to different types of exercises.

Fast twitch fibres tire easily, but are responsible for the fast reflex response associated with coughing, sneezing, etc., and also for providing a maximum voluntary contraction. This is important to enable a woman to quickly and strongly elevate and occlude the urethra prior to a stress-provoking act such as coughing, lifting or sneezing. When providing a strong maximum contraction, the fast twitch fibres also suppress urgency and relax detrusor contractions, thus activating the perineodetrusor inhibitory reflex.

This reflex, which travels from the pelvic floor back to the bladder, 'informs' the detrusor muscle to stop contracting and pushing urine out.

The *slow twitch fibres*, on the other hand, do not tire so readily. They provide a postural tone which generally supports the bladder and the sphincteric action for long periods of time. Pelvic floor weakness will reduce the ability of both of these types of fibres to function in their important role of sustaining continence.

Sexual responses and the pelvic floor muscles

The pubococcygeus has also been referred to as the 'love muscle'. Women with strong pelvic floor muscles seem to enjoy the bonus of good sexual responses. In a study of orgasm, Graber and Kline-Graber (1979) found that orgasm was significantly related to maximum pubococcygeal squeeze pressure.

The pelvic floor muscles are directly responsible for the amount of sensation that a woman feels during intercourse. The lining of the vagina is not well endowed with sensation (you can test this by drawing your finger down the inside surface) and most vaginal sensations come from the pelvic floor muscles that loop around behind the vagina. The pubococcygeus also directly affects the amount of sexual sensation male partners feel (Chiarelli, 1991).

The nerve endings in the muscles respond to being stretched, so the firmer and stronger the muscle is, the more it responds to the erect penis. As the glans of the penis moves back and forth during intercourse, the firm muscles will rhythmically stretch and relax, thus heightening vaginal sensations. The ability to achieve orgasm will be enhanced as pelvic floor muscle strength increases. The pubococcygeus is also responsible for helping to lubricate the vaginal walls during foreplay and intercourse, so, sexually speaking, these muscles play a vital role (Box 17.6).

Making an assessment of the pelvic floor muscles

The role of the nurse is increasing in many spheres of practice and they are nowadays

> **Box 17.6** Effects of strong pelvic floor muscles on sexual response will:
>
> ◆ Increase vaginal lubrication during foreplay/intercourse
> ◆ Increase sexual sensation felt vaginally
> ◆ Increase orgasmic response
> ◆ Give you a better grip on your partner.

expected to undertake new skills. One such skill could be that of making a pelvic floor muscle assessment, thereby avoiding the need for a woman to see her doctor. This type of assessment requires training and you will not understand the principles without adequate instruction. It will be necessary for you to make enquiries about courses in pelvic floor assessment in your area. However, even without extended training it is hoped that by reading this section you will have a better understanding of pelvic floor exercises and be able to advise and help your patients.

Awareness of the pelvic floor muscle and its contraction is best assessed by a digital vaginal examination (Laycock, 1987). The woman can then be shown what is expected from an exercise programme.

Having obtained permission to do a vaginal examination, the women lays supine on the couch, hips flexed and abducted. A gloved, lubricated index finger is inserted 5 cm into the vagina and the rim of the pubococcygeus palpated. This will determine muscle bulk and any asymmetry, and will detect a change in tone as the woman contracts and relaxes the muscle (Laycock, 1992). Next, the index and middle fingers are inserted into the vagina in the antero-posterior (A-P) position with fingers spread apart. When the woman is squeezing and lifting the fingers, you should be able to detect the lift movement of the coccyx towards the pubis and evaluate the squeeze potential of the pubococcygeus (Brink *et al.*, 1989).

The Oxford grading system is widely used by nurses and physiotherapists for assessing pelvic floor muscle strength:

0 = nil, no squeeze
1 = flicker only
2 = weak contraction
3 = moderate contraction
4 = good contraction
5 = strong contraction.

Fatigue assessment

When assessing for muscle fatigue, the length of time the muscle is contracted is recorded in seconds. The woman must be in charge of the muscle's relaxation and note if the contraction has already faded away. If the contraction has faded before you finish counting the seconds, repeat with fewer seconds until the woman consciously relaxes the muscle herself. That will be her starting point for her individual exercise programme.

Example: Moderate contraction (3) held for 4 seconds.

It is then necessary to determine the number of repetitions that can be tolerated to further evaluate endurance.

Example: Moderate contraction (3) held for 4 seconds, relax for 4 seconds, repeated four times.

This individual's starting point would therefore be: four contractions each to the count of 4, relaxing to the count of 4, repeated four times, and this group of four to be repeated as often as possible throughout the day without causing muscle fatigue, i.e. an aching muscle would result.

So far, you have been concentrating on the slow twitch fibres of the muscle which are responsible for the endurance qualities. As the woman progresses and has had time to practise what you have taught her, the next visit will be the time to introduce the 'quick flick' contractions. This re-educates the fast twitch fibres, which are used whenever a maximum voluntary contraction, or speed, is required.

Example: Five 'quick flick' contractions lasting 1 second.

Total exercise programme from above example:

1. Moderate contraction (grade 3)

2. 4-second contraction, 4-second relaxation

3. Repeat this group four times each session

4. Do as many daily sessions as possible

5. Start each session with 3–5 quick flick contractions.

Each woman will have a different starting point according to her own muscle capabilities and this can only be determined from a proper pelvic floor assessment.

Once the pelvic floor assessment is complete and an individual home exercise programme has been discussed, the woman needs to be encouraged to adhere to this programme. Compliance will depend on individual motivation, remembering to do the exercises and trying to fit them in during a busy lifestyle (Dolman, 1995).

Women do not have an innate ability to perform pelvic floor exercises in the Western world,

and as such the quality of the teaching of the exercises is of vital importance. According to Bump *et al.* (1991), some women are unable to locate and contract the proper muscles when given either verbal or written instructions, and this is obviously inadequate preparation for a woman about to pursue a pelvic floor exercise programme. Some women bear down instead of squeezing and lifting. It is also important to eliminate the use of other muscle groups such as the abdominal, glutei and thigh abductors which are often used instead of the pelvic floor muscles.

Dolman (1995) found from a postal survey that a significantly higher proportion of women were doing pelvic floor exercises who had been examined vaginally (71%) compared to those who were not examined vaginally (59%). However, it is not always possible, or desirable by the woman, to do a vaginal examination, and verbal or written instruction in these cases will have to suffice. A guideline that you can print and discuss with your clients is given in Box 17.7.

Alternatives to pelvic floor exercises

What happens when a woman cannot contract the pelvic floor muscles? How can she be helped?

Electrical stimulation of the pelvic floor muscles

Women with no ability to contract the pelvic floor muscles at will, or who find it difficult to identify the muscles, can receive treatment from neuromuscular stimulation. This method of treatment has traditionally been one used by physiotherapists. However, with home devices now purchasable by mail-order for women to self-administer (see Figures 17.6a and 17.6b), with or without a clinician's recommendation, it is necessary for nurses to be made aware of the principles of treatment and to know how to answer enquiries from women in their care.

Principles of electromuscular stimulation
In order for a muscle to contract, impulses pass from the anterior horn cell to the neuromuscular

---

Box 17.7 Guidelines for pelvic floor exercise

1. Sit comfortably with knees slightly apart. Without moving your tummy muscle or bottom, try to squeeze the muscle around the back passage. Pretend you are trying to stop wind from escaping and squeeze and lift the muscle; this tightening should give you a feeling of being lifted away from the chair

2. Now try the same with the front part of the muscle. Again, without moving the tummy and bottom, squeeze and lift the muscle into the vagina. Alternatively, pretend you are on the toilet and want to stop the flow of urine. Moving this front part of the muscle is harder than exercise one above and takes some time to practise

3. Once you can tighten the muscles, pull up as hard as you can and hold for at least 5 seconds, then relax for 5 seconds. Repeat this as often as possible during the day without tiring the muscle

4. Also try to pull up the muscles quickly, a one second flick and then relax. Repeat this five times in conjunction with the exercises in No. 3

5. These two exercises combined will strengthen your pelvic floor muscle and as you progress you will be able to hold the contraction longer and do more repetitions

6. If you are in any doubt about exercising the muscles correctly, please seek advice. You do not want to think you are doing the exercises correctly only to find out years later you have wasted your time

7. Looking after a healthy and strong pelvic floor muscle is a lifelong exercise.

junction where a chemical reaction causes the muscle fibres to shorten. The frequency of these impulses depends on the type of muscle fibre to be supplied, i.e. slow or fast twitch fibres. The slow twitch fibres receive 10–20 pulses per second and the fast twitch fibres receive 30–60 pulses per second (Eccles *et al.*, 1958).

Neuromuscular stimulation 'mimics' a muscle contraction by passing an electrical impulse along the efferent nerves using low frequencies of 10–60 Hz. It is used as a treatment for women who are unable to contract their pelvic floor muscles on command and it aims to teach them the correct action. They will learn voluntarily to contract the muscles with the electrical stimulus.

As well as being a treatment for stress incontinence, neuromuscular stimulation can also be used for treating an unstable bladder which may lead to urge incontinence. By stimulating the pelvic floor and external urethral sphincter via branches of the pudendal nerves (S2, S3, S4), the perineodetrusor inhibitory reflex is also activated, thus reducing bladder instability (see page 505).

There are no side effects to electrical stimulation, although there may be some discomfort as the sensory nerves are activated, so the intensity of the current must be kept just below the patient's tolerance level. This treatment should only be used on women who can understand the procedure and who can verbalize any discomfort. Contraindications for use would be pregnancy, vaginitis, someone with a pacemaker and those with a diagnosis of pelvic malignancy.

It must be emphasized that any woman who cannot voluntarily contract the pelvic floor muscles and is in need of electrical stimulation treatment should be referred to a specialist nurse or physiotherapist. Electrode pads may be placed on the skin suprapubically, inner thigh, perineum or sacrum or a vaginal probe may be placed in the vagina, depending on the woman's preference.

Once a woman can contract her pelvic floor muscles, electrical stimulation will no longer be necessary and this may be a 'once only' treatment. However, if compliance to a pelvic floor exercise programme is not adhered to over the following months or years, a 'top-up' course of electromuscular stimulation may be necessary.

Biofeedback therapy

Biofeedback therapy is simply a means of giving the patient immediate information about a physiological state of a bodily process. A vaginal probe with built-in electrodes (Figure 17.6b) can be inserted and the leads attached to a machine which will record and display the pelvic floor muscle bioelectrical activity when the muscle is contracted and at rest. Known as an electromyography (EMG) this gives immediate visual feedback on how weak/strong the pelvic floor muscle is. Electrodes used can be via the vagina, anus or surface electrodes placed on the skin. Biofeedback signals can be visual or auditory or a combination of the two.

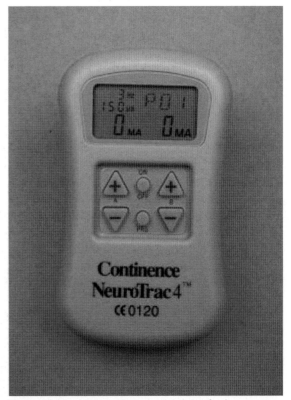

Figure 17.6a NT4 continence stimulator for home use. (Reproduced with permission from De Smit Medical for Verity Medical Ltd.)

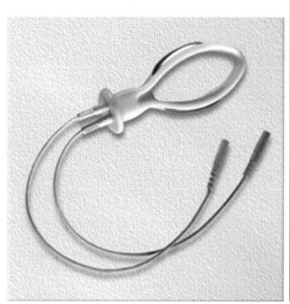
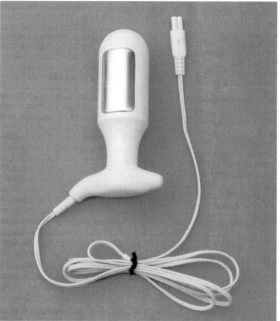

Figure 17.6b, Periform probe (left) and Veriprobe (right) for use with continence stimulator. (Reproduced with permission from De Smit Medical for Verity Medical Ltd.)

This therapy teaches the patient how to isolate the pelvic floor muscle and records the strengthening progress of the exercise programme (see Box 17.8). In particular it records the fatigue/ endurance levels of a contraction, the resting tone of the muscle and the response of the fast twitch muscle fibres. A resting tone of more than 6 microvolts indicates the patient needs to learn to relax the pelvic floor muscle as seen in sensory and motor urinary urgency or idiopathic constipation.

Box 17.8 Phases of pelvic floor development using biofeedback

- ◆ Phase 1: Gives an awareness, identification and coordination of the muscle groups
- ◆ Phase 2: Transition – muscle control develops and strengthening begins
- ◆ Phase 3: Muscle strengthening completed and pelvic innervation improves with symptoms decreasing
- ◆ Phase 4: Muscle tone good – palpation (digital assessment) finds a firmer, bulkier and broader muscle.

This treatment has no side effects and can be used for all types of incontinence or pelvic floor muscle dysfunction. It may be useful, however, to combine this therapy with other treatment modalities. There are home devices that can be purchased (Figure 17.7) so patients can do their own exercises at home and know they are doing them correctly. Biofeedback stimulates motivation and compliance to do the exercises and therefore patients respond quickly to the treatment (Smith and Newman, 1994). Training is necessary for professionals to understand the principles and use of biofeedback (see Resources).

From the above you can see why and how this therapy would be an excellent way to treat a lax vagina especially when this symptom causes sexual problems and can lead to the breakdown of a relationship.

Vaginal cones as an adjunct to pelvic floor exercises

Although vaginal cones are available to buy, recommendations by health care professionals to

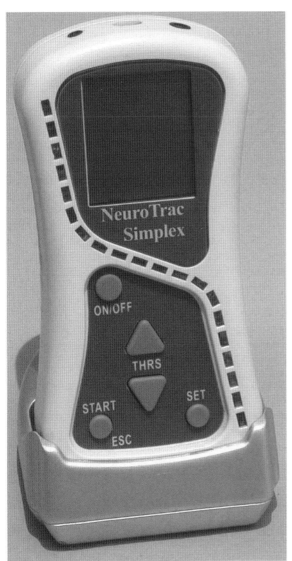

Figure 17.7 Simplex and stand home biofeedback. (Reproduced with permission from De Smit Medical for Verity Medical Ltd.)

use them are less prevalent than 10 years ago. This is due to the fact that a pelvic floor muscle grading (strength) must be grade 3 before a cone can be kept *in situ* to work effectively. Cones are a good adjunct to pelvic floor exercises and can be used as a biofeedback therapy once daily if required. Bo *et al.* (1999) compared pelvic floor exercises, electrical stimulation and vaginal cones for treating women with stress incontinence and found exercises to be a superior mode of treatment. One has to assume that all the women could already contract the muscles and be at least grade 3 on muscle assessment.

Surgery for stress incontinence

Women are better informed today about alternative treatment options for bladder/pelvic floor muscle dysfunction but still surgery may be the only choice in some cases. Rigorous assessment, investigations and urodynamic studies should be done prior to any urogynaecological surgery. Conservative treatments, already discussed, should have been attempted before surgery and many women are now asking for these alternatives. If these fail then she knows she has tried her best and surgery is inevitable.

Details of the surgery for incontinence are discussed in Chapter 19, but there are over 100 different operative procedures. The most commonly used operations are listed in Box 17.9.

Many of the operations are adaptations or modifications of previous procedures showing evidence of the desperation many surgeons

---

Box 17.9 Operations for stress incontinence

Vaginal

◆ Tension-free vaginal tape
◆ Anterior colporrhaphy + urethral buttress (pelvic floor repair)
◆ Urethrocliesis.

Abdominal

◆ Marshall–Marchetti–Krantz
◆ Burch colposuspension.

Combined

◆ Endoscopic bladder-neck suspension, e.g. Stamey, Raz
◆ Slings.

Complex

◆ Neourethra
◆ Artificial sphincter
◆ Urinary diversion.

face in operating on this difficult condition. There is a definite role for surgery for urinary stress incontinence, but it is most important that the first operation that is performed is the correct procedure, as subsequent operations are more difficult and less likely to be successful. The aims of surgery are

> to elevate the bladder neck and proximal urethra into an intra-abdominal position where intra-abdominal pressure will act as an additional closing force. Surgery should also support the bladder neck and align it to the postero-superior aspect of the pubic symphysis which will, in some cases, increase outflow resistance.
>
> (Cardozo *et al.*, 1993, p. 82)

Postoperative complications that may result from surgery for stress incontinence are:

◆ Overactive detrusor (frequency and urgency of micturition)

◆ Voiding difficulties (incomplete emptying of the bladder, poor stream, residual urine which may lead to UTI)

◆ Bladder pain

◆ Dyspareunia

◆ Surgical failure (stress incontinence symptoms might recur either immediately or at a later date).

The success or failure of surgery for urinary stress incontinence lies mainly in the competence and skill of the surgeon. A full explanation of the procedure must be given preoperatively and the chances of success should be honestly discussed so that the woman can make an informed choice before deciding on surgery.

Newer surgical techniques: Tension-free Vaginal Tape (TVT)

A TVT is a modification of the suburethral sling procedure in which a prolene tape, covered by a plastic sheath, is inserted around the mid-urethra without fixation. It is a minimally invasive surgical procedure through the vagina, which may be appropriate for some women with stress incontinence, and it can be performed under local anaesthetic. The surgeon must be proficient in its use and the procedure takes about half an hour. Recovery time is shorter: a day case rather than the longer time with conventional surgery. However, there are few data on its continued effectiveness and complication rate beyond the first few years, although Rezapour *et al.* (2001) reported continence in 80% of patients at a five-year follow-up. Shah (2003) states that although women prefer the minimally invasive surgery, shorter recovery period and ability to return to work quickly, there still remain no data on the theoretical possibility of long-term complications such as erosion of TVT material into the urinary tract. Gynecare manufactures the TVT product and women and health professionals can obtain further information at www.gynecare.com.

Hormonal influences and the menopause

The embryological development of the vagina, trigone and urethra was explained earlier in the chapter so you should understand why oestrogen affects the urethra. In pre-menopausal women when oestrogen levels drop just prior to menstruation, the resting urethral pressure falls, and some women say that their stress incontinence tends to be worse in the week before the period. The urethral wall is soft and convoluted, forming many folds, and when fully oestrogenized creates a watertight seal. When hormone levels fall, the urethral walls become less soft, the folds less pronounced and the closure is less efficient.

In post-menopausal women, the oestrogen levels may take some years to fall, but some women remain well oestrogenized into old age. The lower oestrogen levels after the menopause combined with pelvic floor trauma from pregnancy and childbirth leads to stress incontinence. Lack of oestrogen may cause urethritis and trigonitis, often associated with atrophic vaginitis. This can easily be recognized by looking at the vulva which will appear red, inflamed and often dry. Vaginal dryness means there is a loss of sexual lubrication and intercourse can be uncomfortable and painful.

Some women experience discomfort while passing urine due to the urine being in contact with the inflamed vulva. They may be treated for a urinary infection when in reality they have atrophic vaginitis.

Treatment for atrophic vaginitis is with low-dose oestrogen replacement therapy. Local application of creams, pessaries, tablets or a ring into the vagina at night is often recommended although some older women dislike doing this and find it difficult to use the applicator. Oral hormone replacement therapy may produce side effects such as a monthly bleed which the older woman may not want to tolerate. Oestrogen supplementation improves the vaginal, urethral and trigonal epithelium and leads to a restoration of the pre-menopausal vaginal flora.

A study by Guthrie (2001) found there was no association between the development of incontinence and the transition from pre- to post-menopause. However, she did find that women who had undergone hysterectomy were more likely to experience incontinence than those women who had not had this surgery.

Hysterectomy

A hysterectomy, particularly if accompanied by bilateral oophorectomy, will result in a surgical menopause. If hormone replacement therapy is not commenced the woman will have the symptoms described above, and you may frequently hear women say 'I was alright until I had my hysterectomy'. In addition to the oestrogen depletion following a hysterectomy, postoperative scarring and infection were suggested by Smith *et al.* (1970) as aetiological factors for urinary symptoms. Occasionally urethral obstruction is due to peri-urethral fibrosis and damage to the bladder base and proximal urethra during a total abdominal hysterectomy resulting in scar formation. When the bladder is not emptied completely the woman may have symptoms of needing to void again soon after the initial void: 'I have to go to the toilet again about 2 minutes after I've just been'. The symptom may be frequency of micturition or repeated UTIs. Often a simple dilatation of the urethra will resolve the problem. A women can be taught to self-dilate the urethra using a urethral dilator (AstraTech).

Detrusor overactivity: the overactive bladder

The second most common type of urinary dysfunction in menopausal women is detrusor overactivity, which used to be known as detrusor instability (also referred to as the overactive bladder). It is a condition characterized by involuntary detrusor contractions occurring during bladder filling. The normal inhibiting impulses are not sent from the cortical centre to prevent completion of the sacral reflex arc, and so the bladder begins to contract before micturition is voluntarily initiated (Figure 17.8). The symptoms are usually frequency and urgency, sometimes resulting in urge incontinence, nocturia or even nocturnal enuresis. In the majority of cases there is no known cause and it is called idiopathic

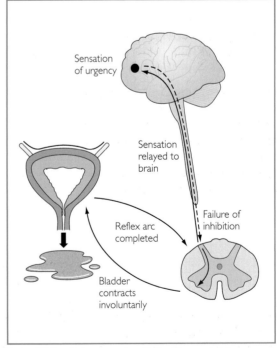

Sensation of urgency

Sensation relayed to brain

Failure of inhibition

Reflex arc completed

Bladder contracts involuntarily

Figure 17.8 Detrusor overactivity (the unstable bladder).

detrusor overactivity. It is sometimes thought that poor bladder control learnt in infancy may be a cause, for example, if the woman was always told as a child to go to the toilet when it was not really necessary. Later in adulthood a woman adopts bad toileting habits by going to the toilet 'in case' rather than waiting for the bladder signals that it needs emptying. When a woman has a dreaded fear of wetting herself and does not know when or where this may happen, it is easy to understand how she may begin to withdraw from social activities. These women learn where all the public toilets are so that they can go shopping without being 'caught out' (see also section on Quality of Life).

> I don't go to my friend's anymore because
> I am so embarrassed about always going to the
> toilet, nobody else seems to need the toilet
> as much as I do.

Women with urge incontinence suffer greater disruption to daily activities than those with stress incontinence. However, in 20% of women the two symptoms coexist. Leaking urine during sexual intercourse and at orgasm is associated with detrusor overactivity as mentioned earlier.

In some women detrusor overactivity may be secondary to an upper motor neurone lesion such as multiple sclerosis and there is increased evidence that detrusor overactivity may occur after surgery for stress incontinence (Cardozo, 1997).

Treatment

First, objective assessment for detrusor overactivity must be confirmed by a urodynamic investigation and other diagnostic tests (see Box 17.10) but some women with mild or intermittent symptoms may be helped with reassurance and simple measures such as:

◆ Explanation of how the bladder should function

◆ Reducing fluid intake if in excess of 2 litres

◆ Avoiding tea, coffee or alcohol which are bladder stimulants

◆ Retraining the bladder to hold more urine, i.e. increase the interval time between toileting.

Bladder retraining

This technique can be very successful when used properly and it is important that you understand the principles of bladder retraining before advising your clients.

The most important element for success is to use the correct regime for each individual person and their situation. A prior assessment is essential to identify those who will benefit from bladder retraining. Other contributing factors such as UTI and constipation must be treated first. A frequency/volume chart needs to be recorded by the individual for a week as this will show the extent of the problem. Every time she goes to the toilet she will use a jug to measure the amount of urine passed. No special 'chart' is needed, simply a plain piece of paper recording day-to-day frequency and volume (Box 17.11).

After explaining the function of the bladder and its ability to hold urine, the client is encouraged to increase the interval time between voiding by not answering the first signal from the bladder as it is filling and by contracting the pelvic floor muscles to suppress detrusor contractions. The 'urgency' feeling should diminish and the client can 'hold on' for longer periods.

After 4 weeks another chart can be recorded and compared to the base-line chart to check the reduction in frequency episodes and to note the increased volumes of urine being voided. Bladder retraining can take as little as 2 weeks or as long as 6 months to show some improvement.

Electrical stimulation for the overactive bladder

Treatments for an overactive bladder (symptoms of urgency and frequency) with electrical stimulation

---

Box 17.10   Diagnostic investigations

◆ Urodynamic investigations
◆ Ultrasound
◆ Micturating cystography
◆ X-ray: kidneys, ureters, bladder
◆ Intravenous urography
◆ Cystourethroscopy.

Box 17.11 Example of a frequency/volume chart			
Day 1	**Day 2**	**Day 3**	**Day 4, etc.**
7 am/200 ml	6.15/220 ml	7.15/150 ml	7 am/220 ml
7.30/50 ml	7 am/20 ml	7.30/30 ml	7.45/40 ml
8 am/125 ml	7.45/50 ml	8 am/100 ml	8 am/50 ml
9 am/–	9 am/125 ml	9.30/–	9 am/30 ml
10.30/–	11 am/–	11 am/120 ml	10 am/–

have been shown to be effective (Lewey, 1999). A low frequency of 10–20 Hz is administered for 20 minutes a day by using the home device as mentioned on page 500. This should only be considered after assessment by an experienced clinician and where follow-up appointments monitor the patient's progress. There is little research evidence at the present time to say the length of time or even the frequency and duration of treatment, but from clinical experience 6–8 weeks is required on a daily basis. There seems to be a requirement for a 'top-up' with this treatment after 2 years. Most patients prefer this mode of treatment which has no side effects to the medication approach, although a few patients may need a combination of these therapies.

EMG/biofeedback techniques

Most women have difficulty isolating the pelvic floor muscle to exercise it effectively. A method becoming more popular in this country for teaching the exercises is biofeedback (see page 499). Biofeedback is also used for urological conditions, e.g. obstruction caused by an inability to relax pelvic floor muscles, pelvic floor dysfunction in women which causes vaginal pain, vaginismus and vulvodynia.

Physiotherapists and trained specialist nurses may offer biofeedback in a clinical setting but home devices are available (Figure 17.7) which women can purchase (de Smit Medical) as long as they have been recommended by a clinician.

If there is little improvement after 3 months women feel frustrated so the next stage is a referral for urodynamic investigation to diagnose detrusor overactivity. If confirmed, bladder retraining should be used in conjunction with a low-dose anticholinergic drug (oxybutynin). You will need to warn your client about the side effects of these drugs, the most common of which is a dry mouth. Some women will not tolerate this. Occasionally constipation and blurred vision can affect the elderly. The side effects of oxybutynin are dose related and 3 mg twice a day causes fewer problems than 5 mg twice a day, but of course may not be effective!

Once the bladder has been retrained using the combined drug therapy and bladder retraining schedule, a reduction in drug dosage can commence until drugs are no longer required. Much support and encouragement is required from you to help your client succeed with bladder retraining, particularly if you have to retrain someone who has lived with years of bad toileting habits.

In severe cases of detrusor overactivity (e.g. every 20 minutes, 24 hours a day) surgery may be indicated. The bladder can be overdistended with water while the patient is under anaesthetic, thus producing ischaemic nerve damage which reduces the nerve stimulation to the bladder. A bladder retraining programme should follow this procedure.

More drastic surgery is a clam augmentation cystoplasty, in which the bladder is divided and augmented with a section from the large bowel or ileum. All cystoplasties produce mucus which can be kept less viscous by a high fluid intake, but the reduction in bladder contraction may mean the patients have difficulty in voiding. Straining to void or the use of intermittent self-catheterization will probably be required to empty the bladder.

Voiding difficulties

Voiding difficulties may be due to a weak bladder contraction (hypotonic detrusor contraction) or an outflow obstruction, or the two causes may coexist. Some of the causes have already been mentioned in this chapter under overflow incontinence on page 492.

General measures

◆ If drugs with anticholinergic side effects are being taken, try to withdraw them if possible, e.g. anticholinergics, tricyclic antidepressants

◆ Encourage the woman to double void, i.e. when she thinks she has emptied the bladder, wait 30–50 seconds and bear down using the abdominal muscles to try to cause another bladder contraction. This may prevent residual urine and a UTI

◆ A change in voiding position may help the bladder to empty completely if there is a problem after incontinence surgery or a hysterectomy

◆ The woman may need to learn intermittent self-catheterization after each void until the residual is less than 100 ml, then the procedure can stop. Detrusor hypotonia may be the result of acute retention, i.e. following epidural anaesthesia or general anaesthetic

◆ Cholinergic drug therapy, e.g. distigmine bromide, may help chronic voiding difficulties. These drugs stimulate bladder contractions. Response to treatment must be monitored by measuring the post-micturition urinary residual

◆ Where there is longstanding detrusor hypotonia the only treatment may be intermittent self-catheterization. This is preferable to an indwelling catheter as the incidence of UTI is much lower and a more normal lifestyle can be resumed.

Intermittent catheterization

As the name suggests, this involves introducing a catheter into the bladder intermittently to remove any residual urine, then removing the catheter so the woman is catheter-free between catheterizations. The catheter used for single use is a Jacques or Nelaton plastic catheter Charrier 10/12. In a hospital the procedure must be

strictly aseptic but in the home environment the woman learns a clean technique.

This technique is only used when the woman has a persistent residual urine volume greater than 100 ml and is experiencing problems of overflow incontinence and/or recurrent bladder infections. A competent urethral sphincter mechanism is required to maintain continence.

The techniques must be discussed fully with the woman and the final choice whether to proceed lies with her. Booklets are available for teaching this procedure (from Astra Tech or Hollister Ltd), but dexterity and good eyesight are important factors towards the success of the technique. Good teaching by a competent nurse will enhance the chances of success with this technique.

Most women are not aware of the position of the urethral meatus and many find that touching themselves in that area is not acceptable. The psychological aspect of this technique needs full discussion.

Assessing female bladder dysfunction

Before you can advise women complaining of any bladder dysfunction you must take an accurate and detailed history of the problem. You must also have a basic knowledge of the subject and understand the significance of her answers. The history is a tool to aid diagnosis and to help in planning treatment and care and it provides a baseline from which to monitor progress. It will also highlight when referral to another discipline is necessary.

Key points for assessment

History taking and recording:

◆ Relevant medical, surgical and obstetric history

◆ Urinary symptoms and date of onset

◆ Related circumstances or events precipitating incontinence

◆ Current medication

◆ Bowel habit

◆ Attitude to problem (patient, carer or staff)

◆ Support services used

◆ Environmental/living conditions

◆ Aids/appliances used.

Frequency/volume charts:

◆ How much urine is lost (Box 17.11)

◆ Day/night frequency

◆ Baseline chart of incontinent episodes

◆ Fluid intake – amount and type.

Physical examination and tests:

◆ Urinalysis

◆ Mobility/dexterity

◆ Hearing and eyesight

◆ Mental alertness

◆ Abdominal, rectal and vaginal examinations

◆ Residual urine

◆ Pad test (if indicated).

Investigations that can be performed by nurses are summarized in Box 17.12. Most of these will be familiar to you and others are described in detail elsewhere in this chapter. Since 2000, a care pathway (Bayliss, 2000) for dealing with urinary incontinence has been developed and implemented in most primary and secondary Trusts. Nurses are trained at a basic level of bladder/ bowel knowledge regarding symptoms and are able to perform first-level interventions, e.g. urinalysis, pelvic floor exercises, fluid/

Box 17.12 Investigations nurses can perform

◆ Urinalysis
◆ Mid-stream specimen of urine if required
◆ History of condition and assessment
◆ Vaginal examination for prolapse or vaginitis
◆ Vaginal examination for pelvic floor muscle action
◆ Rectal or abdominal examination for constipation
◆ Post-micturition residual urine (in/out catheter)
◆ Dry/wet pad test
◆ Bladder charting for frequency/volume (see Box 17.11).

---

dietary advice, bladder retraining. If there is a variation from the normal parameters measured by evidence-based symptomatology (a symptom chart is provided) then the assessor refers on to the appropriate person for more experienced assessment and treatment, i.e. continence services, physiotherapist, urologist, gynaecologist, etc. This saves the woman having an unnecessary or inappropriate referral.

Pad test – a simple technique

This test can be used to quantify the degree of urinary incontinence and to verify that there is incontinence. A dry pad is pre-weighed, in grams, and then weighed wet. Any increase in weight will indicate the degree of incontinence. As a guide, 1 g is equivalent to 1 ml of urine. Therefore, if a pad weighs 95 g when dry and then 125 g when wet, the urine loss is 30 ml. In the standard test the patient drinks 500 ml of fluid and then wears the pre-weighed dry pad while certain activities are carried out, e.g. walking, jumping, coughing, etc. The pad is then re-weighed and the urine loss estimated. More recently it has been suggested that a 24-hour home pad test is more representative as the woman can carry out her normal activities while wearing the pre-weighed pad.

Specialist investigations

Investigations must be tailored to the individual's needs (Boxes 17.10 and 17.12) and referral to specialist centres may be required to complete the assessment and final diagnosis.

There has long been a fragmented and inadequate continence service for patients, resulting in going from one person to another and not getting the appropriate treatment or advice. In 1998 a working group was set up by the parliamentary under secretary of state for the Department of Health (DoH) to look at continence services and advise on guidance. From this group *Good Practice In Continence Services* was published (DoH, 2000). The key recommendations included the principles for service commissioning, the components of service delivery, approaches to service organization, and tools to improve service provision.

Some Trusts are beginning to report on how an interdisciplinary integrated service for continence care has been developed (Logan and Proctor, 2003), resulting in a best practice approach thus benefiting patients in their care. With the demands that modern health care brings and the challenges of local health strategies, a comprehensive continence service package needs to be in place.

Prevention is better than cure

There are many opportunities for nurses in the community and in hospital environments to approach the subject of bladder problems with women. The conversation can take place casually while assessing or advising them on other issues. You can give women a chance to talk about and maybe admit to bladder problems in a friendly atmosphere, but you must be able to understand the meaning of their symptoms.

Asking the right questions at the right time will often be a relief to the woman that the subject has been mentioned and taken seriously rather than glossed over. During cytology, family planning and well-woman clinics you could ask 'have you noticed an increase in the number of times you go to the toilet each day?' A typical question to ask at a chest clinic could be 'do you leak urine during a coughing attack?' Pelvic floor muscle exercise can be mentioned at any clinic and should be part of your routine vocabulary. Key points are listed in Box 17.13.

> **Box 17.13   Key points to help you help your client**
>
> ◆ Teach pelvic floor exercises at all stages of a woman's life from puberty onwards
> ◆ Where possible, assess pelvic floor muscle function by doing a vaginal examination
> ◆ Use every opportunity to explain *why* pelvic floor muscle exercises are important. Discuss the advantages of a strong, healthy pelvic floor
> ◆ Remember, most urinary incontinence can be avoided if a woman understands bladder function and exercises her pelvic floor muscles throughout her life.

Conclusion

The disruption of normal daily and social activities due to the symptoms of urinary incontinence has a devastating effect on women. The psychological aspect has not been fully discussed within this chapter, but I am sure you can perceive for yourself the range of feelings, including anger, experienced by most women who suffer from incontinence.

The sad part about incontinence is that this distressing situation can be prevented. Eighty-five per cent of women can be cured if their symptoms are treated in the early stages.

There are many instances in a woman's life when she is in contact with a nurse and every opportunity should be used by you to open the lines of communication about pelvic floor function. Nurses working in pre-conceptual care, family planning, ante- and postnatal clinics, well-woman clinics, cytology, gynaecology in/out patients – the list is endless – have daily occasions when they can broach the subject.

It is hoped that this chapter will help you to take on the role of trying to prevent incontinence, thus ensuring that your clients are fully informed of the advantages of strong pelvic floor muscles. Try to remember that a woman with urinary incontinence frequently feels that she has lost her femininity and sexuality.

> **Ideas for personal and professional development**
>
> ● Contact your local continence services to find out if care pathways have been implemented and how this affects you and your clients
> ● Arrange a visit to your local continence advisor. Do women always need to be referred by a health professional or can they refer themselves?
> ● Devise an 'at risk' list for your practice or department, showing the potential causes of incontinence in women
> ● Further your interest by monitoring your clients who have sexual problems as a result of weak pelvic floor muscles

- Attend a local study day on bladder/bowel problems which includes TVT techniques and post-operative nursing care
- With some extra knowledge you may want to participate in the development of integrated continence services in your Trust.

Patient education points

- Incontinence is very common problem in women, and can affect many aspects of life
- It is never too late to start pelvic floor exercises
- Display patient leaflets on 'pelvic floor exercises' and have available a leaflet explaining 'bladder retraining'
- Advertise the Continence Foundation helpline number 0845 345 0165 and your local continence service's contact number
- Have information about web sites that are dedicated to urinary/faecal incontinence available.

RESOURCES

Association for Continence Advice

Winchester House, Kennington Park,
  Cranmer Road, The Oval,
  London SW9 6EJ
Tel: 020 7820 8113
www.aca.uk.com

Continence Foundation

307 Hatton Square, 16 Baldwins Gardens,
  London EC1N 7RJ
Tel: 020 7404 6875
Helpline: 0845 345 0165 (Mon–Fri
  9.30 am–1.00 pm)
www.continence-foundation.org.uk
Provides information and education for
  professionals and public.

Incontact

United House, North Road, London N7 9DP
Tel: 020 7700 7035
www.incontact.org
An organization for people with incontinence.
  Produces a quarterly magazine, organizes

study days and is a strong consumer group, testing the usefulness of new products that manage incontinence.

Interstitial Cystitis Support Group

76 High Street, Stony Stratford,
  Bucks MK11 1AK
Tel: 01908 569169
www.interstitialcystitis.co.uk

RCN Continence Forum

RCN, 20 Cavendish Square,
  London W1M 0AB

Informative web sites

There are so many to choose from that it is impossible to mention them all here. For example an MSN search on incontinence and the quality of life will give you 30,470 to read!
www.medscape.com
www.gynecare.com
www.pelvicfloor.com
www.drdonnica.com The First Name in
  Women's Health relating to incontinence
www.rcn.org.uk
www.doh.gov.uk
www.nice.org (search for TVT)

Suppliers

Astra Tech Ltd

Brunel Way, Stonehouse, Gloucestershire
  GL10 3SW
Tel: 01453 791763
www.astratechuk.com
Provides Lofric intermittent catheters, urethral
  dilators. Prescription service to home.

Coloplast Ltd

Peterborough Business Park, Peterborough,
  Cambridgeshire PE2 6FX
Tel: 01733 392000
Manufacturers of containment products.

de Smit Medical Ltd

30 Highfields Close, Stoke Gifford,
  Bristol BS34 8YB
Tel: 01179 697865
E-mail: sales@desmitmedical.com
www.desmitmedical com

Distributor for pelvic floor electrical stimulator and biofeeback equipment for home use. Organizes study days for this equipment and has many other continence-related products for purchase by mail order.

Hollister Ltd

Rectory Court, 42 Broad Street, Wokingham, Berkshire RG40 1AB

Tel: 01189 895009

www.hollister.com

Manufacturers of intermittent catheters, sheaths, urine bags, faecal collector and stoma products which are on the drug tariff.

Neen Mobilis Healthcare Group

100 Shaw Road, Oldham, Lancashire OL1 4AY

Tel: 0161 678 0233

www.neenhealth.com

Provides electrical stimulator and biofeedback equipment, probes, educator (for pelvic floor muscle treatment) and booklet 'Women's Waterworks'.

Shiloh Healthcare

Park Mill, Bleasdale Street, Royton, Oldham OL2 6PZ

Tel: 0161 624 5641

Provides washable products which manage incontinence for adults and children.

Further reading

ABRAMS, P., KHOURY, S. and WEIN, A. (eds) (1999) Incontinence, 1st International Consultation on Incontinence, Monaco, 28 June–1 July. ISBN 1 898452 25 3.

CARDOZO, L., CUTNER, A. and WISE, B. (1993) *Basic Urogynaecology*. Oxford: Oxford Medical Publications.

CARDOZO, L.D. (ed.) 1997 *Urogynaecology: The King's Approach*. London: Churchill Livingstone.

GETLIFFE, K. and DOLMAN, M. (1997) *Promoting Continence: A Clinical and Research Resource*. Edinburgh: Elsevier.

LAYCOCK, J. and HASLAM, J. (eds) (2002) *Therapeutic Management of Incontinence and Pelvic Pain*. London: Springer.

MUNDAY, A.R., STEPHENSON, T.P. and WEIN, A.J. (eds) (1994) *Urodynamics: Principles, Practice and Application*, 2nd edn. Edinburgh: Churchill Livingstone.

For patients

CASTLEDEN, C.M. and DUFFIN, H. (1991) *Staying Dry: Advice for Sufferers of Incontinence*. Quay Publishing.

DOREY, G. (2003) *Make it or Fake it!* A self-help guide for women: using your pelvic floor muscles to achieve sexual function. Available from de Smit Medical Ltd, 30 Highfields Close, Stoke Gifford, Bristol BS34 8YB.

FADER, M. and NORTON, C. (1994) *Caring for Continence: A Care Assistant's Guide*. Better Care Guides. Hawker Publications.

MARS, P. (1990) *In Control – Help with Incontinence*. London: Age Concern.

NEEN HEALTHCARE. Women's Waterworks. Available from de Smit Medical Ltd (as above).

References

ABRAMS, P., BLAIVAS, J.G., STANTON, S.L. and ANDERSON, J.T. (1990) The standardisation of terminology of lower urinary tract function. *British Journal of Obstetrics and Gynaecology* **6**(Suppl):1–16.

ALLAN, E. (1998) Interstitial cystitis. *Nursing Standard* **12**(38):43–6.

ALLEN, R.E. and WARRELL, D.W. (1987) The role of pregnancy and childbirth in partial denervation of the pelvic floor. *Neurology and Urodynamics* **6**(3):183–4.

BAYLISS, V., CHERRY, M., LOCKE, R. and SALTER, L. (2000) Pathways for continence care: background and audit. *British Journal of Nursing* **9**(9):590–6.

BLATHERWICK, N.R. and LONG, M.L. (1923) Studies of urinary acidity: the increased acidity produced by eating prunes and cranberries. *Journal of Biological Chemistry* **57**:815–18.

BO, K., HAGEN, R.H., KVARSTEIN, B. *et al.* (1991) Effects of two different degrees of pelvic floor muscle exercises. *Journal of the Association of Chartered Physiotherapists in Obstetrics and Gynaecology* **69**:12–17.

BO, K., TALSETH, T. and HOLME, I. (1999) Single blind, randomised controlled trial of pelvic floor exercises, electromuscular stimulation, vaginal cones, and no treatment in management of genuine stress incontinence in women. *British Medical Journal* **18**(7182):487–93.

BODEL, P.T., COTRAN, R. and KASS, E. (1959) Cranberry juice and the antibacterial action of hippuric acid. *Journal of Clinical Medicine* **56**(4):881–7.

BRINK, C.A., SAMPSELLE, C.M., WELLS, T.J. *et al.* (1989) A digital test for pelvic muscle strength in older women with urinary incontinence. *Nursing Research* **38**(4):196–9.

BUMP, R.C., HURT, W.G., FANTL, J.A. and WYMAN, J.F. (1991) Assessment of Kegel pelvic muscle exercise performance after brief verbal instruction. *American Journal of Obstetrics and Gynecology* **165**(2):322–9.

CARDOZO, L., CUTNER, A. and WISE, B. (1993) *Basic Urogynaecology*. Oxford: Oxford Medical Publications.

CARDOZO, L.D. (ed) (1997) *Urogynaecology: The King's Approach*. London: Churchill Livingstone.

CARDOZO, L.D. and CUTNER, A. (1993) Is disturbed bladder function after pregnancy normal? *Maternal and Child Health* 180–3.

CARR, A.J. and HIGGINS, I.J. (2001) Are quality of life measures patient centred? *British Medical Journal* **322**:1357–60 (Education and Debate).

CHIARELLI, P.E. (1991) *Women's Waterworks: Curing Incontinence*. Gore & Osment.

COMMITTEEE ON SAFETY OF MEDICINES (2003) *Current Problems in Pharmacovigilance* **29**:8.

DAVIS, K. and KUMAR, D. (2003) Pelvic floor dysfunction: a conceptual framework for collaborative patient-centred care. *Journal of Advanced Nursing* **43**(6):555–68.

DoH (DEPARTMENT OF HEALTH) (2000) *Good Practice in Continence Services*. London: DoH.

DOLMAN, M. (1995) Remedial action. *Nursing Times* **91**(24) (Continence supplement).

DOLMAN, M. (1998) Cystitis: alleviating symptoms. *Women's Health* **3**(3):26–8.

DOLMAN, M.E. (1992) Midwives' recording of urinary output. *Nursing Standard* **6**(27):25–7.

DOLMAN, M.E. and CHASE, J. (1996) Comparison between the Health Belief Model and Subjective Expected Utility Theory: predicting incontinence prevention behaviour in post-partum women. *Journal of Evaluation in Clinical Practice* **2**(3):217–22.

DOREY, G. (2003) *Make it or Fake it!: A Self-help Guide for Women* booklet. ISBN 0-9545393-0-3.

ECCLES, J.C., ECCLES, R.M. and LUNDBERG, A. (1958) The action potentials of the alpha motorneurones supplying fast and slow muscles. *Journal of Physiology* **142**:275–91.

GOMER-JONES, E. (1963) Non-operative treatment for stress incontinence. *Clinics in Obstetrics and Gynaecology* **6**:220–35.

GOSLING, J. (1979) The structure of the bladder and urethra in relation to function. *Urologic Clinics of North America* **6**(1):31–8.

GRABER, B. and KLINE-GRABER, G. (1979) Female orgasm: role of pubococcygeus muscle. *Journal of Clinical Psychiatry* **40**:348–51.

GUTHRIE, J.R. (2001) Natural menopause not a significant risk factor for urinary incontinence. *Obstetrics and Gynaecology* **98**:628–33.

HILTON, P. (1988) Urinary incontinence during sexual intercourse: a common, but rarely volunteered symptom. *British Journal of Obstetrics and Gynaecology* **95**:377–81.

IRAVANI, A. (1988) Causes, diagnosis and treatment of bacterial infections of the urinary tract. *Comprehensive Therapy* **14**(11):49–53.

KEGEL, A. (1948) Progressive resistive exercise in the functional restoration of the perineal muscles. *American Journal of Obstetrics and Gynecology* **56**:238–48.

KELLEHER, C.J., CARDOZO, L.D., KHULLAR, V. and SALVATORE, S. (1997) A new questionnaire to asses the quality of life of urinary incontinent women. *British Journal of Obstetrics and Gynaecology* **104**:1374–9.

LAYCOCK, J. (1987) Graded exercises for the pelvic floor muscles in the treatment of urinary incontinence. *Physiotherapy* **73**(7):371–3.

LAYCOCK, J. (1992) Pelvic floor re-education for the promotion of continence. In Roe, B. (ed.) *Clinical Nursing Practice: The Promotion and Management of Continence*. New York: Prentice Hall, Chapter 5.

LAYCOCK, J., FARRAGHER, D., GARDNER, J. *et al.* (1992) Standardisation of physiotherapy: clinical practice in the management of female urinary incontinence. In Roe, B. (ed.) *Clinical Nursing Practice: The Promotion and Management of Continence*. New York: Prentice Hall.

LEWEY, J. (1999) Electrical stimulation of the overactive bladder. *Professional Nurse* **15**(3):211–14.

LOGAN, K. and PROCTOR, S. (2003) Developing an interdisciplinary integrated continence service. *Nursing Times* **99**(21):34–7.

MUNDY, A.R. (1984) Clinical physiology of the bladder, urethra, and pelvic floor. In Mundy, A.R., Stephenson, T.P. and Wein, A.J. (eds) *Urodynamics: Principles, Practice and Application*. Edinburgh: Churchill Livingstone, pp. 14–25.

NICOLLE, L.E. and RONALD, A.R. (1987) Recurrent urinary tract infection in adult women: diagnosis and treatment. *Infectious Disease Clinics of North America* **1**(4):793–806.

NICOLLE, L.E., HARDING, G.K., PREIKSAITIS, J. and RONALD, A.R. (1982) The association of urinary tract infection with sexual intercourse. *Journal of Infectious Diseases* **146**:579–83.

NORTON, C. (1986) *Nursing for Incontinence*. Beaconsfield: Beaconsfield Publications.

NORTON, P.A. (1990) Prevalence and social impact of urinary incontinence in women. *Clinical Obstetrics and Gynaecology* **33**(2):295–7.

REZAPOUR, M., FALCONER, C. and ULMSTEN, U. (2001) Tension free vaginal tape (TVT) in stress incontinence women with intrinsic sphincter deficiency (ISD) – a long-term follow-up. *International Urogynecolgy* **2**(Suppl):S12–14.

ROYAL COLLEGE OF PHYSICIANS (1995) Report of a working party: *Incontinence – Causes, Management and Provision of Services*. London: RCP.

SCHMIDT, R.D. and SOBATA, A.E. (1988) An examination of the anti-adherence activity of cranberry juice on urinary and non-urinary bacterial isolates. *Microbias* **55**:173–81.

SHAH, J. (2003) Stress incontinence: which urodynamic studies and surgery? *Trends in Urology Gynaecology and Sexual Health* July/August:30–2.

SMITH, D.A. and NEWMAN, D.K. (1994) Basic elements of biofeedback therapy for pelvic floor muscle rehabilitation. *Urologic Nursing* **14**(3):130–5.

SMITH, P., ROBERTS, M. and SLADE, N. (1970) Urinary symptoms following hysterectomy. *British Journal of Urology* **42**:3–9.

SUTHERST, J. and BROWN, M. (1980) Sexual dysfunction associated with urinary incontinence. *Urology International* **35**:414–16.

THOMAS, T.M., PLYMAT, K.R., BLANNIN, J. and MEADE, T.W. (1980) Prevalence of urinary incontinence. *British Medical Journal* **281**:1243–6.

WEIL, A., REYES, H., ROTTENBERG, R.D. *et al.* (1983) Effect of lumbar epidural anaesthesia on lower urinary tract function in the immediate postpartum period. *British Journal of Obstetrics and Gynaecology* **90**:428–32.

18: Common Gynaecological Problems

Gilly Andrews and Jill Steele ◆

OBJECTIVES

This chapter should help you understand:

◆ The anatomy and physiology of the female reproductive system ◆

◆ How to recognize some of the disorders which women encounter during their reproductive lives ◆

◆ How to respond supportively ◆

◆ The alternative methods available for women for whom orthodox treatment is not working or is not acceptable ◆

◆ That things are not always what they seem and that it is important to be aware of hidden problems and unspoken anxieties. ◆

Introduction

In order to appreciate why gynaecological problems occur and how they may affect women it is essential that you have an understanding of the anatomy of the female reproductive system and the physiology of menstruation. Without this basic knowledge it will be difficult for you to educate your patients so that they can understand what is happening to their bodies throughout the month.

Gynaecological problems are common and are frequently interrelated. They are often complicated by events in a woman's life that may have nothing at all to do with gynaecology. In this chapter they have been grouped so that you will think of the problem as it affects your client rather than as a problem on its own. Some problems you will come across frequently in your clinical practice, others are more unusual, whilst some you may never meet. You should try to remember that although a problem may seem 'routine' to you, your patient may view it very differently and may require sensitive discussion and support.

Anatomy and physiology of the reproductive system

The female reproductive system consists of the pelvic organs: the uterus and cervix, the vagina, two ovaries, two Fallopian tubes; and the external genitalia. The pelvis is the name given to the basin-shaped structure formed by the ilium, the sacrum and the coccyx at the back and the symphysis pubis (the joint between the pubic bones) at the front (Figure 18.1).

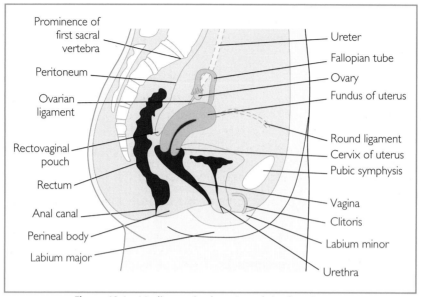

Figure 18.1   Median sagittal section of the female pelvis.

Uterus

During the reproductive years, the uterus is normally the size and shape of a small pear. It is made up of the fundus, body and cervix (Figure 18.2). The uterus has three distinct layers:

◆ *Endometrium* This is the uterine lining which varies in thickness both between individual women and also at different stages in the menstrual cycle. It grows in each cycle and is largely shed during menstruation

◆ *Myometrium* This middle layer contains the muscle fibres which run both transversely and longitudinally to allow the uterus to accommodate a growing baby and to produce the strong contractions necessary for the baby to be born. The uterus may enlarge when fibroids are present, depending on their size

◆ *Peritoneum* This is the serous layer which forms the outer covering of the uterus, apart from the lower anterior segment where the uterus lies in close proximity to the bladder and the peritoneum is reflected over the bladder.

The uterus usually lies in an anteverted position but in 20% of women it is retroverted without causing any problems. The broad ligament, round ligament and utero-sacral ligament help to maintain the uterus in its anteverted, anteflexed position. Having said this, the uterus is by no

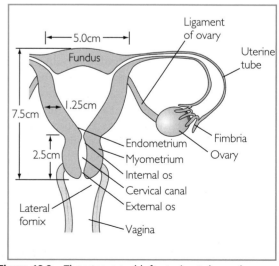

Figure 18.2   The uterus and left uterine tube and ovary.

means 'fixed' and will alter position slightly when the bladder is full and rise to an almost upright position in the pelvis during sexual arousal and orgasm.

Cervix

The cervix of the uterus is situated partly above the vagina and partly within it. The cervix is 2–3 cm long and opens into the uterus via the cervical isthmus or internal os. The isthmus dilates and becomes part of the uterus during labour. The external os at the lower end is normally closed and plugged with mucus which protects the uterus from infection. It dilates and opens up completely during labour.

The endocervical canal is lined with columnar epithelium and connects the internal and external os. The outer cervix in the vagina is covered with squamous epithelium up to the external os. The junction of these two types of cells forms the transformation zone where the abnormal cell changes, known as cervical intraepithelial neoplasia (CIN), take place (see Chapter 13).

The cervix undergoes the same cyclical changes as the uterus but the endocervical mucosa is relatively thin compared with the endometrium and so does not bleed. The cervical glands secrete mucus that is thin after menstruation, profuse at the time of ovulation and thick after ovulation.

Fallopian tubes

Two Fallopian tubes join the uterus just below the fundus, or upper part of the uterus. Each tube is 10–14 cm long and opens out into a funnel-shaped structure of small, finger-like projections which is called the infundibulum or fimbriated end. One fimbria of each tube is slightly longer than the rest and is attached by its tip to one of the two ovaries which lie close to the ends of the tubes. The tubes are mobile to enable them to pick up ova. At ovulation the fimbriae wrap around the adjacent ovary.

The function of a tube is to carry the fertilized ovum along its three parts:

- ◆ The ampulla (where fertilization usually takes place)
- ◆ The isthmus
- ◆ The interstitial section where the tube joins the cornu of the uterus.

The epithelial lining is coated with fine, hair-like, mobile processes called cilia which waft the ovum along the tube.

Ovaries

Ovaries are normally similar in size and shape to an almond. The surface is usually irregular. At birth the ovaries contain some 2–3 million follicles. Most of these develop incompletely and regress before puberty, although the number left is well in excess of those needed for childbearing. During the years of fertility with regular menstruation a woman will ovulate about 400 times. Each follicle contains an oocyte which, if matured, will be released as an ovum ready for fertilization by a sperm. Ovulation occurs 14 days before the onset of menstruation and therefore mid-cycle in the usual 28-day cycle. The ovaries form part of the endocrine system and secrete the hormones oestrogen and progesterone and small amounts of testosterone in response to stimulation by the gonadotrophins secreted by the anterior pituitary gland.

The vagina

The vagina is a tubular structure connecting the uterus to the external genitalia. It is about 8 cm long. Normally the anterior and posterior walls lie in contact. They are lined with mucous membrane and lie in folds (rugae) which make the vagina capable of distending to accommodate a baby in childbirth.

The pockets caused by the insertion of the cervix into the vagina are called the anterior, posterior and lateral fornices (singular, fornix). Cervical swabs and smears are taken from the external os and high vaginal swabs from the fornices.

During the reproductive years the vagina is kept moist by mucus from the cervix and from glands.

Transudation of fluid into the vagina during sexual arousal also has a lubricating effect on the tissues.

Under the influence of oestrogen, glycogen is produced which, when fermented by the Doderlein's bacilli (a form of lactobacillus which normally inhabits the vagina), produces lactic acid. This helps to keep the vagina free from infection by maintaining an acid balance in the vagina with a pH of 3.4–4.5. The growth of other bacteria is inhibited.

In the absence of oestrogen, or when there is trauma or haemorrhage, the vagina becomes more susceptible to infection. This can happen after childbirth, before puberty, after the menopause and when antibiotics are taken and the acid balance is disturbed, or the hormonal status changed, e.g. whilst taking the contraceptive pill. The vaginal orifice is the midline opening of the vagina. In the young girl it is incompletely closed by the hymen, a thin fold of tissue covered with squamous epithelium. There is a variable opening for blood to escape during menstruation. It is stretched during sexual intercourse and the first coitus usually causes slight bleeding. The hymen is virtually destroyed during childbirth.

The pelvic floor is the name given to the group of muscles that support the organs in the pelvis. They run from front to back and side to side so the effect is of a sling or hammock with openings in the middle for the urethra, vagina and the rectum. The perineal body is a fibromuscular node between the vagina and the anus with attachments to eight muscles. If the perineum is damaged in childbirth it can lead to later problems of weakness in the pelvic floor. Teaching your clients, especially after childbirth and also those approaching their middle years, how to do regular pelvic floor exercise before their muscles lose tone may help prevent such problems as prolapse and stress incontinence (see Chapter 17).

The external genitalia are depicted in Figure 18.3.

The normal menstrual cycle

Menstruation is the cyclical activity involving the partial shedding of the endometrium. It usually occurs every 21–35 days with a 28-day cycle being regarded as normal. While many women do have a 5/28-day cycle, variations of a few days are common. This is how a period is usually described in the patient's notes, with 5 representing the days of bleeding and 28 the length of the cycle (i.e. from the first day of one bleed to the first day of the next). If the cycle is irregular you may see it written as, for example, 5–7/26–32. Longer variations can be worrying and shorter cycles troublesome.

Variations in cycle length are most common at either end of the reproductive years but can occur at any time when ovulation may be delayed, e.g. by a change in body weight, stress or disease. A vegetarian diet has been known to disrupt cycle length when adopted for the first time but this settles as the body adjusts to the change (Balen, 1993).

The menstrual cycle (Figure 18.4) is controlled by the hypothalamus and the anterior pituitary gland with feedback pathways between the brain and the ovaries involving circulating levels of oestrogen. When gonadotrophin-releasing hormone (GnRH) is released from the hypothalamus

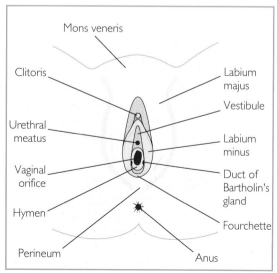

Figure 18.3 The external genitalia.

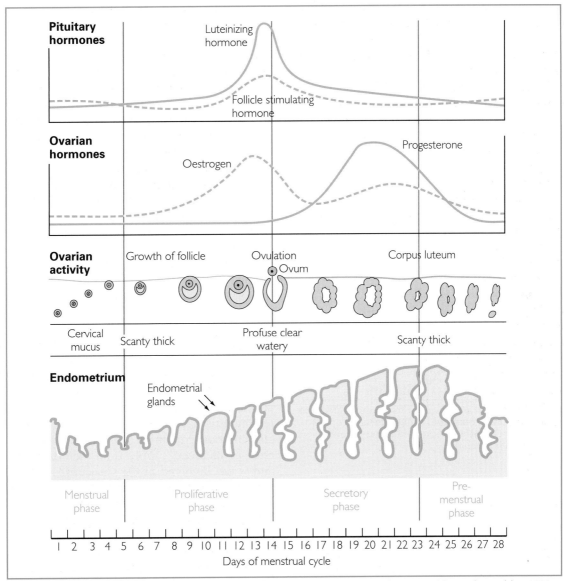

Figure 18.4 Schematic description of menstruation and ovulation. (Modified from Scambler and Scambler, 1993, with permission.)

the anterior pituitary is stimulated to release first follicle-stimulating hormone (FSH) then luteinizing hormone (LH). FSH starts activity within one or other ovary and stimulates a few sensitized follicles to mature. Oestrogen is released from these follicles and one dominant follicle progresses to maturity while the others

are subject to atresia (this is the degenerative procedure that affects most ovarian follicles). The mechanism is complex but as the oestrogen level reaches a peak there is a surge of LH from the anterior pituitary gland which causes the ripened follicle to rupture and release the ovum (Figure 18.5).

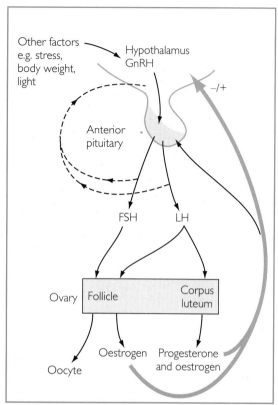

Figure 18.5 Possible pathways controlling the release of female reproductive hormones (GnRH, gonadotrophin-releasing hormone; FSH, follicle-stimulating hormone; LH, luteinizing hormone).

Ovulation occurs about 30 hours after the LH surge. Some women experience pain which may be sharp or of a cramp-like nature. It may last for a day or two and is sometimes replaced by a dull ache. Known as *mittelschmerz*, the cause of this pain is unknown, but is thought to be due to irritation of the peritoneum by the fluid and blood that come from the ruptured follicle.

When ovulation occurs the follicle collapses, becoming the corpus luteum which secretes progesterone. Oestrogen and progesterone are responsible for the changes that take place within the uterus during the menstrual cycle:

◆ Proliferative or follicular phase

◆ Ovulation

◆ Secretory or luteal phase

◆ Menstruation.

During the proliferative phase, the stroma and glands in the endometrium are regenerated in a process of thickening from the basal layer which remains after the previous menstruation (now about 0.5 mm thick). Usually 10–14 days long, the proliferative phase will vary in length where the cycle is irregular.

Ovulation and the start of the secretory phase usually occur 14 days before the onset of menstruation. Progesterone continues the thickening process and produces secretions to fill the endometrial glands ready for the fertilized ovum. The endometrium will be 5–6 mm thick before menstruation, but again this varies between women and it can be several millimetres thicker than this. The thickness of the endometrium can be measured by pelvic ultrasound.

If fertilization does not take place, the corpus luteum normally degenerates into a corpus albicans. As the corpus luteum function decreases, a fall in progesterone occurs which causes changes in the endometrium. Spasm of the arterioles occurs in the basal layer of the endometrium. The resulting ischaemia leads to shedding of the endometrium down to the basal layer which receives its blood supply from the artery below and is not involved in the vasoconstriction. The mechanism is similar to that which is involved in cardiac ischaemia.

Menstruation has begun on day 1 of the menstrual cycle. Bleeding usually lasts 4–5 days with a normal range of 1–7 days. Normal blood loss is estimated to be 30–40 ml with bleeding in excess of 80 ml being described as menorrhagia. Eighty per cent of menstrual loss is blood, with less than 25% consisting of endometrial tissue, tissue fluid and mucus. The blood contains minimal fibrinogen and does not clot, although rapid bleeding can result in clot formation within the uterine cavity before the blood is seen in the vagina.

Nurses should be aware of the different cultural attitudes to menstruation and the importance attached by many women to the cleansing effect of a regular show of menstrual blood. At the same time many nationalities use a colloquial word which supports the view that menstrual blood is polluting and unclean – 'the curse' in the UK, 'avadi' (polluted) in India, 'kotoran' (dirt) in Java.

Despite this, menstruation is regarded as a symbol of youth, fertility and usefulness and the menopause is an event that many women contemplate with dismay (Snowden and Christian, 1983).

Menarche

Menarche, the onset of periods, is being reached at an increasingly early age. The normal range in the UK is now 10–16, with some girls starting as early as 9 years old. The onset of periods can be delayed by intensive sport and physical activity and it seems that a critical weight needs to be reached for menarche to occur. A normal body mass index (BMI) is 20–25; amenorrhoea is common when the BMI is 19 or below (see also pages 41 and 161).

Occasionally precocious puberty may happen before 8 years with the first period before 10. For children, identification with a peer group is important and having periods before the rest of your friends can be frightening and confusing and may well lead to teasing or bullying. During the first year or two the cycles may be anovular. Because of this, periods though free from pain may be heavy or irregular. This can be distressing and possibly alarming both to a young girl and her parents. Preparation for the event at such a young age needs careful, sympathetic handling and many mothers find this a difficult task. You may be able to help both the child and her parents by offering support and reassurance.

We can only hope that with increasing openness about sexual matters the situation described by Deutsch (1944), where mothers were so inhibited that they found it easier to talk to their daughters about conception, pregnancy and birth than menstruation, has improved so that young girls are no longer quite so unprepared as they were then.

The menopause

The menopause (the last period) marks the end of the female reproductive life and normally

SCENARIO

Jean, now aged 37, described her introduction to menstruation. She was 10 years old when her periods started – the first in her class.

'I was reading in my bedroom when I felt my pants were wet and sticky. I found that I was bleeding. I can remember feeling terrified and I started screaming. My parents came rushing up stairs. My father was sympathetic but taken aback. My mother told me to stop being stupid and making such a noise – it was only my periods and every one has them. I did not know what she was talking about and was convinced that I was going to die. She showed me some sanitary towels and told me to go to the chemist to buy some for myself. He was a man and I felt embarrassed although I didn't know why. It was the chemist who explained what was happening to me and told me about menstruation. I have always had trouble with periods – I don't know if that is why.'

occurs between 45 and 55 years of age, with an average age of 51 (Chapter 16).

Once a woman in this age group has had 6 months without a period she is usually defined as post-menopausal, although she may have a further period. If this happens, it must be differentiated from post-menopausal bleeding, which may be a symptom of serious disease such as carcinoma of the endometrium.

Women experience the menopause in different ways. Periods may stop suddenly, gradually, or there may be problems with irregular and/or heavy bleeding. The menopause may be welcomed if the woman has experienced problems with menstruation, but more often it raises feelings of regret and misgiving. The menopause may come at a time when there are other problems in her life, such as children leaving home, ageing parents to worry about, possible redundancy for herself or her partner. It will certainly mean that she can no longer have a child without assisted reproduction techniques. On the other hand she will be free to enjoy her sexuality with no fear of pregnancy. With correct information, this stage of a woman's life can be very positive and active, but unfortunately many women do not know where to find such information. You, as a nurse, can offer advice and support and may be the person she feels able to ask for help at this potentially difficult time of her life.

Menstrual problems

Menstrual disorders are among the 10 conditions most frequently seen by the GP (Scambler and Scambler, 1993). Common menstrual problems include:

◆ Menorrhagia

◆ Amenorrhoea

◆ Oligomenorrhoea

◆ Dysmenorrhoea

◆ Dysfunctional uterine bleeding

◆ Inter-menstrual bleeding (IMB)

◆ Irregular periods/irregular bleeding.

Because menstruation is not a subject that is generally talked about, it can be difficult for a woman to realize she has a problem. She may seek help and advice from a doctor or nurse for a number of reasons. The pattern of her periods may have changed and be causing her concern. She may be experiencing pain or she may be subject to stresses in her life which are affecting her tolerance towards menstruation which she has hitherto regarded as normal.

Menorrhagia

Menorrhagia occurs in about 10% of women and is usually regarded as bleeding in excess of 80 ml. The bleeding may be heavy or prolonged, or both. In young women occasional heavy periods do not require investigation, but any marked change in menstrual pattern in an older woman should be investigated thoroughly.

Causes

Common causes of menorrhagia are listed in Box 18.1.

Uterine fibroids (Figure 18.6). Uterine fibroids occur in 25% of women over 40. They are benign, oestrogen-dependent growths of fibrous and

Box 18.1 Causes of menorrhagia
◆ Fibroids
◆ Polyps
◆ Endometrial hyperplasia
◆ Intrauterine contraceptive device (IUD)
◆ Underactive thyroid gland
◆ Psychosomatic causes
◆ Endometriosis and adenomyosis
◆ Polycystic ovaries
◆ Pelvic inflammatory disease
◆ Blood coagulation disorders
◆ Endometrial carcinoma and cervical carcinoma.

muscular tissue. They can occur singly but are usually multiple. Much of the time they do not cause any problem but if they are in the submucous layer, distorting the endometrium, then menstruation may be heavier. If the fibroid protrudes into the endometrium enough to stretch and thin it, inter-menstrual bleeding may occur and there may be a vaginal discharge. Occasionally, submucous fibroids develop into polyps which may reach the cervix and will cause dysmenorrhoea and severe menorrhagia.

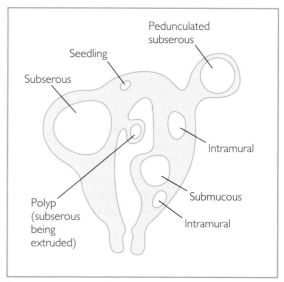

Figure 18.6 Uterine fibroids. (Reproduced from Steele, 1985, with permission.)

Fibroids do not usually cause pain but may cause symptoms of pressure on the bladder or the bowel.

Malignant change within a fibroid is rare.

Endometrial polyps. These are benign growths which protrude into the cavity of the uterus. They are common, vary in size and there may be several. Inter-menstrual bleeding, a vaginal discharge, or increased bleeding during a period are all possible symptoms. Some polyps are asymptomatic. They are removed during a hysteroscopy and curettage, which is a minor procedure (see page 550).

Endocervical polyps are also common, usually benign, and may cause discharge or intermenstrual bleeding.

Endometrial hyperplasia. Disruption of the balanced levels of oestrogen and progesterone can occur as a woman approaches the menopause, when she may find her periods become irregular both in length and in the amount of bleeding that she experiences. Some cycles will be anovular and the period may be very heavy, due to excessive thickening of the endometrium. Urgent medical intervention may be indicated. It is important to exclude serious disease and establish a diagnosis. This will usually be done with the help of a pelvic ultrasound and endometrial sampling before treatment is started, as once hormones have been given the histology of the sample will be affected.

Intrauterine contraceptive device. Periods may become heavier after the insertion of an intrauterine contraceptive device (IUD). This usually settles in 2 or 3 months and the bleeding and any associated pain may be helped by one of the non-steroidal anti-inflammatory group of drugs such as mefenamic acid (Guillebaud *et al.*, 1978). If menorrhagia continues, the device may have to be removed. IUDs are generally not recommended for women with heavy or painful periods.

The intrauterine system (IUS) (see Chapter 11), a small, plastic T-shaped frame containing the progestogen levonorgestrel, has been one of the most significant advances in contraception and gynaecology in recent years. Unlike the IUD it does not cause heavier periods and is particularly suitable for women who suffer from menorrhagia and dysmenorrhoea, as these

symptoms will be reduced (Barrington and Bowen Simpkins, 1997).

Underactive thyroid. This condition is easy to miss as the symptoms may be masked by the menorrhagia. As well as having no energy and feeling more tired than usual (both common symptoms of menorrhagia), the woman may be overweight and complain of being unable to lose this weight. Diagnosis is confirmed by a blood test and the treatment will be replacement thyroxine.

Hyperthroidism may also cause menstrual disorders and amenorrhoea.

Psychosomatic causes. Life events, such as a recent bereavement, break-up of a relationship or redundancy, can be traumatic enough to disturb normal endocrine function and contribute to menorrhagia. Long-term stressful situations at home or at work can have the same effect. It is quite possible for the woman herself not to be aware of the connection, therefore such events may well not be mentioned while she is with the doctor. Most patients hesitate to 'waste the doctor's time'.

Time spent with you following the consultation with an opportunity to discuss different treatment options, may provide the helpful environment needed for your client to discover the underlying cause of her problem and consider ways of dealing with it.

In some cases the present difficulty seems relatively small and the stress belongs to an event or situation from the past, maybe even from childhood, which was repressed at the time. Such problems will probably need specialist help from a clinical psychologist, skilled psychotherapist or counsellor and must certainly be resolved before major surgery such as hysterectomy is considered.

Endometriosis. See page 539.

Polycystic ovaries. See page 527.

Pelvic inflammatory disease. See page 531.

Blood coagulation disorders, e.g. thrombocytopaemia will cause menorrhagia.

Endometrial carcinoma. This occurs most commonly after the menopause with about three-quarters of sufferers being over the age of 50. At present there is no screening test for this disease so it is especially important to advise all women to seek medical advice without delay if they have any post-menopausal bleeding, or irregular bleeding around the time of the menopause.

Carcinoma of the cervix. This is usually preceded by dysplasia of the cervix and cervical intraepithelial neoplasia (CIN grade I–III), which can be detected by cervical cytology and colposcopy (see Chapter 13).

The woman may be asymptomatic or may complain of:

◆ Abnormal bleeding: post-coital, intermenstrual, post-menopausal bleeding, or menorrhagia

◆ Discharge which may be offensive or blood-stained

◆ With advanced disease, a fistula or pain.

Other causes. Women who have been sterilized may complain of heavier periods. This is particularly noticeable in women who have been taking the combined contraceptive pill prior to their sterilization procedure. While there is no evidence that modern methods of sterilization cause menorrhagia, sometimes the perception of heavier periods may be due to the psychological disturbance caused by menstruation when fertility has been removed (Pearce, 1991).

Other conditions and diseases can contribute to menorrhagia, sometimes because of the medication needed, such as anti-clotting drugs (e.g. warfarin) for the patient who has had heart-valve replacement surgery. Menorrhagia may make a pre-existing condition such as rheumatoid arthritis or lupus erythematosus more difficult to cope with. Because it is not always possible to find compatible drugs, patients in this situation may be recommended to consider hysterectomy and be referred to a gynaecologist for an opinion. You may be able to offer extra support while a decision is reached.

Dysfunctional uterine bleeding. Frequently no explanation for menorrhagia will be found and it will be described as dysfunctional uterine bleeding. This means that, despite all the research into the subject, scientists have still not fully identified the cause of the disturbance.

Clearly the woman's perception of her situation is important and it is not helpful for her to be dismissed by medical staff because she is not anaemic or because no abnormality in the pelvis has been found. This effectively discounts what for her is a major problem.

Assessment of menorrhagia

Assessment of menorrhagia is for the most part subjective although researchers have long recommended scientific measurement (Haynes *et al.*, 1977) because of the variability of a woman's idea of her own blood loss (Chimbira *et al.*, 1980). The equipment for this is not available to most practices or hospital departments but Waytt *et al.* (2001) showed that using a menstrual pictogram provided a simple way of measuring menstrual blood loss. By careful listening, a nurse or doctor can form a good idea of the situation by finding out:

◆ If her nights are disturbed and if the sheets need changing

◆ If she has to wear towels as well as tampons and how frequently she has to change them

◆ If she passes clots and/or experiences flooding

◆ If her activities are restricted during menstruation.

However, there are clinicians who argue that this is not a satisfactory way of assessing the problem (Fraser *et al.*, 1984).

Some women overestimate the amount they are losing during menstruation, but the nature of a woman's job or employment can make loss of a small amount seem intolerable and she may need help in understanding and managing the situation. A 2-hour spell of duty at a supermarket checkout where unscheduled breaks to change a towel or tampon are frowned on can cause great anxiety. 'Flooding', the rapid loss of blood, can be particularly embarrassing and is not always related to a total heavy loss. A board meeting in a City office where all the other directors are men may be difficult for the woman trying to cope with menorrhagia while striving to resist being made to feel inadequate.

> **Box 18.2** Investigations for menorrhagia
>
> ◆ *Blood tests* These will determine hormonal and endocrine status, also anaemia
> ◆ *Pelvic ultrasound* The ovaries can be seen and the thickness of the endometrium estimated. Polyps, fibroids or other tumours may be noted and measured
> ◆ *Endometrial biopsy* This can be done as an outpatient procedure using a pipelle or vabra (see also page 549)
> ◆ *Hysteroscopy and biopsy* Hysteroscopy alone can be done as an outpatient procedure, without anaesthetic, allowing examination of the endometrium and a biopsy if appropriate
> ◆ *Laparoscopy* This allows inspection of the pelvic organs.

Investigations

Women with known or suspected pathology will be referred to a gynaecologist for an opinion. Investigations may be necessary to confirm the diagnosis and exclude serious disease (Box 18.2).

Treatment

This may be medical or surgical and will depend on the diagnosis and the preference of the patient (Box 18.3).

The Royal College of Obstetricians and Gynaecologists (1999) found only 58% of women

> **Box 18.3** Treatment for menorrhagia
>
> **Medical options**
> ◆ Reassurance
> ◆ Hormonal treatment
> ◆ Non-hormonal drugs
> ◆ Prostaglandin inhibitors
> ◆ Anti-fibrinolytic agents
> ◆ Iron
> ◆ Removal of IUD
> ◆ Insertion of the intrauterine system (IUS).
>
> **Surgical options**
> ◆ Endometrial resection
> ◆ Endometrial ablation
> ◆ Hysterectomy
> ◆ Myomectomy.

received medical therapy before referral to a specialist and issued guidelines for the initial management of menorrhagia. Two recent studies (Kupperman *et al.*, 2004; Hurskainen *et al.*, 2004) have shown that despite aggressive medical management most women with menorrhagia, unrelated to pregnancy or malignancy, will eventually need surgery and will undergo additional suffering by forestalling more definitive treatment. Roy and Bhattacharya (2004), in a literature review to compare the efficacy and tolerability of different medical treatments for menorrhagia, conclude that there is a general lack of an evidence-based approach, marked variation in practice and continuing uncertainty regarding the most appropriate therapy.

Hormonal treatment. If there are no contraindications the combined oral contraceptive pill is effective at reducing menstrual blood loss.

The levonorgestrel-releasing intrauterine system, releasing 20 µg of levonorgestrel daily into the uterine cavity, rendering the endometrium inactive, is also effective. Not only does it provide effective contraception, but it also reduces menstrual blood loss by 80% (Andersson and Rybo, 1990) and has now gained a licence in the UK for the treatment of idiopathic menorrhagia.

In an emergency the bleeding may be controlled by giving moderately high doses of progestogen. Oral medroxyprogesterone acetate (MPA) (Provera), norethisterone (Primolut N) or dydrogesterone (Duphaston) should be effective but are disappointing in the majority of cases (Coulter *et al.*, 1995). It takes 48 hours or more for progestogens to become effective. If the bleeding does not respond to treatment by then it may be necessary for the woman to have a hysteroscopy and curettage to remove some of the thickened endometrium. The curettage will not have a lasting effect and she will normally be prescribed further hormonal treatment. Usually this will be a progestogen taken from mid-cycle or from day 5 of the cycle. If there are no contraindications she may prefer to take the combined oral contraceptive pill instead. Treatment will usually only be needed for 3 or 4 cycles until the hormonal balance is restored.

Women who become anaemic will need maintenance courses of iron until the situation has improved.

Danol (danazol) inhibits ovarian activity in a similar way with different side effects which are dose-dependent. Low-dose treatment is worth trying as it may improve menorrhagia. It can be given for longer than the GnRH analogues (usually 9 months). Side effects are a problem and they can be unpleasant – including weight gain, depression, hirsutism, acne and voice changes. Danol is not the treatment of choice for singers as changes to the voice may be permanent. Other side effects are temporary. Although periods may be suppressed with danol, some form of contraception (not hormonal) must be used during treatment. This is especially important when danol is used because of the possibility of masculinization of a female fetus should pregnancy occur.

Hormones in the GnRH analogues group will control the cycle by preventing ovulation through intervention at the pituitary level, e.g. leuprorelin acetate (Prostap). Women using these drugs may experience a surge of oestrogen initially which can cause extra or heavier bleeding but, once ovarian suppression is achieved, menstruation will be minimal or non-existent. A temporary menopausal state will be induced by taking the drug. It is worth warning your client that she will experience menopausal symptoms such as hot flushes, night sweats and dryness in the vagina. This situation is reversible and as soon as treatment stops the hormone levels will return to normal.

Some women find this treatment unpleasant and may decide to discontinue, while others welcome the break from heavy periods and would like to be able to continue for longer. The treatment is expensive and for short-term use only because of the effect of oestrogen withdrawal on bone density, leading to osteoporosis. It is particularly useful for reducing the size of fibroids before surgery and the thickness of the endometrium before an endometrial resection. Some forms of GnRH analogues are taken nasally by sniffing (buserilin), others are given by injection (goserilin). One injection lasts a month.

Non-hormonal treatment. Anti-prostaglandin synthetase inhibitors (also called non-steroidal anti-inflammatory drugs) can be useful in controlling menorrhagia and are effective analgesics. They are a large group which includes mefenamic acid, naproxen and ibuprofen. To avoid gastrointestinal upset always advise patients using drugs from this group to take the tablets with food.

The anti-fibrinolytic agents aminocaproic acid and tranexamic acid can be effective in reducing menorrhagia, particularly when an IUD is thought to be the problem. Ethamsylate, a haemostatic agent, has a similar effect.

Surgical options. Surgical options are discussed in Chapter 19. Fibroids are particularly common in African women and if hysterectomy is being considered as a possible method of treatment, it is vital that the woman and her partner, if she wishes, should be included in the discussion. In many cases the ability to have children is most important and without sufficient counselling and time to reflect, the woman could accept a cure for her distressing symptoms which might leave her relationship in pieces.

Amenorrhoea

Amenorrhoea is classified as primary or secondary and is defined in the Oxford Concise Medical Dictionary as 'the absence or stopping of the menstrual periods'.

Primary amenorrhoea

This refers to the delayed onset of periods or menarche. Puberty, which is the onset of sexual maturity, may or may not be delayed. Some causes are listed in Box 18.4.

Whether the cause of the delay is endocrinological or congenital, it will be a source of concern and distress for the parents, and as time progresses for the young woman as well. A mother may appreciate the opportunity to talk to a nurse about amenorrhoea before involving her daughter in the process of investigations. Figures vary, but the incidence of endocrine disorders being the cause of primary amenorrhoea is in the order of 40% (Ross and Vandewiele, 1985). Ninety-five per cent of girls menstruate before they are 16. In the absence of the development of any secondary sexual characteristics (breast development indicates that the gonads are active and producing oestrogen), investigation may be justified at 14 but this will depend on the family history and the level of anxiety shown by the parents and the young woman. Delayed puberty is often familial or constitutional and will need no treatment other than time. Primary ovarian failure or dysfunction of the hypothalamus or anterior pituitary will need to be excluded (Brook, 1985).

Management of primary amenorrhoea is specialized and the young woman will usually be referred to the care of an endocrinologist or a gynaecologist with a particular interest in paediatric gynaecology and/or endocrinology.

The commonest cause of ovarian dysgenesis (the ovaries develop and then fail) is Turner's syndrome. This is a chromosomal abnormality in which spontaneous menstruation and development of secondary sex characteristics are rare.

Turner's syndrome is treated with the administration of oestrogen to establish breast development. Oestrogen is essential for growth and bone development and for maintaining health in the female. If it is not produced or its production is inhibited then hormone replacement at an early age is indicated. If the patient has a uterus, hormone replacement therapy (HRT) including

a progestogen will achieve a monthly bleed and maintain the health of the endometrium. The chances of a normal pregnancy are small.

In cases of *androgen insensitivity syndrome* (AIS) (or testicular feminization syndrome) the girl will look female and will have normal breast development but no pubic or axillary hair. She will have no uterus and only a short vagina. Fortunately this is a rare condition but, when it does occur, skilled ongoing support for the young woman and her family are essential in order to achieve a successful psychological and sexual adjustment to a complex situation (Goodall, 1991).

Occasionally, investigations for primary amenorrhoea will reveal functioning ovaries but an absent uterus, with or without a vagina. Sometimes an adequate vagina can be obtained by indentation and stretching of the skin. If this is not possible, a vaginoplasty may be performed. This is a major operation and the constructed vagina will stenose if not dilated artificially or by coitus. Again, careful counselling and support will be needed for the young woman and her parents. The mother particularly may feel guilty in these circumstances and the relationship with her daughter may be put under great strain.

Local support groups for these conditions are starting to be formed. Up-to-date information can be obtained from the organization Contact-A-Family and the AIS support group (see Resources).

Fortunately cases such as that described in the Scenario are rare, but they are highly specialized, difficult areas of female health. Minto *et al.* (2003) found 90% of women with AIS had sexual difficulties and concluded that clinical services for the management of intersex conditions should be multidisciplinary and aim to optimize the woman's physical and psychological health. This is best provided by a hospital where all the resources needed are available on one site, and there is good communication between all carers, particularly the general practitioner.

Cryptomenorrhoea is a physical cause of primary amenorrhoea where menstrual blood is

SCENARIO

Lucy, a 19-year-old in her first year at university, was referred to the gynaecologist because she was unable to have sexual intercourse and attempts at penetration were distressingly painful for her. She was accompanied by her anxious, distressed mother. Examination was not possible and so Lucy was admitted for an examination under anaesthetic and a laparoscopy. She had been having periods and had developed as a normal female.

At this stage Lucy asserted her independence as a young adult and requested that she should be told the results of the investigations. She would then tell her parents, and any further conversations with them were to be in her presence. This caused considerable consternation within the family but Lucy's wishes were respected. Laparoscopy confirmed the findings of the ultrasound scan which had shown two ovaries and a uterus. The examination under anaesthetic (EUA) revealed that there was no practical vagina present, just a small track through which menstrual blood could escape. Initially Lucy was angry and refused to see the psychologist to whom she was referred for an assessment. After some weeks of silence, however, she phoned to say that she would like to return for treatment and that she would see the psychologist first.

The vaginal opening was enlarged surgically and when the tissues had healed Lucy was taught how to gently stretch her new vagina with dilators. The instructing nurse and Lucy got on well together and Lucy was able to talk about some of the issues that were bothering her. Her partner was supportive and understanding and together they went for psychosexual counselling. Her relationship with her parents changed to one where Lucy was treated as an adult, capable of making her own decisions.

> **Box 18.5** Causes of secondary amenorrhoea and oligomenorrhoea
>
> ◆ Pregnancy
> ◆ Eating disorders
> ◆ Stress, emotional upset
> ◆ Strenuous exercise
> ◆ Pituitary tumour or hyperprolactinaemia
> ◆ Uterine adhesions (Asherman's syndrome)
> ◆ Polycystic ovary syndrome
> ◆ Premature ovarian failure
> ◆ Radiotherapy and chemotherapy.

that she is known to have produced gonadotrophins and must therefore have ovaries, a uterus and a vagina. Investigations are therefore less extensive. Some causes of secondary amenorrhoea and oligomenorrhoea (i.e. infrequent menstruation with gaps of 6 weeks or longer) are listed in Box 18.5.

Pregnancy. The most common cause of secondary amenorrhoea is pregnancy, sometimes overlooked by the woman herself.

Lactation may prolong amenorrhoea when breastfeeding is frequent and demand-led.

SCENARIO

Dina, a 41-year-old woman with a history of infertility and no children, went on holiday to Baghdad to visit her family for three months. While there she developed severe abdominal pain and was admitted to hospital. She gave birth to a healthy 3.75 kg baby girl.

unable to escape from the uterus either because of a transverse vaginal septum or an imperforate hymen. Both are rare conditions but will require surgical intervention.

The symptoms are cyclical pain with lower abdominal swelling. Surgery is usually straightforward although the Fallopian tubes may have been damaged by retrograde menstruation (the menstrual blood flows backwards up the tube).

Secondary amenorrhoea

This refers to absence of menstruation for 6 months in a woman who has previously menstruated. The fact that she has a menstrual history means

Eating disorders. Being underweight can delay menarche or, at a later age, can cause secondary amenorrhoea (Adams *et al.*, 1986). Fat should comprise at least 17% of body weight for the onset and maintenance of regular menstruation to be achieved (Frisch *et al.*, 1973). Anorexia nervosa and bulimia are both psychosomatic illnesses where the individual has a disturbed pattern of eating which is linked to a disturbed body image (see page 161). If psychological treatment is successful and a satisfactory body mass index can be attained, regular menstruation will return.

It has been suggested that dieting is an aetiological factor in the onset of bulimia (Treasure, 1990).

There are many women for whom weight and body image become an obsession. Dieting is big business and for over a decade the fashionable figure has been slim not fat. It is perhaps not surprising that eating disorders are so common and that some women who present in the infertility clinic are unable to conceive because their low weight is suppressing regular menstruation. (Obesity can have a similar effect.)

A brief period of amenorrhoea may result from psychological stress and emotional upset (Franks, 1987). Unless associated with a marked loss in weight it is unlikely to last longer than two or three cycles. Hypothalamic GnRH secretion is temporarily disturbed.

Strenuous exercise. Athletes, particularly runners, are more prone to oligomenorrhoea and amenorrhoea than the general population. The combination of stress, intensive exercise and weight loss appears to be the factor that affects GnRH secretion. Ballerinas and other dancers, where height, weight and shape can influence their career prospects, are also more likely to experience amenorrhoea. Puberty and menarche may be later than average because of a low body mass index.

Ballerinas are also susceptible to eating disorders. Low levels of circulating oestrogen over an extended period can result in osteoporosis and scoliosis (Warren, 1983). Stress fractures and soft tissue injuries are the result of the osteoporotic changes and lower than normal levels of collagen. Intensive exercise in these circumstances can only slightly compensate for the oestrogen deficiency. Appropriate counselling is needed and in some cases dietary advice. When the body weight is increased, menstruation usually resumes.

Kazis and Iglesias (2003) describe the female athlete triad, a syndrome consisting of disordered eating, amenorrhea and osteoporosis. This syndrome is increasing in prevalence as more women are participating in sports at a competitive level. Adolescents particularly may be at risk because it is during this crucial time that females attain their peak bone mass. Treatment of the female athlete triad is initially aimed at increasing calorie intake and decreasing physical activity until normal menstruation returns.

Hyperprolactinaemia. This is a disruption of the normal secretion of prolactin from the pituitary. It is most commonly due to a tumour but may occasionally be a symptom of polycystic ovary syndrome (PCOS). If due to PCOS the woman will not be short of oestrogen but if a tumour is present she will show symptoms of low oestrogen.

Hypothyroidism must be excluded and treatment will be according to the diagnosis.

Asherman's syndrome. This is a condition where intrauterine adhesions are formed following vigorous curettage or a severe intrauterine infection (including tuberculosis). While the full syndrome is rare, it is not unusual to see cases where adhesions restrict the growth of the endometrium causing menstrual irregularities and subfertility.

Treatment where possible is by hysteroscopic division of adhesions (Magos, 2002) followed by a course of oestrogen or a cyclical oestrogen/progestogen preparation. Sometimes steroids are given for 3 weeks and an IUD may be inserted temporarily to prevent further adhesions forming.

Polycystic ovary syndrome (PCOS). About 20% of women have polycystic ovaries (Polson *et al.*, 1988), whilst about 5-10% have additional symptoms and have PCOS (Franks, 1995).

Polycystic ovaries contain at least 10 small cysts and can be observed on a pelvic ultrasound scan (Figure 18.7). Normally these cysts (partially developed eggs that were not released) do not cause any problem.

A woman has PCOS when she has other symptoms in addition to the cysts on the ovaries, such as:

◆ Irregular periods
◆ Acne

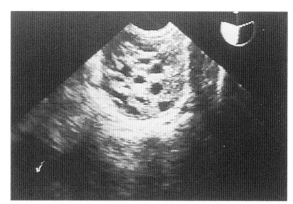

Figure 18.7 Polycystic ovaries. (Photograph courtesy of Organon Laboratories.)

◆ Hirsutism

◆ Tendency to be overweight

◆ Pelvic pain

◆ Possible infertility

◆ Recurrent miscarriage

◆ Insulin resistance.

Diagnosis is confirmed by trans-vaginal ultrasound scan and a blood test to confirm raised LH and/or raised testosterone levels.

The cause of PCOS is not known although it may be that the ovary does not secrete the right balance of hormones which causes an abnormal feedback to the pituitary gland. The pituitary then releases high amounts of LH in an attempt to correct the problem. In recent years it has become clear that PCOS is closely related to a problem with insulin. In PCOS there is a resistance of the cells in the body to insulin, so the pancreas makes more insulin to try and compensate. The excessively high levels of insulin have an effect on the ovary, preventing ovulation and causing a rise in testosterone levels. There is also a hereditary element in some families.

The hormonal imbalance leads to either irregular ovulation or anovulation, resulting in oligomenorrhoea and occasionally amenorrhoea. With irregular ovulation the chances of conception are reduced. If she does become pregnant, a woman with PCOS has an increased risk of miscarriage, probably because the high level of LH affects development of the ovum and the implantation of the embryo in the wall of the uterus.

Raised testosterone levels from the ovary and metabolism of oestrogen in fat may cause both acne and hirsutism. These are embarrassing symptoms and women with unwanted hair have to cope with additional expenditure on depilatory creams or electrolysis.

Weight control is often a problem for women with PCOS and they will be asked to diet in order to achieve a satisfactory weight-to-height ratio. In fact, some women only have symptoms as their weight increases. Just as being underweight can affect ovulation, so obesity can have a similar effect and has to be considered when fertility treatment is being contemplated. Any encouragement that you can give to a woman to enable her to reduce weight before she is seen and investigated in hospital will help to make treatment more likely to succeed.

PCOS is treated by establishing control of and regularizing ovarian activity.

For women who have no wish to become pregnant, the oral contraceptive pill is the easiest solution. Ovarian activity is suppressed and a regular withdrawal bleed achieved. Pills vary in strength and progesterone content and experimentation may be needed to find the best one for an individual. A pill containing cyproterone acetate is beneficial for those who mainly complain of acne and hirsutism. A short course of a GnRH analogue will control symptoms in the short term, but, as mentioned earlier, cannot be used for longer than 6 months. In the hyperandrogenic woman an anti-androgen such as cyproterone acetate can be given. Acne often responds quickly with this treatment but any effect on hirsutism will take some months.

Metformin, an 'insulin-sensitising agent' used in Type 2 diabetes, lowers the blood sugar level thereby reducing the excessively high insulin levels and has increasingly been used in the treatment of PCOS. Harborne *et al.* (2003), whist acknowledging that there were modest benefits in the published studies with metformin, urged caution in prescribing this medication until more studies have been completed. Metformin is not licensed for PCOS, and therefore women must be adequately counselled before starting therapy.

Drugs to induce ovulation, e.g. clomiphene citrate, will be used when infertility is a problem; although spontaneous ovulation may occur when excess weight is lost. Sometimes surgical intervention is indicated as an alternative to ovarian stimulation. A minimally invasive technique known as laparoscopic ovarian diathermy, 'ovarian drilling', or laser laparoscopy has shown good pregnancy rates. The beneficial endocrinological and morphological effects of ovarian drilling appear to be sustained for up to nine years with most patients (Amer *et al.*, 2002).

Premature ovarian failure. The most commonly accepted definition of premature ovarian failure is the cessation of periods before the age of 40 years (Abdalla, 1993) (see also page 465) and can happen as early as the late teenage years.

The condition affects 1% of women, and in Britain the numbers are estimated to be in excess of 110,000. The news of premature ovarian failure triggers the emotions and feelings of bereavement and the young woman will require understanding and careful counselling from all involved. She will need to be given time to understand and come to terms with her feelings of acute loss and disbelief. Hopes of fertility without medical intervention are very unlikely. Occasionally a pregnancy will occur with or without treatment, but the outlook is poor.

In many cases the reason for the early ovarian failure will not be known. The woman will have been referred to the clinic with amenorrhoea. She may have had occasional periods with longer spells without bleeding. Some possible causes are listed in Box 18.6.

Resistant ovary syndrome is a relatively rare condition which may be an autoimmune disorder. The patient has amenorrhoea, high FSH and LH levels indicating a post-menopausal state but the ovary still contains follicles.

Premature ovarian failure is investigated with blood tests for FSH, LH, oestradiol and ovarian antibodies, and a pelvic ultrasound scan. An ovarian biopsy could confirm the absence of follicles but is rarely done because of the likelihood of causing antibodies and adhesion formation. If there

---

Box 18.6 Causes of premature ovarian failure

- ◆ Surgery
  - ◆ Hysterectomy with oophorectomy
  - ◆ Hysterectomy with conservation of the ovaries
- ◆ Iatrogenic
  - ◆ Radiotherapy
  - ◆ Chemotherapy
- ◆ Natural causes
  - ◆ Genetic factors
  - ◆ Autoimmune disease
  - ◆ Infection
- ◆ Unknown.

---

are no follicles there will be no further activity from the ovaries.

The only way that a young woman with premature ovarian failure can contemplate a family, apart from adoption, is by oocyte donation and *in vitro* fertilization (IVF) or gamete intra-fallopian transfer (GIFT) (see Chapter 10). These options need to be approached with caution and should not even be considered until the woman and her partner are both strong enough to be able to cope with the investigations, medication and interventions involved. But most of all they have to be strong enough to accept the disruption of their sexual privacy and the disappointment of no baby should the procedure fail.

Women with premature ovarian failure will be advised to take HRT to prevent the long-term consequences of oestrogen deficiency such as osteoporosis. Taking HRT may not be an easy decision and you may be able to help by talking it through with her and explaining the reasons and benefits. Occasionally the combined oral contraceptive pill may be prescribed. Although taking 'the pill' normalizes the woman with others of her peer group, the oestrogens used are synthetic and at a higher dose than required. Additionally, as it is only taken for 3 weeks out of 4, the skeleton will lose out on optimal protection against osteoporosis, and symptoms such as hot flushes and night sweats can return in the pill-free week.

Beverley, a 32-year-old woman who had been married for 8 years, came to the clinic asking for advice about her periods, which had been infrequent since she stopped taking the oral contraceptive pill 7 months previously. She and her husband wanted to start a family. Taking her history the nurse learnt that she had been treated for Hodgkin's disease with chemotherapy 10 years ago and again for a recurrence 5 years later.

At no time had it been suggested to Beverley that her fertility might be affected. Blood tests and a pelvic ultrasound scan confirmed the diagnosis of premature ovarian failure.

Beverley had several sessions with the counsellor in which she expressed her sadness, anger, feelings of guilt and resentment that she had had no counselling before chemotherapy nor been given any hint of the possibility of ovarian failure. On the contrary, she had been prescribed the pill so that she would avoid the risk of pregnancy until her body had time to recover from the effects of the second course of treatment. The irony of the situation made it more difficult to accept. Investigation showed that it was possibly the first treatment that had caused the damage. Beverley was encouraged to tell her doctor at the next check-up how she was feeling, and eventually agreed to start HRT.

Her husband joined her for counselling and they discussed their future hopes and plans, including the possibility of life without children. She obtained information about infertility treatment which she shared with her counsellor. There followed a period of no contact and then a phone call came to say that she was on a waiting list for IVF (with ovum donation).

HRT will quickly relieve the immediate symptoms of oestrogen deficiency so that the woman will regain some of her former sense of well-being.

There is still concern about the effect of long-term HRT on the breasts and the small increase in the risk of developing breast cancer (Writing Group for the Women's Health Initiative Investigators, 2002; Million Women Study Collaborators, 2003). Breast awareness should be encouraged, but it is generally agreed that with premature ovarian failure the benefits of HRT outweigh the risks, except perhaps in those with a strong family history of carcinoma of the breast.

Dysmenorrhoea

Dysmenorrhoea is painful menstruation. Many women experience some discomfort with the onset of a period, but dysmenorrhoea is more severe, with pain often felt in the lower back and radiating down the tops of the legs.

Primary dysmenorrhoea

Primary dysmenorrhoea occurs within 1 or 2 years of the onset of menstruation (the first cycles are usually anovular and not painful). Primary dysmenorrhoea affects most women throughout the menstrual years but improvement is more likely in women who have children. Dysmenorrhoea severe enough to cause absence from work occurs in less than 5% of women (Weissman *et al.*, 2004).

It is thought that prostaglandins, present in the uterus in large numbers during menstruation, cause the pain. Other possible causes that may need to be considered include pelvic inflammatory disease, congenital abnormalities and endometriosis.

Symptoms associated with severe dysmenorrhoea include:

◆ Nausea/vomiting
◆ Pallor/fainting
◆ Headache/migraine
◆ Bowel disturbance
◆ Bladder irritability.

Treatment. Primary dysmenorrhoea can be treated with an anti-prostaglandin synthetase inhibitor such as mefenamic acid, ibuprofen, or naproxen to lessen the pain. Treatment must be started as soon as the period starts. An alternative is the combined oral contraceptive pill, which will suppress ovulation and reduce the amount of blood lost. Occasionally the symptoms are so severe that a hysteroscopy is performed to exclude pathology within the uterus. A laparoscopy may also be needed, as endometriosis has been found to occur as early as 3–4 years after the onset of menstruation (Hoshiai *et al.*, 1993).

If symptoms persist and you have a good relationship with your client she may indicate that she would like to talk to you about the pain and the difficulty it causes her. If still at school she may be under undue pressure, perhaps related to her own wish to succeed. There may be problems at home or difficulty with a relationship. Tension affects perception of pain and she may find some relief when given the opportunity to talk freely with someone who is outside her circle of friends and family. You can also offer practical advice on managing pain. Sometimes pain is soothed by cuddling a hot-water bottle whilst others find that exercise encourages the release of endogenous endorphins which have natural analgesic properties.

Secondary dysmenorrhoea

Secondary dysmenorrhoea occurs later in life and is related to acquired disorders such as pelvic inflammatory disease, endometriosis and adenomyosis (endometriosis occurring in the myometrium). Less commonly, it is caused by uterine fibroids, cervical stenosis, psychological factors or an IUD.

The treatment will depend on finding the underlying cause of the pain.

Pelvic inflammatory disease (PID). This is infection or inflammation in the pelvis and is usually an ascending infection via the cervix (Box 18.7). The infection tends to centre on the Fallopian tubes or the endometrium with varying involvement of the peritoneum and surrounding structures, e.g. the ovary. It may be acute, subacute or chronic. Estimates from industrialized countries indicate an annual incidence of PID of 9.5–14 cases per 1000 women in their fertile years (Mårdh *et al.*, 1996). In the USA PID is the most common cause of hospitalization of reproductive-age women (Velebil *et al.*, 1995).

A woman with acute PID may present with

◆ Pyrexia, headache, malaise

◆ Lower abdominal pain, usually bilateral

◆ Vaginal discharge

◆ Dyspareunia

◆ Abnormal bleeding (e.g. heavier than normal).

Occasionally, she may have late onset of nausea and vomiting (in appendicitis the vomiting is usually an early symptom).

Box 18.7	Causes of pelvic inflammatory disease

◆ Ascending infection, usually sexually transmitted (often *Gonorrhoea* or *Chlamydia*)

◆ After surgery: curettage, termination of pregnancy, hysteroscopy, hysterosalpingography

◆ Transperitoneal: appendicitis or abdominal surgery

◆ Blood-borne infection, e.g. tuberculosis. This is rarely seen in the UK but the incidence may be increasing.

The onset of symptoms often coincides with the start of a period, and the lower abdominal pain is at its worst during or sometimes immediately after a period. Examination of the patient will reveal a tender abdomen and occasionally a mass may be felt. In severe, acute PID there may be signs of peritonitis. Pelvic examination will be very painful. A mass felt in one of the fornices will usually indicate that an abscess has formed.

Investigations for PID include vaginal, urethral and cervical swabs for culture, blood tests (white cell count and ESR) and pelvic ultrasound scan. Laparoscopy is the only reliable way to confirm the diagnosis. The pelvis can be inspected and swabs taken from any site of infection.

Inflammation with no infection is usually due to pelvic surgery, haemorrhage or endometriosis.

Once diagnosed, the patient with PID may be admitted to hospital or she may stay in the care of her GP or be treated by the department of genitourinary medicine. Rest is essential. Antibiotic coverage will be given for at least 2 weeks, probably using two different antibiotics, and the earlier antibiotics are given the better. The aim is to cure the condition in the acute stage and to prevent it from recurring and becoming chronic. Her partner should be encouraged to attend a genitourinary clinic for swabs and treatment.

After one attack of PID the patient is vulnerable to further episodes. She should have been warned about this and you will be able to reinforce the advice to take life quietly until she has had time to recover fully. This will include avoiding energetic sexual activity. Barrier methods of contraception are protective. Explanation is needed that the risk of the disease becoming chronic is quite high and brings with it the scenario of future problems with fertility, pain, menstrual problems and dyspareunia.

You can also provide the understanding and sympathy which she will need. As well as the condition being painful and unpleasant there are additional feelings of guilt and self-reproach, particularly if the disease has been sexually transmitted, fear of future attacks and also implications for her fertility. She may feel resentment if the disease has been transmitted by her regular partner and will need help in managing the situation in which she finds herself. It may be helpful to suggest seeing a counsellor or therapist. You will find it useful if you know what resources are available in your area and the method of referral, e.g. self-referral, or by the nurse or doctor.

Salpingitis. This is an infection or inflammation in the Fallopian tubes and is commonly caused by *Chlamydia*. Seen through the laparoscope the tubes appear red, swollen and oedematous. At this stage the openings into the uterus are still patent and if successfully treated with antibiotics there will probably be no long-term damage. Tubal patency will be maintained.

If the disease progresses to subacute salpingitis a tubo-ovarian abscess or a pyosalpinx will have developed.

With chronic salpingitis the lumen of the tube becomes blocked at the fimbrial end with fluid in the tube. This is a hydrosalpinx. Hydrosalpinges cause infertility and pain and are usually associated with dyspareunia. The patient may also complain of dysuria.

If, after treatment with antibiotics, a pyosalpinx or tubo-ovarian abscess does not resolve it may have to be drained or the tube removed.

In severe cases, where the pain, misery and disruption of PID is affecting quality of life to such an extent that it has become disabling, hysterectomy with removal of both tubes may be considered an appropriate option. The ovaries could remain if unaffected but if they are removed oestrogen replacement should be given.

Clearly this is a big decision for any woman to make, especially in the light of the emotional agenda that often accompanies the onset of PID. To have reached the stage of considering major surgery, much suffering will have already been endured. The chance to talk the issues through with an informed and sympathetic nurse before coming to a decision may help her to feel she is more in control of the situation.

One of the major considerations will be future fertility. If the infection has been controlled but she has been left infertile, the option of IVF remains. After a hysterectomy she will have no hope of having children unless by surrogacy.

Even if a hysterectomy is what she wants, as her family may be complete or she may not want children, it is still important that she has an opportunity to explore her feelings with a nurse or counsellor before surgery. Feelings of loss after the operation are better coped with when they are recognized beforehand. It is one thing to decide that they do not want children but quite another to know that the option no longer exists.

Toxic shock syndrome (TSS). This is an infection caused by the bacteria *Staphylococcus aureus* which can enter the body via the vaginal wall from a tampon which has been left in too long, or was contaminated before insertion. Tampons should be changed about every 4 hours and one with reduced absorbency used if changing is not necessary. Damage to the membrane lining can be caused by a fingernail, a tampon applicator, or a tampon inserted with difficulty into a dry vagina. TSS is rare (an average of 18 cases are notified annually) but can be fatal. The symptoms are severe and include a sore throat, pyrexia, rash, diarrhoea, aching muscles and inflamed, sore eyes. Early diagnosis and removal of the tampon are essential. An appropriate antibiotic will be prescribed.

Pelvic pain

Some of the causes of pelvic pain have already been discussed and will be mentioned again. There are many gynaecological reasons for such pain but sometimes it may be related to other systems of the body, such as the urinary tract, intestinal tract or musculoskeletal system, or to a systemic disorder (porphyria) or psychosomatic causes.

Pelvic pain is a complex subject and can be acute or chronic (Box 18.8).

Acute pelvic pain associated with pregnancy

This is pain that starts suddenly with little if any prior warning. It is usually caused by ectopic pregnancy, miscarriage or degenerating fibroids.

Ectopic pregnancy

An ectopic pregnancy is a pregnancy occurring outside the uterus. Ninety-five per cent occur in one or other tube. In the UK there are around 11,000 cases of ectopic pregnancy per year with an incidence 11.5 per 1000 pregnancies (Tay *et al.*, 2000). Ectopic pregnancy is the fourth most common cause of maternal death during pregnancy, and accounts for about 10% of maternal deaths in the UK (HMSO, 1994).

The most common sites are the ampulla and the isthmus of the Fallopian tube and the cornual angle of the uterus. A pregnancy may less commonly be implanted on the interstitial section and the fimbriated end of the tube and rarely on the ovary and cervix or in the abdominal cavity, and is often the result of fibrosis or damage to the cilia in the tube following salpingitis. IVF carries an increased risk of ectopic pregnancy.

Other contributing factors include:

◆ IUD or progestogen-only pill
◆ Tubal surgery, including sterilization
◆ Postpartum or post-abortion infection
◆ Tuberculosis
◆ Low-grade pelvic inflammatory disease
◆ Congenital abnormality of the upper Mullerian duct (this forms the Fallopian tube)
◆ Endometriosis
◆ Uterine fibroids in or near the cornu
◆ Previous ectopic pregnancy (there is a 10% risk of a second ectopic occurring).

Depending on the site of the implantation the patient's symptoms will vary. If the event occurs within 4–6 weeks of her last period she may not realize she is pregnant. As most ectopic pregnancies are tubal, the space available for the developing ovum will affect the time before the woman has symptoms. She may or may not have had amenorrhoea or a minimal bleed coinciding with an expected period.

Diagnosis of an intact ectopic pregnancy can be difficult. Symptoms usually include lower abdominal tenderness or discomfort on one side and vaginal bleeding. If it is not recognized and treated, a tubal pregnancy has three possible outcomes:

1. *Tubal mole* The ovum separates. It is surrounded by blood which forms a clot. It may be reabsorbed or be expelled from the fimbriated end as a tubal abortion

2. *Tubal abortion* Haemorrhage is followed by separation of the ovum from the wall which is then passed from the fimbriated end into

the peritoneal cavity. Very rarely the pregnancy may continue in the abdominal cavity. The ovum implants or re-implants on a site such as the external surface of the uterus which has an adequate blood supply to sustain the developing fetus

3. Tubal rupture The trophoblast erodes the wall of the tube. This is followed by severe haemorrhage.

A woman with tubal rupture may not realize that she is pregnant but often will have missed one or two periods and may be feeling tenderness and tingling in her breasts. Presentation is sudden and the condition serious (Box 18.9 and page 556).

A diagnosis of ectopic pregnancy can be confirmed using a serum βhCG pregnancy test, which is accurate two weeks after conception, and a pelvic ultrasound scan or a transvaginal scan. Bimanual examination may reveal the site of the pain and any tender mass, but this has to be done with utmost care, as not only is it possible to rupture an ectopic pregnancy, it is also likely to be extremely painful.

Surgical treatments may be radical (salpingectomy) or conservative (usually salpingostomy) and they may be performed by laparoscopy or laparotomy. Salpingectomy is the treatment of choice if the Fallopian tube is extensively damaged as there is a high risk of recurrent pregnancy in that tube (Tay et al., 2000). Methotrexate, a folic acid antagonist, is used for medical management in patients before rupture who are haemodynamically stable (Jimenez-Caraballo and Rodriguez-Donoso, 1998).

In some cases of tubal abortion the ovum and debris will be reabsorbed without intervention.

The patient will be admitted to hospital for observation while the βhCG levels fall.

An ectopic pregnancy is a distressing event, calling for supportive skills and understanding. As well as having lost the pregnancy, the woman will have to come to terms with the fact that there is an increased risk of subsequent pregnancies being ectopic as well. She will be understandably apprehensive when she next realizes she is pregnant until implantation can be confirmed by pelvic ultrasound scan. If she has had previous pelvic inflammatory disease she may experience feelings of guilt or anger which will complicate her adjustment to the situation. Grieving is an important part of healing and your awareness of this can help you encourage the process and relieve the guilt.

Early miscarriage

Miscarriage or spontaneous abortion is the loss of a pregnancy before the fetus is legally viable at the 24th week of pregnancy. It is estimated that about 25% of pregnancies end in miscarriage during the first trimester (Pearce, 1991), due to a variety of causes (Box 18.10). In a three-year period 11 women died following a spontaneous abortion in the UK, whilst six died from post-abortion sepsis (Hibbard et al., 1994).

Pregnancy is divided into three trimesters – the first trimester refers to the first 12 weeks and it is during this period that early miscarriage or spontaneous abortion occurs. Miscarriage risk decreases as the pregnancy continues. Many women think that the word abortion refers to

---

Box 18.9 Symptoms of tubal rupture

◆ Sudden severe pain
◆ Vaginal bleeding
◆ Shoulder tip pain when lying down caused by irritation of the diaphragm by blood in the peritoneal cavity
◆ Pallor and signs of shock and blood loss
◆ Distended abdomen due to bleeding.

Box 18.10 Causes of early miscarriage

◆ Blighted ovum – an empty sac, no fetus
◆ Fetal abnormality of chromosomal origin
◆ Uterine abnormality – fibroids, divided septum
◆ Maternal disease – renal problems, diabetes, Listeria, tuberculosis, syphilis, rubella if infection between 4 and 8 weeks
◆ Endocrine problems – high LH levels, raised androgen levels may affect fetus and implantation
◆ Chorionic villus sampling – about 2% around 8–12 weeks.

a pregnancy that has been terminated deliberately. It has been suggested that the term 'miscarriage' should be used when referring to a spontaneous abortion and it is important for nurses to appreciate that, for most women in these circumstances, the word 'abortion' adds to their distress.

Bleeding will occur after a period of amenorrhoea where pregnancy is either suspected or has been confirmed. If, on gentle digital examination, the cervical os is found to be closed, a pelvic ultrasound scan should be arranged as soon as possible to confirm whether the fetal heartbeat is present and whether the pregnancy is still viable.

The only symptom of threatened miscarriage is bleeding. The likelihood of this pregnancy continuing is good and it is usually advisable for the woman to rest in bed until 24 hours after any bleeding has stopped. Opinions vary as to whether intercourse should be avoided until the second trimester.

With an inevitable or incomplete abortion the os will be found to be open on vaginal examination. The bleeding will be heavier with clots. Miscarriages of this kind before 6 weeks are often complete with the fetus and placenta being expelled together and the woman may not realize that she was pregnant.

Later than this, although many abortions are complete, it is more likely that the placenta will be left behind. The bleeding and uterine contractions can be so painful that they are comparable with labour pains (Weideger, 1975). Management of a spontaneous first trimester miscarriage can be surgical with an evacuation of the retained products of conception (ERPC) (see also page 556) or expectant management. Luise *et al.* (2002) in a study to evaluate the uptake of expectant management found that women preferred less intervention and 81% of women had a successful outcome without surgical intervention.

The differential diagnosis between a ruptured ectopic pregnancy and an incomplete abortion can be difficult to make. If the pain is one-sided it is more likely to be due to an ectopic pregnancy, while the pain felt during an incomplete abortion is central lower abdominal.

Many women are unaware that miscarriage is a common event and feel isolated and distressed in their misery at losing the pregnancy. Even in the early weeks miscarriage is felt as a great loss and a bereavement, and the support needed will be of the same quality as that offered after an ectopic pregnancy. Because for many women miscarriage is not something they have anticipated, these feelings can be bewildering. A woman struggling to come to terms with the event will welcome the chance to talk to you and the use of open-ended questions may help her to find a way of expressing her feelings. Too often follow-up in the community is haphazard and she has to cope alone in the best way she can. It can help to put her in touch with a support group.

Degenerating fibroids (red degeneration)
This is the most important complication of fibroids during pregnancy. Usually the woman will be known to have fibroids which will provide a clue to the diagnosis. The onset of symptoms is often sudden and can include severe pain localized over the fibroid, and possible vomiting with a raised temperature and pulse rate. If there is no improvement after 24 hours of treatment with analgesics, bed-rest and a local application of heat, then the diagnosis will be reconsidered.

Acute gynaecological pain

Onset of pain will be sudden. There will probably be no previous similar history. Possible causes include the onset of PID, ruptured corpus luteum, torsion of an ovarian cyst (associated with vomiting and bleeding), rupture of an ovarian cyst, and *mittelschmertz* (ovulation pain).

PID, ruptured corpus luteum and torsion of an ovarian cyst all feature in the differential diagnosis of an ectopic pregnancy which must be considered if there is any possibility of the woman being pregnant, even though there is no history of amenorrhoea or unusual vaginal bleeding.

Investigations to establish a diagnosis include:

◆ Pelvic examination
◆ Pregnancy test
◆ Pelvic ultrasound scan
◆ Laparoscopy.

Treatment will be conservative except where bleeding into the peritoneum occurs when the bleeding point will have to be ligated. The twisted ovary or cyst may have to be removed. If the ovary is still viable an ovarian cystectomy will be performed.

Chronic pelvic pain

Chronic pelvic pain is one of those conditions that causes a 'heartsink' reaction in the GP and the nurse as the patient comes through the surgery door. This is because it is a condition that can persist over many years, causing considerable disability. Despite extensive investigation and treatment, sometimes the onset and cause of the pain cannot be identified.

Various disorders cause chronic pelvic pain (see Box 18.8). Whilst some of the clinical causes have already been discussed, endometriosis, ovarian cysts and uterine prolapse will be discussed in greater length at the end of this chapter. It is worth remembering that patients presenting with chronic pelvic pain run the risk of being over-investigated or inappropriately treated. Sometimes the problem turns out to have a psychological origin.

Some points to consider when a client presents with chronic pelvic pain are:

◆ Are there any previous life events or unresolved problems that may be relevant?

◆ Why is the woman seeking help now?

◆ What is the effect on her relationships or family life?

◆ What is the effect on her ability to work?

Diastasis Symphysis Pubis (DSP)

DSP means an abnormally wide gap between the two pubic bones at the symphysis pubis joint. It usually occurs following pregnancy when progesterone will have softened the ligaments. After delivery the gap between the pubic bones will usually close but in cases of DSP there is gap of 1 cm or more.

This gap can cause chronic pain over the symphysis pubis joint which can also be felt in the hips, groin and may radiate down the inner thighs.

Diagnosis is by X-ray or ultrasound. Management is usually by analgesia, anti-inflammatory drugs and physiotherapy. Referral to a pain clinic may be helpful.

Psychological causes

Sometimes, chronic pelvic pain turns out to be functional – i.e. no physical cause can be found for the symptoms. This may be difficult for a woman to accept and all your listening and counselling skills will be needed to help her come to terms with her problem.

Considerable research has been done into the psychological aspects of women who have pelvic pain but the incidence of unexplained pain varies. One of the most comprehensive studies found that about two-thirds of the women presenting with pelvic pain had no obvious pathology to explain it (Gillibrand, 1981).

A history taken carefully and with time for the woman to talk may reveal unsuspected problems which at first might seem quite unrelated. With experience you will begin to recognize the external factors that can make the perception of pain more intense. For instance, she may have been sexually abused as a child and be showing signs of the unresolved consequences (see Chapter 5).

What you do when you have identified these stressful situations is another matter. To some extent this will depend on what confidence you have in your own counselling skills, what other resources are available and the complexity of the problem.

It is important for health care professionals, listening in depth to the worries and problems of clients, to have access to another member of staff to talk to if needed – rather in the way a counsellor will have a recognized support system. Such a system of clinical supervision not only benefits you by sharing a problem that could become overwhelming, but enables you to look at aspects of the problem in a different light in order to help your client. This does not involve breaking a confidence but gives you a useful sounding-board. Other people's problems when off-loaded on to you can feel quite stressful, and to be of further use to your client you have to avoid taking those problems home with you. It is important to remember that nobody should attempt to undertake a therapeutic counselling role until trained to do so.

If you are genuinely interested in your clients and show that you have time to listen, then you may well find yourself hearing some distressing information (Tschudin, 1991). Your response can trigger further confidences, but you should be aware of your own clinical boundaries and limits in dealing with such patients and not 'hang on' to a problem when you are out of your depth. This will certainly not help you or your client. Awareness that this may happen will enable you to plan your strategy of referral in advance of it being needed. Ideally it is helpful if you have a regularly updated list of local agencies, support groups and counsellors which can be shared by all members of the health care team. Comments from previous clients who have used the resources are also very helpful.

Other things can affect the perception of pain and previously unresolved life events can intensify the effect of pain without the sufferer being aware of what is happening to her (Holmes and Rahe, 1967). Some examples of such 'events' are:

- ◆ Bereavement – either recent or unresolved from the past
- ◆ Disturbed family relationships
- ◆ Marital problems
- ◆ Employment problems
- ◆ Stressful lifestyle
- ◆ Abuse
    - ◆ A violent relationship
    - ◆ Child abuse
    - ◆ Sexual abuse
    - ◆ Rape.

The suggestion that there may be a psychological element to pain is something that many of us find difficult to understand or accept. Your client may resist the idea that her pain is anything other than completely physical. Before you can help her to find a way acceptable to her of coping with the pain and making the perception of it less intense, you will have to convince her that you believe her, that you care about her problem and that you are on her side. Let her know that you do

SCENARIO

Carol was referred to the gynaecologist for advice about PMS. The nurse taking her history soon realized that the symptoms she was describing did not fit the definition of PMS. She was encouraged to talk about the issues in her life that put pressure on her, and about her relationships and her job. There were no obvious contributing factors although she was clearly not happy but did not appear to understand why. Carol was then asked to think back to her childhood. Had she been happy at school? Had she had any lengthy period of separation, e.g. in hospital? She described a stable family background and there was no apparent answer as to why she was having the symptoms she described.

There was a spell of silence, broken only when Carol began to talk about a single episode of sexual abuse which had happened to her when she was 11. She had felt guilty at the time, not really understanding what had happened but knowing that it was wrong and that she hated it. She had never talked about it before. It seemed that her first sexual relationship had triggered the onset of her 'PMS' symptoms.

Carol agreed to see the clinical psychologist. There was a 3-week delay before her first appointment. The nurse, concerned about her in the meantime, phoned to see how she was coping. She said that she had cried a lot and that having started to talk about it she could not stop. She was looking forward to seeing the psychologist and wished she had had the opportunity to reveal the event before.

The psychologist reassured the nurse that Carol would be able to cope with her distress while waiting, knowing that an appointment had been made.

not think the pain is in her mind, and if she is referred, for example to a psychologist, reassure her that you and her doctor are not trying to get rid of her and you will always be happy to see her again. Anything less than this does not justify the trust she has already put in you by confiding in you. The fact that she has been able to talk about and identify areas of her life that are hurting her may leave her feeling vulnerable and sensitive.

The help you will be able to suggest for your client will depend on what is available locally and the impression you have from her as to what is acceptable and what she will feel comfortable with. Supportive therapies such as relaxation techniques, hypnotherapy, acupuncture, massage with aromatherapy, reflexology or shiatsu may be available and may appeal to your client (Wells and Tschudin, 1994).

You will probably want to discuss the problem with the doctor involved who may have ideas on this. It is sometimes useful to ask yourself why has your client come for help *now*. For example, feelings attached to a previous termination of pregnancy may have been repressed or denied at the time. Still unresolved, these feelings will continue to cause unhappiness which can be disregarded by the patient until a totally unrelated event proves to be the last straw which makes her seek help. The termination will not be the cause of the pain but will affect her perception of it.

Feelings attached to a bereavement can intensify pain and referral to a bereavement counsellor or CRUSE may be the place to start (see Resources).

In some cases of PID or endometriosis the pain can become incapacitating. Major surgery such as hysterectomy and removal of both ovaries and tubes may be suggested as the only solution. Allowing your client to vent her feelings of anger or guilt may help her in the process of recognition that relief may be available to her.

Your ability to appear receptive to clients and then hear what they are saying will depend on your professional communication skills. Books are available which, although often targeted at doctors and medical students, contain suggestions on how these skills may be improved which apply equally well to nurses (Davis and Fallowfield, 1991).

Referral to a psychologist or counsellor with an interest in gynaecological pain may be acceptable to your client and help her to come to terms with the situation and to decide how to cope in the future.

Much has been written during the last 30 years on helping relieve pelvic pain where investigations have failed to reveal any identifiable gynaecological disorder or pathology (Pearce and Beard, 1984). A 'model of pain' may be agreed upon with the patient before the psychologist takes a history (Erskine and Pearce, 1991). Such a history will include past episodes of pain and any psychosexual experiences. A pain diary can be kept and brought to the next appointment.

Clients are often resistant to accepting a referral of this kind and may need time to think about it. Some will be referred to a hospital pain clinic.

Dyspareunia

Many conditions can give rise to painful intercourse or dyspareunia, which is clearly a distressing symptom not only for the woman but also for her partner.

Dyspareunia can be defined as either *deep* – referring to problems within the pelvis – or *superficial* – relating to pain or discomfort at or near the introitus. The causes are listed in Box 18.11.

Whatever the cause of dyspareunia it will be made worse by dryness in the vagina. This may be due to a physiological lack of oestrogen, as happens after the menopause, or in response to fear of pain which can inhibit lubrication. Whatever the

---

Box 18.11   Causes of dyspareunia

Deep dyspareunia

- Endometriosis
- Pelvic inflammatory disease
- Adhesions
- Prolapsed ovary in the pouch of Douglas (usually associated with a retroverted uterus)
- Ovarian cyst.

Fibroids rarely cause pain but may make intercourse uncomfortable.

Superficial dyspareunia

This occurs with most vaginal and vulval infections and irritations.

- Vaginal atrophy
- Vaginitis
- Vaginismus – muscle tension or spasm in the lower third of the vagina that prevents penetration
- Painful perineal scar
- Bartholin's cyst
- Vulvodynia – pain in the vulva which is triggered by intercourse and which often remains unexplained.

cause it is helpful to suggest a topical lubricant such as KY jelly to apply until treatment takes effect. 'Replens' is a non-hormonal vaginal moisturizer which you can safely recommend to the post-menopausal woman complaining of a lack of lubrication. It should be used three times a week, and multiple applications restore the pH to the normal physiological range found in pre-menopausal women.

Dyspareunia needs to be taken seriously as it is the cause of much unhappiness. It can be a pre-cursor to vaginismus, which will prevent the woman having intercourse or using tampons. The cause may be physical or psychological, or a combination, and may need expert help from a psychosexual counsellor or a psychologist. A sensitive nurse may become aware of the woman's difficulty in this area when carrying out a speculum examination. Careful counselling and steps taken to alleviate the cause will help to avoid the onset of vaginismus.

Bartholin's cyst

Bartholin's glands lie on each side of the vulva with a duct that opens at the vaginal introitus. They are susceptible to infection by sexually transmitted infections and also the general organisms such as staphylococci and Escherichia coli. If the duct becomes blocked the mucus secretions that lubricate the vaginal opening during intercourse are unable to drain and a cyst forms. Sometimes the cyst may resolve, or resolve and recur with sexual arousal. The usual treatment is excision of part of the wall of the gland (marsupialization) (see page 555).

If the gland is infected, an abscess will occur which is extremely painful (Bartholin's abscess). The treatment is admission to hospital, marsupialization and antibiotic therapy.

Endometriosis

Endometriosis is the presence of tissue histologically similar to the endometrium which is outside the uterine cavity. Endometriosis is most commonly found on the ovary. It also occurs on the outside of the uterus, on the utero-sacral and broad ligaments and the peritoneum. Other less common sites include the bowel wall, the bladder, cervix, vagina, vulva, and umbilicus and in scar tissue. It occasionally, but rarely, occurs in the lung.

There are three accepted theories as to why endometriosis occurs. It is generally agreed that none of these provide the complete answer (Olive and Schwartz, 1993).

1. *The transplantation theory* This was first proposed in the 1920s. During menstruation some blood mixed with cells flows backwards up the tubes and escapes into the peritoneal cavity. This is called 'retrograde menstruation'. Since then it has been widely established by laparoscopy that this is a common event in normal menstruating women. The unknown factor is why some women and not others develop endometriosis

2. *Involvement of the autoimmune system* has been suggested

3. The role of *peritoneal fluid* is also being researched (Ramey and Archer, 1993).

The endometrial deposits outside the uterus are subject to the same hormonal changes, so during menstruation it will continue to function in the same way as the endometrium lining the uterus. The blood released has no way of escape and is reabsorbed into the bloodstream. The inflammation caused gives rise to scarring which, if extensive, forms adhesions that distort the normal anatomy in the pelvis.

Another puzzling thing about endometriosis is that the symptoms experienced by the woman do not necessarily reflect the degree of the disease. Patients with minimal disease can have considerable pain and dyspareunia, while some women with severe endometriosis do not have symptoms that upset them unduly.

Endometriosis has been classified by the American Fertility Society into four stages according to severity:

Stage I = minimal

Stage II = mild

Stage III = moderate

Stage IV = severe.

> **Box 18.12   Symptoms of endometriosis**
>
> ◆ *Dysmenorrhoea* The pain tends to last throughout the period and may get worse towards the end rather than tailing off
> ◆ *Menorrhagia* Patients with endometriosis often find their periods start with 2 or 3 days spotting of dark blood and that their periods are heavy
> ◆ *Dyspareunia*
> ◆ *Infertility* About a third of known cases are affected. This may be the only symptom.

In severe endometriosis the ovaries, Fallopian tubes, uterus and bowel are stuck together and may be fixed by dense adhesions. An ovary may be out of position on the back of the uterus or in the pouch of Douglas. This gives rise to deep dyspareunia with pain persisting for several hours. The partners of women who suffer from endometriosis are affected by the fact that they initiate the pain and this frequently has a harmful effect on the sexual side of the relationship. Release of an ovum and subsequent passage through the tube in such circumstances may be difficult and the woman may have problems with conception.

Some symptoms of endometriosis are listed in Box 18.12. Some women also experience tiredness and depression.

Diagnosis

Initial diagnosis of endometriosis is by pelvic examination which may reveal tenderness and nodularity. Pelvic ultrasound scan is not very helpful although it can pick up an ovarian cyst which may be an endometrioma.

Diagnosis is confirmed by laparoscopy. The deposits may be seen as tiny black spots or larger cysts known as 'chocolate cysts' from the appearance of altered blood. Depending on the stage of development of the disease the colour of the deposits ranges from almost colourless, through pink, to red, to purple and then black when endometriosis is long-standing.

Treatment

Medical treatment

Endometriosis rarely occurs after the menopause and then only in women taking HRT. Pregnancy has a limiting, often curative, effect on the disease but, even if a baby is wanted, infertility may be one of the symptoms of the disease. Medical treatment therefore is based on suppressing ovarian function, as was described earlier in treatment of menorrhagia (page 523). The difference between various medical treatments is in their side effects, with some treatments being more acceptable than others.

Non-steroidal anti-inflammatory drugs such as ibuprofen and mefenamic acid for pain relief.

The combined contraceptive pill. The pill can be successful in the treatment of mild cases, particularly when contraception is also needed. It is particularly effective when the tricycling method is used (page 270).

Progestogens. Norethisterone, dydrogesterone or medroxyprogesterone acetate given in high doses will have the same hormonal effect as a pregnancy. The side effects are symptoms similar to those of PMS, and breakthrough bleeding may be a problem.

Danol (danazol). This may be used for up to 9 months and where the side effects (discussed earlier) are tolerated can dampen down the endometriosis. It may well recur when the normal menstrual cycle is re-established although some women find their symptoms are improved.

GnRH analogues. These are effective in suppressing the disease but can only be taken in the short term because of the risk of osteoporosis.

Alternative and complementary therapies. Many women report an improvement in their symptoms when they take vitamins, mineral trace elements or herbal remedies. It is an area of therapy that has not attracted research but the interest in these sorts of cures for PMS has encouraged endometriosis sufferers to try them. Mood swings, vaginal dryness and cramp-like pain are all reported to have been relieved by oil of evening primrose. The B vitamins (particularly B_6) and trace elements such as zinc and magnesium are also found to be effective. Without the support of reputable scientific studies, the part played by the placebo effect in these treatments is unknown. It will be helpful if you have knowledge of some of the alternatives available and can advise your client where she can go for more information if she expresses an interest (see Chapter 4).

Endometriosis is similar to chronic pelvic pain in that some women suffering from the disease may have taken a long time to find a doctor to make the diagnosis. Your client may wish to discuss her progress with you. It can be therapeutic and reassuring for her to find a professional who understands and is willing to listen. She may have had to curtail her social activities and her quality of life may have suffered. Dyspareunia can have a disastrous effect on a relationship. Unfortunately, symptoms may persist in some patients even after the disease has been successfully treated and laparoscopy reveals no further evidence of active disease.

Surgical treatment

Women who do not respond to the above therapies or are unable to tolerate the side effects should be referred to a gynaecologist and may require surgical intervention (Prentice, 2001).

Techniques using local ablative treatment, with diathermy or laser laparoscopes, have been developed with mixed reports of success. Sutton *et al.* (1994) found the benefit greater in women with the most severe disease. There is less recovery time needed when micro-surgical techniques are used but the equipment is expensive and availability is limited. Consequently many women have to undergo major surgery. The problem of recurrence may remain although treatment with suppressive therapy prior to surgery may be helpful in this respect.

Hysterectomy and bilateral salpingo-oophorectomy may be considered as the final option available to the woman who has suffered pain and its consequences over a number of years (Mathur and Fox, 2003). The implications are similar to those discussed for women with chronic pelvic pain. The decision to have surgery may come as a relief, but again it is wise if you help the patient to examine her feelings about fertility beforehand.

Ovarian cysts

There are many types of ovarian cysts. The most common types are described in Box 18.13.

Ovarian cysts are often asymptomatic and the woman may not consult the doctor until the cyst is large and causing pressure symptoms such as abdominal distension, interference with normal

---

Box 18.13 Ovarian cysts

Distension or non-neoplastic cysts

◆ *Follicular cysts* These are common and usually single. They seldom grow to be larger than 5 cm in diameter and most are discovered incidentally during a pelvic ultrasound scan or laparoscopy. Most regress spontaneously and require no treatment

◆ *Corpus luteum cysts* These may be associated with amenorrhoea and can occur in the pregnant or non-pregnant woman. They usually regress, but occasionally rupture, when the symptoms may be similar to those of an ectopic pregnancy. The pain, which can be severe, is usually short-lived. A pelvic ultrasound scan may help in making the diagnosis, if this is in doubt

◆ *Theca lutein cysts* These are multilocular and associated with hydatidiform mole

◆ *Cystic neoplasms* These occur between the menarche and the menopause

◆ *Serous cystadenoma* This is an epithelial cyst which may be simple or multilocular. Usually not larger than 15 cm in diameter, it may be bilateral

◆ *Mucinous cystadenoma* These are common and can grow to an enormous size. They are multilocular in structure and contain mucus which may be thick or thin. If a mucinous cyst ruptures, the rare condition myxoma peritonei may occur. Large collections of mucinous material accumulate in the peritoneal cavity and progressively spread, even after removal

◆ *Benign cystic teratomas, or dermoid cysts* These occur most commonly in young women, and again may grow to a large size. They are derived from germ cells. The cysts are covered in a firm, fibrous capsule and may contain sebaceous material, hair, teeth, bone, cartilage, thyroid and neural tissue and gastrointestinal mucosa. Dermoid cysts are heavy and are susceptible to torsion.

micturition, altered bowel habit, dyspareunia and pelvic or epigastric discomfort.

Pain will be a symptom of rupture or torsion of a cyst.

All cysts larger than 5 cm in diameter will usually be removed as soon as possible because of the risk of malignancy. Benign cysts are usually resected in younger women leaving as much ovarian tissue intact as possible. Cysts occurring in the peri- and post-menopausal woman must always be investigated, and a hysterectomy with bilateral salpingo-oophorectomy will be advised if malignancy cannot be excluded. If you are involved in helping a woman make this difficult decision, if she is already taking or considering HRT it is worth remembering she will be able to take oestrogen replacement without progestogen. This will be a positive aspect of surgery to discuss with her.

Carcinoma of the ovary

There is as yet no safe and reliable screening method to detect this cancer, which remains a silent and deadly disease. There is often no pain or discomfort until the tumour is quite advanced, when the woman may present with loss of weight and ascites. Some cases may be detected earlier when the woman is found to have an adnexal mass on abdominal examination.

Carcinoma of the ovary is responsible for about 4000 deaths in England and Wales each year. This is about the same number as the combined deaths from cervical and endometrial cancer. Every year nearly 2% of women develop cancer of the ovary. A small percentage of ovarian cancers have a genetic link.

The incidence is higher in women in their fifties and sixties and among single and nulliparous women. Pregnancy and the oral contraceptive pill both have a protective effect and it is thought that repeated ovulation without any gaps may be responsible for the development of this cancer.

A pelvic ultrasound scan, with a laparoscopy if the findings are doubtful, will aid diagnosis. A serum tumour marker assay, CA125, may also be performed but false positives can occur.

Women with ovarian cancer should be seen by expert teams based in cancer centres, and if surgery is needed it should be carried out by specialist gynaecological oncologists, according to guidance by the NHS Executive (NHS Centre for Reviews and Dissemination, 1999). The most important prognostic factor is the stage and distribution of the disease at the time of diagnosis. Generally the prognosis is poor and surgery will usually be followed by radiotherapy or chemotherapy. Unfortunately many women with this disease present late and the survival rate is only about 30%, irrespective of the grading of the tumour (see also Chapter 19).

Uterine prolapse

Uterine prolapse can cause symptoms of pelvic pain or ache, backache, urinary symptoms and dyspareunia. It occurs because of inadequacy of the muscles or ligaments of the pelvic floor. It may be due to pregnancy and delivery, atrophy due to oestrogen deficiency, or intra-abdominal pressure. Occasionally it is seen in women with no children and so presumably a congenital factor, such as an unusually large vagina, may be involved as well. Pelvic floor exercises in the puerperium and later in life when muscle tone decreases are aimed at preventing this from happening. In all types of prolapse the woman will have a bulge into the vagina. Further than this she may be asymptomatic or have minimal problems.

There are three degrees of uterine prolapse:

◆ *1st degree* The cervix does not reach the introitus
◆ *2nd degree* The cervix descends to the introitus
◆ *3rd degree* The cervix is below the introitus.

In extreme cases the uterus prolapses right outside the vagina. This is called a *procidentia*.

Other types of prolapse can still occur after hysterectomy. These include the following:

◆ *Vault prolapse* The vaginal vault prolapses

◆ *Cystocele* The bladder bulges through a weakness in the anterior vaginal wall

◆ *Cysto-urethrocele* The urethra is involved as well. The symptoms reflect problems with the bladder and include: difficulty emptying the bladder, recurrent cystitis, stress incontinence and dyspareunia

◆ *Enterocele* The upper third of the posterior vaginal wall is covered by peritoneum and lies adjacent to the pouch of Douglas. A weakness may result in a hernia, usually containing bowel or omentum

◆ *Rectocele* This is a prolapse in the middle third of the posterior wall which lies adjacent to the rectum. The woman may have backache and a dragging feeling in the pelvic floor. A rectocele can cause dyspareunia and a heavy 'bearing down' sensation. If the perineal body is damaged, the rectocele will extend lower down the vaginal wall. (A rectal prolapse may be associated with vaginal prolapse and cystocele but is a separate condition in which the rectum prolapses through the anal sphincter.)

Treatment

Treatment for a prolapse will depend on the nature of the symptoms and how the woman herself views them and their effect on her life. Any decision to operate should be made only when the nature of the surgery and the likely outcome of the procedure has been fully explained and discussed with the patient. Full recovery time varies considerably with repair operations. She will need time to consider the implications of surgery in the light of her present symptoms and to discuss these with her partner or family. You may be involved in helping her come to a decision.

If she is elderly and unfit for an operation, she may be fitted with a ring pessary. These are changed every 4–6 months and work quite well in this situation by supporting the pelvic organs, although vaginal tissues may become irritated and sore. Intermittent courses of vaginal oestrogen help to prevent atrophic changes, infection, inflammation and discharge.

Conclusion

This chapter can only be an introduction to some of the common gynaecological problems you will meet. Often women seeking help may be embarrassed and confused by the changes that they are aware of in their bodies. You may be the first person your patient can talk to about her problems and difficulties. Once a diagnosis has been made, a knowledge of the implications of a condition may enable you to support and reassure her, if this is what she needs from you.

Often people do not ask for help because they do not realize that they have a problem. This is especially true where pain is involved and it is not easy helping in such cases. Sometimes it can be distressing, which is why you need to consider the support available to you in your working environment. Finding an empathetic listener can be the first step your patient takes in coming to terms with a difficult situation.

Ideas for personal and professional development

● Visit your local gynaecological out-patient clinic to see the variety of problems encountered. Research the disorders that you come across to enable you to give up-to-date advice to your patients

● Find out where your nearest early pregnancy assessment unit is and arrange a visit. How do women access this service and what ongoing support is given?

● Research the treatment options for menorrhagia or chronic pelvic pain and then compile a simple fact sheet for women on how they can cope with the problem

● Gynaecological problems are frequently interrelated with other problems and life events. Start a reflective diary on women that you see with a gynaecological problem. Try and view your clients holistically and find out what has made them seek advice at this moment in time.

Patient education points

- Menstrual problems are very common and assessment of blood loss is highly subjective. Keep a record of how many pads or tampons are used in a day and at night, and whether any clots are present

- If irregular bleeding is a nuisance, try and keep a menstrual diary of spotting, bleeding and pain and bring this diary with you when you next visit a health professional

- Many gynaecological problems can now be sorted with medication, rather than surgery

- The levonorgestrel intrauterine system, as well as providing effective contraception, has a beneficial effect on painful and heavy periods and premenstrual syndrome, and appears to be protective against pelvic inflammatory disease.

Resources

Androgen Insensitivity Syndrome Support Group (AISSG UK)
PO Box 429, Oldham, Lancs OL4 4ZT
www.medhelp.org/www/ais

British Association for Counselling and Psychotherapy
BACP House, 35–37 Albert Street, Rugby CV21 2SG
www.bacp.co.uk

Contact-a-Family
209–211 City Road, London EC1V 1JN
Tel: 020 7608 8701
Helpline: 0808 808 3555
www.cafamily.org.uk
For families who care for children with any disability or special need.

Cruse Bereavement Care (Head office)
Cruse House, 126 Sheen Road, Richmond TW9 1UR
Tel: 020 8939 9530
Helpline: 0870 167 1677
www.crusebereavementcare.org.uk

Will provide local addresses and numbers for bereavement counselling.

Daisy Network
PO Box 183, Rossendale BB4 6WZ
www.daisynetwork.org.uk
A support group for women suffering from a premature menopause.

National Endometriosis Society
50 Westminster Palace Gardens, Artillery Row, London SW1P 1RR
Tel: 020 7222 2781
Helpline: 0808 808 2227
www.endo.org.uk
Offers support and advice to endometriosis sufferers.

Turner's Syndrome Society
12 Irving Quadrant, Hardgate, Clydebank G81 6AZ
Tel: 01389 380385
www.tss.org.uk

Verity (Polycystic Ovaries Self Help Group)
The Grayston Centre, 28 Charles Square, London N1 6HT
www.verity-pcos.org.uk

Vulval Pain Society
PO Box 7804, Nottingham NG3 5ZQ
www.vul-pain.dircon.co.uk

Westminster Pastoral Foundation
23 Kensington Square, London W8 5HN
Tel: 020 7361 4800
www.wpf.org.uk
Self-referral for counselling. There is usually a waiting list for those over 25.

Further reading

BARCLAY, C.S. (1998) *Obstetrics and Gynaecology in Primary Care: The Primary Care Handbook and Aide Memoire.* Salisbury: Quay Books.
BROOME, A. and WALLACE, L. (eds) (1984) *Psychology and Gynaecological Problems.* London: Tavistock Publications.
DAVIS, H. and FALLOWFIELD, L. (eds) (1991) *Counselling and Communication in Health Care.* Chichester: John Wiley.
HARRIS, C. and CAREY, A. (2000) *PCOS: A Women's Guide to Dealing With Polycystic Ovary Syndrome.* London: Thorsons.

MACKAY, E.V., BEISCHER, N.A., COX, L.W. and WOOD, C. (1992) *Illustrated Textbook of Gynaecology*, 2nd edn. Sydney: W.B. Saunders/Baillière Tindall.

RIZK, B. and ABDALLA, H. (2003) *Fast Facts: Endometriosis*, 2nd edn. Oxford: Health Press.

SCAMBLER, A. and SCAMBLER, G. (1993) *Menstrual Disorders*. London: Routledge.

STUDD, J. and EDWARDS, L. (eds) (1997) *Hysterectomy and HRT*. London: RCOG.

SUTHERLAND, C. (2001) *Women's Health: A Handbook for Nurses*. Edinburgh: Churchill Livingstone.

TSCHUDIN, V. (1991) *Counselling Skills for Nurses*, 3rd edn. London: Baillière Tindall.

WELLS, D. (ed.) (2000) *Caring for Sexuality in Health and Illness*. Edinburgh: Churchill Livingstone.

WELLS, R. and TSCHUDIN, V. (eds) (1994) *Wells' Supportive Therapies in Health Care*. London: Baillière Tindall.

References

ABDALLA, H.I. (1993) Oocyte donation. In Asch, R.H. and Studd, J.W.W. (eds) *Annual Progress in Reproductive Medicine*. Carnforth, Lancs: Parthenon Publishing.

ADAMS, J., POLSON, D.W. and FRANKS, S. (1986) Prevalence of polycystic ovaries in women with anovulation and idiopathic hirsutism. *British Medical Journal* **293**:355.

AMER, S.A., BANU, Z., LI, T.C. and COOKE, I.D. (2002). Long-term follow-up of patients with polycystic ovary syndrome after laparoscopic ovarian frilling: endocrine and ultrasonographic outcomes. *Human Reproduction* **17**(11):2851–7.

ANDERSSON, J.K. and RYBO, G.B. (1990). Levonorgestrel-releasing intrauterine device in the treatment of menorrhagia. *British Journal of Obstetrics and Gynaecology* **97**:690–4.

BALEN, A. (1993) Amenorrhoea – causes and consequences. In Asch, R.H. and Studd, J.W.W. (eds) *Annual Progress in Reproductive Medicine*. Carnforth, Lancs: Parthenon Publishing.

BARRINGTON, J.W. and BOWEN SIMPKINS, P. (1997) The levonorgestrel intrauterine system in the treatment of menorrhagia. *British Journal of Obstetrics and Gynaecology* **104**:614–16.

BROOK, C.D.G. (1985) Management of delayed puberty. *British Medical Journal* **290**:657.

CHIMBIRA, T.H., ANDERSON, A.B.M., NAISH, C. *et al.* (1980) Reduction of menstrual blood loss by danazol in unexplained menorrhagia: lack of effect of placebo. *British Journal of Obstetrics and Gynaecology* **87**:1152.

COULTER, A., KELLAND, J., PETO, V. and REES, M.C. (1995) Treating menorrhagia in primary care. An overview of drug trials and survey of prescribing practice. *International Journal of Technology Assessment in Health Care* **11**:456–71.

DAVIS, H. and FALLOWFIELD, L. (1991) Evaluating counselling communication. In Davis, H. and Fallowfield, L. (eds) *Counselling and Communication in Health Care*. Chichester: John Wiley.

DEUTSCH, H. (1944) *The Psychology of Women*. New York: Grune & Stratton.

ERSKINE, A. and PEARCE, S. (1991) Pain in gynaecology. In Davis, H. and Fallowfield, L. (eds) *Counselling and Communication in Health Care*. Chichester: John Wiley.

FRANKS, S. (1987) Primary and secondary amenorrhoea. *British Medical Journal* **294**:815.

FRANKS, S. (1995). Polycystic ovary syndrome. *New England Journal of Medicine*. **333**:853–61.

FRASER, I.S., McCARRON, G., MARKHAM, R. *et al.* (1984) A preliminary study of factors influencing perception of menstrual blood loss volume. *American Journal of Obstetrics and Gynecology* **149**:788.

FRISCH, R.E., REVELLE, R. and COOK, S. (1973) Components of weight at menarche and the initiation of the adolescent growth spurt in girls: estimated total water, lean body weight and fat. *Human Biology* **45**:469.

GILLIBRAND, P.N. (1981) The investigation of pelvic pain. Communication at the Scientific Meeting on 'Chronic pelvic pain – a gynaecological headache'. Royal College of Obstetrics and Gynaecology, London.

GOODALL, J. (1991) Helping a child to understand her own testicular feminisation/Y chromosome. *Lancet* **337**:33.

GUILLEBAUD, J., ANDERSON, A.B.M. and TURNBULL, A.C. (1978) Reduction by mefenamic acid of increased menstrual blood loss associated with intrauterine contraception. *British Journal of Obstetrics and Gynaecology* **85**:53.

HARBORNE, L., FLEMING, R., LYALL, H., NORMAN, J. and SATTAR, N (2003) Descriptive review of the evidence for the use of metformin in polycycstic ovary syndrome. *Lancet* **361**:1894–901.

HAYNES, P.J., HODGSON, H., ANDERSON, A.M. *et al.* (1977) Measurement of menstrual blood loss in patients complaining of menorrhagia. *British Journal of Obstetrics and Gynaecology* **84**:763.

HIBBARD, B.M., ANDERSON, M.M., O'DRIFE, J. *et al.* (1994) *Maternal Mortality Report: Report on the Confidential Enquiries into Maternal Deaths in the United Kingdom 1988–1990*. London: HMSO.

HMSO (1994) *Report on Confidential Enquiries into Maternal Deaths in the UK*. London: HMSO.

HOLMES, T.H. and RAHE, R.H. (1967) Social events readjustment rating scale. *Journal of Psychosomatic Research* **11**:213.

HOSHIAI, H., ISHIKAWA, M., SAWATARI, Y. *et al.* (1993) Laparoscopic evaluation of the onset and progression of endometriosis. *American Journal of Obstetrics and Gynecology* **169**:714.

HURSKAINEN, R. *et al.* (2004). Clinical outcomes and costs with the levonorgestrel-releasing system or hysterectomy for treatment of menorrhagia: randomized trial 5-year follow-up. *Journal of the American Medical Association* **291**(12):1456–63.

JIMENEZ-CARABALLO, A. and RODRIGUEZ-DONOSO, G. (1998). A six-year clinical trial of methotrexate therapy in the treatment of ectopic pregnancy. *European Journal of Obstetrics and Gynaecology* **79**:167–71.

KAZIS, K. and IGLESIAS, E. (2003). The female athlete triad. *Adolescent Medicine* **14**(1):87–95.

KUPPERMAN, M. (2004). Effect of hysterectomy vs. medical treatment on health-related quality of life and sexual functioning: the medicine or surgery (MS) randomized trial. *Journal of the American Medical Association* **291**(12):1447–55.

LUISE, C., JERMY, K., MAY, C. *et al.* (2002) Outcome of expectant management of spontaneous first trimester miscarriage: observational study. *British Medical Journal* **324**:873-5.

MAGOS, A. (2002). Hysteroscopic treatment of Asherman's syndrome. *Reproductive Biomedicine Online* **4**(Suppl 3):46–51.

MÅRDH, P.A., MÖLLER, B., PAAVONEN, J. and WESTRÖM, L. (1996) Pelvic inflammatory disease. In Mandel, L.G. and Rein, M.F. (eds) *Atlas of Infectious Diseases*, Vol V. Philadelphia: Churchill Livingstone, Chapter 5.

MATHUR, R. and FOX, R. (2003) Bilateral oophorectomy and hormone replacement therapy for women with endometriosis. In Studd, J.W.W. (ed.) *Progress in Obstetrics and Gynaecology*, Vol 15. Edinburgh: Churchill Livingstone, Chapter 20.

MILLION WOMEN STUDY COLLABORATORS (2003) Breast cancer and hormone replacement therapy in the Million Women Study. *Lancet* **362**:419–27.

MINTO, C.L., LIAO, K.L., CONWAY, G.S. and CREIGHTON, S.M. (2003) Sexual function in women with complete androgen insensitivity syndrome. *Fertility and Sterility* **80**(1):157–64.

NHS CENTRE FOR REVIEWS AND DISSEMINATION (1999) *Improving Outcomes in Gynaecological Cancers: Guidance for Commissioners of Cancer Services.* Effective Health Care Bulletin No. 5(3). York: University of York.

OLIVE, D.L. and SCHWARTZ, L.B. (1993) Endometriosis. *New England Journal of Medicine* **328**:1759.

PEARCE, J.M. (1991) Spontaneous abortion. In Varma, T.R. (ed.) *Clinical Gynaecology.* London: Edward Arnold.

PEARCE, S. and BEARD, R.W. (1984) Chronic pelvic pain. In Broome, A. and Wallace, L. (eds) *Psychology and Gynaecological Problems.* London: Tavistock Publications.

POLSON, D.W., ADAMS, J., WADSWORTH, J. *et al.* (1988) Polycystic ovaries – a common finding in normal women. *Lancet* **1**:870.

PRENTICE, A. (2001) Endometriosis. *British Medical Journal* **323**(7304):93–5.

RAMEY, J.W. and ARCHER, D.F. (1993) Peritoneal fluid: its relevance to the development of endometriosis. *Fertility and Sterility* **60**:1.

ROSS, G.T. and VANDEWIELE, R. (1985) The ovary. In Wilson, J.D. and Foster, D. (eds) *Textbook of Endocrinology.* Philadelphia: W.B. Saunders.

ROY, S.N., and BHATTACHARYA, S. (2004). Benefits and risks of pharmacological agents used for the treatment of menorrhagia. *Drug Safety* **27**(2):75–90.

ROYAL COLLEGE OF OBSTETRICIANS AND GYNAE-COLOGISTS (1999) *The Management of Menorrhagia in Secondary Care.* London: RCOG.

SCAMBLER, A. and SCAMBLER, G. (1993) Menstrual disorders. In Fitzpatrick, R. and Newman. S. (eds) *The Experience of Illness Series.* London: Tavistock/Routledge.

SNOWDEN, R. and CHRISTIAN, B. (eds) (1983) *Patterns and Perceptions of Menstruation.* A World Health Organization International Study. Beckenham: Croom Helm.

STEELE, S.J. (1985) *Gynaecology, Obstetrics and the Neonate.* London: Edward Arnold.

SUTTON, C.J., EWEN, S.P., WHITELAW, N. and HAINES, P. (1994) Prospective, randomised, double-blind controlled trial of laser laparoscopy in the treatment of pelvic pain associated with minimal, mild and moderate endometriosis. *Fertility and Sterility* **62**:696–700.

TAY, J.I., MOORE, J. and WALKER, J.J. (2000) Regular review: ectopic pregnancy. *British Medical Journal* **320**:916–19.

TREASURE, J.L. (1990) Anorexia nervosa. In Studd, J.W.W. (ed.) *Progress in Obstetrics and Gynaecology*, Vol 8. Edinburgh: Churchill Livingstone.

TSCHUDIN, V. (1991) *Counselling Skills for Nurses*, 3rd edn. London: Baillière Tindall.

VELEBIL, P., WINGO, P.A., XIA, Z., WILCOX, L.S. and PETERSON, H.B. (1995) Rate of hospitalization for gynecologic disorders among reproductive age women in the United States. *Obstetrics and Gynecology* **86**:764–9.

WARREN, M.P. (1983) Effects of under-nutrition on reproductive function in the human. *Endocrinology Reviews* **4**:363.

WAYTT, K.M., DINNOCK, P.M., WALKER, T.J. and O'BRIEN, P.M. (2001) Determination of menstrual blood loss. *Fertility and Sterility* **76**(1):125–31.

WEIDEGER, P. (1975) *Female Cycles.* London: Women's Press.

WEISSMAN, A.M., HARTZ, A.J., HANSEN, M.D. and JOHNSON, S.R. (2004) The natural history of primary dysmenorrhoea: a longitudinal survey. *British Journal of Obstetrics and Gynaecology* **111**(4):345–52.

WELLS, R. and TSCHUDIN, V. (eds) (1994) *Wells' Supportive Therapies in Health Care.* London: Baillière Tindall.

WRITING GROUP FOR THE WOMEN'S HEALTH INITIATIVE INVESTIGATORS (2002) Risks and benefits of estrogen plus progestin in healthy post-menopausal women: principal results from the Women's Health Initiative randomised controlled trial. *Journal American Medical Association* **288**:321–33.

19: Gynaecological Investigations and Surgery

Lisa Lee ◆

OBJECTIVES

This chapter should help you understand:

◆ The most common gynaecological operations and investigations currently performed ◆

◆ What women will experience whilst in hospital and during recovery at home ◆

◆ How to investigate the sexual aspects of surgery and discuss both practical and emotional issues ◆

◆ The importance of being aware of recent surgical developments and research within the field of women's health ◆

◆ The impact of government policy on the provision and access to health care ◆

◆ The changes within the organization and management of gynaecological cancers ◆

◆ The importance of the role of the nurse before, during and after gynaecological investigations and treatment. ◆

Introduction

The specialism of gynaecology is one of many areas of medical and nursing care that is constantly undergoing review and resulting in the change of practice. This is influenced primarily by the advances in surgical technology, leading to the introduction of a wider variety of procedures that are less invasive and, more importantly, more acceptable to women. Expectations of health care outcomes are continuing to rise with the access to health information via the internet, media, associations and support groups. Therefore it is vital that *all* health care professionals recognize the need to provide care and information that is relevant, evidence based and, most importantly, up to date.

Surgery on any part of the body can cause preoperative anxiety, and gynaecological surgery (however minor and routine a procedure may be) is no exception. A woman's anxieties relating to gynaecological problems are unique. Not only does she worry about vaginal examinations, but impending surgery also poses a threat to her concept of body image, her role as a woman and mother, her sexuality and her relationship with her partner (Broome and Wallace, 1984). Therefore the provision of emotional and psychosexual support for women and their partners throughout and following any procedure is vital to physical and psychological well-being.

Therefore in line with the NHS Plan (Department of Health (DoH), 2000a) gynaecological nurses must strive to ensure that the patient is central to care that is provided. The planning of any care pathway must reflect a streamlining of processes that women should undergo before having definitive treatment and, ultimately, that women have choice.

547

Gynaecological outpatient procedures

Ultrasound

Ultrasound is the first-line management for many gynaecological investigations such as pelvic pain, pelvic masses, dysfunctional uterine bleeding, menorrhagia, postmenopausal bleeding and problems related to early pregnancy. Ultrasound is used as a means of examining various organs of the body by means of high-frequency sound waves. These form pictures on a screen and a large number of abnormalities can be detected. Ultrasound scans are performed in a variety of departments: the diagnostic imaging department, gynaecology outpatient clinics, rapid access clinics and inpatient wards with a mobile scanner.

The Royal College of Obstetricians and Gynaecologists recommended (RCOG, 2000) that all gynaecology units should provide an early pregnancy assessment unit. Bigrigg and Read (1991) outline the benefits of such units in that they provide a streamlined service for women with bleeding or pain during pregnancy, therefore improving the quality of care. Units are able to provide assessment, diagnostic, counselling and support services to women within an allocated appointment. Central to these units is access to ultrasonography. Prior to the development of these units it was common practice for women presenting to accident and emergency departments to be admitted to an inpatient bed and then have a long wait for an ultrasound scan. Therefore the improvement in quality can be demonstrated with these units. From a government policy perspective, these units are vital in diverting patient admission via accident and emergency departments in achieving the current '4-hour wait' target as stated in the NHS Plan (DoH, 2000a).

Transabdominal ultrasound scan

The woman can prepare for the scan by drinking one and a half litres of fluid (not carbonated drinks) during the 2 hours before the appointment to enable the bladder to fill. A very full bladder feels uncomfortable but is important as it helps to push the uterus and ovaries into a better position for examination.

A cold gel is applied to the woman's abdomen, which helps the sound waves to pass into the abdomen by forming a good contact with the skin. A small scanning device (abdominal transducer) is then pressed firmly against the abdominal wall and is moved backwards and forwards across the abdomen to produce a picture on the nearby screen. The picture is built up from the differing times echoes take to bounce back from structures of varying density. The scanning room is darkened so that the images on the screen are more clearly visible.

The procedure takes between 5 and 10 minutes and is not painful but may be uncomfortable. This is because the clinician has to press firmly against the abdomen and full bladder in order to produce a clear picture. Once the scan has been performed, the bladder can be immediately emptied. The results of the scan are then explained to the woman.

Transvaginal ultrasound scan

This type of scan facilitates a much clearer view of the pelvic organs than a transabdominal ultrasound scan. The tip of a round-edged probe is inserted into the vagina. The probe is covered by a condom which is changed for each patient. A full bladder is not required for this procedure, making it easier for the clinician and certainly more comfortable for the patient. The scan cannot harm a pregnancy.

Colour flow Doppler scan

This is performed as a transvaginal scan but also involves the use of colour flow Doppler to identify blood flow through the pelvic organs. It has been suggested that these scans could be used to detect malignant conditions when previously not detected by ordinary ultrasound. However, in the detection of endometrial cancer colour flow, Doppler offers no significant benefits over the transabdominal scan (Vuento et al., 1999).

Further uses of ultrasound

◆ Ultrasound guidance for procedures such as cyst aspiration and insertion of drainage systems such as paracentesis and supra-pubic catheters

◆ Ultrasound guided biopsy of tissue to deter-mine pathology to aid staging procedures in the management of suspected gynaecological malignancies

◆ Transvaginal ultrasound guided aspiration of pelvic abscesses (Corsi *et al.*, 1999)

◆ Follicular tracking, egg collection and embryo transfer procedures during fertility treatments

◆ Measurements of bladder volume, which is less invasive and reduces the risk of intro-ducing infection compared to the insertion of a urinary catheter

◆ Three-dimensional ultrasound of the ure-thral sphincter for incontinence investigation (Athanasiou *et al.*, 1999)

◆ Sonohysterography – insertion of saline into the uterine cavity via a fine catheter under ultrasound guidance to examine the endometrium (Jorizzo *et al.*, 1999).

Endometrial biopsy

This can be undertaken in the outpatient setting without the need for a general anaesthetic. However, it is not suitable for nulliparous women, and women should be informed that they will experience some discomfort during the procedure. Two types of instruments are used to obtain a biopsy:

◆ *Pipelle* – a fine-bore catheter inserted into the endometrial cavity via the cervix to sample the endometrium

◆ *Vabra aspirator* – a sharp curette instrument connected to suction is used in the same way as a pipelle to obtain a biopsy of the endometrium.

Developments in gynaecological assessment procedures for dysfunctional uterine bleeding demonstrate how this procedure is undertaken as part of endometrial assessment during hys-teroscopic procedures (see hysteroscopy, page 550). Endometrial biopsy alone, however, has several associated risks, primarily that it is performed blind, and therefore has a high rate of false nega-tive results and also the biopsy can cause severe discomfort for some women (Akande, 2003).

Infertility investigations

Hysterosalpingogram (HSG)

A hysterosalpingogram is an X-ray examination of the female genital tract and takes about 15–20 minutes. It is a diagnostic aid and demon-strates internal uterine abnormalities, such as fibroids, bicornuate uterus and occasionally cervical incompetence. The test also illustrates the site of tubal occlusion in cases of infertility. If the Fallopian tubes are patent, radio-opaque dye will spill into the pelvic cavity. However, in many cases of infertility, the usefulness of this procedure has now been superseded by the 'laparoscopy and dye' test, which gives more detail about the nature of the tubal occlusion.

Women should be advised that period-type pains may be felt afterwards for which parace-tamol may be taken. Slight vaginal bleeding is common which may be mixed with a small amount of clear sticky fluid – the liquid used in the test. The woman should be escorted home and should rest as needed.

Hysterosalpingo-contrast sonography

This procedure is used to detect tubal defect and tubal blockage indicated by infertility problems. It can also demonstrate any irregularity within the uterine cavity. It has an advantage over HSG in that it does not expose the woman to X-rays, and, as it requires ultrasound guidance, it allows the pelvic organs to be assessed at the same time.

The procedure involves the insertion of a speculum to visualize the cervix through which a fine catheter is passed under vaginal ultrasound guidance. The catheter is held in place by a bal-loon. A solution of galactose-based echo contrast medium is injected into the uterine cavity via the catheter. The solution is inserted until the ultra-sound identifies the solution in the tubes or iden-tifies a blockage in one or both Fallopian tubes. Occasionally the woman may experience vasova-gal symptoms, usually due to instrumentation of and insertion of the catheter through the cervix.

Following the procedure the woman should be given mild analgesia if needed, informed that she will experience a milky white discharge and may also have some spotting that day. She should also be accompanied home and should rest as needed.

Minor gynaecological surgery

This section gives an outline of the procedures that are undertaken routinely as an outpatient or as a day-case; occasionally some women will require an overnight stay usually due to co-morbidities or social support. The baseline procedures will be initially described and, due to the advancements in minimally invasive surgery, concurrent treatments will be discussed later in this section.

Hysteroscopy

This procedure has superseded dilatation and curettage (D and C) as the most common minor gynaecological procedure. It should be offered as first-line surgical treatment for women presenting with dysfunctional bleeding (Pinion *et al.*, 1994). It is performed under a general or local anaesthetic. It involves the insertion of a small fibre-optic telescope into the uterine cavity via the cervix. The uterus is filled with gas or fluid to enable the gynaecologist to view the cavity. Nagele *et al.* (1996) demonstrated that using normal saline compared to carbon dioxide provided the gynaecologist with better views, shorter operating times and improved patient acceptability. The uterine cavity is visualized on a monitor allowing the surgeon to undertake endometrial biopsies.

Prior to discharge the woman should be given the following advice:

◆ Light vaginal bleeding may occur; if it becomes heavy or offensive she should contact her GP

◆ Use sanitary towels not tampons due to the neck of the cervix being dilated

◆ Abdominal cramps may be experienced; these can be relieved with analgesia such as paracetamol

◆ Do not drive for 48 hours if procedure was performed under general anaesthetic

◆ Resume sexual activity when comfortable for both partners

◆ Return to work within 1–2 days if fit

◆ Contact number should problems occur.

Davidson and Dubinsky (2003) state that 'hysteroscopy is likely to become the new gold standard in the future because of its ability to visualize directly the endometrium and perform directed biopsies as indicated'. The use of hysteroscopy within the outpatient setting has seen a rapid increase in service provision. This cannot be solely attributed to clinical or patient preference but also in conjunction with national guidance. This can be demonstrated with treatment targets set out within the National Cancer Plan (DoH, 2000b), and the formation of cancer centres, cancer units and rapid access or one-stop diagnostic clinics. This guidance focuses on optimizing patients' treatment pathways whist acknowledging evidence-based practice and fundamentally providing patient choice alongside accurate informed consent. The advantages of a one-stop clinic for post-menopausal bleeding are that ultrasonography, hysteroscopy, endometrial biopsy and haematological tests can be performed at the one attendance by the same clinician. In comparison, referral to a traditional gynaecology clinic required more hospital visits before eventually being put on a waiting list for a hysteroscopy with potential time delays from referral to diagnosis.

Bain *et al.* (2002) outlined that whilst outpatient diagnostic hysteroscopy did not influence clinical management it may give more reassurance. A study by Abu *et al.* (2001) found women were consistently more positive about their experience in a one-stop clinic compared to attending a traditional gynaecology clinic.

Current hysteroscopic techniques and developments for the treatment of menstrual disorders

When medical treatment fails to alleviate menorrhagia, the alternative minimally invasive technique of endometrial ablation is recognized as an effective alternative to hysterectomy (O'Connor and Magos, 1996). Over the past 15 years there have been many different types of endometrial resection and ablation techniques. The principle of these techniques is to remove hysteroscopically the lining of the uterus. There are a number of different ablative instruments that have been introduced and trialled since the introduction of the conventional transcervical resection of the endometrium (TCRE) which was pioneered in Oxford in 1987.

It is important to provide clear and concise information to women regarding treatment options and reinforce the fact that unlike hysterectomy, ablation does not guarantee amenorrhoea and women may require further surgery at a later date. However, a long-term study by the Aberdeen Endometrial Ablation Trials Group (1999), comparing endometrial ablation to hysterectomy, has shown that hysterectomy was avoided in 76% of women with dysfunctional bleeding.

Prior to any ablation women are usually given drugs such as Zoladex, a gonadotrophin-releasing hormone (GnRH) analogue or Danazol. They are given with the aim of reducing the thickness of the lining of the endometrium.

Current endometrial ablative procedures

- ◆ *Endometrial laser ablation (ELA).* This involves the passage of a small Nd:YAG laser (Nd:YAG = neodymium:yttrium aluminium garnet) into the uterus and heating the endometrium with laser energy. This can be time-consuming and the laser is very expensive and is viewed as a first-generation ablative technique.
- ◆ *Roller-ball.* This involves a small 25-mm oval-shaped roller-ball electrode that is passed, via a resectoscope, quickly over the surface of the uterus. A diathermy blade may be used to cut away the base of the polyps or fibroids.

These electrical techniques are all performed while fluid is circulated through the uterus.

The resectoscope is attached to a hysteromat pump which irrigates and expands the uterine cavity with glycine 1.5% irrigation fluid. This fluid is a nonconductive, transparent medium through which the gynaecologist maintains visibility whilst operating. The fluid, blood and debris are drawn out by suction into a separate container. Due to the intrauterine pressure the fluid can be absorbed, causing dilational hyponatraemia (low sodium) and fluid overload. During the procedure a precise fluid balance is maintained. If an excess of 200 ml is absorbed the procedure is quickly finished and the patient is given a diuretic.

There were concerns regarding the safety of these procedures and their complication rates due to the lack of frequency with which surgeons performed them. However, the MISTLETOE study (minimally invasive surgical techniques, laser, endothermal or endoresection) (Overton *et al.*, 1997) showed that these procedures were performed widely with low morbidity and mortality. It also stated that some forms of resection were safer than others and this has led to the development of further ablative devices.

Second-generation endometrial ablative techniques

Radiofrequency endometrial ablation (RaFEA)

An intrauterine probe is inserted via the cervix into the uterine cavity. The probe tip emits radiofrequency energy at a recognized medical frequency (27.12 MHz). The probe, in conjunction with an abdominal diathermy plate, creates an electric field around the active probe tip sufficient to cause rapid movement of water molecules in surrounding cells. This creates sufficient localized heating to destroy the surrounding endometrium. A temperature of between 63 and 65°C is required to destroy the endometrium and the basal layer on which it regenerates. The advantage of RaFEA is that it does not require the gynaecologist to visualize the uterine cavity, thereby removing the need for large volumes of flushing medium which can cause fluid overload and pulmonary oedema.

Microwave Endometrial Ablation (MEA)

Under either general or local anaesthesia a microwave applicator is inserted into the uterine cavity. A microwave frequency of 9.2 GHz is applied to the whole of the uterine cavity, limiting tissue destruction to no more than 6 mm. The procedure takes approximately 3 minutes. The advantage of MEA is that there is no need to use uterine distension fluids, therefore reducing the risk of fluid overload compared to first-generation ablative procedures. Seymour *et al.* (2003) have demonstrated that MEA performed under local or general anaesthesia is a highly acceptable treatment for menorrhagia. Seymour *et al.* state that an advantage of MEA is the ability to use the system within a dedicated outpatient setting using local anaesthesia – a quality outcome for women, eliminating the need for hospital admission and a general anaesthetic.

Cavaterm thermal balloon ablation

A disposable silicone balloon catheter is inserted into the uterine cavity. The balloon is filled with 1.5% glycine up to a maximum 30 ml and a balloon pressure is measured until a pressure of 200 mmHg is obtained via a central computerized unit. The fluid in the balloon is heated to a preset temperature of 75°C and maintained for 15 minutes. The balloon is then deflated and removed. A study comparing Nd:YAG laser endometrial ablation with the Cavaterm system concluded that the second-generation device is easier to use and achieves similar results to those with a more skill-dependent device (Hawe *et al.*, 2003).

Versapoint bipolar electosurgery system

This system supplies bipolar energy for dissection, vaporization, coagulation and cutting. Normal saline via a constant pressure pump is used to maintain uterine distension. The Versapoint electrode is inserted into the uterine cavity via a hysteroscope. Bipolar energy is delivered to the electrode tip to carry out the above treatments. Research into the efficacy of Versapoint is ongoing; however, studies are highlighting the benefits of the use of bipolar energy and normal saline. Together they reduce the risk of fluid overload and electro-thermal injury. As well as carrying out ablative techniques, the system can be used to remove fibroids and polyps, and to dissect adhesions and septa.

Endometrial Laser Interstitial Thermotherapy (ELITT)

This involves the Gynelase system, consisting of a tabletop diode laser and a disposable handset. Hysteroscopic inspection of the uterine cavity is performed; three laser fibres are inserted into the light diffuser handset which is inserted into the uterus. The handset is advanced to the fundus of the uterus and the handset opened out to form a butterfly wing contour that conforms to the shape of the uterine cavity. The laser fibres are pre-programmed to deliver and transmit laser light in all directions. The cycle lasts for 7 minutes:

◆ 20 W of energy are delivered for 90 seconds

◆ 18 W for the next 90 seconds

◆ 16 W during the final 240 seconds.

Jones *et al.* (2001) found that the ELITT system is easy to use, with a short learning curve, and is associated with a low complication rate. The amenorrhoea rate was consistent with other second-generation devices.

Advice to women. Light bleeding is usually experienced for several days, followed by a watery discharge which may continue for 2–3 weeks. Sanitary towels rather than tampons should be used to reduce the risk of infection. Menstrual bleeding usually decreases progressively during the next two to three periods. Slight cramping pelvic pain may be experienced for several hours that should be relieved by paracetamol or voltarol. Any temperature or offensive-smelling discharge is suggestive of infection and medical advice should be sought.

Sexual intercourse may be resumed when the vaginal bleeding has ceased. Pregnancy is unlikely in those women whose periods become lighter or disappear, but sterility cannot be guaranteed so contraception remains necessary; some hospitals offer women a simultaneous laparoscopic sterilization. Women usually return to work within 1–2 weeks.

Menopausal women using hormone replacement therapy still need to take cyclical progestogen with their oestrogen, as small patches of endometrium may remain in the uterus and these may be subject to excessive growth (hyperplasia) if the oestrogen is not opposed by progestogen.

Laparoscopy

Laparoscopy may be described as the direct visualization of the pelvic organs with a fibre-optic light and a telescope-like instrument, known as a laparoscope. This procedure is usually performed as a day-case. However, depending on diagnosis, there are now many procedures that previously would have been treated with the conventional laparotomy that are now undertaken laparoscopically, e.g. laparoscopic hysterectomy.

Under general anaesthesia the woman is catheterized and placed in the Trendelenburg's position. The table is tilted downwards to allow the upper abdominal contents to fall away from the pelvic organs. A small incision is made below the umbilicus and 2–3 litres of carbon dioxide is introduced into the abdominal cavity. This produces a pneumoperitoneum, which helps to displace the intestines, and allows the pelvic and abdominal organs to be viewed easily via the laparoscope. A second instrument is inserted through a small incision near the upper pubic hairline.

At the end of the operation the carbon dioxide is expelled by abdominal pressure and the small incisions may be sutured or steristrips applied. Any remaining gas is absorbed over the next few days.

You should warn the woman that she might feel bloated and have an aching pain around the shoulders following a laparoscopy. This is quite usual and is caused by the carbon dioxide in the abdomen irritating the phrenic nerve. Paracetamol and hot peppermint water can give relief. Occasionally, opiate analgesia is necessary. Sometimes the incisions may bleed or ooze a little but an ordinary plaster should be sufficient covering. If they become painful or produce an offensive-smelling discharge, medical advice should be sought.

It normally takes a woman a few days to recover fully from a laparoscopy and she should resume normal activities and work when she feels ready. Sexual intercourse may be resumed when she feels comfortable.

Laparoscopic procedures
This section outlines the variety of procedures that are now routinely carried out laparoscopically.

Diagnostic laparoscopy. This is used to investigate pelvic pain or previously unexplained infertility. Outcomes may reveal endometriosis, pelvic infection, ovarian cysts, adhesions, hydrosalpinx, pyosalpinx, ectopic pregnancy, polycystic ovaries and fibroids.

Laparoscopy and dye. Methylene blue dye is injected through the cervix into the uterus and observed to detect the patency of the Fallopian tubes that could be causing infertility.

Laparoscopic salpingectomy. Removal of part or a complete Fallopian tube (often because of an ectopic pregnancy or a blockage caused by infection or disease).

Laparoscopic salpingostomy. Opening of a Fallopian tube to remove an ectopic pregnancy (see page 557).

Laparoscopic adhesiolysis/salpingolysis. This is the division of adhesions (scar tissue) that are causing organs to adhere together. It enables the surgeon to mobilize pelvic organs in an attempt to increase the chances of fertility. A synthetic material may be placed in the pelvis such as Interceed (Ethicon: Johnson & Johnson) that breaks down to provide a protective material to prevent further adhesions forming in the initial healing period.

Laparoscopic lymph node sampling. Removal of either bilateral inguinal lymph nodes or paraortic lymph nodes for the staging of gynaecological malignancies.

Laparoscopic sterilization. The Fallopian tubes are occluded/blocked by clips or lasering or may be cut. Occasionally it may be necessary to perform a mini laparotomy to perform the sterilization if the Fallopian tubes cannot be clearly visualized.

Laser laparoscopy. The word 'laser' refers to light amplification by stimulated emission of radiation. The carbon dioxide laser vaporizes tissue so that malignant or unwanted tissue, such as adhesions and endometriosis, may be removed painlessly and completely under the enhanced vision of the laparoscope.

The laser has a sealing effect on the blood vessels and the risk of bleeding is greatly reduced. The Nd:YAG laser is an exceptional coagulator which delivers an invisible beam near to the infrared region of the spectrum.

Laser laparoscopy may be used to treat endometriosis and polycystic ovarian disease (see Chapter 18). In the latter case it replaces the old-fashioned wedge resection which was often followed by spontaneous ovulation. Cauterization and multiple ovarian biopsy have also been used to mimic a wedge resection, but can cause formation of adhesions and haematomas. Using a laser, multiple holes in the ovary are made causing drainage of the subcapsular cysts which contain high levels of androstenedione. This will lead to a rise in follicle-stimulating hormone (FSH) secretion and ultimately spontaneous ovulation should occur. The laser drill technique results in about 60% of patients returning to spontaneous ovulation, and the remaining 40% will usually respond to clomiphene, even though they were resistant to it before surgery. Although the effect is usually temporary, it allows 'a window of opportunity' for women to attempt conception without having to resort to expensive infertility options.

Current developments

Laparoscopic surgery to treat conditions that previously required the traditional laparotomy is now routinely performed. Studies have shown that in terms of operating time laparoscopic procedures are less predictable than open surgery (Shushan *et al.*, 1999). However, the laparoscopic approach enhances patient satisfaction by offering reduced postoperative pain, smaller incisions, shorter length of stay and faster recovery times. Therefore the impact of continuing developments within this field of gynaecology can only enhance the quality of life for women.

The following laparoscopic procedures can also be carried out due to the use of surgical instruments such as Ultracision-Harmonic Scalpel (Ethicon: Johnson & Johnson). This is a multifunctional instrument that allows surgeons to make incisions to tissue, by simultaneously cutting tissue and sealing blood vessels. This provides the potential for reduced tissue damage and can result in faster recovery and less patient scarring.

Laparoscopic oophorectomy/ovarian cystectomy myomectomy. Following preoperative diagnosis usually by ultrasound scan, the laparoscope is used to remove ovaries, ovarian cysts and fibroids.

Laparoscopic hysterectomy, colposuspension and staging procedures. Previous editions highlighted the development of these surgical techniques. The type of surgery, incidence and comparative studies with traditional open laparotomy are discussed later in the chapter according to the appropriate procedure.

Cystoscopy

A cystoscopy is a minor operative procedure that takes about 15 minutes and allows a thorough examination of the bladder. It is performed under a general or local anaesthetic.

This operation is carried out to investigate the cause of recurrent urinary tract infections, the presence of blood in the urine and as part of a staging process for cervical cancer. A small polyp may also be removed from the bladder during the procedure, or a carbuncle at the urethral entrance. A fine telescope-like instrument – a cystoscope – with a light source is inserted into the urethra and passed along into the bladder. This enables the gynaecologist to view the inside of the bladder, and a biopsy may be taken if necessary. Occasionally, a woman may have a urethral catheter inserted at the end of the procedure.

Cystoscopy is performed as a day-case or as an outpatient. It is important that the woman has passed urine before she goes home. Initially there may be blood in the urine due to bleeding from the biopsy site. If the woman has a catheter she will usually stay in overnight. The catheter will be removed in the morning and once she has passed urine she may go home. A bath or shower may be taken but bubble baths or perfumed bath oils are not recommended. Most women will feel well enough to return to work and their usual activities within 1–2 days.

It is probably advisable to refrain from sexual intercourse following cystoscopy for up to a week to avoid infection or trauma to the urethra. A vaginal lubricant may reduce friction. Women should also be advised to empty their bladder before and after intercourse. The woman should be told to see her GP if she experiences any uncomfortable urinary symptoms.

Marsupialization of a Bartholin's abscess

The Bartholin's glands, which lubricate the vulva, lie behind the vestibule. The duct can become blocked, giving rise to a painless swelling, which becomes palpable, called a Bartholin's cyst. The cyst may become infected resulting in a painful Bartholin's abscess which is often initially noticed during sexual intercourse. The abscess can be extremely painful and appear hot, red and swollen. The woman may have difficulty in walking, be unable to sit down and is reluctant to pass urine.

It is preferable not to excise the gland because it provides lubrication for sexual intercourse. Instead, marsupialization is performed (from the Greek *marsipos* = bag). The abscess is opened to facilitate drainage and the walls of the abscess are sutured to the surrounding skin to leave a large orifice to facilitate drainage of the pus (see Figure 19.1). A new duct forms as healing occurs. During the operation a swab will be taken for microscopy, culture and sensitivity, and antibiotics may be prescribed. The cavity is loosely packed with ribbon gauze impregnated with an antiseptic solution such as proflavin.

This operation is often performed as an emergency and women usually go home 24 hours later, once they have passed urine. The vaginal pack will be removed either by the nurse or by the woman herself. This can be helped by sitting in a soothing bath of warm water. Regular use of a bath, shower or bidet is important to keep the

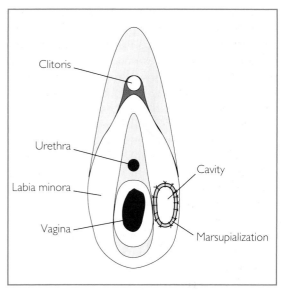

Figure 19.1   Marsupialization of Bartholin's abscess.

area clean. A hair dryer can be used instead of a towel for drying. Antibiotics are not given routinely unless infection is proven. It is probably advisable not to have sexual intercourse for 2 weeks following the operation to avoid re-infection and to allow the area to heal.

Pregnancy loss

All health professionals must remember that pregnancy loss encompasses not only miscarriage but also ectopic pregnancies and terminations for fetal abnormality. The care that is given is paramount to a woman and her partner's well-being. Despite the increase of research into the effects of early miscarriage, there still remains criticism of health professionals. Prettyman (1995) points out the lack of awareness and support during and after hospital admission for a miscarriage. It is also vital to provide support to the partners of the women, understanding their needs and assisting them to fulfil a supportive role (Miron and Chapman, 1994).

Miscarriage
With enhanced ultrasonography and the availability and access to early pregnancy assessment units, scanning is usually the diagnostic method.

In the case of an inevitable miscarriage the woman may be in pain and bleeding, whilst those with a missed miscarriage may not have either of these symptoms and can be even more distressed to discover their baby has stopped growing and died.

Women are particularly sensitive at this time and appreciate health professionals recognizing their loss as significant and as a real baby (not as a 'fetus'). It is also vital not to use terms such as 'complete abortion' which are commonly used in medical textbooks; RCOG (2000) guidance emphasizes the use of the word miscarriage to replace abortion. Nurses have the opportunity to educate junior medical staff, who often do not know how to deal with the psychological aspects of pregnancy loss. Women not only need physical and emotional support at this time but they require information to be given clearly, honestly and in a sensitive manner.

Research in Sweden has shown that expectant management (i.e. no surgical intervention) in selected cases of spontaneous miscarriage has a similar outcome to an evacuation of the retained products of conception (ERPC) (Nielsen and Hahlin, 1995). Some women prefer to miscarry spontaneously and some prefer to have another scan a week later as they find it hard to come to terms with the death of their baby. Therefore development of pregnancy assessment units provides women with alternative choices (Moulder, 1998) for their management.

Surgical intervention. An ERPC is carried out to remove any remaining tissue that might cause infection or excessive bleeding. Again, the language you use is important and it is advisable that you do not refer to it as a D and C or a 'scrape', since this can understandably upset some women. An ERPC is usually performed under general anaesthesia, although some hospitals do offer a spinal block or local anaesthesia.

These operations are often performed at the end of a booked theatre list or placed on a CEPOD (Confidential Enquiry into Peri-Operative Deaths) list. It is vital that nursing staff provide women and their partners with regular information regarding the rationale for delays in surgery. This is also pertinent as women are often nil by mouth for excessive periods of time and for some women an intravenous infusion may be appropriate.

It could be assumed that as most acute services provide day surgery units, and with the development of day treatment centres (NHS Plan; DoH 2000a), there should be structured pathways in place to provide care for women who need an ERPC. These settings would allow the direct booking of a dedicated theatre slot that would ensure an improved quality service for women.

Discharge advice. The advice for women following an ERPC is similar to the advice given following a hysteroscopy. Women who have had a miscarriage are only in hospital for a short time so it is important that relevant discharge advice is given. It is good practice to provide written discharge advice; if this is not available, booklets by the Miscarriage Association can be given. Some hospitals provide support groups; if not, again, the Miscarriage Association will provide details of the nearest group for women and their partners.

Vaginal bleeding may continue for 7–10 days but should not be heavier than a normal period. Women should contact their GP if the bleeding becomes heavier or they develop an offensive discharge. Breast tenderness may be a problem, especially if the miscarriage occurred later in the pregnancy, and women should be warned as this can be a distressing problem for them. A well-supporting bra will help reduce discomfort but it is not usually felt that medication is necessary.

There is no evidence to suggest that women cannot try to conceive immediately following a miscarriage; however, psychologically it may be beneficial for women to wait for two menstrual periods to have occurred. A follow-up appointment is not usually offered unless the woman has had three consecutive miscarriages, or has a miscarriage in the second trimester of pregnancy.

Ectopic pregnancy

The word 'ectopic' comes from the Greek *ektopos*, meaning 'misplaced', and an ectopic pregnancy occurs when the fertilized ovum implants and develops outside the uterus. Approximately 1 in 200 pregnancies are ectopic and the condition is discussed more fully in Chapter 18.

A woman with a suspected ectopic pregnancy should always be treated as a gynaecological emergency since this condition is potentially life-threatening. Despite medical advances in the past decade there has been no decrease in the number of women dying from an ectopic pregnancy. This is because the sudden rupture of the Fallopian tube can lead to a massive intra-peritoneal haemorrhage.

Some women arrive in a state of collapse in the accident and emergency department requiring resuscitation, blood transfusions, and immediate surgery by laparoscopy or laparotomy.

Laparoscopic treatment of an ectopic pregnancy

With the development of minimally invasive surgical techniques, it has been possible to treat unruptured ectopic pregnancies laparoscopically. Forceps may be used to 'milk' the pregnancy from the tube, or the tube may be irrigated via a suprapubic cannula and also by hydrotubation through the cervix to flush out any remaining products of gestation. Alternatively, linear salpingostomy (opening of the tube) may be carried out using a laser to open carefully the tube and remove the pregnancy. Aspiration under ultrasound control may be possible in some hospitals.

Women consenting to a laparoscopy should be warned of the possibility of the procedure proceeding to a laparotomy.

Laparoscopy proceeding to laparotomy

This will be carried out when an ectopic pregnancy is diagnosed or in hospitals where scanning and βHCG radioassay are not available at all times. If an ectopic pregnancy is visualized via the laparoscope, the gynaecologist may proceed to a laparotomy and remove the damaged tube (salpingectomy) and the remainder of the pregnancy. Any bleeding will be stopped and a Redivac drain and urinary catheter may be inserted.

Medical management of ectopic pregancy

This involves the administration of a single dose intramuscular injection of methotrexate. Methotrexate is a folic acid antagonist that induces dissolution of trophoblastic tissue. Parker et al. (1998) state that this treatment results in a high failure rate, prolonged follow-up with serious complications and side effects. However, Sowter et al. (2001) state that although methotrexate is a less effective treatment than laparoscopic salpingotomy, it is well tolerated. It should only be offered as an alternative to surgery to women with mild symptoms and who present with low serum βHCG concentrations. Larger randomized clinical trails of medical management of ectopic pregnancy are required with particular regard to the use of multiple dose intramuscular methotrexate (Farquhar, 2003).

Psychological aspects of an ectopic pregnancy

Women are often very distressed when an ectopic pregnancy is diagnosed, particularly if they were using contraception (commonly the IUD or progestogen-only pill) and had not even realized they were pregnant. Conversely, a couple may have been trying to conceive for many years, have had a previous ectopic, or are on an infertility programme such as IVF, ICSI, GIFT or ZIFT. An ectopic pregnancy in these situations is even more distressing.

Women and their partners should receive sensitive care and be given an opportunity to discuss their concerns. Information about the Miscarriage Association may be helpful and staff should remember that ectopic pregnancy not only involves feelings of loss and bereavement, but also involves major surgery. Women attending the author's pregnancy loss support group who have experienced an ectopic pregnancy have expressed feelings that they were seen as 'a post-operative patient' and would have welcomed the opportunity to discuss their pregnancy loss.

Women usually remain in hospital for 2–3 days following laparotomy and 1–2 nights following laparoscopy. The woman's rhesus status will be ascertained before she goes home.

Sexual intercourse may be resumed once any bleeding has stopped. It is probably advisable for the couple to wait until one or two normal periods have occurred before trying for another pregnancy. Contraception should therefore be discussed (preferably not the IUD or progestogen-only pill) and this conversation can provide a starting point for discussion of any sexual concerns.

Aftercare following loss of a pregnancy

Psychosexual support. Loss of a pregnancy or baby, for whatever reason – miscarriage, intrauterine death, stillbirth, ectopic pregnancy and termination of pregnancy – can all cause psychological problems for the woman and her partner for some time after the event. Guilt is a common feeling and it can take a very sympathetic partner to help a woman through this time.

Miscarriage may create problems with self-concept, inner feelings of failure, loss of faith in her physical body, and other conflicts in the marriage and family relationships. Some studies indicate a serious increase in marital conflict after the loss of a pregnancy. Peppers and Knapp (1980) attribute some of this difficulty to what they term 'incongruent bonding' where the mother has had the biological bonding experience of carrying her child, while the father's process has been on a mental, intellectual level. Couples often experience sexual difficulties after the loss of a pregnancy and may not understand the relationship between these difficulties and their loss (Schiff, 1977).

Some couples may avoid intercourse as it evokes memories of the baby's conception. Others may be fearful of another pregnancy too soon, and be unwilling to trust contraception. Physically the couple may feel too exhausted from the emotional grief to begin to contemplate a sexual relationship. For those who are fearful of intercourse and are therefore tense and anxious, it is advisable that they take their time to begin a sexual relationship again, and to understand that other expressions of love, such as cuddling, can be just as fulfilling as the act of intercourse.

Rhesus status. After a pregnancy loss, whether a miscarriage or an ectopic pregnancy, it is crucial that the woman's rhesus status is checked to prevent haemolytic disease of the newborn. The rhesus factor is found in the red blood cells of 85% of the population (rhesus positive), the other 15% are rhesus negative. If a woman with rhesus negative blood becomes pregnant by a man with rhesus positive blood, the fetus may have rhesus positive blood. A small amount of blood will pass into the woman's blood which will form antibodies. If the woman continues with the pregnancy, there will be no harm to the fetus, but if she becomes pregnant again by a rhesus positive man, the woman's body will 'attack' the fetus. This will either cause a miscarriage or the child will be born with haemolytic disease of the newborn and will require a full exchange of blood. Rhesus disease may be prevented by the injection of 'Anti-D' which destroys any rhesus positive cells that have entered a woman's bloodstream. It therefore prevents the woman's body from making the antibodies, but must be given within 72 hours of the pregnancy finishing.

Major gynaecological surgery

Most minor gynaecology surgery is carried out in a designated day surgery unit unless the woman has predisposing medical problems indicating an overnight stay or her body mass index (BMI) is over the accepted limit for the unit. Day treatment centres (NHS Plan; DoH, 2000a) are not restricted by the above and can be the base for carrying out both minor and major surgery. However, adherence to stringent care pathways is fundamental to the continuation of high standards of women's health care, as postoperative care will not necessarily be carried out in a designated gynaecology ward.

Therefore the majority of surgery carried out within the inpatient setting is major surgery, usually with hospitalization longer than over 2 days. Lengths of stays have shortened drastically over the last few years. Once again, this can be related to the advancement in surgical technique, for example laparoscopic assisted vaginal hysterectomy. Many surgeons now use dissolvable suture material, so women rarely stay in hospital just to have their sutures removed. Patient choice also plays a large part in early discharge and women are usually keen to regain independence. It must be added that pressure on the utilization of beds is a national problem, and it is important to ensure that women are not discharged too early. This does not ease the bed problem because premature discharge can on occasion lead to an increase in readmissions.

This section outlines the types of gynaecological surgery that are routinely performed, the pre- and postoperative care, and discusses the impact of this type of surgery for women.

Pre-assessment

There has been an abundance of research carried out over the past 25 years that stresses the importance of reducing anxiety of patients by the provision of accurate and detailed information. This concept is paramount for women undergoing gynaecological procedures. Many women may have been on a waiting list for a significant amount of time, their symptoms may have changed, or they may have developed other medical problems which could lead to cancellation of the operation. This in turn causes stress to the woman and her family, having planned their lives around the operation, and it is a wasted operation slot that could have been utilized for another patient.

A pre-assessment clinic allows the woman a dedicated time to discuss her impending operation and gives the nurse an opportunity to provide information on all aspects of the procedure without interruption. Any potential medical problems can be investigated and treated prior to the operation. This would not always be possible if the woman was admitted one day prior to surgery. Written information that backs up the verbal information should be given. This should include precise information about the proposed surgery, the various methods of analgesia administration, and postoperative advice to include available social support agencies and gynaecology support groups.

A women can then review this information in her own time, discuss it with her family and contact the ward if any questions arise. It is important that all health professional use words that women understand, i.e. womb instead of uterus, 'removal of your ovaries' rather than oophorectomy. Prior to all major gynaecological procedures women should be informed of the following risks:

◆ There is always a very small risk of adverse reaction attached to a general anaesthetic whatever the operation

◆ Bowel or bladder damage can occur, but very rarely

◆ Chest infections are more likely if the woman is prone to them or smokes heavily – try to cut down smoking if unable to give up

◆ Urine infections may occur after the operation

◆ The risk of wound infections or deep vein thrombosis increases if overweight – weight loss should be encouraged prior to surgery.

Hysterectomy

The most commonly performed major gynaecological operation in the UK continues to be a hysterectomy (Thakar *et al.*, 2002) with more than 65,000 undertaken in 1995 (Maresh *et al.*, 2002). A hysterectomy usually involves the removal of the uterus and its neck, the cervix. There are various types of hysterectomy (see Figure 19.2). The types of surgical procedure have increased with continuing development and use of minimal access surgery (MAS). These varying procedures are discussed at the end of this section. It is important that the woman knows which procedure she is having. The type performed will depend on the reason for the hysterectomy (Box 19.1).

Total abdominal hysterectomy
This involves the removal of the uterus and cervix through a transverse incision in the abdomen just above the pubic bone: a Pfannenstiel or 'bikini-line' incision. Some women may require a vertical incision where there is a large abdominal swelling or a previous scar.

Bilateral salpingo-oophorectomy
This refers to the removal of both Fallopian tubes and ovaries and is often performed at the same time as a total abdominal hysterectomy – particularly where there is evidence of disease or if the woman is approaching the menopause or is already post-menopausal.

Bhavnani *et al.* (2003) demonstrated the lack of preoperative information that women were

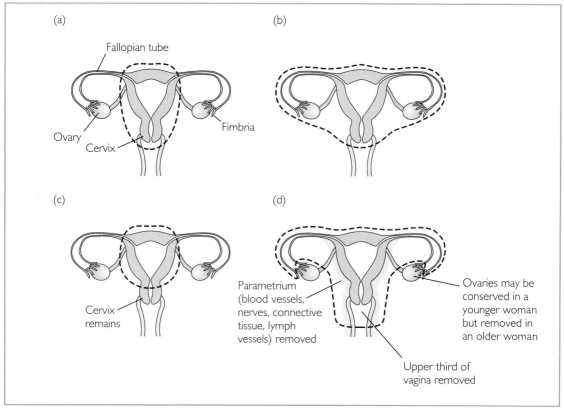

Figure 19.2 Types of hysterectomy. (a) Total abdominal hysterectomy; (b) total abdominal hysterectomy with bilateral salpingo-oophorectomy; (c) subtotal hysterectomy; (d) Wertheim's hysterectomy.

given regarding prophylactic oophorectomy (i.e. the removal of healthy ovaries). Their qualitative interviewing study showed that women's main concerns were the short-term impact of oophorectomy, i.e. the sudden onset of menopausal symptoms and the use of HRT. They also found that there was little acknowledgement of the increased risk of coronary heart disease and osteoporosis associated with an early menopause.

Conversely, as would be expected, the study found that the main reason expressed for a prophylactic oophorectomy was the risk of ovarian cancer if the ovaries remained.

Therefore it is vital that all medical staff ensure that women are given concise, relevant verbal and written preoperative information. This will ensure that women feel that a collaborative process has occurred regarding the decision to undergo oophorectomy.

Subtotal hysterectomy

This involves the removal of the uterus leaving the cervix behind. This type of hysterectomy is growing in popularity due to media speculation that keeping the cervix retains sexual pleasure, and due to the effect of the surgical method that is undertaken in comparison to total abdominal hysterectomy. Thakar *et al.* (2002) showed that women showed similar effects on sexual and pelvic organ function following both subtotal and abdominal hysterectomies. Roovers *et al.* (2003) found that sexual pleasure improves after hysterectomy, sexual problems present before surgery are less common after surgery, and that sexual well-being does not depend on the surgical procedure.

Box 19.1 Reasons for hysterectomy

◆ Painful or irregular periods or episodes of unexplained vaginal bleeding

◆ Previous ablative surgery that has not improved quality of life

◆ Fibroids that can cause pain, heavy bleeding and occasionally pressure on other pelvic organs, e.g. the bladder

◆ Uterine prolapse which may interfere with bladder and bowel function

◆ Severe endometriosis – a condition where the endometrium grows in other parts of the body, such as the ligaments of the uterus or ovaries, causing inter-menstrual bleeding, dysmenorrhoea and dyspareunia

◆ Chronic pelvic pain caused by pelvic infection

◆ Gynaecological cancers of the vagina, cervix, endometrium, Fallopian tubes or ovaries

◆ Occasionally a hysterectomy is performed in an emergency, e.g. in instances of postpartum haemorrhage or following a gynaecological procedure where haemostasis cannot be maintained.

Radical Wertheim's hysterectomy

This operation is an extended hysterectomy where the uterus, ovaries, Fallopian tubes, adjacent pelvic tissue, lymph ducts and the upper third of the vagina are removed. This is necessary in cases of advanced cervical and endometrial cancer. The ovaries may be conserved in a younger woman (ovariopexy – the ovaries are suspended in the abdominal cavity).

Vaginal hysterectomy

This involves the removal of the uterus through the vagina, with conservation of the ovaries. A vaginal hysterectomy is usually performed where there is a prolapse of the uterus. Contraindications to vaginal hysterectomy include a bulky uterus (larger in size than a 14-week pregnancy), and suspected or known malignancy. Women may refer to this type of hysterectomy as a 'suction hysterectomy', although this is not an accurate description. There will be no abdominal scar.

Laparoscopic hysterectomy

This is discussed at the end of this section on hysterectomies.

Physical aspects of hysterectomy

Preoperative care. Dependent on the hospital admission policy, women may be admitted the evening prior to surgery or on the day of surgery, depending on the time of the operation.

◆ Ensure that the woman is not constipated; if this is the case then aperients should be administered

◆ A pubic shave, performed by either the woman herself or her nurse

◆ In most hospitals, women are measured for special support (anti-embolism) stockings which help prevent deep vein thrombosis, and given anti-coagulation injections (e.g. Clexane) until full mobility is resumed

◆ Reiterate pre- and postoperative care and advice.

New patients are usually introduced to each other and Wilson-Barnett (1975) found that patients derive considerable support from one another.

The woman may find during her stay in hospital that a ward round takes place, which not only includes members of the medical team, but also several medical students. All women have the right to refuse to be part of the teaching round or to be examined vaginally by medical students. At some hospitals women may sign a consent form for medical students to perform vaginal examinations while they are in theatre under general anaesthesia. It is not always possible to ensure that a female doctor examines a woman but it is worth asking beforehand if this is what she would prefer. A nurse should always chaperone any doctor.

Postoperative care. Surgery takes approximately 45 minutes; ensure that women are aware that they will wake up in the recovery area in the theatre.

Women *may* have the following:

◆ Oxygen administered via a face mask or nasal cannula aiding dispersal of anaesthetic agents. If an epidural or patient-controlled analgesia (PCA) is used, then the oxygen remains *in situ* until the devices are discontinued

◆ Analgesia can also be administered by intramuscular injection, e.g. with morphine sulphate

◆ Anti-emetics as Stemeti prochlorperazine (Stemetil), metoclopramide (Maxolon) or cyclizine may be given for nausea and vomiting

◆ An intravenous infusion, especially following abdominal surgery as the bowel has been mobilized: this remains for about 24 hours until bowel sounds are established

◆ A blood transfusion must be in progress if there has been excessive blood loss during surgery

◆ A Foley urinary catheter to rest the bladder following surgery and, importantly, for patient comfort

◆ A Redivac drain near the incision site; this drain has a suction that removes excess blood from the operation site and prevents haematoma formation.

◆ Women who have had a vaginal hysterectomy may have a 'vaginal pack' (a length of ribbon gauze soaked in proflavin antiseptic cream), which is inserted in the vagina rather like a large tampon instead of a Redivac drain.

Day 1 Postoperatively. Nursing staff must remember the individuality of their patients and the following should act as a guide to recovery but is in no way prescriptive.

◆ The following day the woman will be encouraged to sit out of bed and will be assisted to have a wash. Many women should be able to walk to the bathroom and take a bath

◆ When bowel sounds are heard, the woman can start sipping water and gradually progress to a light diet. Her intravenous infusion will then be removed

◆ A urinary catheter (if present) will be removed according to surgeon choice. In the author's department, the nursing staff found that by removing the catheter at 22.00 hours there was a decrease in the number of urinary retention post catheter removal. This could be attributed to the fact that the patient would go to sleep as usual, wake in the morning and pass urine as normal. In comparison, women who had their catheter removed during the daytime would then spend the day worrying as to whether they would be able to pass urine. This would often lead to recatheterization, an increase in the risk of a urinary track infection and potentially an increased length of stay in hospital. Sometimes women contract urinary tract infections following hysterectomy and these will be treated with antibiotics. It is important that the woman empties her bladder fully and squeezes out the last few drops. Some women who are prone to urinary tract infections find drinking cranberry juice an effective prophylaxis (see page 491).

The Redivac drain is removed when drainage is minimal and although not very painful, this will feel like a sharp tugging sensation which lasts for a few seconds.

Subsequent days. Women should be able to walk around without too much discomfort. Diclofenac Sodium (volatarol) suppositories are frequently used for analgesia alongside oral analgesics due to its anti-inflammatory properties. Women may worry about 'bursting their stitches' and need reassurance that this is not possible since there are several strong layers beneath the skin.

Many women experience griping 'wind' pain after the operation which can cause considerable discomfort. Hot peppermint water sipped slowly may help, and some doctors prescribe enteric-coated peppermint oil capsules (Colpermin) which are excellent. Walking around and sitting in a warm bath may also help.

Constipation can be a problem and glycerine suppositories, milpar, fybogel or senokot are all remedies that can be offered.

It is very common for women to feel emotional following surgery and many women find themselves in tears for no apparent reason. They should be reassured that this is a normal reaction and will pass, although some women do experience similar feelings again on leaving hospital. Hormone replacement therapy will help many women, particularly those who are peri-menopausal and those who have had a bilateral salpingo-oophorectomy, but there may be many more subtle reasons for this feeling of depression.

Most transverse wounds tend to have dissolvable sutures that need to be trimmed before discharge, which is usually between 3 and 5 days post-surgery. Vertical wounds tend to have interrupted silk or prolene sutures and these stay in for 7–10 days. These women can be discharged around 5 days post-surgery and can go to their GP to have them removed.

Psychological aspects of hysterectomy

All major surgery has implications for an altered body image but the removal of a uterus can alter a woman's self-image and essentially her perceived femininity. The uterus is a symbol of reproduction and without it, and the associated menstruation, a woman may well feel she is less of a sexual being.

To many women the suggestion of having a hysterectomy provokes fear and horror due to the misconceptions and old wives' tales surrounding this particular operation. In fact, the ancient Greeks believed the uterus (*hystero*) to be the source of all emotions; hence the words 'hysteria' and 'hysterectomy'.

Women have often heard from relatives and friends prophecies of doom which make them wonder if a hysterectomy will cause them to grow hair on their face, gain weight, become unattractive to their sexual partners and, above all, lose all their own desires and feelings of pleasure. Some mistakenly believe that the vagina is sewn up at the vulva, and others think that a uterus is necessary for orgasm.

Naturally the role of the nurse is of utmost importance, to uncover anxieties and fears, to correct any myths and misconceptions and to give clear, accurate advice. Unfortunately, instead of the detailed information women require, they are often only given brief hints about 'not lifting', and important concerns such as when to resume sexual activity are neglected. Webb (1985) in her study of gynaecology nurses found that although nurses did talk to their patients and were aware that hysterectomy patients feared 'losing their womanhood', they interpreted this as referring only to patients' sex lives and not to the wider aspects of sexuality, self-concept and self-esteem. Selby (see Chapter 5) states that sometimes it takes as much courage for nurses to overcome their inhibitions as it does for the patient to raise sexual matters.

Some women do not realize they will no longer have periods following a hysterectomy, and in pre-menopausal women the cessation of menses and loss of fertility must be addressed and accurate information about hormone replacement therapy given (see Chapter 16). Those women who suffered from premenstrual syndrome and think that a hysterectomy will cure this problem may well find that cyclical symptoms persist following hysterectomy if the ovaries have been conserved, leading to the term 'ovarian cycle syndrome' (Backstrom *et al.*, 1981). The implications of oophorectomy can also be misunderstood and Williamson (1992) comments that some women believe that they will die at an earlier age if their ovaries are surgically removed.

Certain ethnic groups find hysterectomy particularly hard to accept and nurses should be aware of the impact this operation may have on different cultures and communities. West Indian women view menstruation as a cleansing act, ridding the body of impurities and are reluctant to have a hysterectomy. Some also fear they will be 'less of a woman' in the eyes of their men, who may be tempted to look for another 'whole woman'. For this reason they may not wish their partner or family to know exactly what operation they are having, and all staff should respect their right to confidentiality.

The cultural role of Muslim women is dependent on their fertility and, again, it may be difficult for both partners to come to terms with surgery. It can be of enormous value if you find time for discussion about impending surgery, not only with the woman but also with her partner and other members of the family.

Williams (1986) revealed that women wanted specific advice to aid recovery and this was frequently lacking. Gould (1986) found that all the women in her study stated spontaneously that they were glad of the opportunity to talk to the researcher about their experiences and feelings, indicating an unmet need and a lack of support by hospital staff. In Gould's (1986) study, ward nurses often expressed surprise that women's recovery from hysterectomy should be a topic worthy of investigation in view of its 'routine' nature and apparent lack of problems. Careful documentation of events after discharge from hospital suggested that many problems did, in fact, exist and women would have worried less if they had been adequately prepared.

It is vital that all nurses, whether in hospital or primary care, realize how patients' home circumstances and need for information vary, and these must be assessed individually when care is planned. There is also a national network of hysterectomy support groups (see Resources) and practice nurses could develop small support groups to meet the needs of their patients.

Discharge advice following hysterectomy and other major gynaecological surgery

Women normally stay in hospital for 3–5 days following major gynaecological surgery, and should be encouraged to go home when they feel ready to do so. Unfortunately, pressure on hospital beds means discharge is often too early. It is important that the whole family, particularly the woman's partner, understands what she can and cannot do whilst she is recovering at home. The discharge information given prior to surgery should be reiterated throughout the stay and prior to discharge with an assurance that she can ring the ward for advice at any time.

Bleeding. There may be a vaginal discharge for up to 4 weeks which will turn from red to a pale brown colour. If it becomes heavier, brighter in colour or offensive-smelling, medical advice should be sought. Occasional red spotting may occur when stitches fall out. Sanitary towels rather than tampons should be used.

Resting. It is important that the woman should rest sufficiently during the first 2 weeks. However, it should be emphasized that this does not mean going home to bed. Women should be encouraged to be up and dressed and that they can go up and down stairs and walk as they feel able. It is common to suddenly feel tired and

exhausted, or occasionally have strange sensations in the abdomen (sometimes described as 'pinging elastic').

Exercise. Exercise is important and many gynaecology units have a dedicated physiotherapist who will teach appropriate exercises for patients to begin and then continue at home. It is advisable to go for short walks, increasing gradually to 45 minutes by 6 weeks after the operation. Swimming may be resumed after about 4 weeks if vaginal bleeding has stopped. Cycling and other light exercise may also be resumed at this stage.

Housework. No housework should be performed for the first 2 weeks but, after this, light chores can be safely done. It is very important to avoid lifting anything heavy for the first 4 weeks and very heavy items, such as shopping, wet laundry, full bin bags or toddlers, should not be lifted for at least 3 months. When anything is lifted it is important to remind the woman to bend her knees, keep her back straight and hold the object close to her. This avoids straining her abdomen.

Diet. Many women have heard that they will gain weight or develop 'middle-age spread' following hysterectomy. This is a myth and any weight gain is due to an increased calorie intake combined with a lack of exercise. It is advisable to eat a variety of foods, including fresh fruit and vegetables to avoid constipation. Some women find prune juice (available at some supermarkets and health food shops) effective. Other preventative measures such as drinking at least eight glasses of water per day and taking high fibre foods are also recommended.

Work. Some women feel able to return to work 6–8 weeks following surgery, while others may feel the need to take further time off. Obviously some jobs are more strenuous than others and women should judge for themselves when they feel ready. Some employers may allow women to return on a part-time basis initially, which is an ideal way to readjust to the demands of a job. Rarely, some women may take up to a year to feel completely fit.

Sexual intercourse. Generally speaking it takes about 6 weeks to feel both physically and emotionally ready to resume intercourse after major gynaecological surgery, and most gynaecologists recommend this time interval before attempting intercourse. In any event, hysterectomy patients should certainly be advised to wait until any vaginal bleeding has stopped to prevent the risk of infection. The woman's partner should understand the importance of being gentle initially, to avoid undue trauma to the area. Tissue strength is adequate by this time, and the risk of infection is virtually non-existent in the presence of complete healing.

Even before the 6 weeks, however, you could advise the couple that other forms of sexual expression may be explored. Two weeks or so after surgery clitoral stimulation to orgasm without intercourse can be resumed, as can other methods for satisfying the partner, short of intercourse. Many women find that experiencing orgasm for the first time after surgery is best done alone through masturbation (Williamson, 1992). This allows them to take their time, tune in to any new sensations and experience an orgasm without the pressures of their partner. Barback (1975) recommends self-stimulation as a very reassuring strategy that can be recommended to women who do not object to the idea of masturbation, because it confirms their potential to reach orgasm.

The hormonal effects of oophorectomy, i.e. reduced oestrogen and testosterone, may cause loss of libido, vaginal atrophy and reduction of vaginal lubrication. This may be overcome by hormone replacement therapy or locally applied oestrogen cream. Vaginal dryness may also be helped by using an over-the-counter lubricant which will reduce chafing and discomfort, and increase sensitivity.

Sexual anxieties following hysterectomy. Blundell (1829), who performed the first hysterectomy in Britain in 1828, commented: 'the continuance of sexual desires – is very remarkable'. Many women fear that they will become 'frigid' following a hysterectomy and they can be assured that this is not correct. Some women feel more relaxed about lovemaking when there is no risk of pregnancy, and those undergoing hysterectomy for fibroids or endometriosis may find sexual intercourse less painful and more enjoyable than before. A study by Rhodes *et al.* (1999) has shown

that sexual functioning improved overall after hysterectomy and that sexual activity increased and problems with sexual functioning decreased.

However, Shingleton and Orr (1987) stress that if surgery is perceived as 'mutilating' it is likely to become damaging rather than restorative. The woman who expects hysterectomy to decrease her sexual excitability and enjoyment often exhibits a self-fulfilling prophecy when she experiences decreased libido postoperatively. Women who depend on their gynaecological illness to secure relief from sexual commitments to their partners may develop anxiety if they believe the removal of the source of their symptoms will lead to the expectation that they will become more responsive sexually (Shingleton and Orr, 1987). Thus, surgery may constitute a threat to the relationship in opposing ways.

In general, however, the single most significant factor in postoperative sexual behaviour is pretreatment sexual adjustment. The woman who has had a satisfying sexual relationship prior to surgery is likely to resume such a relationship postoperatively, while those with sexual problems preoperatively will find them likely to continue, not cease, following surgery.

Although postoperative tenderness may persist for as long as 12 weeks postoperatively, the couple need to resume their sexual relationship in some form as soon as possible. You could talk to them about different positions for intercourse in order to avoid abdominal or vaginal discomfort. Hysterectomy usually includes removal of the cervix, which can slightly decrease the length of the vagina, but not to the extent of limiting intercourse. A change in position may be more comfortable initially such as female astride or 'legs together'.

The character of orgasm for women who have had a hysterectomy may change. This is due to the lack of any uterine contractions, but does not usually affect overall satisfaction, as discussed above.

Laparoscopic hysterectomy

The following are performed laparoscopically.

Laparoscopic assisted vaginal hystectomy (LAVH). The laparoscope is used to assist the upper part of the vaginal hysterectomy; it enables the surgeon to visualize the uterine pedicles and ligate the uterine arteries, reducing the risk of bleeding. The uterus is removed vaginally.

Total laparoscopic hysterectomy (TLH). The hysterectomy is performed completely using the laparoscope without any form of vaginal surgery. The uterus and cervix are either removed via the vagina or via a small abdominal incision.

Laparoscopic subtotal hysterectomy. The hysterectomy is performed laparoscopically, removing the uterus but leaving the cervix *in situ*; the uterus is removed via a small abdominal incision.

As discussed, the traditional methods for performing a hysterectomy are either by the abdominal or vaginal route. Garry *et al.* (2004) state that laparoscopic hysterectomy is a relatively new approach to hysterectomy and is infrequently performed in the UK. Maresh *et al.* (2002) found that in 1995 only 3% of 37,000 hysterectomies in the VALUE national hysterectomy study were performed laparoscopically. Garry *et al.* (2004) and Sculpher *et al.* (2004) have produced the results of both studies investigating both the actual surgical procedures of conventional abdominal or vaginal hysterectomy compared to laparoscopic hysterectomy.

Garry *et al.* (2004) found that in the eVALuate study (two parallel randomized trials, one comparing laparoscopic with abdominal hysterectomy, the other comparing laparoscopic with vaginal hysterectomy) that with laparoscopic hysterectomy patients experience less pain, have a shorter length of stay and have a quicker recovery. However, with laparoscopic hysterectomy there was an increase in the incidence of complications compared with the abdominal approach. Laparoscopic hysterectomy is also associated with a significantly longer operating time compared to the traditional methods. Sculpher *et al.* (2004) found that laparoscopic hysterectomy is not cost effective relative to vaginal hysterectomy and its cost effectiveness relative to the abdominal procedure is finely balanced. Therefore it can be seen that the place of this form of minimal access surgery in current gynaecological practice remains controversial (Garry, 2002).

Postoperative care. Nursing care is as described under laparoscopic surgery (see page 553). The length of hospital stay is variable. Some women are fit for discharge on the day of surgery whilst others may need to stay in hospital for 24–48 hours following surgery.

Myomectomy

A myomectomy is a major operation to remove fibroids from the uterus. A fibroid (also known as myoma or leiomyoma) begins as a single cell in the endometrium of the uterus, which multiplies to become a mass of muscle and fibrous connective tissue. Most fibroids are no larger than a pea but they can grow to the size of a grapefruit. Fibroids (see Chapter 18) seem to occur more frequently in West Indian and West African women, although the reason for this is not clear.

It is not entirely clear why fibroids develop although it has been thought that they are hereditary. Their growth is dependent on oestrogen since they tend to grow faster during pregnancy and shrink after the menopause. Before a myomectomy, a woman is often prescribed Zoladex (goserelin) to suppress the release of oestrogen and cause the fibroids to shrink.

It is important that women are reassured that fibroids are benign tumours of connective tissue. In very rare cases a fibroid may turn into a fast-growing malignant tumour (leiomyosarcoma) and a hysterectomy will be performed.

Reasons for myomectomy

Small fibroids are asymptomatic and treatment is not required. However, where diagnosis of the pelvic mass is in doubt, where the mass is larger than the size of a 16-week pregnancy, or where there are unpleasant symptoms, surgery is advised.

Menorrhagia is a common problem caused by the larger area of endometrium that is shed at menstruation. Large fibroids may press on the bowel causing constipation, or on the bladder causing urinary frequency or retention.

How it is performed

A myomectomy involves the 'shelling out' of the fibroids and is preferable for women who still want children. If no further pregnancies are desired then a hysterectomy may be the operation of choice.

Lewis and Chamberlain (1991) consider the risks of a straightforward myomectomy or a hysterectomy are about equal but, if a large number of fibroids are present, myomectomy can be more difficult with a risk of considerable haemorrhage at surgery. Women should always be aware of the risk that if bleeding cannot be controlled a hysterectomy will be performed. A vertical incision is usually necessary.

Postoperative care

See the above discussion on postoperative care for hysterectomy. In addition the following should be noted:

◆ Women will often return to the ward with a blood transfusion and therefore this operation is not always suitable for women who do not accept the transfusion of blood, e.g. Jehovah's Witnesses

◆ An increased risk of febrile morbidity compared to hysterectomy

◆ The length of stay is usually 5–7 days compared to that of a hysterectomy

◆ There is a risk of the formation of a haematoma and adhesions may develop between the intestines and the suture lines on the uterus. The suture line may weaken the wall of the uterus, requiring a Caesarean section for subsequent births.

Discharge advice is similar to the advice given for women who have undergone hysterectomy. Myomectomy is associated with significant morbidity and difficulty in long-term management because of high recurrence rates (Visvanathan, 2003). Some gynaecologists recommend that a woman tries to become pregnant during the first 3–6 months following surgery, before fibroids have had a chance to recur. There should be no problems sexually once the scar has healed and any bleeding has stopped. However, it is worth mentioning that a woman with multiple fibroids may have had a full feeling during intercourse and she may now experience an 'empty sensation' once the fibroids are removed.

Recent developments for the treatment of fibroids

Laparoscopic myomectomy

The removal of subserous and intramural fibroids during laparoscopy has increased with better patient selection, the improvement of laparoscopic skills, microsurgical technique and advanced equipment such as morcellators to break up the fibroid tissue (Vivasanathan, 2003). Vivasanathan also outlines the advantages of this procedure, i.e. reduced postoperative pain, shorter length of stay, reduced adhesions and a quicker return to normal activity. Women must be informed of the possibility of the procedure converting to a laparotomy if complications arise during the laparoscopy. Nursing care is as discussed in laparoscopic surgery.

Uterine Artery Embolization (UAE)

The procedure involves the insertion of a catheter into the femoral artery and, using fluoroscopy guidance, the catheter is passed through a series of blood vessels until it reaches the uterine artery. A solution of polyvinyl alcohol particles is then injected into the artery: this solution is carried in the blood until the particles stick in the arterial branches, causing a permanent blockage of blood flow to the fibroid. This embolization causes the fibroids to shrink, therefore producing significant improvements in symptoms and in some cases resolution of symptoms (Goodwin et al., 1997).

Women must be informed that this procedure requires admission to hospital for 24–36 hours, as the main postoperative side effect is pain that often needs opiate relief. A more long-term side effect is the vaginal expulsion of submucosal fibroids (Berkowitz et al., 1999).

There were three reported cases of death from UAE: two from sepsis and one from pulmonary embolism. Therefore, in the UK, the Royal College of Radiologists and RCOG in 2000 recommended that all cases of UAE must be part of a primary research programme and be registered with the Safety and Efficacy Register for New Interventional Procedures (RCOG, 2001).

Surgery for vaginal prolapse and urinary incontinence

Prior to undergoing any form of surgery to correct prolapse or urinary incontinence, it is vital to carry out rigorous investigations into symptoms and cause. A woman will not be satisfied with her treatment if, despite being cured of her stress incontinence, she develops detrusor instability (Chaliha and Stanton, 1999). The aims of continence surgery are discussed in Chapter 17.

Vaginal and abdominal surgery for prolapse

The most common vaginal repair operations include anterior colporrhaphy (anterior repair), posterior colporrhaphy (posterior repair) and the Manchester repair which is not so frequently performed these days.

Anterior colporrhaphy

An anterior repair is carried out to cure a cystocele or cystourethrocele with or without stress incontinence. The anterior vaginal wall is incised and a triangular portion of vaginal skin from below the external urethral opening to the front of the cervix is excised. One or two sutures are placed deep around the bladder neck. The edges of the wound are sutured together to provide extra support for the bladder and urethra.

Posterior colporrhaphy

This procedure is used to repair a rectocele, or a rectocele and enterocele. A triangular portion of posterior vaginal wall, with its apex at the mid-vaginal level and its base at the introitus, is removed by an inverted T incision to expose the levator ani muscles. These muscles are brought together with one to two interrupted sutures,

closed in a Y-shape to avoid narrowing the entrance to the vagina. The operation also involves the excision of any enterocele and repair of the perineal body (perinorrhaphy).

Manchester repair

This operation is not so common, and involves amputation of the cervix and shortening of the cardinal ligaments, in addition to an anterior repair.

Sacrospinous fixation

This is a procedure to correct vaginal vault prolapse. Vaginal vault prolapse occurs in 0.2% to 43% of women who have had a hysterectomy (Toozs-Hobson *et al.*, 1998). A traditional approach to treating this prolapse was a pelvic floor repair; however, this does not support the vault. This procedure supersedes that approach. The sacrospinous fixation involves fixation of one side of the vaginal vault to the sacrospinous ligaments. The operation has the advantage over the procedure described immediately below in that it can be performed at the same time as repair of other prolapse and has a faster recovery time.

Sacrocolpopexy

This is also a procedure to correct vaginal vault prolapse and is performed through an abdominal incision rather than by the vaginal approach. It involves the retroperitoneal tunnelling with the passage of a sling from the sacral promontory to the vaginal vault. It appears that this form of surgery gives a better resting position of the vagina. It does carry a minimal risk of bleeding from the presacral vessels.

Both sacrospinous fixation and sacrocolpopexy appear to be superior to the pelvic floor repair in that they have lower failure rates, cause less sexual dysfunction and have low complication rates. If genuine stress incontinence is present on urodynamic assessment, a colposuspension should be performed with either of the procedures. Sacrocolpopexy is more suitable to perform for recurrent prolapse, as previous scarring and shortening of the vagina may make fixation more difficult to achieve.

Preoperative care. The preoperative care is very similar to that of women undergoing vaginal hysterectomy. Again, all women will require a full explanation of the proposed surgery, and discharge planning should commence at the time of admission, since these patients are often elderly.

Repair operations take about 45 minutes. On return to the ward a woman can expect:

◆ An intravenous infusion

◆ A vaginal pack

◆ A urethral catheter (occasionally suprapubic).

Drinking is often resumed later in the day provided any nausea has passed.

Following vaginal repair surgery:

◆ The vaginal pack will be removed the following day

◆ The urinary catheter will be removed in the first couple of days

◆ Pain can be a particular problem for those women who have had a posterior repair.

Regular opiate injections will be given initially and Voltarol suppositories are very effective in reducing inflammation and pain:

◆ Ice packs can be useful, or advising the woman to change her position in bed, e.g. to lie on her stomach, and the physiotherapist may have helpful advice

◆ Women need reassurance as the pain and discomfort initially appear to be worsening due to the bruising 'coming out' and the fact that she is probably moving around more than on the day after the operation.

Discharge advice. This is similar to the advice given for women who have undergone hysterectomy. However, more care needs to be taken to avoid constipation or straining bowel motions. For this reason, health education and discharge advice is crucial. Some women may like to hold a sanitary towel supporting the perineum when they first have their bowels open. Women undergoing repair procedures need to be told about their internal sutures since no external wound is visible and they may not understand why precautions about lifting, etc., are necessary.

Surgery for genuine stress incontinence

Surgery for genuine stress incontinence should only be contemplated when urethral sphincter incompetence has been demonstrated objectively by urodynamic studies and conservative treatments have failed (Chaliha and Stanton, 1999). Women should be given the following information when discussing surgery:

◆ Voiding difficulties may be experienced; this may result in the woman being discharged with a suprapubic catheter *in situ*

◆ Very occasionally a woman will need to be taught intermittent self-catheterization (ISC)

◆ The operation may not be curative and incontinence may return to some degree, resulting in a repeat procedure.

Marshall-Marchetti-Krantz (vesico-urethropexy)

This operation is performed through a suprapubic incision. The urogynaecologist inserts a urethral catheter to help identify the bladder neck and cuts into the retropubic space. The tissues at the side of the urethra are sutured to the periosteum behind the symphysis pubis so the bladder neck is re-elevated above the urethrovesicular junction.

Burch colposuspension

The number of treatments for genuine stress incontinence increases each year, but the Burch colposuspension remains the gold standard to which all operations are compared (Cardozo *et al.*, 1999). This is similar to the above procedure. The sutures inserted on either side of the bladder neck and urethra are passed through the paravaginal fascia, which becomes elevated and is sutured to the ileopectinal ligaments. As well as raising the urethra and bladder neck to restore the urethrovesicular junction, this procedure elevates the vaginal vault, so any coexisting anterior vaginal wall prolapse is simultaneously repaired.

The results of both these suprapubic operations are better than those for traditional anterior colporrhaphy with bladder neck buttress.

The first operation for stress incontinence is the one most likely to succeed, so it is important that the best operation is performed first. Most suprapubic operations in current use produce a subjective cure rate in excess of 85% in patients undergoing their first operation for correctly diagnosed stress incontinence (Cardozo, 1993, unpublished). Subsequent surgery may have to be performed on a vagina that is less mobile and where there is fibrosis of the urethra. In such cases a Sling operation or an endoscopic bladder neck suspension, such as the Stamey or Raz procedure, may be easier to perform and more effective.

Physical aspects of abdominal continence surgery. The pre- and postoperative care is very similar to that of any major gynaecological operation.

The operation takes approximately 45 minutes. On return to the ward a woman can expect:

◆ An intravenous infusion

◆ A Redivac drain

◆ A suprapubic catheter will be used, rather than a urethral (Foley) catheter, to avoid the risk of urinary tract infection. A suprapubic catheter is a fine plastic tube, which is inserted through the abdomen just above the wound and has a plastic disc with four sutures attached to the abdominal skin to prevent it from falling out.

Depending on the urogynaecologist's preference the suprapubic catheter will be left to drain freely for 1–2 days. After this time a 'suprapubic clamping regime' will commence to test whether normal bladder function has returned. On the first day the catheter is usually clamped for a period of around 6 hours to observe whether the woman can pass urine urethrally. After this time the clamp is released and the residual that drains into the bag is measured. Initially the residual may be larger than the amount of urine passed urethrally; when the residual is less than approximately 100 ml the catheter may be removed. This is a painless procedure and the small hole in the abdomen heals quickly without the leakage of urine that women might expect.

The regime used in different hospitals does vary and initially can appear complicated. Time and patience is required whilst explaining to the woman about clamping and measuring residuals. Women are usually taught how to clamp their own catheter, empty the drainage bag using their own individual jugs and record their own fluid balance measurements.

Women often need considerable encouragement, especially when they compare themselves with other patients who may be progressing with the regime more rapidly. Occasionally women are unable to pass urine urethrally due to excessive trauma during surgery, and these women may go home with their suprapubic catheter *in situ*. They can either give their bladder a rest at home, or they may continue with the suprapubic clamping regime where the familiar home environment often produces better results. They are taught to strap their catheter correctly, how to use a leg bag during the day and how to change to an overnight bag when necessary. Some district nurses will supervise a clamping regime.

In rare instances of women being unable to pass urine urethrally after at least a month following surgery, intermittent self-catheterization will be taught (see page 506).

Laparoscopic colposuspension

The above procedure is performed laparoscopically and has the advantage of smaller incisions, less discomfort and faster recovery times. However, despite a quicker recovery, laparoscopic colposuspensions take longer to perform and are associated with an increased rate of surgical complications and are more expensive. Trials have also demonstrated that laparoscopic colposuspensions show similar or lower continence rates in comparison to the open Burch colposuspension (Fatthy *et al.*, 2001; Summitt *et al.*, 2000).

Tension-free Vaginal Tape (TVT) colposuspension

This is a procedure that is performed under general, local or spinal anaesthesia. Two small incisions are made in the abdomen, and one in the vagina just beneath the urethra. A small channel is dissected on each side of the urethra, and an instrument is used to place a piece of tape under the urethra. The tape rests tension free under the urethra like a hammock supporting during straining so there is no leakage of urine. The surgeon asks the woman to cough following the procedure to check that the bladder is continent. Usually there is no problem passing urine but a Foley catheter may be left *in situ* for a short period. Some units teach self-catherization before the procedure in case the woman has difficulty passing urine whilst at home. Discharge is either the same day or the following day. She is told to refrain from heavy lifting and sexual intercourse for 4 weeks to allow the incisions in the vagina to heal. The stitches in the vagina will come out in small pieces.

Ward and Hilton (2002) state that surgery with TVT is associated with more operative complications than colposuspension, but colposuspension is associated with more postoperative complications and a longer recovery. It has also been found that TVT is a cost-effective alternative to colposuspension (Manca *et al.*, 2003).

Sexual anxieties following continence surgery. It is important that the sexuality of women over 60 is not ignored but addressed in the same manner as for young women. Older women may be even less likely to initiate discussions about sexual concerns and you should act as a sensitive facilitator and advocate for her. You should ascertain whether she is still sexually active and the doctors should be aware of this when they are suturing near the introitus, to prevent future dyspareunia.

Sexuality in the elderly is difficult to discuss and Griffiths (1988) states that there are two main reasons for this. First, nurses have historically not been trained to cope with sexuality. Their own sexuality is 'suppressed and repressed' with the aim of 'purity' and 'asexuality', and they suffer from sexism and stereotyping at work. Second, the elderly themselves are reluctant to verbalize their sexual feelings, for fear of being seen as depraved or lecherous. It is vital that each woman is treated as an individual and such assumptions are not made.

It is probably wise for women to wait 6 weeks before attempting full sexual intercourse to prevent bruising to the urethra. Extra lubrication can be used. If a suprapubic catheter is in place, it need not interfere with intercourse, especially if

a leg bag is used, or the tube is clamped and spigotted. A high standard of hygiene should be maintained to prevent infection and both partners should wash around the genital area before and after intercourse.

Gynaecological cancers

Within England and Wales cancers of the ovary, endometrium and cervix are the fourth, fifth and sixth most common sites after breast, lung and bowel cancer. The diagnosis of a gynaecological cancer will affect a woman's physical well-being, and the psychological effects of surgery and adjuvant treatment can have a devastating effect on self-esteem, body image, relationships and sexual function. However, the number of these cancers within the population is small: ovarian cancer has an incidence rate of 20 per 100,000 and endometrial and cervical cancer an incidence rate of below 15 per 100,000 (Office for National Statistics, 1998).

In 1999 the National Cancer Guidelines Steering Group published *Improving Outcomes in Gynaecological Cancers* in response to the acknowledgement that nationally the treatment for gynaecological cancers was fragmented and lacked structure. This guidance became known as the Cancer Outcome Guidance (COG) and further acknowledged that the numbers of gynaecological malignancies were low in volume in comparison to other tumour groups: for example, 50% fewer occurrences than for breast cancer. The recommendations that have since developed are the formation of two levels of treatment provision: diagnostic and assessment at cancer units (district general hospitals) and definitive treatment at cancer centres (teaching hospitals with specialist multi-professional gynaecological oncology teams).

In 2000 the government made cancer a top policy priority with the publication of the NHS Cancer Plan (DoH, 2000b). The plan is a long-term strategy to prevent, diagnose and treat cancer; to reform the way cancer services are delivered; to standardize care; and to improve patient experience. The plan has facilitated the formation of cancer networks throughout the country, with the emphasis on collaborative partnerships and multidisciplinary working.

Women with a suspected gynaecological malignancy should be referred on an urgent fast track proforma and it is a government target that women are seen within 2 weeks and that time from referral to definitive treatment should not exceed 62 days.

Ovarian cancer

Diagnosis of ovarian cancer is often difficult, due to the vagueness of the symptoms, which can include increasing abdominal distension, abdominal discomfort, backache, change in bowel habit, fatigue and weight loss. These symptoms can be attributed to a number of other conditions and can often lead to a delay in the diagnosis of ovarian cancer. Irritable bowel syndrome is often given as the cause of presenting symptoms. Many women and their partners express frustration that they have been ignored regarding their symptoms and nurses must be prepared to cope with these emotions and be able to understand them.

Diagnosis

◆ Measurement of Ca 125, CEA and CA 199 serum tumour markers

◆ Pelvic and abdominal ultrasound +/− CT, MRI scan.

The tests together are more likely to distinguish between a benign and malignant tumour.

Treatment

First-line treatment for ovarian cancer is surgery. If the tumour is contained within the ovary, where possible, a total abdominal hysterectomy, bilateral salpingo-oophorectomy and omentectomy are performed. For a woman with early disease and where preservation of fertility is a major issue, unilateral oophorectomy can be performed. However, in most women the disease is advanced and in these cases debulking surgery is performed to remove as much tumour as is possible. Occasionally the tumour may involve the

bowel, requiring varying degrees of bowel resection and the formation of a colostomy. It is important that the woman is informed of this possibility when treatment is initially discussed.

Pre- and postoperative care is fundamentally the same as discussed for major gynaecological surgery. However, due to the possible bowel involvement, more aggressive bowel preparation is given, e.g. picolax and postoperatively a nasogastric tube may be *in situ* and, as previously stated, a colostomy. The psychological effects of this additional surgery on the woman's well-being will be discussed later in the section.

Chemotherapy

Unless early disease is found, most women will be offered chemotherapy and this may be followed by interval debulking of the tumour.

The correct definition of chemotherapy is the specific treatment of disease by the administration of chemical compounds, including sulphonamides and antibiotics. It is often misused to imply treatment only by the use of cytotoxic agents.

The treatment of cancer is by cytotoxic chemotherapy. The word cytotoxic literally means 'cell poisoning' and this is precisely what these drugs do. Cytotoxic drugs work by disrupting the process of cell division through a direct effect on DNA.

There are numerous side effects from chemotherapy because cytotoxic chemotherapy cannot distinguish between cancerous cells and normal cells which are also dividing rapidly. Cytotoxic agents therefore produce unavoidable damage to normal proliferating tissues, such as bone marrow, lymphoid tissue and the epithelial lining of the intestinal tract. Unlike radiotherapy, which is used to attack local and regional disease when the target has been identified, cytotoxic chemotherapy is chosen to attack systemic disease and is useful for metastatic disease or after surgery when microscopic disease may be present. It has a major role in the palliative care of advanced and recurrent gynaecological malignancies.

A balance has to be achieved between killing malignant cells and allowing regeneration and recovery of normal healthy cells. For this reason, chemotherapy is usually given intravenously every 3–4 weeks for a period of 6 months. Some chemotherapy drugs are given orally.

Clinical trials to compare different drug regimes, the effects on morbidity and mortality take long periods of time. However, their results enable women to be offered optimum treatment options. Different regimes are used depending on the type and advancement of the tumour. Results of a large number of trials have shown that platinum-based combination chemotherapy offers improved survival rates among women with advanced ovarian cancer.

The current 'gold standard' combination chemotherapy for first-line treatment is paclitaxel/carboplatin. Paclitaxel/cisplatin can be used but causes more severe side effects; and if paclitaxel is not tolerated, carboplatin alone can be used. If women relapse with their cancer other drugs may be used such as Topotecan, Etoposide, Caelyx and Doxyrubicin.

Both paclitaxel and carboplatin are administered intravenously. Paclitaxel is given over 3–4 hours and carboplatin over 30–60 minutes.

Side effects of chemotherapy. Women should be given information regarding the drugs that they are given and the potential side effects that can affect physical (see Box 19.2), psychological and sexual quality of life. It is important that the woman and her family are given contact numbers so that they do not feel isolated between treatment cycles. Ovacome is a support group run by women who have had or have ovarian cancer and is an excellent resource for women and their families (see Resources).

Psychological/sexuality issues. The impact of surgery, with or without chemotherapy, for women with ovarian cancer is enormous. The 5-year survival rate is often low and the fear of relapse if in remission is great. Therefore nurses must understand issues related to the treatments in order to provide informed support and advice to women and their families. Petersen and Quinlivan (2002) state that spending time talking to patients may represent better value for money than incorporation of the newest and increasingly more expensive chemotherapy regimens. The side effects of chemotherapy alone can cause immense loss of

---

Box 19.2   Physical side effects of chemotherapy

◆ Nausea and vomiting – this is very common following chemotherapy. The duration of these side effects is dependent on the drugs used, though not usually longer than 1 week following a treatment cycle. The following anti-emetics are currently used: granisetron or ondansetron can be given by injection following the chemotherapy, dexamethasone is usually given in reducing doses for 1–4 days, and metoclopramide will be given to take as needed when at home. Nausea is enhanced by the smells of food and cooking; women can be advised to eat cold foods or pre-prepared meals. Ginger has anti-emetic properties, so women could be advised to try sipping ginger beer

◆ Reduction in bone marrow function – this can result in women being prone to infection, anaemia, fatigue, breathlessness and bruising. Occasionally the bone marrow does not recover sufficiently in time for the next dose so the treatment is delayed. Women should be informed that they should contact their treatment centre if they develop any infections

◆ Hair loss – this is rare with carboplatin, common with topotecan and ectoposide, whereas paclitaxel induces the complete loss of all body hair. It starts to occur about 2 weeks after the first treatment and may be rapid. All patients should be given information regarding wigs. Women should be reassured that their hair will regrow once their treatment has been completed

◆ Appetite suppression – can be caused by nausea, temporary taste changes, mouth ulcers and fatigue. Women should be treated for each symptom and advised to eat little and often. Referral to a dietician should be made if problems persist

◆ Peripheral neuropathy – this can be temporary or long term. Women may experience numbness, tingling, pins and needles in their hands and feet. This is caused by the effect of the drugs on the nervous system

◆ Tinnitus – can be caused by high dose carboplatin and may also result in the loss of hearing of high-pitched noises. This can be long term

◆ Diarrhoea – can occur following topotecan.

---

body image; alopecia although temporary can have a profound effect on self-esteem. Loss of libido can be a result of the physical side effects of chemotherapy but also attributed to the loss of fertility from surgery. Younger women, who have undergone unilateral oophorectomy to preserve fertility, often find that the chemotherapy has affected their fertility, and obviously this has a major impact on their body image and role as a woman. Women and their partners must have the opportunity to discuss these issues; this support can be provided by nurse specialists and advising of resources such as Ovacome or BACUP (see Resources).

Endometrial cancer

Endometrial cancer is most commonly found in post-menopausal women. It is usually detected at an early stage because the primary symptom is vaginal bleeding.

Diagnosis

Women should be able to attend an outpatient rapid access clinic, where the following diagnostic tests can be performed:

◆ Transvaginal ultrasound – to assess the thickness of the endometrium. If a tumour is seen the scan can assess the depth of myometrial invasion and therefore the potential for lymph node involvement. Smith-Bindman *et al.* (1998) found that transvaginal ultrasound is an accurate way of excluding endometrial cancer
◆ Hysteroscopy – see page 550
◆ MRI scan.

Treatment

First-line treatment for the majority of women with endometrial cancer is surgery. Total abdominal hysterectomy, bilateral salpingo-oophorectomy (TAH/BSO) and lymphadenectomy in many cases is the only treatment needed. However, the depth of invasion through the myometrium and grade of tumour will indicate the need for adjuvant radiotherapy. There is no evidence to suggest that adjuvant chemotherapy is beneficial for women with endometrial cancer.

Pre- and postoperative care is the same as discussed for major gynaecological surgery.

Cervical cancer

See Chapter 13 to understand the initial diagnosis and treatment of cervical cancer. Landoni *et al.* (1997) have shown that women with early cervical cancer can be treated with surgery or radiotherapy.

Surgery

Women diagnosed with invasive cancer of the cervix, where cone biopsy has failed to excise the tumour, completely undergo a radical hysterectomy with pelvic lymphadenectomy (Wertheim's hysterectomy). This usually involves a TAH/BSO, removal of the upper third of the vagina and pelvic lymph node clearance. Some women undergo ovarian conservation, if they want to retain fertility and for hormonal issues. These women must be informed that although retained ovaries can continue hormonal function, a high incidence of premature ovarian failure has been noted (Anderson *et al.*, 1993).

Pre- and postoperative care is similar to that of major gynaecological surgery. Due to the more radical nature of this surgery, the following may apply:

◆ A Foley catheter is left *in situ* for about 5 days to allow any swelling around the urethra to subside
◆ Redivac drains may be left *in situ* for a few days to drain any excessive lymphatic fluid.

Adjuvant therapy

Histology of the Wertheim's hysterectomy may necessitate the need for adjuvant therapy. Conventional therapy was a combination of external beam radiotherapy and brachytherapy delivered to the inside of the vaginal vault. However, research from five randomized, controlled trials has shown that concurrent chemoradiotherapy using Capstan can significantly improve survival rate, although this treatment does cause more adverse side effects (Rose *et al.*, 1999; Keys *et al.*, 1999; Morris *et al.*, 1999; Peters *et al.*, 2000; Whitney *et al.*, 1999).

Radical trachelectomy and pelvic lymph node dissection

This is a treatment that is performed to allow preservation of fertility for women with early-stage cancer of the cervix. Smith *et al.* (1997)

describe the procedure as being similar to a radical hysterectomy and lymphadenectomy. However, the ovarian vessels are not ligated and following lymphadenectomy and skeletonization of the uterine arteries, the cervix, parametrium and vaginal cuff are excised. The residuum of the cervix is then sutured to the vagina and the uterine arteries are re-anastamosed.

Although to date numbers are small, Covens *et al.* (1999) have reported that the procedure appears to have similar efficacy to the radical hysterectomy. Shepherd *et al.* (2001) found that on present short-term evidence radical trachelectomy and pelvic node dissection appears to be a safe method of treatment in a highly selected group of women with very early invasive carcinoma of the cervix. This is important in the management of women where fertility is of major psychological importance and has the potential of being conserved.

Vulval cancer

Carcinoma of the vulva accounts for 5% of all cases of genital cancer in women. It is most often seen in elderly women, aged over 60 years. The most common malignancy of the vulva is squamous cell carcinoma, which accounts for 95% of all vulval cancers.

The traditional surgery for invasive vulval cancer was 'en bloc' technique: this involved the extensive excision of the vulval tissue, often including the clitoris; bilateral lymph node groin dissection; and the removal of a substantial amount of tissue over the mons pubis. This surgery is extremely mutilating and involves a long hospital stay due to delayed wound healing, skin grafts and decreased mobility caused by the wounds; hence, a high morbidity rate.

The gold standard for surgical treatment of vulval cancer is the triple incision vulvectomy. The groins are dissected with individual incisions and the vulval area is excised without the need for removing a large amount of pubic tissue. This is still a mutilating procedure but results in less morbidity. Siller *et al.* (1995) have shown that there is no significance in the survival and recurrence rates of the two procedures.

However, due to the immense psychological impact of these procedures, the procedure that is less mutilating should be the preferred option.

For women who are not fit for radical surgery, a wide local tumour excision can be performed. Nurses should remember that women will regard this surgery as a form of mutilation regardless of the less radical method of excision.

Nursing care

The general principles of nursing care are the same as for all major gynaecological surgery along with the following:

◆ The operation will take 2–4 hours. Regular injections of opiate analgesia will be given or an epidural may be in progress. A blood transfusion may be required due to excessive blood loss and intravenous fluid replacement is always necessary, since fluid loss is considerable during this complicated operation. After the initial drowsiness and nausea, drinking and eating may gradually be resumed. A low-fibre diet is necessary to avoid bulky stools and straining.

◆ A urethral (Foley) catheter will be in place to ensure infection of the wound does not occur from spilling of urine, or that urinary retention does not occur due to peri-urethral tissue being bruised during the operation. The catheter will remain *in situ* for 7–10 days while healing occurs. Occasionally one-third to a half of the urethra may be removed; however, spontaneous voiding is possible. Some women find that urine no longer flows out in a steady stream, so they need to be taught how to squat and sit back slightly to avoid wetting their legs or the floor.

◆ Two Redivac drains are inserted into the groins to prevent haematoma formation and will remain *in situ* for 7–10 days. There will be a non-adhesive dressing over the stitched areas, often held together by a bandage between the legs. Depending on the gynaecologist the bandages may be kept on for up to 4 or 5 days to allow undisturbed healing to occur. If the dressings do become very soiled they will be changed and the area will be irrigated with normal saline or a gentle antiseptic solution. It can then be dried thoroughly using a hair dryer. The sutures are usually removed about 10 days following surgery. The groin wounds and vulval area should be observed closely for signs of infection or breakdown, and treated with antibiotics if needed.

Adjuvant therapy

Radiotherapy can be given to women where the lymph nodes dissected during surgery are positive to tumour. To date, research into the use of chemotherapy and concurrent chemoradiotherapy for the treatment of primary disease is limited.

Psychological effects of vulvectomy

All patients facing vulvectomy require psychologically sensitive nursing care. A full sexual history and assessment should be made, and at all times the woman's partner should be included, if possible. They should both be encouraged to discuss any sexual concerns preoperatively and should be given clear explanations about the surgery and its implications.

Obviously, women may find it difficult to look at their new altered appearance and it is advisable they try to do so before going home. If possible, the woman should look with the help of a mirror, in her own time, but with her nurse present if she prefers. Many women in this age group are not used to looking 'down below' so you should act sensitively. This sensitive approach can really only occur if the nurse has already built up a relationship with the woman and her partner and discussed sexual concerns. It may be better to wait until the stitches are removed since they can make the scarring look worse. Many women find it hard to visualize what the scar will look like. Due to the fatty, stretchy nature of vulval skin, the remaining skin can be stretched to leave a very neat scar. They need to be warned that because the labia have been removed, the opening of the vagina will be more visible. If the clitoris has been removed the area will now be flat skin, without the usual folds of the vulva. The groin may feel tight at first if lymph nodes

have been removed and some women describe this feeling of tightness between their legs 'as though a sanitary towel is being pulled upwards'.

Women usually stay in hospital for 1–2 weeks and discharge planning from the time of admission is essential. Unfortunately, there is no special support group for vulvectomy patients, like the Hysterectomy Support Group or Mastectomy Association, but BACUP (see Resources) is a very helpful organization, and health care professionals can network between old and new patients.

Total pelvic exenteration (TPE)

This extensive operation is used as a curative procedure in the treatment of certain types of pelvic malignancy, the most notable being recurrent cancer of the cervix. The surgery involves removal of the rectum and distal sigmoid colon, the urinary bladder, all reproductive organs and the entire pelvic floor, and necessitates the formation of both a urostomy and a sigmoid colostomy. These women, as with vulvectomy patients, require considerable nursing and a sensitive approach to their care in order to facilitate their recovery and rehabilitation. This surgery can take most of a day to perform, especially if it involves organ reconstruction such as the transposition of the gracilis muscle to reconstruct the vagina.

The nursing care depends on the degree of exenteration, and the patient will spend the first 24–48 hours in a high-dependency unit. This can provide women's partners with increased anxiety and every effort should be made to keep them informed of the procedure and condition of their partner. The length of stay for these procedures is dependent on the surgery and each woman's physical and psychological recovery.

Radiotherapy

Radiotherapy is used for some women where disease is too advanced for surgery or surgical removal of a tumour is incomplete. It is also used for adjuvant treatment in women diagnosed with high-grade cancer following first-line surgery.

Radiotherapy is the use of ionizing radiation to destroy cancer cells by inhibiting their ability to divide and proliferate. As radiation passes through a tissue, some of its energy is transferred to the cells of that tissue, causing ionization. This results in chemical changes which lead to cellular damage or death. The target of the radiation and, indeed, damage is DNA and therefore the greatest effects are seen during mitosis when the amount of DNA is doubled.

It is usually necessary to divide the calculated tumour lethal dose into smaller doses (fractionation) to prevent acute radiation exposure. This allows both normal and cancer cells to attempt repair between consecutive treatments.

Radiotherapy for endometrial cancer

There are ongoing studies to compare the use of external beam radiotherapy with lymphadenectomy and TAH/BSO alone (ASTEC Trial commenced 1998 and continues to recruit patients). There are two types of radiotherapy that are used and there is no evidence to indicate which of the following should be used.

External beam radiotherapy

An external source is specifically focused on to the tumour, which is about 100 cm from the source of ionizing radiation. Gamma rays or electrons are used – depending on which is felt to be the most appropriate. The treatment is usually given 5 days a week for 5–6 weeks. Each treatment lasts a few minutes. It is important to explain the fractionation process to women as they often have to travel relatively long distances and they find it quite arduous.

Vault brachytherapy

The radioactive source is positioned via small ovoid applicators at the vault of the vagina. The aim of brachytherapy is to deliver a dose of radiation as close as possible to the parametria and the proximal parts of the uterosacral ligaments. This treatment is usually given 2–3 times, lasts a few minutes and is often given in conjunction with external beam radiotherapy.

Radiotherapy for cervical cancer

Radiotherapy as adjuvant therapy is, as above, both external beam and radiotherapy. If the radiotherapy is being given for advanced disease or palliation of symptoms, the brachytherapy source is inserted into the uterine cavity or into the tumour mass.

Selectron

This is a type of intracavity therapy using a remote control radioactive microsource, such as 'microselectron'. Under general anaesthesia hollow applicators are inserted and positioned correctly in the uterus, and ovoids are placed in the fornices. All the sources have tubes attached through which the radioactive material can be inserted. A remote afterloading system will deliver radioactive caesium pellets into the applicators in the patient by a pneumatic system using compressed air, after the staff have left the radiation-protected treatment area. If it is necessary to enter the room for nursing care, the sources are automatically withdrawn from the patient and stored in the machine. A scintillation counter measures the amount of radiation being received by the rectum and checks it is acceptable. If the bladder and rectum receive excessive irradiation, severe cystitis or proctitis will develop, possibly leading to necrosis and fistula formation.

Side effects of radiotherapy

Radiotherapy can result in a wide range of physical side effects (see Box 19.3), which, in turn, can have a profound effect on the psychosexual function of women and their partners. Women should be fully informed of the side effects of radiotherapy. Unlike chemotherapy where many of the side effects are transitory, radiotherapy can cause long-term problems. Booklets outlining treatment and side effects are available from BACUP and cancer centres such as the Royal Marsden Hospital, London.

Psychosexual anxieties following surgery and radiotherapy

Sexual dysfunction is common following radical pelvic surgery and tends to remain a chronic problem (Corney et al., 1993). This is often linked to the side effects of radiotherapy (chronic fatigue, diarrhoea, tender scars, pain and alopecia resulting in embarrassment), which all contribute

Box 19.3 Physical side effects of radiotherapy

◆ Hair loss – pubic hair within the treatment field will gradually fall out; this is temporary and will normally grow back after treatment

◆ Skin irritation – skin within the treatment field may become inflamed and sore during treatment. Women should be advised to have warm rather than hot baths or showers and not to use perfumed products such as bubble bath. They can be advised to dust the area lightly with baby powder. Clothing should be loose, so women should be advised to avoid wearing tight belts and tight underwear

◆ Bowel dysfunction – women may experience diarrhoea or loose stools due to the effect of radiation on the bowel mucosa. They should be encouraged to avoid high fibre foods and vegetables and ensure they drink plenty of fluids. Drugs such as immodium can be given to alleviate symptoms

◆ Bladder dysfunction – women may experience cystitis, urinary tract infections, urgency or frequency due to the effect of radiation on the bladder mucosa. They should be encouraged to drink at least 2 litres of fluid a day and inform their doctor of these symptoms

◆ Vaginal changes – radiotherapy renders the vaginal mucosa dry, causing it to be easily traumatized, stenosed and less stretchable. Women can be taught to use vaginal dilators (see text)

◆ Ovulation failure – radiotherapy results in an almost immediate premature menopause for those women who are not post-menopausal.

to making sexual intercourse difficult. Surgery and radiotherapy may cause damage to the sacral nerves, causing neurological changes to sensory perception within the genital area, resulting in an alteration to sensation.

Radiotherapy can result in temporary or permanent sexual dysfunction. It is important that women understand they are not a danger to their partner and that no radiation remains inside the body, and their cancer cannot be passed on during sexual intercourse.

Radiotherapy may cause the fragile tissues in the genital area to become more fibrotic and lose their elasticity. This fibrosis will not disappear and scar tissue at the surgical site within the vagina will not engorge and stretch as well during intercourse as other genital tissue. Vaginal fibrosis can also cause vaginal shortening and narrowing.

Vaginal dilators, lubricants and new intercourse positions may relieve dyspareunia and preserve vaginal function. Sexual activity should be encouraged during this time and ideally should occur at least once per week. This not only helps the couple to maintain a sense of sexual normality but also preserves the patency of the vagina which could be threatened by adhesions. Fear of pain from friction, fibrosis, or even the sensation that semen can cause should not be reasons for abstaining. You should discuss these anxieties with your patients and if problems exist you could suggest using lubricants, vaginal dilators and condoms to ameliorate them.

Even women who have no sexual partners can take steps to maintain vaginal function through masturbation, which increases blood circulation to the pelvis and vagina, or through use of a dildo or vaginal dilator. Without these precautions adhesions, fibrosis or loss of elasticity can result and corrective surgery may become necessary. Corney et al. (1993) also state that the mutilating effect of vulvectomy and exenterative surgery has resulted in some women never resuming sexual intercourse.

The psychosexual implications of vulvectomy are of utmost importance since genitals are intimately associated with a woman's sexuality, body image, gender identity and general quality of life. Excision of the clitoris is likely to reduce greatly sensation and sexual arousability, and orgasm is rare (Wabrek and Gunn, 1984). The scarred tissue at the remaining vaginal opening can be insensitive to penetration, or hypersensitive to friction. Removal of the pelvic lymph nodes can result in oedema of the legs, which can cause embarrassment, and excision of fatty tissue can cause pain on sitting.

A woman who has undergone a vulvectomy should be advised that she may resume intercourse when she feels ready, probably 4–12 weeks following surgery. Couples should be advised to compensate for loss of perineal sensation by exploring other erotic areas – breasts, buttocks and thighs (Lamb, 1985). Massage, mutual masturbation and oral sex may be advised if penetration is not possible. Wallace (1987) recommends encouraging patients to use fantasy material, such as explicit accounts of female sexual experiences in books such as *My Secret Garden* by Nancy Friday.

Limited hip abduction is advisable for the first 4–6 weeks to avoid putting undue stress on the groin and perineal sutures. Some women find it difficult to abduct their thighs and couples need to find the most comfortable position for lovemaking. A pillow under the woman's thighs may be helpful. The missionary position may be especially painful for the woman due to the deep penetration. It has to be remembered that couples may need explicit advice and information rather than vague generalizations about intercourse, since people's sexual experiences vary immensely.

Although such detailed discussion may or may not be accomplished by all nurses, depending on their personal expertise and degree of comfort, it is important not to neglect the issue of the patient's altered sexuality, since this will only reinforce the fallacy that her sexual role is over.

The role of the nurse is imperative in the support of women and their partners. Information relating to the effects of surgery and adjuvant therapy should be discussed prior to commencement of any treatment. Jusenius (1991) states that 'nurses are accessible to women undergoing evaluation and care for gynaecological cancer. In building a caring, therapeutic relationship, nurses can assess the woman's needs, convey accurate information about treatment effects and support adaptations to changes wrought by disease or its treatment'. Waterhouse and Metcalfe (1991) also found that a large number of patients expressed wishes that the nurses would initiate the discussion of their sexual concerns.

Follow-up for women is 3-monthly for 1 year, 6-monthly for 2 years, then yearly until 5 years following surgery. Follow-up often alternates between the centre and unit. Women find these visits reassuring although there is no evidence that the visits have any effect in detecting any recurrence, as it is usually the woman who contacts the hospital if she has developed symptoms of recurrence.

Conclusion

This chapter has described the investigations and surgical procedures that are routinely performed for gynaecological conditions. There has been a great move towards the use of minimally invasive surgery, with the constant evolution of new techniques. These procedures should be seen in the context in which they are often performed: to alleviate symptoms, not with the aim of cure. Major gynaecological surgery continues to be the mainstay of the care carried out on a general gynaecology ward. Reduction in lengths of stay and patient expectation reinforces the need for good communication, encompassing all aspects of women's health. Nurses should endeavour to recognize the diverse needs of each individual and understand the impact of gynaecological surgery on their physical and psychological wellbeing. Unfortunately, all health professionals still do not openly discuss sexuality but it is hoped that with support and guidance this vital area of women's health care will be encompassed.

Undoubtedly, with the aid of modern technology and with the aim of treating conditions that are less debilitating, new adaptations of current gynaecological procedures will continue. Nurses must be encouraged to be proactive and to see the procedures being performed, which can only enhance the care and information given to women and their families.

> ### Ideas for personal and professional development
>
> - All gynaecology nurses should ensure that they experience a variety of inpatient and outpatient settings and observe surgical procedures in the operating theatre
>
> - Develop an in-depth knowledge and rationale for specific procedures. For example, colposuspension: visit a urodynamics clinic, carry out a nursing assessment of a particular admission and observe the operation. Finally, write a brief case study of the patient to demonstrate an understanding of the procedure, incorporating all aspects of nursing care
>
> - Research the need for and develop a patient information leaflet for a specific condition or procedure within your clinical area
>
> - Liaise with your designated cancer centre using your gynaecology oncology nurse specialist to arrange a visit to observe an outpatient clinic and/or a radiotherapy department

Patient education points

● With new advances in technology there are a number of minimally invasive treatment options for menorrhagia

● Are you aware as a gynaecology nurse of the diverse number of websites and support groups that are available to women and their partners? Research these and choose those that offer sound evidence-based information to help inform your patients

● Loss of a pregnancy can cause psychological problems for the woman and her partner

● Teach a patient to manage their own catheter following discharge, discussing the rationale

● Hormone replacement therapy following a hysterectomy and oophorectomy in a pre-menopausal woman is important in providing symptom relief.

Resources

Amarant Trust
5 Sycamore Street, London EC1Y 0SR
Helpline: 01293 413000
www.amarantmenopausetrust.org.uk
Menopause and HRT charity. Provides details of lists of well woman clinics and menopause clinics. Helpline staffed by specialist nurses.

ARC (Antenatal Results and Choices)
73 Charlotte Street, London W1T 4PN
Helpline: 020 7631 0285
www.arc-uk.org
Support and information for parents during antenatal screening/testing, awaiting results and diagnosis of foetal abnormality. Available Mon–Fri, 10 am–5 pm. Answerphone after hours.

BACUP
3 Bath Place, Rivington Street,
  London EC2A 3JR
Tel: 020 7696 9003
Helpline: Freephone 0808 8001234
www.cancerbacup.org.uk
Counselling service. Information on all aspects of cancer. Booklets available on all types of cancer, encompassing physical and emotional issues.

British Pregnancy Advisory Service
Austy Manor, Wootton Wawen, Solihull,
  West Midlands B95 6BX
Tel: 0845 304 030
www.bpas.org

Cancer During Pregnancy
Tel: 020 8942 8759
Telephone support service for women that are diagnosed with cancer during pregnancy, or their relatives.

Continence Foundation
307 Hatton Square, 1 Baldwins Gardens,
  London EC1N 7RJ
Tel: 0845 345 0165
www.continence-foundation.org.uk

Daisy Chain
PO Box 183, Rossendale BB4 6WZ
www.daisynetwork.org.uk
Support group for women suffering premature menopause due to ovarian failure.

Endometriosis
www.endometriosis.org
The endometriosis society provides support and information for women and their families.

Gynae C
1 Bolingbrooke Road, Swindon,
  Wiltshire SN2 2LB
Tel: 01793 338885
www.communigate.co.uk/wilts/gynaec
Support for women diagnosed with gynaecological cancer, from women that have or had cancer themselves.

Hysterectomy Association
60 Redwood House, Charlton Down,
  Dorchester, DT2 9UH
www.hysterectomy-association.org.uk/
  index.htm

Hysterectomy support groups
c/o Women's Health, 52 Featherstone Street,
  London EC1Y 8RT
Tel: 020 7251 6333

Helpline: 020 7251 6580
E-mail: womenshealth@pop3.poptel.co.uk
Provides contact numbers for local support
  groups.

Infertility Network UK
Charter House, 43 St Leonards Road,
  Bexhill-on-Sea, East Sussex TN40 1JA
Tel: 01424 732361
www.infertilitynetworkuk.com
National infertility support network.

Jo's Trust
www.jotrust.co.uk
Support group for women diagnosed with
  cervical cancer, information regarding
  treatment, radiotherapy, chemotherapy,
  counselling and related issues.

Lymphoedema Support Group
St Luke's Crypt, Sydney Street, London SW3
  6NH
Tel: 020 73514480
www.lymphoedema.org
Provides support and information for women
  with lymphoedema.

Macmillan Cancer Relief
Tel: 0845 601 6161

Miscarriage Association
c/o Clayton Hospital, Northgate,
  Wakefield, West Yorkshire WF1 3JS
Tel: 01924 200795
Helpline: 01924 200799
www.the-ma.org.uk
Excellent support group for women who have
  suffered a pregnancy loss. Provides leaflets
  and newsletters. Includes support for women
  who have experienced an ectopic pregnancy.

National Endometriosis Society
Suite 50, Westminster Palace Gardens, 1–7
  Artillery Row, London SW1P 1RL
Tel: 020 7222 2776
www.endo.org.uk

National Osteoporosis Society
Camerton, Bath BA2 0PJ
Tel: 01761 471771
www.nos.org.uk

**National Society of Gynaecological
  Oncology Nurses**
Tel: 0208 383 3317
Specialist gynaeoncology nurses' information
  and support group for all health
  professionals.

NHS Direct
Tel: 0845 4647
www.nhsdirect.nhs.uk
Health information on the internet.

Ovacome
Elizabeth Garrett Anderson Hospital,
  Huntley Street, London WC2E 6DH
Tel: 020 7380 9589
www.ovacome.org.uk
National support group for women diagnosed
  with ovarian cancer; excellent quarterly
  newsletter and website detailing all aspects
  of treatments and support.

Polycystic Ovarian Syndrome Group
30 Charlton House, Charlton Street,
  London NW1 1HH

Radical Vulvectomy Support Group
Tel: 01977 640234
Support for women with vulval cancer.

Recurrent Miscarriage Clinic
St Mary's Hospital, Praed Street,
  London W2 1PG
Tel: 020 7258 0285

Royal Marsden Hospital
203 Fulham Road, London SW3 6JJ
Tel: 020 7352 8171
www.royalmarsden.org

**SAFTA (Support around Termination
  for Abnormality)**
73–75 Charlotte Street, London W1P 1LB
Tel: 020 7631 0280

SANDS (Stillbirth and Neonatal Death Society)
28 Portland Place, London W1B 1LY
Helpline: 020 7436 5881
www.uk-sands.org

Thrombosis Advice
www.schollflights.co.uk or www.yeoman.org.uk

For information, advice and supplies of stockings.

Vulval Pain Society
PO Box 514, Slough, Berkshire SL1 2BP

Women's Health Concern
PO Box 2126, Marlow, Bucks SL7 2NB
Tel: 01628 483612
www.womens-health-concern.org
Enclose SAE.

Further reading

CLARK, J. (1993) *Hysterectomy and the Alternatives*. London: Virago.
GOULD, D. (1990) *Nursing Care of Women*. Hertfordshire: Prentice Hall.
HUNTER, M. (1994) *Counselling in Obstetrics and Gynaecology*. Leicester: BPS Books.
JOHNSON, L.E. (1987) *Intimacy. Living as a Woman After Cancer*. Toronto: NC Press.
LAMBERT, H.E. and BLAKE, P.E. (1992) *Gynaecological Oncology*. Oxford: Oxford University Press.
MEERABEAU, L. and DENTON, J. (1995) *Infertility, Nursing and Caring*. London: Scutari Press.
MOULDER, C. (1995) *Miscarriage: Women's Experiences and Needs*, 2nd ed. London: Pandora Press/Harper Collins.
MOULDER, C. (1998) *Understanding Pregnancy Loss, Perspectives and Issues in Care*. Hampshire: Macmillan Press.
NATIONAL CANCER GUIDELINES STEERING GROUP (1999) *Improving Outcomes in Gynaecological Cancers: The Manual*. London: NHS Executive, Department of Health.
NATIONAL CANCER GUIDELINES STEERING GROUP (1999) *Improving Outcomes in Gynaecological Cancers: The Research Evidence*. London: NHS Executive, Department of Health.
OAKLEY, A., McPHERSON, A. and ROBERTS, H. (1990) *Miscarriage*, revised edn. Harmondsworth: Penguin.
REGAN, L. (1997) *Miscarriage, What Every Woman Needs To Know*. London: Bloomsbury.
SHAW, R.W., SOUTTER, W.P. and STANTON, S.L. (2003) *Gynaecology*. Edinburgh: Churchill Livingstone.
SUTHERLAND, C. (2001) *Women's Health: A Handbook for Nurses*. Edinburgh: Churchill Livingstone.
THOMAS, J. *Supporting Parents when a Baby Dies: Before or Soon After Birth*, 2nd edn. Published privately. Available from: Mrs J. Brown, 1 Millside, Riversdale, Bourne End, Bucks SL8 5EB.
WALTON, I. (1994) *Sexuality and Motherhood*. Cheshire: Books for Midwives.

References

ABERDEEN ENDOMETRIAL ABLATION TRIALS GROUP (1999) A randomised trial of endometrial ablation versus hysterectomy for the treatment of dysfunctional uterine bleeding: outcome at four years. *British Journal of Obstetrics and Gynaecology* **106**:360–6.
ABU, J.I., HABIBA, M.A., BAKER, R., HALLIGAN, A.W.F., NAFTALIN, N.J., HSU, R. and TAUB, N. (2001) Quantitative and qualitative assessment of women's experience of a one-stop menstrual clinic in comparison with traditional gynaecology clinics. *British Journal of Obstetrics and Gynaecology* **108**(9):993–9.
AKANDE, V.A. and VYAS, S.K. (2003) Questioning the ubiquity of outpatient endometrial sampling in the management of menstrual disorders. *BJOG: An International Journal of Obstetrics and Gynaecology* **110**(11):971–4.
ANDERSON, B., LAPOLLA, J., TURNER, D., CHAPMAN, G. and BULLER, R. (1993) Ovarian transposition in cervical cancer. *Gynecologic Oncology* **78**:2229–35.
ATHANASIOU, S., KHULLAR, V., BOOS, K., SALVATORE, S. and CARDOZO, L. (1999) Imaging the urethral sphincter with three-dimensional ultrasound. *Obstetrics and Gynecology* **94**(2):295–301.
BACKSTRÖM, T., BOYLE, H. and BAIRD, D.T. (1981) Persistence of symptoms of premenstrual tension in hysterectomised women. *British Journal of Obstetrics and Gynaecology* **88**:530–6.
BAIN, C., PARKIN, D.E. and COOPER, K.C. (2002) Is outpatient diagnostic hysteroscopy more useful than endometrial biopsy alone for the investigation of abnormal uterine bleeding in unselected premenopausal women? *BJOG: An International Journal of Obstetrics and Gynaecology* **109**(7):805–11.
BARBACK, L.G. (1975) *For Yourself. The Fulfilment of Female Sexuality*. New York: Signet/Doubleday.
BERKOWITZ, R., HUTCHINS, F. and WORTHINGTON-KIRSCH, R. (1999) Vaginal expulsion of submucosal fibroids after uterine artery embolisation. A report of three cases. *Journal of Reproductive Medicine* **44**(4):373–6.
BHAVNANI, V. and CLARKE, A. (2003) Women awaiting hysterectomy: a qualitative study of issues involved in decisions about oophorectomy. *BJOG: An International Journal of Obstetrics and Gynaecology* **110**(2):168–74.
BIGRIGG, M.A. and READ, M.D. (1991) Management of women referred to early pregnancy assessment unit: care and cost effectiveness. *British Medical Journal* **302**(6776):577–9.
BLUNDELL, J. (1829) Extirpation of the uterus. *Lancet* **215**.
BROOME, A.K. and WALLACE, L.M. (eds) (1984) *Psychology and Gynaecological Problems*. London: Tavistock.
CARDOZO, L., HEXTALL, A., BAILEY J. and BOOS, K. (1999) Colposuspension after previous failed incontinence surgery: a prospective observational study. *British Journal of Obstetrics and Gynaecology* **106**:340–4.
CHALIHA, C. and STANTON, S.L. (1999) Complications of surgery for genuine stress incontinence. *British Journal of Obstetrics and Gynaecology* **106**:1238–45.
CORNEY, R., CROWTHER, M., EVERETT, M., HOWELLS, A. and SHEPHERD, J. (1993) Psychosexual dysfunction in women with gynaecological cancer following pelvic surgery. *British Journal of Obstetrics and Gynaecology* **100**:73–8.
CORSI, P., JOHNSON, S., GONIK, B., McNEELEY, S. and DIAMOND, M. (1999) Transvaginal ultrasound-guided aspiration of pelvic abscesses. *Infectious Diseases in Obstetrics and Gynaecology* **7**(5):216–21.

COVENS, A., SHAW, P., MURPHY, J. *et al.* (1999) Is radical trachelectomy a safe alternative to radical hysterectomy for patients with stage 1A-B carcinoma of the cervix? *Cancer* 86(11):2273–9.

DAVIDSON, K.G. and DUBINSKY, T.J. (2003) Ultrasonographic evaluation of the endometrium in postmenopausal vaginal bleeding. *Radiologic Clinics of North America* 41(4):769–80.

Department of Health (2000a) *The NHS Plan. A Plan for Investment, A Plan for Reform*. London: Department of Health.

Department of Health (2000b) *The NHS Cancer Plan*. London: Department of Health.

FARQUHAR, C. (2003) Author's reply. A six year audit of the management of ectopic pregnancy. *Australian and New Zealand Journal of Obstetrics and Gynaecology* 43(3):225.

FATTHY, H., EK HAO, M., SAMAHA, I. and ABDALLAH, K. (2001) Modified Burch colposuspension: laparoscopy versus laparotomy. *Journal of the American Association of Gynecologic Laparoscopists* 8:99–106.

GARRY, R. (2002) The benefits and problems associated with minimal access surgery. *Australian and New Zealand Journal of Obstetrics and Gynaecology* 42(3):239–44.

GARRY, R., FOUNTAIN, J., MASON, S., NAPP, V., BROWN, J., HAWE, J., CLAYTON, R., ABBOTT, J., PHILLIPS, G., WHITTAKER, M., LILFORD, R. and BRIDGEMAN, S. (2004) The eVALuate study: two parallel randomised trials, one comparing laparoscopic with abdominal hysterectomy, the other comparing laparoscopic with vaginal hysterectomy. *British Medical Journal* 328:129–34.

GOODWIN, S., VEDANTHAM, S., McLUCAS, B., FORNO, A. and PARRCLLA, P. (1997) Preliminary experience with uterine artery embolisation for uterine fibroids. *Journal of Vascular and Interventional Radiology* 8:517–26.

GOULD, D. (1986) Hidden problems after a hysterectomy. *Nursing Times* 82(23):43–6.

GRIFFITHS, E. (1988) No sex please, we're over sixty. *Nursing Times* 84(1):34–5.

HAWE, J., ABBOTT, J., HUNTER, D.J., PHILLIPS, G. and GARRY, R. (2003) A randomised controlled trial comparing the Cavaterm endometrial ablation system with the Nd:YAG laser for the treatment of dysfunctional uterine bleeding. *British Journal of Obstetrics and Gynaecology* 110(4):350–7.

JONES, K., ABBOTT, J., HAWE, J., SUTTON, C. and GARRY, R (2001) Endometrial laser intrauterine thermotherapy for the treatment of dysfunctional uterine bleeding: the first British experience. *British Journal of Obstetrics and Gynaecology* 108(7):749–53.

JORIZZO, J., RICCO, G., CHEN, M. and CARR, J. (1999) Sonohysteroscopy: the next step in the evaluation of the abnormal endometrium. *Radiographics* 19:117–30.

JUSENIUS, K. (1991) Sexuality and gynecologic cancer. *Cancer Nursing* 4(6):479–84.

KEYS, H., BUNDY, B., STEHMAN, F. *et al.* (1999) Cisplatin, radiation and adjuvant hysterectomy compared with radiation and adjuvant hysterectomy for bulky stage 1B cervical carcinoma. *New England Journal of Medicine* 340:1154–61.

LAMB, M. (1985) Sexual dysfunction in the gynaecological oncology patient. *Seminars in Oncology Nursing* 1(1):9–17.

LANDONI, F., MANCO, A., COLOMBO, A. *et al.* (1997) Randomised study of radical surgery versus radiotherapy for stage 1b-1a cervical cancer. *Lancet* 350:535–40.

LEWIS, T.L.T. and CHAMBERLAIN, G.V.P. (1991) *Gynaecology by Ten Teachers*. London: Edward Arnold.

MANCA, A., SCULPHER, M.J., WARD, K. and HILTON, P. (2003) A cost-utility analysis of tension-free vaginal tape versus colposuspension for primary urodynamic incontinence. *BJOG: An International Journal of Obstetrics and Gynaecology* 110(3):255–62.

MARESH, M.J.A., METCALFE, M.A., McPHERSON, K., OVERTON, C., HALL, V., HARGREAVES, J., BRIDGMAN, S., DOBBINS, J. and CASBARD, A. (2002) The VALUE national hysterectomy study: description of the patients and their surgery. *BJOG: An International Journal of Obstetrics and Gynaecology* 109(3):302–12.

MIRON, J. and CHAPMAN, J. (1994) Supporting men's experiences with the event of their partners' miscarriage. *Canadian Journal of Nursing Research* 26(2):61–72.

MORRIS, M., EIFEL, P., Lu, J. *et al.* (1999) Pelvic radiation with concurrent chemotherapy for locally advanced cervical cancer. *New England Journal of Medicine* 340:1137–43.

MOULDER, C. (1998) *Understanding Pregnancy Loss, Perspectives and Issues in Care*. Hampshire: Macmillan Press.

NAGELE, F., BOURNAS, N., O'CONNOR, H., BROADBENT, M., RICHARDSON, R. and MAGOS, A. (1996) Comparison of carbon dioxide and normal saline for uterine distension in outpatient hysteroscopy. *Fertility and Sterility* 65(2):305–9.

NATIONAL CANCER GUIDELINES STEERING GROUP (1999) *Improving Outcomes in Gynaecological Cancers: The Research Evidence*. London: NHS Executive, Department of Health.

NIELSEN, S. and HAHLIN, M. (1995) Expectant management of first-trimester spontaneous abortion. *Lancet* 345:6–8.

O'CONNOR, H. and MAGOS, A. (1996) Endometrial resection for the treatment of menorrhagia. *New England Journal of Medicine* 335(3):151–6.

OFFICE FOR NATIONAL STATISTICS (1998) Cited in: Management of gynaecological cancers 1999. Effective health care. *NHS Centre for Reviews and Dissemination* 5(3).

OVERTON, C., HARGREAVES, J. and MARESH, M. (1997) A national survey of the complications of endometrial destruction for menstrual disorders: the MISTLETOE study. Minimally Invasive Surgical Techniques – Laser, Endo Thermal or Endoresection. *British Journal of Obstetrics and Gynaecology* 104(12):1351–9.

PARKER, J., BISITIS, A. and PROIETTO, A.M. (1998) A systematic review of single-dose intramuscular methotrexate for the treatment of ectopic pregnancy. *Australian and New Zealand Journal of Obstetrics and Gynaecology* 38(2):145–50.

PEPPERS, L.G. and KNAPP, R. (1980) *Motherhood and Mourning*. New York: Praegar.

PETERS, W., LIU, P., BARRETT, R. *et al.* (2000) Concurrent chemotherapy and pelvic radiation therapy compared with pelvic radiation therapy alone as adjuvant therapy after radical surgery in high-risk early-stage cancer of the cervix. *Journal of Clinical Oncology* 18(8):1606–13.

PETERSEN, R.W. and QUINLIVAN, J.A. (2002) Preventing anxiety and depression in gynaecological cancer: a randomised controlled trial. *BJOG: An International Journal of Obstetrics and Gynaecology* 109(4):386–94.

PINION, S.B., PARKIN, D.E., ABRAMOVICH, D.R. *et al.* (1994) Randomised trial of hysterectomy, endometrial laser ablation and transcervical endometrial resection for dysfunctional uterine bleeding. *British Medical Journal* **309**(6960):979–83.

PRETTYMAN, R. (1995) The psychological sequelae of miscarriage. *Maternal and Child Health* **20**(6):207–9.

RHODES, J., KJERULFF, K., LANGENBERG, P. and GUZINSKI, G. (1999) Hysterectomy and sexual functioning. *Journal of the American Medical Association* **282**(20):1934–41.

ROOVERS, J.W.R., VAN DER BOM, J.G., HUUB VAN DER VAART, J. and HEINTZ, A.P.M. (2003) Hysterectomy and sexual wellbeing: prospective observational study of vaginal hysterectomy, subtotal abdominal hysterectomy and total abdominal hysterectomy. *British Medical Journal* **327**:774–8.

ROSE, P., BUNDY, B., WATKINS, E. *et al.* (1999) Concurrent cisplatin-based radiotherapy and chemotherapy for locally advanced cervical cancer. *New England Journal of Medicine* **340**:1144–53.

ROYAL COLLEGE OF OBSTETRICIANS AND GYNAE-COLOGISTS (2000) The Management of Early Pregnancy Loss (25). www.rcog.org.uk/guidelines.

ROYAL COLLEGE OF OBSTETRICIANS AND GYNAE-COLOGISTS (2001) Clinical Recommendations on the Use of Uterine Artery Embolisation in the Management of Fibroids. Report of a Joint Working Party. www.rcog.org.uk/guidelines.

SCHIFF, H. (1977) *The Bereaved Patient.* New York: Crown.

SCULPHER, M., MANCA, A., ABBOTT, J., FOUNTAIN, J., MASON, S. and GARRY, R. (2004) Cost effectiveness analysis of laparoscopic hysterectomy compared with standard hysterectomy: results from a randomised trial. *British Medical Journal* **328**:134–7.

SEYMOUR, J., WALLAGE, S., GRAHAM, W., PARKIN, P. and COOPER, K. (2003) The cost of microwave endome-trial ablation under different anaesthetic and clinical settings. *BJOG: An International Journal of Obstetrics and Gynaecology* **110**(10):922–6.

SHEPHERD, J.H., MOULD, T. and ORAM, D.H. (2001) Radical trachelectomy in early stage carcinoma of the cervix: outcome as judged by recurrence and fertility rates. *British Journal of Obstetrics and Gynaecology* **108**(8):882–5.

SHINGLETON, H.M. and ORR, L.W. (1987) *Cancer of the Cervix: Diagnosis and Treatment.* Edinburgh: Churchill Livingstone.

SHUSHAN, A., MOHAMED, H. and MAGOS, A. (1999) How long does laparoscopic surgery really take? Lessons learned from 1000 operative laparoscopies. *Human Reproduction* **14**(1):39–43.

SILLER, B., ALVAREZ, R., CONNER, W. *et al.* (1995) T2/3 vulva cancer: a case control study of triple incision versus enbloc radical vulvectomy and inguinal lymphadencc-tomy. *Gynecologic Oncology* **57**:335–9.

SMITH, J., BOYLE, D., CORLESS, D. *et al.* (1997) Abdominal radical trachelectomy: a new surgical technique for the conservative management of cervical carcinoma. *British Journal of Obstetrics and Gynaecology* **104**(10):1196–200.

SMITH-BINDMAN, R., KERLIKOWSKE, K., FELDSTEIN, V. *et al.* (1998) Endovaginal ultrasound to exclude endometrial cancer and other endometrial abnormalities. *Journal of the American Medical Association* **280**:1510–17.

SOWTER, M.C., FARQUHAR, C.M, PETRIE, K.J. and GUDEX, G. (2001) A randomised trial comprising single dose systemic methotrexate and laparoscopic surgery for the treatment of unruptured tubal pregnancy. *British Journal of Obstetrics and Gynaecology* **108**(2): 192–203.

SUMMIMITT, R.L. Jr., LUCENTE, V., KARRAM, M., SHULL, B. and BENT, A. (2000) Laparoscopic versus open Burch colposuspension: a randomised clinical trial. *Journal of Obstetrics and Gynaecology* **43**:584–93.

THAKAR, R., AYERS, S., CLARKSON, P., STANTON, S. and MANYONDA, I. (2002) Outcomes after total versus subtotal hysterectomy. *New England Journal of Medicine* **347**:1318–25.

TOOZS-HOBSON, P., BOOS, K. and CARDOZO, L. (1998) Management of vaginal vault prolapse. *British Journal of Obstetrics and Gynaecology* **105**:13–17.

VISVANATHAN, D., BOWN, S.G. and CUTNER, A.S. (2003) Review of the conservative surgical management of uterine fibroids. *Reviews in Gynaecological Practice* (in press).

VUENTO, M., PIRHONEN, J., MAKINEN, J. *et al.* (1999) Screening for endometrial cancer in asymptomatic post-menopausal women with conventional and colour Doppler sonography. *British Journal of Obstetrics and Gynaecology* **106**:14–20.

WABREK, A.J. and GUNN, J.L. (1984) Sexual and psychological implication of gynaecological malignancies. *Journal of Gynaecologic and Neonatal Nursing* **13**(6): 371–5.

WALLACE, C. (1987) Sexual adjustment after radical genital surgery. *Nursing Times* **83**(51):41–3.

WARD, K. and HILTON, P. (2002) Prospective multicentre randomised trial of tension-free vaginal tape and colpo-suspension as primary treatment for stress incontinence. *British Medical Journal* **325**:67.

WATERHOUSE, J. and METCALFE, M. (1991) Attitudes toward nurses discussing sexual concerns with patients. *Journal of Advanced Nursing* **16**(9):1048–54.

WEBB, C. (1985) *Sex, Nursing and Health.* Chichester: Wiley.

WHITNEY, C., SAUSE, W., BUNDY, B. *et al.* (1999) Randomised comparison of fluorouracil plus cisplatin versus hydroxyurea as an adjuvant to radiation therapy in stages IIB-IVA carcinoma of the cervix with negative para-aortic lymph nodes. *Journal of Clinical Oncology* **17**:1339–48.

WILLIAMS, H.A. (1986) Nurse attitudes towards sexuality in cancer patients. *Oncology Nursing Forum* **13**(12):39–43.

WILLIAMSON, M.L. (1992) Sexual adjustment after hys-terectomy. *Journal of Gynaecologic and Neonatal Nursing* **21**(1):42–7.

WILSON-BARNETT, J. (1975) Factors affecting patients' response to hospitalization. *Journal of Advanced Nursing* **3**:221–8.

Glossary

Adenomyosis: endometrium which is found within the uterine myometrium.

Adnexa: appendages (the ovaries and Fallopian tubes).

Amenorrhoea: absence of menstrual periods.

Amniocentesis: sampling and examination of the amniotic fluid in early pregnancy. A diagnostic test for chromosomal abnormality.

Androgens: hormones that produce male characteristics in either sex.

Anorexia nervosa: a condition in which the sufferer diets drastically to lose real or imagined weight: 'the slimmers' disease'.

Antiretrovirals: drugs that are active against the retrovirus family that HIV belongs to.

Atrophy: wasting away through lack of use or nutrition.

Atrophic vaginitis: wasting away through lack of oestrogen in vagina tissues causing dryness and inflammation.

Autonomic reaction: under the control of the sympathetic and parasympathetic nerves which control involuntary muscles and glandular secretion over which there is no conscious control.

Bartholin's glands: vestibular glands which lie on either side of the vaginal orifice.

Bone density: a measure of the amount of mineral (mainly calcium) in bone.

Bulimia: a condition in which the sufferer binges on large quantities of food, and then vomits, as a means of losing real or imaginary weight.

Caruncle: a small fleshy lump at the urethral opening.

Cautery: the application of searing heat by a hot instrument, an electric current or other means such as a laser. Cold cautery is cauterization by carbon dioxide, also called cryocautery.

Chorioamnionitis: inflammation of the membranes, the amnion (fetal surfaces) and the chorion.

CIN: cervical intraepithelial neoplasia.

Climacteric: the years around the menopause, before and after the final period, when menopausal symptoms are being experienced.

Coitus interruptus: a method of contraception in which the male withdraws his penis before ejaculation.

Collagen: part of the skin and bone in which calcium is deposited.

Colporrhaphy: repair of the vaginal wall due to lax pelvic floor muscles or following trauma, e.g. childbirth.

Colposcopy: examination of the cervix and vagina using an instrument called a colposcope.

Continuous combined HRT: a form of hormone replacement therapy in which oestrogens and progestogens are both taken continuously.

Corpus luteum: a yellow mass which develops in the ovarian follicle after ovulation and rupture of that follicle.

CVS: chorionic villus sampling by removal of a piece of early placental tissue to detect chromosomal abnormality.

Cystocele: prolapse of the bladder into the vagina caused by laxity of the anterior abdominal wall.

Detrusor: smooth muscle of the urinary bladder made up of longitudinal fibres that form the external layer of the muscular coat of the bladder.

Detrusor instability: a condition in which the detrusor contracts either spontaneously or on provocation during bladder filling while the patient tries to inhibit micturition.

Dysuria: difficulty or a burning sensation when passing urine.

Dyspareunia: painful sexual intercourse.

Dysplasia: abnormal development; often noted on cervical smear reports referring to abnormal cells.

Ectopic pregnancy: implantation of the zygote outside the uterus, usually in the Fallopian tube.

Ectropion or ectopy: when the squamo-columnar junction of the cervix is on the ectocervix and looks red in appearance (used to be termed an 'erosion').

Endometrial hyperplasia: non-cancerous over-growth of the endometrium.

Endometriosis: abnormal growth of endometrial tissue outside the uterine cavity.

Endometrium: the lining of the uterus.

Enterocele: formed by the prolapse of the pouch of Douglas through the upper part of the vaginal vault.

Fibroid: non-cancerous muscle growth in the uterine wall.

Fornix: (plural = fornices). The recesses at the top of the vagina in relation to the cervix: anterior, posterior or lateral.

HCG: human chorionic gonadotrophin; a hormone secreted early in pregnancy. Pregnancy tests are based on the detection of HCG.

Hydatidiform mole: disordered development of the zygote resulting in a rapidly growing cystic mass.

Hydrosalpinx: distension of the Fallopian tubes with fluid.

Hypotonic detrusor contraction: a weak bladder contraction which may result in incomplete emptying of the bladder.

Koilocytes: cells invaded by wart virus; a term usually seen on cervical smear reports.

Libido: sex drive, interest in sex.

Leucoplakia: development of white or greyish patches on the vulva; these may become malignant.

Leucorrhoea: non-pathological, excessive white vaginal discharge.

Menarche: onset of menstruation.

Menorrhagia: heavy menstrual bleeding.

Micturition: the act of passing urine, also called urination.

Missed abortion: the embryo or fetus dies but it is not expelled by the uterus.

Mittelschmerz: pain caused by ovulation.

Neuromuscular stimulation: a process of passing an electrical current along the efferent nerves at low frequencies in order to elicit a muscular contraction.

Oligomenorrhoea: infrequent menstrual periods or very light vaginal loss at time of normal menses.

Osteoporosis: a disease in which bone becomes so porous, brittle and fragile that it breaks very easily.

PID: pelvic inflammatory disease.

Procidentia: complete prolapse of the uterus into the vagina.

Pyosalpinx: the presence of pus in the Fallopian tube.

Rectocele: prolapse of the rectum into the vagina caused by laxity of the posterior vaginal wall.

Residual urine: a volume of urine remaining in the bladder after micturition.

Seroconversion: the development of certain antibodies that can be detected in the circulation. In an HIV infected person, seroconversion relates to the production of anti-HIV antibodies.

Skene's glands: a pair of glands which open into the posterior urethral orifice of the female.

Spinnbarkeit: clear thin 'elastic' cervical mucus at the time of ovulation.

Stress incontinence: involuntary leakage of urine when intra-abdominal pressure is raised, e.g. when coughing or laughing.

TOP: termination of pregnancy.

Trigone: a triangular area of smooth muscle of the bladder between the opening of the ureters and the orifice of the ureters.

Trimester: a third; usually referring to the first, second and third three months of pregnancy.

Tachyphylaxis: in the case of HRT this is a condition in which some women with implants experience a return of menopausal symptoms even though their blood oestrogen levels are normal or high.

Urethrocele: where the urethra bulges through the anterior vaginal wall.

Vaginismus: spasm of the vagina which is so severe as to prevent digital or penile penetration.

Index